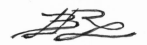

Edward C. Stafne, D.D.S., F.A.A.O.R.

Emeritus Senior Consultant and Formerly Head,
Department of Dentistry, Mayo Clinic and Mayo
Foundation, and Emeritus Professor of Dentistry and
Oral Surgery, Mayo Graduate School of Medicine
(University of Minnesota), Rochester, Minnesota.

Joseph A. Gibilisco, D.D.S., M.S.D., F.A.C.D., F.I.C.D.

Chairman, Department of Dentistry, Mayo Clinic and
Mayo Foundation, and Professor of Dentistry,
Mayo Medical School, Rochester, Minnesota.

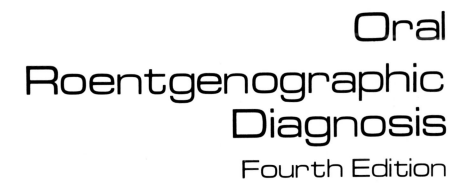

Oral Roentgenographic Diagnosis

Fourth Edition

W. B. SAUNDERS COMPANY, Philadelphia, London, Toronto

W. B. Saunders Company: West Washington Square
Philadelphia, PA 19105

1 St. Anne's Road
Eastbourne, East Sussex BN21 3UN, England

1 Goldthorne Avenue
Toronto, Ontario M8Z 5T9, Canada

Library of Congress Cataloging in Publication Data

Stafne, Edward C

Oral roentgenographic diagnosis.

Includes bibliographies and index.

1. Mouth — Radiography.   2. Teeth — Radiography.
   I. Gibilisco, Joseph A., 1924– joint author.   II. Title.

RK309.S73 1975   616.3′1′0757   74-9440

ISBN 0-7216-8547-1

Listed here is the latest translated edition of this book together
with the language of the translation and the publisher.

German (4th edition) — Medica Verlag, Stuttgart, Germany

Spanish (4th edition) — Editorial Medica Panamericana,
            Buenos Aires, Argentina

Oral Roentgenographic Diagnosis   ISBN 0-7216-8547-1

Last digit is the print number: 9   8   7

CONTRIBUTORS

ROGER E. CUPPS, M.D., M.S. (Radiology)

Consultant, Division of Therapeutic Radiology, Mayo Clinic and Mayo Foundation, and Assistant Professor of Radiology, Mayo Medical School, Rochester, Minnesota.

EUGENE E. KELLER, D.D.S., M.S.

Consultant, Department of Dentistry, Mayo Clinic and Mayo Foundation, and Instructor in Dentistry, Mayo Medical School, Rochester, Minnesota.

STANLEY A. LOVESTEDT, D.D.S., M.S., F.A.C.D.

Senior Consultant, Department of Dentistry, Mayo Clinic and Mayo Foundation, and Professor of Dentistry, Mayo Medical School, Rochester, Minnesota.

BRUCE A. LUND, D.D.S., M.S.

Consultant, Department of Dentistry, Mayo Clinic and Mayo Foundation, and Assistant Professor of Dentistry, Mayo Medical School, Rochester, Minnesota.

CHARLES M. REEVE, D.D.S., M.S., F.A.C.D.

Consultant, Department of Dentistry, Mayo Clinic and Mayo Foundation, and Assistant Professor of Dentistry, Mayo Medical School, Rochester, Minnesota.

PHILLIP J. SHERIDAN, D.D.S., M.S.

Consultant, Department of Dentistry, Mayo Clinic and Mayo Foundation, and Instructor in Dentistry, Mayo Medical School, Rochester, Minnesota.

DAN E. TOLMAN, D.D.S., M.S., F.A.C.D.

Consultant, Department of Dentistry, Mayo Clinic and Mayo Foundation, and Assistant Professor of Dentistry, Mayo Medical School, Rochester, Minnesota.

EASTWOOD G. TURLINGTON, D.D.S., M.S., F.A.C.D.

Consultant, Department of Dentistry, Mayo Clinic and Mayo Foundation, and Assistant Professor of Dentistry, Mayo Medical School, Rochester, Minnesota.

MARVIN M. D. WILLIAMS, Ph.D., A.A.C.R.

Emeritus Consultant, Department of Physiology and Biophysics, Mayo Clinic and Mayo Foundation, and Emeritus Professor of Biophysics, Mayo Graduate School of Medicine (University of Minnesota), Rochester, Minnesota.

Dedicated to the Late

DR. CHARLES HORACE MAYO

whose early interest in and support of dentistry did much to establish a closer relationship between medicine and dentistry.

PREFACE
to the
Fourth Edition

This revision has afforded us the opportunity to introduce five distinguished authors. Their contributions markedly strengthen the text. Dr. Roger E. Cupps, a therapeutic radiologist, has prepared the chapter "Effects of Irradiation Upon the Teeth and Their Supporting Structures." Dr. Eugene E. Keller, an oral surgeon, has revised and expanded the chapter "Oral Roentgenographic Manifestations of Systemic Disease." Dr. Bruce A. Lund, an oral surgeon, has assumed the responsibility for revising the chapter "Nonodontogenic Tumors of the Jawbones," and Dr. Phillip J. Sheridan and Dr. Charles M. Reeve, periodontists, have completely rewritten the chapter "Periodontal Disease." Many of the figures used in previous editions have been replaced with films that illustrate points more vividly. A substantial number of panoramic views of the teeth and jaws have also been included with this edition. For several years we have been making extensive use of such panoramic roentgenograms, not only in the Department of Dentistry but also in response to referrals from the Departments of Plastic Surgery, Otorhinolaryngology, and Diagnostic Roentgenology.

We have continued to cite references by the name and date system. As in previous editions, a bibliography is appended after each chapter. The articles referred to usually provide a more detailed and involved coverage of the subject than is presented in the chapter, and many of the references contain comprehensive bibliographies in themselves. They should be helpful to those who wish to obtain additional knowledge of the subject.

A positive diagnosis often can be made only from the roentgenographic evidence; however, it again must be emphasized that in many instances a diagnosis cannot be considered final until the radiologist, pathologist, and clinician are in basic agreement. This applies particularly to abnormal changes in the bone pattern and to lesions of the jaws that frequently may have similar roentgenographic appearances. An awareness of the limitations of the roentgenographic evidence is therefore extremely important.

We are grateful to all the contributing authors for their careful and generous cooperation in this revision and to other members of the staff of the Department of Dentistry who have provided us with valuable material that

v

otherwise would not have come to our attention. We are especially indebted to Bernard K. Forscher of the Section of Publications, who has edited the manuscript for this edition, and to Mrs. Betty Calkins, who prepared the manuscript submitted to the publishers. We also are indebted to Mr. James F. Martin, Head of the Section of Photography, and to Mr. Robert C. Benassi, Head of the Section of Medical Graphics, for the preparation of the photographic and schematic material. To Mr. Carroll Cann, Dental Editor of the W. B. Saunders Company, we extend our thanks and appreciation for his helpful advice and suggestions.

It continues to be our goal to provide a single volume on dental roentgenology that will be appropriate for the student as an introduction to the subject and for the clinician as a useful reference.

EDWARD C. STAFNE
JOSEPH A. GIBILISCO

PREFACE
to the
First Edition

In the preparation of this volume I have had at my disposal a large volume of roentgenograms that have been accumulated over a period of some 33 years. Since these roentgenograms were made in the Department of Dentistry and Oral Surgery of a medical clinic, the majority of them concern patients suffering from systemic disease. This material has given me the opportunity to observe and study the oral roentgenographic manifestations of many varied disease entities, and has demonstrated that the roentgenographic patterns of the jaws are as frequently diagnostic of systemic disease as are lesions of the oral soft tissues. It was chiefly with the view of demonstrating some of the characteristic oral roentgenologic findings of systemic disease that I undertook the preparation of this book.

Since a great deal of material illustrative of local conditions was also available, I decided to include some of this material, too, and thereby provide a more comprehensive coverage of the field of oral roentgenology. I hope, therefore, that this volume will be of particular value to dentists, especially those who choose oral roentgenology as a specialty of their profession, and to general roentgenologists as well.

In a broad sense the subject matter covered is anatomic landmarks, anomalies and conditions peculiar to the teeth themselves, pathologic calcifications of the hard and soft tissues, infections, cysts and tumors of the jaws, and oral roentgenographic manifestations of systemic disease. In dealing with tumors of the jaws I selected in most instances illustrations from patients in whom the lesion had been diagnosed on the basis of microscopic examination. Following the discussion of tumors is a chapter dealing with the effects of irradiation upon the teeth and their supporting structures.

In addition to identifying a condition that is revealed by the roentgenographic examination, I have discussed its significance and, in some instances, offered suggestions as to its treatment.

In order to conserve space and to present all illustrations in an upright position across the page, some of the illustrations have been reduced from a 16- or 18- to a 10-film mount; in each of these instances the condition could be illustrated adequately by the smaller number of films. In other cases, only one side of the jaws is illustrated, particularly if the opposite side exhibited similar features. In illustration of many of the conditions dealt with, only the standard intraoral dental roentgenogram is shown, with the realization that often it does not give all the desired information as to the extent and limits of the condition, and that either occlusal or extraoral views, or both, are indicated as well. Some conditions present a variable picture, depending on the stage of their development, and in many of these more than one illustration is shown to demonstrate the variations.

I am grateful to the many persons who have contributed to the preparation of the manuscript for this volume. Among these are my secretary, Mrs. Myrtle Simon, who aided materially in the assembly of the original manuscript; Dr. Carl M. Gambill, who edited the manuscript, and other members of the Section of Publications, who prepared the manuscript in its final form for submission to the publisher; and Mr. Leonard Julin and Mr. Ervin Miller, of the Section of Photography, who prepared the prints used for illustration.

For the provision of valuable material that otherwise would not have come to my attention I am indebted to my colleagues in the Section of Dentistry and Oral Surgery: Drs. S. A. Lovestedt, R. Q. Royer, R. J. Gores, and J. A. Gibilisco. They have made many excellent suggestions in the preparation of this volume.

To the staff of the W. B. Saunders Company I am grateful for much helpful advice.

E. C. Stafne, D.D.S.

CONTENTS

ANATOMIC LANDMARKS

In the interpretation of the roentgenogram one must first have a knowledge of the normal, realizing that there are wide structural variations that are within normal limits. Particularly does this apply to the trabecular pattern of bone which presents a variable picture depending on the size of the bone, size of its medullary space, and thickness of its cortex. It also varies with use, disuse, and the age of the patient. With disuse and advanced age the trabeculations tend to become more sparse and less coarse in structure.

Anatomic landmarks are by no means all demonstrable in any given roentgenogram; as a matter of fact, there are those that are visualized in a small percentage of cases only. One therefore should become familiar with them so that they can be identified and interpreted correctly when they are visualized. McCauley (1945) contributed an excellent article dealing with anatomic landmarks.

The component structures of the tooth and its supporting tissues usually are well defined and can be demonstrated best in younger persons (Fig. 1–1). The enamel, which is the densest of the hard structures of the tooth, is seen as a very radiopaque band that covers the coronal portion and tapers to a fine edge at the cervical margin of the tooth. The dentin, which exhibits a lesser degree of radiopacity than does enamel, accounts for the largest portion of the hard structures of the tooth. The cementum, which covers the surface of the root of the tooth, has a lesser degree of radiopacity than dentin, but is discernible

only when it has undergone hyperplasia. The pulp chamber and the root canal are visualized as a continuous radiolucent space in the center of the tooth which extends from the coronal portion to the apex of the root. The lamina dura, which represents the wall of the alveolar tooth socket, is seen as a radiopaque line which follows a course parallel to the root of the tooth. The periodontal-membrane space is depicted by a fine radiolucent line that is situated between the lamina dura and the root of the tooth. The cortical bone on the crest of the alveolar ridge is continuous with the lamina dura.

The largest number and variety of anatomic structures appear in dental roentgenograms made of the maxillary teeth. In the maxilla more structures are present adjacent to the alveolar process, and added to these are the superimposed

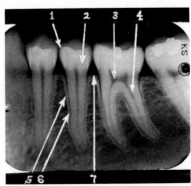

Figure 1–1 Anatomy of the tooth and its supporting structures. Key: *1*, enamel; *2*, dentin; *3*, pulp chamber; *4*, root canal; *5*, lamina dura; *6*, periodontal-membrane space; and *7*, cortical bone on crest of alveolar ridge.

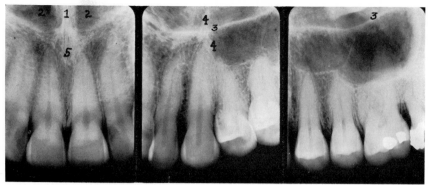

Figure 1–2   Anatomic structures of the anterior and premolar regions of the maxilla. Key: *1*, nasal septum; *2*, nasal fossae; *3*, floor of the nasal fossa as it extends posteriorly; *4*, anterior wall of the maxillary sinus; and *5*, nasal spine.

structures of the face and palate. Some of the structures that may appear in roentgenograms of the incisors, canines, and premolars are shown in Figure 1–2. Anatomic features of the maxillary molar region are dealt with in the chapter on the maxillary sinus.

NUTRIENT CANALS

The nutrient canals referred to here are those that contain blood vessels and nerves that supply the teeth, interdental spaces, and gingivae. In the roentgenogram they are evidenced by radiolucent lines of fairly uniform width which sometimes exhibit radiopaque borders.

The nutrient canals of the mandible are more often visualized in the roentgenogram than are those of the maxilla, and, because of its large size, the mandibular canal is seen in a high percentage of cases, particularly that portion of it which extends from the mandibular foramen to the mental foramen. In its course forward from the region of the mental foramen it becomes reduced in size and, as a result, that portion of it is not often visible. The canal varies greatly in size and in its location in relation to the roots of the teeth. It often loosely proximates and may come in contact with the roots of the third molar, and sometimes it follows a path that also is in proximity to the roots of the premolars and the first and second molars (Fig. 1–3).

Nutrient canals that arise from the mandibular canal are those that extend upward into the interdental space, and those that extend directly to the periapical foramina of the root of the tooth. The latter canals are very small and are rarely visualized in the roentgenogram. Those that lead to the foramina of the posterior teeth may be seen in instances in which the bone trabeculae are sparse, and they are evidenced by fine radiopaque lines which represent the walls of the canal (Fig. 1–4).

The interdental canals are seen more often in the anterior regions of the mandible, and particularly in patients in whom the alveolar process is very thin. In rare instances the canals that lead to the apical foramina are also faintly visible in this region (Fig. 1–5). In the edentulous mandible the interdental canals become increasingly prominent (Fig. 1–6).

Of the nutrient canals of the maxilla that supply the teeth and their supporting

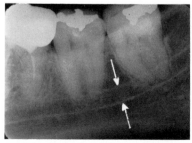

Figure 1–3   Mandibular canal as seen in the molar region.

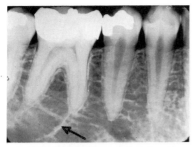

Figure 1–4 Nutrient canals leading to periapical foramina of the posterior teeth as evidenced by radiopaque lines extending down from the apex of the roots.

structures, the canal or groove that the posterior superior alveolar artery occupies is the one that is most often visualized. It is situated in the lateral wall of the maxillary sinus, and is seen as a curved radiolucent line of fairly uniform width. From its point of origin on the posterior aspect of the maxilla, it extends forward and downward as far as the premolar region where it takes a course upward toward the nasal fossa (Fig. 1–7). If the antral wall is very thin, a network of minute canals that extend from it to the alveolar process and other parts of the antral wall may be visible.

In the anterior region of the maxilla the nutrient canals that are occupied by terminal branches of the anterior superior alveolar artery are seldom visualized when the teeth are present, although the interdental canals often come into view when the jaw becomes edentulous. The interdental canals may, however, be sufficiently large to be seen clearly, and in some instances foramina from which branches emerge to the external surface of the maxilla are seen as small radiolucent areas between and at about the level of the root apexes of the teeth (Fig. 1–8).

ANTERIOR PALATINE (INCISIVE) CANAL

The incisive canal through which the nasopalatine nerves and the anterior branch

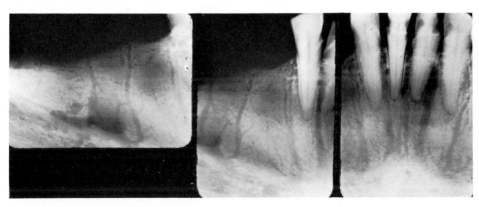

Figure 1–5 Vertical radiolucent lines are interdental nutrient canals in the anterior region of the mandible. Canals that lead directly to the apical foramina are also faintly visible.

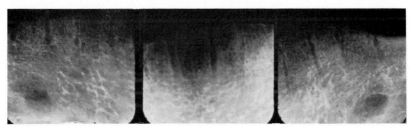

Figure 1–6 Interdental nutrient canals in the anterior region of an edentulous mandible. Both mental foramina are also clearly visible.

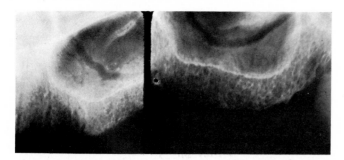

Figure 1–7 Canal that contains the posterior superior alveolar artery.

of the descending palatine vessels pass is not always visualized in the roentgenogram. It varies greatly in width and length, and when seen it is evidenced by two radiopaque lines which extend downward, one from the floor of each nasal fossa, and which depict the lateral walls of the canal. These lines tend to converge and they fade out imperceptibly at the lateral borders of the anterior palatine foramen (Fig. 1–9).

FORAMINA

ANTERIOR PALATINE (INCISIVE) FORAMEN

The anterior palatine foramen through which the nasopalatine nerve and vessels emerge is situated in the anterior portion of the midline of the palate. Its anterior border may closely approach the crest of the alveolar ridge, or it may be situated at some distance posterior to it. As seen in the roentgenogram, its image therefore varies in relation to the roots of the incisor teeth, and ranges from a position near the crest of the alveolar ridge to one that may be at

the level of the apex of the roots (Fig. 1–10). In some instances its image may be superimposed on the apex of the root of the central incisor when roentgenograms of the adjacent teeth are made, and it may then be mistaken for a periapical lesion (Fig. 1–11). It is almost always elliptical in shape and variable in size. A cyst of the incisive canal with which it may be confused has a well-defined border and tends to be round.

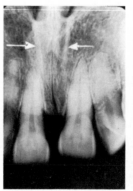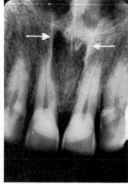

Figure 1–9 Anterior palatine (incisive) canals, the lateral borders of which are depicted by the two radiopaque lines that extend downward from the nasal fossae.

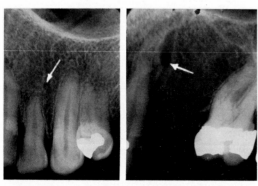

Figure 1–8 Interdental nutrient canals of the maxilla showing foramina through which branches of their contents emerge to the external surface.

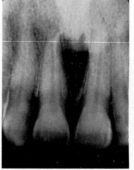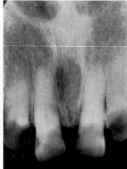

Figure 1–10 Anterior palatine (incisive) foramen. Two illustrations showing varied positions in relation to the crest of the alveolar ridge.

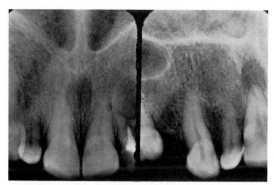

Figure 1–11 Anterior palatine (incisive) foramen that is situated at a high level and that becomes superimposed on the root of the central incisor when a roentgenogram of the adjacent teeth is made *(right)*.

SUPERIOR FORAMINA OF THE INCISIVE CANAL

Foramina through which the nasopalatine nerves and branches of the descending palatine vessels pass downward into the incisive canal are most often visualized in roentgenograms made of the maxillary lateral incisors and canines, and when the central rays are directed onto the film at a high vertical angle. They are seen as rounded radiolucent areas situated adjacent to the nasal septum and in the anterior region of the floor of each nasal fossa (Fig. 1–12).

MENTAL FORAMEN

The mental foramen through which the mental nerve and blood vessels emerge is seen as an oval or round radiolucent area in the mandibular premolar region. Its location varies in relation to the roots of the premolar teeth and its image may be seen inferior to, at the same level as, or superior to the apex of a root. It may be situated directly opposite either of the premolars, or between them (Fig. 1–13). Its image may be superimposed on the apex of the root of a tooth, in which event it may be mistaken for a periapical lesion. In some instances the mandibular canal can be seen extending directly to the foramen (Fig. 1–14). An intact lamina dura, when visualized, should serve to differentiate them. Evidence of the mental foramen is not always visualized in the roentgenogram.

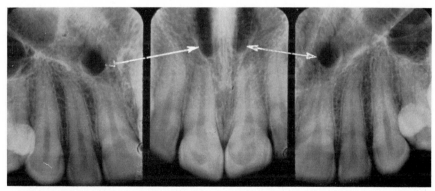

Figure 1–12 Superior foramina of the incisive canal. Bilateral and evidenced by round radiolucent areas in the floor of the nasal fossae and near the nasal septum.

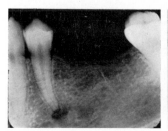
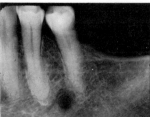
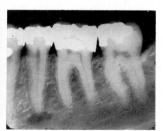

Figure 1–13 Mental foramen. Three illustrations showing its varied position in relation to the roots of the premolar teeth.

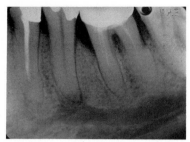

Figure 1–14 Large mandibular canal which extends directly to a mental foramen situated near the apex of a second premolar.

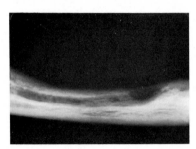

Figure 1–15 Mental foramen situated near superior border of edentulous mandible.

Sweet (1942) estimated that in about 50 per cent of patients it is demonstrable in routine roentgenographic examination, and that it is in evidence more often in the edentulous mandible. If the alveolar bone has undergone marked resorption and atrophy, it may be situated near the superior border of the ridge (Fig. 1–15).

LINGUAL FORAMEN

The lingual foramen through which a branch of the incisive artery emerges is situated on the lingual surface of the mandible at the symphysis. It is evidenced by a small radiolucent dot which is brought into prominence by a radiopaque circle that surrounds it and represents the genial tubercles (Fig. 1–16).

RIDGES, PROCESSES, AND TUBERCLES

These structures are radiopaque and, with the exception of the zygomatic process which is almost constantly present, they are by no means always visible in dental roentgenograms.

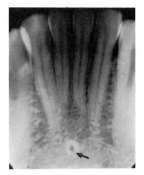

Figure 1–16 Lingual foramen seen as a small round radiolucent area in the midline and below the roots of the mandibular central incisor teeth.

EXTERNAL OBLIQUE RIDGE

The external oblique ridge is a continuation of the anterior border of the ramus that passes forward and downward over the outer surface of the body of the mandible to the mental ridge. It is visualized as a radiopaque line of varied width and density which passes anteriorly and across the molar region (Fig. 1–17). In the edentulous mandible where the alveolar process has undergone complete resorption, it may assume a position that is at the level

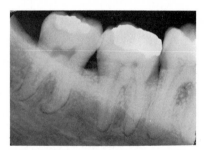

Figure 1–17 External oblique ridge.

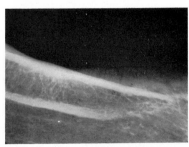

Figure 1–18 External oblique and mylohyoid ridges in the edentulous mandible where the external oblique ridge is situated near the superior border.

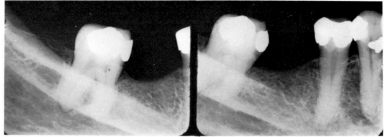

Figure 1–19 Mylohyoid ridge, the image of which runs parallel to and below the external oblique ridge.

of the superior border of the mandible (Fig. 1–18).

MYLOHYOID (INTERNAL OBLIQUE) RIDGE

The mylohyoid ridge begins on the medial and anterior aspect of the ramus and extends downward and forward diagonally on the lingual surface of the mandible toward the lower border of the symphysis. It varies greatly in size and, since its posterior portion is the most prominent, it is most often visualized where it crosses the retromolar and molar regions. It may be evidenced by a radiopaque line which varies from one that is very faint and narrow to one that is very broad and dense. Its course forward usually is on a lower level than that of the external oblique ridge, and its image is sometimes superimposed on the roots of the molar teeth (Fig. 1–19). The inferior border of a broad, dense ridge may be even and well defined. In the event that there also is an abnormally deep depression of the mandibular fossa, the bone seen inferior to the ridge appears to be abnormally radiolucent and may mistakenly be thought to represent a cystic condition (Fig. 1–20).

MENTAL RIDGE

The mental ridge is situated on the anterior aspect and near the inferior border of the mandible. It varies in prominence and extends from the premolar region to the symphysis. It is visualized as a radiopaque line that appears below the apices of the roots of the anterior teeth and that usually takes an upward turn as it approaches the symphysis. In some instances the image of the ridge may be superimposed on the roots of the teeth (Fig. 1–21).

ZYGOMATIC PROCESS AND MALAR BONE

The zygomatic process of the maxilla arises on the lateral surface directly above the first molar region. It may have a broad or narrow base, and it extends away from the surface in an upward direction of varied degree. In dental roentgenograms it is usually seen as an inverted radiopaque loop which represents the cortex of the inferior aspect of the process. The malar bone, which is a continuation of the zygomatic process and extends posteriorly, is seen as a shadow of lesser and more uniform radiopacity (Fig. 1–22). Superimposition of these structures often can be avoided

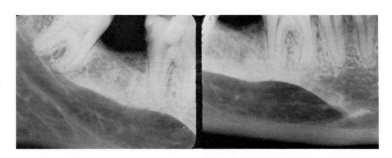

Figure 1–20 A prominent mylohyoid ridge and a deep mandibular fossa may produce a picture that may be mistaken for that of a cyst.

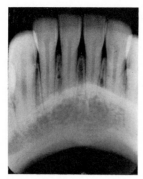

Figure 1–21 Mental ridge which is evidenced by the radiopacity that extends across the mandible and is superimposed on the roots of the anterior teeth.

by altering the vertical angulation of the central rays in making the exposure.

CORONOID PROCESS

The image of the coronoid process of the mandible often appears in periapical roentgenograms made of the molar region of the maxilla. As the mouth is opened, the process moves forward, and therefore it comes into view most often when the mouth is opened to its fullest extent at the time the exposure is made. It is evidenced by a

tapered or triangular radiopacity which may be seen below or, in some instances, superimposed on the molar teeth and maxilla (Fig. 1–23). If its superimposition on the maxilla reduces the diagnostic value of the roentgenogram, another view should be made in which the opening of the mouth is held to a minimum when the exposure is made. This measure invariably avoids superimposition of the process on the maxilla.

HAMULAR PROCESS

The hamular process is a bony projection that arises from the sphenoid bone and extends downward and slightly posteriorly. In the roentgenogram its image is seen in proximity to the posterior surface of the tuberosity of the maxilla. It varies greatly in length, width, and shape from patient to patient. It usually exhibits a bulbous point, but sometimes the point is tapered (Fig. 1–24).

GENIAL TUBERCLES

Genial tubercles are situated on the lingual surface of the mandible at a point about midway between the superior and inferior borders. There are four of them, two of which are situated on each side and adjacent to the symphysis. Although usually relatively small, they may be fairly large and extend outward from the surface as spinous processes (Fig. 1–25). In some instances such a prominent bony projection may interfere with the successful wearing of an artificial denture.

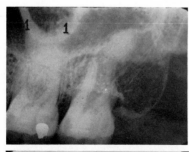

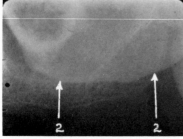

Figure 1–22 *Above,* Zygomatic process *(1)* superimposed on the roots of the teeth. *Below,* Zygomatic process superimposed on the edentulous jaw. The radiopacity that extends posteriorly from the zygomatic process is the malar bone *(2)*.

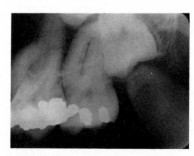

Figure 1–23 The coronoid process is the tapered radiopaque structure that extends upward and forward toward the upper jaw.

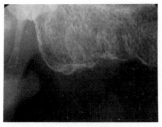 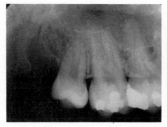 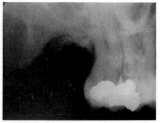

Figure 1–24   Hamular process, the image of which is seen posterior to the tuberosity of the maxilla. The three illustrations shown demonstrate variable lengths and shapes of the process.

NASOLACRIMAL DUCT

The orbital entrance of the naso-lacrimal duct is almost always visualized in occlusal views of the palate. It is seen as a fairly large, rounded, radiolucent area superimposed on the posterior region of the hard palate, and at the junction of the images of the medial wall of the maxillary sinus and the lateral wall of the nasal fossa (Fig. 1–26). From the superimposition of its image in this location on the palate, and near the greater palatine foramen, it may be misinterpreted as being the latter structure.

MISCELLANEOUS STRUCTURES

An anatomic variation that is evidenced by a fairly well-circumscribed radiolucent area which may be mistaken for a pathologic condition is that sometimes seen in the mandibular incisor region. In these instances the jaw is very thin in this region and there is almost no medullary space. Good visualization of the nutrient canals is a constant feature, and this serves to differentiate it from a pathologic condition (Fig. 1–27).

The distance between the nasal fossae and the roots of the anterior teeth varies greatly. In some instances the fossae may be situated at some distance from the teeth, and their images do not appear on the dental roentgenogram. On the other hand, abnormally large nasal fossae may encroach upon and cause divergence of the roots of the central incisors (Fig. 1–28).

The tooth germ, when seen prior to the onset of calcification of the tooth, is evidenced by a well-defined round or oval area of uniform radiolucency (Fig. 1–29).

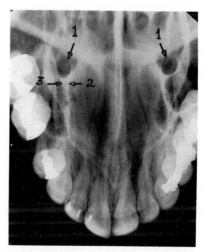

Figure 1–25   Genial tubercle. Occlusal view showing tubercles that have converged to form a spinous process on the lingual surface of the mandible.

Figure 1–26   Nasolacrimal ducts superimposed on the posterior surface of the hard palate. Key: *1*, orbital entrance to duct; *2*, lateral wall of nasal fossa; and *3*, medial wall of maxillary sinus.

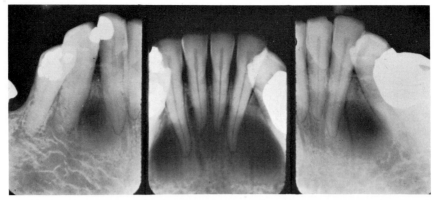

Figure 1–27 Marked radiolucence in the incisive region that occurs when the mandible is very thin. It may be mistaken for a pathologic condition.

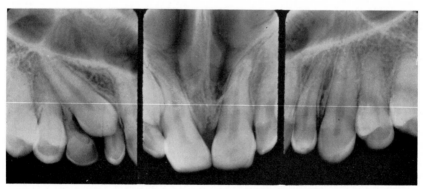

Figure 1–28 Low nasal fossae with divergence of the roots of the central incisors.

The formation of the germ of second premolars and third molars is often retarded in relation to the chronologic age of the patient, and cases have been noted in which roentgenographic evidence of the tooth bud of third molars had not appeared until after the patient had reached 20 years of age. In this event the bud might be interpreted as being a cyst.

A dentin papilla that is superimposed on the image of the mandibular canal may

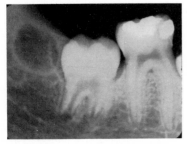

Figure 1–29 Tooth germ of the mandibular third molar in a patient 10 years of age.

produce an area of marked radiolucence. This most often occurs with the development of the second and third molars, and should not be mistaken for a periapical lesion (Fig. 1–30).

THE STYLOHYOID CHAIN

The stylohyoid chain consists of the styloid process of the temporal bone, the lesser cornu or horn of the hyoid bone, and the connection, usually the stylohyoid ligament, between these two. It develops from the cartilage of the second branchial or hyoid arch, also known as Reichert's cartilage. In many mammals this cartilage gives rise to a series of four bony parts (Kingsley, 1925), variously called tympanohyal, stylohyal, epihyal, and ceratohyal (or tympanohyal, stylohyal, ceratohyal, and hypohyal), and some or all of these names are also used in describing the embryology of the chain. In man, the tympanohyal is

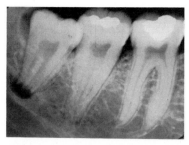

Figure 1–30 Dentin papilla of the mandibular third molar superimposed on the mandibular canal.

said to fuse with the petrous part of the temporal bone and with the stylohyal to form the styloid process; the epihyal (or ceratohyal) cartilage normally degenerates (Hamilton et al., 1945), or its blastema may apparently even fail to chondrify (Keibel and Mall, 1910), but its covering fibrous sheath persists as the stylohyoid ligament; and the hypohyal (or ceratohyal) persists as the lesser cornu of the hyoid bone (Wilder, 1923). Variation in the ossification and fusion of these various parts can lead, however, to marked variation in the appearance of the chain.

The normal styloid process is a cylindric spur of bone that usually tapers gradually toward a pointed free extremity. It varies much in length, usually being from 5 to 50 mm long, and it often varies also in thickness, form, and shape (Fig. 1–31). It is apparently impossible, as a rule, to establish how much of the styloid process

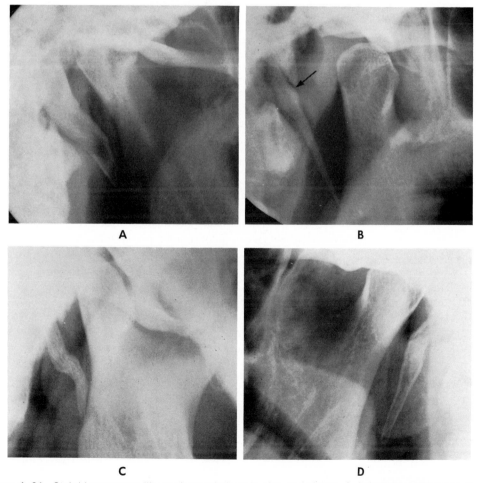

A   B

C   D

Figure 1–31 Styloid processes illustrating variations in size and shape. *A,* A thick heavy process. *B,* A long thin process with bony enlargement which probably represents the junction of the tympanohyal and stylohyal parts of the styloid process. *C* and *D,* Process with marked curvatures. (Reproduced with permission from Stafne, E. C. and Hollinshead, W. H.: Roentgenographic Observations on the Stylohyoid Chain. Oral Surg., Oral Med. & Oral Path. *15:*1195–1200 [Oct.] 1962.)

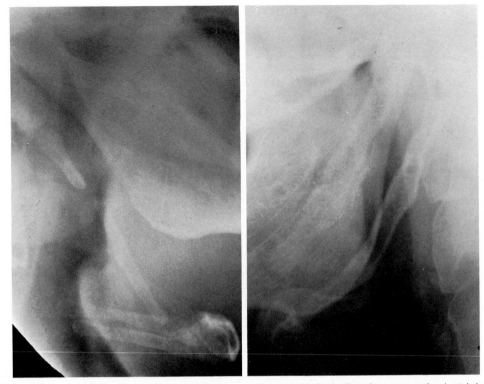

Figure 1–32 *Left,* A case in which the ossified parts of the chain, including the tympanohyal, stylohyal, and epihyal elements, have remained separate. The tympanohyal is abnormally large and bulbous. *Right,* Unusually large solid bony rod of irregular thickness. The image of a similar one on the opposite side is superimposed on the mandibular ramus. (Reproduced with permission from Stafne, E. C. and Hollinshead, W. H.: Roentgenographic Observations on the Stylohyoid Chain. Oral Surg., Oral Med. & Oral Path. *15*:1195–1200 [Oct.] 1962.)

has been contributed by the tympanohyal, how much by the stylohyal, and how much, if any, by the epihyal. However, not infrequently there is a bony enlargement, generally believed to represent the junction of the tympanohyal and stylohyal parts, not far from the base of the process (Fig. 1–31*B*). From this enlargement the distal part usually continues in a straight line, but in some instances it may change direction to form a process that has a marked curvature (Fig. 1–31*C* and *D*). Occasionally, moreover, a long styloid process consists of three unfused parts (Fig. 1–32, *left*), and the proximal two then rather obviously represent tympanohyal and stylohyal elements.

The stylohyoid ligament, the normal representative of the epihyal link of the chain, is a band of connective tissue which is attached to the free extremity of the styloid process and extends to the lesser horn (cornu) of the hyoid bone. As already intimated, the ligament may be partially

represented by bone, most often at its proximal extremity, or in some instances it is completely or almost completely replaced by bone. There is much variation in both the length and width of this element when it is ossified, and there may or may not be clear evidence as to its point of junction with the styloid process proper (Figs. 1–32, 1–33, and 1–34).

This ossification should not be considered a degenerative change depending on age, for most of the striking cases observed by Dwight (1907) occurred in persons less than 31 years of age. In most cases, also, the bar of bone formed is much larger than the stylohyoid ligament and therefore could not have resulted from degenerative changes in that. In such instances, it seems obvious that part of the epihyal portion of Reichert's cartilage persisted rather than degenerated, and subsequently became ossified just as did other members of the chain. While reference to a long styloid process as having had its length added to by

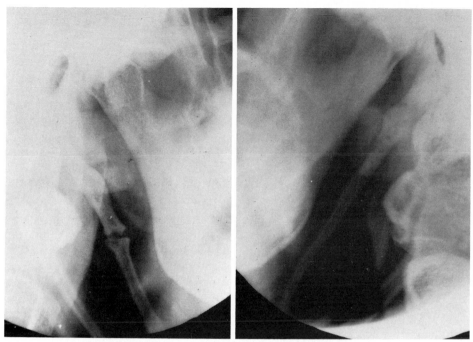

Figure 1–33   Bilateral ossified epihyal (ceratohyal) element of chain. *Left,* Epihyal part is not fused with the tip of the styloid process. The broad jointlike junction is not an infrequent occurrence. *Right,* Ossified epihyal part is continuous with the styloid process. (Reproduced with permission from Stafne, E. C. and Hollinshead, W. H.: Roentgenographic Observations on the Stylohyoid Chain. Oral Surg., Oral Med. & Oral Path. *15*:1195–1200 [Oct.] 1962.)

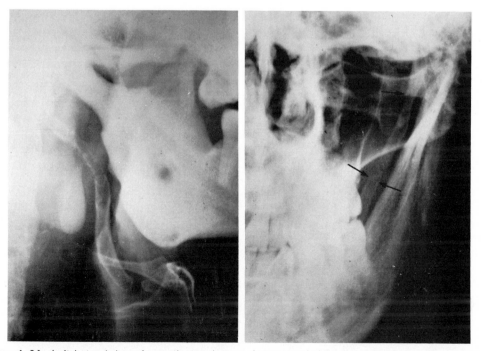

Figure 1–34   *Left,* Lateral view of a continuous bony rod composed of the three proximal elements of the chain and extending to the lesser cornu of the hyoid bone. *Right,* Anteroposterior view of the bony rod *(arrows)* shown at left. (Reproduced with permission from Stafne, E. C. and Hollinshead, W. H.: Roentgenographic Observations on the Stylohyoid Chain. Oral Surg., Oral Med. & Oral Path. *15*:1195–1200 [Oct.] 1962.)

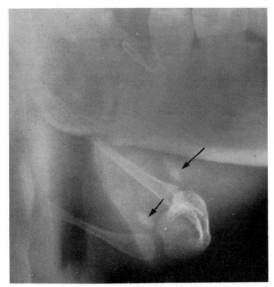

Figure 1–35 Lesser horns or cornua *(arrows)* of the hyoid bone. These represent the hypohyal (also called ceratohyal) element of the stylohyoid chain. (Reproduced with permission from Stafne, E. C. and Hollinshead, W. H.: Roentgenographic Observations on the Stylohyoid Chain. Oral Surg., Oral Med. & Oral Path. *15*:1195–1200 [Oct.] 1962.)

"ossification of the stylohyoid ligament" is readily understandable therefore, it may be misleading in the sense that it implies that the ligament first formed, and later ossified. There is no justification for referring to this condition as "calcification of the stylohyoid ligament," a not uncommon term, since the distal parts of long styloid processes are always true bone.

The lesser horns (Fig. 1–35) usually ossify a few years after birth, and are typically small nodules of bone united to the body of the hyoid bone by fibrous tissue and to the greater horns of the hyoid bone by fibrous tissue or tiny synovial joints. They, like the styloid process, may, however, be markedly elongated by fusion with an ossified portion of what should have been a distal part of the stylohyoid ligament.

Where ossification of all segments of the chain occurs, the condition is more often bilateral. Even then, however, it is not uncommon to find considerable departure from symmetry in details such as thickness and length of the parts, and their relation to one another. Often the three proximal elements of the chain are fused into a continuous bony rod (Fig. 1–34); sometimes all four parts are fused. In rare instances the ossified parts of the chain remain separate (Fig. 1–32, *left*) but are held together by fibrous tissue continuous with the periosteum. Particularly large solid bony rods are shown on the right in Figure 1–32. The photographs shown in Figure 1–36 may clarify further some of the points that have been discussed concerning the stylohyoid chain.

A styloid process that projects against the tonsillar region or farther forward in the palatal region may be a source of pain or other symptoms referable to the throat. The pain has been described as a dull ache,

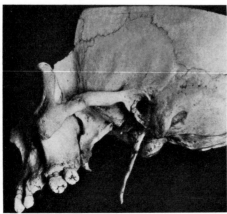 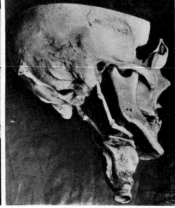

Figure 1–36 *Left,* An abnormally long styloid process with a very prominent tympanohyal segment. *Right,* Bilateral ossification of the three proximal parts of the stylohyoid chain. The parts are not fused with one another. (Reproduced with permission from Dwight, T.: Stylo-hyoid Ossification. Ann. Surg. *46*:721–735, 1907.)

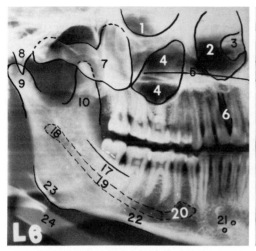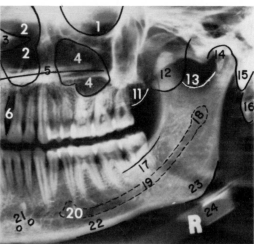

Figure 1–37 Anatomic landmarks as visualized on the Panorex film (dried specimen). Key: *1,* orbital cavity; *2,* nasal cavity; *3,* inferior concha; *4,* maxillary sinus; *5,* palatal process of maxilla; *6,* incisive canal; *7,* azygomatic arch and malar process; *8,* angular spine of the sphenoid bone; *9,* condylar process of the mandible; *10,* coronoid process of the mandible with superimposition of the zygomatic arch; *11,* tuberosity of the maxilla; *12,* lateral pterygoid plate with superimposition of the coronoid process of mandible and zygomatic arch; *13,* coronoid notch; *14,* glenoid fossa; *15,* styloid process; *16,* mastoid process; *17,* oblique ridge of the mandible; *18,* mandibular foramen; *19,* mandibular or inferior alveolar canal; *20,* mental foramen; *21,* genial tubercles; *22,* inferior border of the mandible; *23,* angle of the mandible; *24,* Panorex chin rest.

neuralgic pain, and lancinating pain that extends to the ear, all of which may be aggravated by swallowing. Also there may be a sensation of fullness, and of food having lodged in the throat and necessitating frequent swallowing (Eagle, 1949; Donohue, 1959).

Treatment for the relief of pain is entirely operative. Fracture of the process sometimes affords relief; however, partial amputation appears to be the method of choice. Removal of the entire process is unnecessary, and would seem to be contraindicated because of the muscular attachments closer to its base, and the relation of the base to the facial nerve.

ANATOMIC STRUCTURES AS SEEN IN PANOREX VIEWS

Most of the prominent anatomic landmarks that appear on the Panorex film are shown in Figure 1–37.

REFERENCES

Donohue, W. B.: Styloid Syndrome. Canad. Dent. A. J. *25:*283–286 (May) 1959.

Dwight, T.: Stylo-hyoid Ossification. Ann. Surg. *46:*721–735, 1907.

Eagle, W. W.: Symptomatic Elongated Styloid Process: Report of 2 Cases of Styloid Process—Carotid Artery Syndrome with Operation. Arch. Otolaryng. *49:*490–503 (May) 1949.

Hamilton, W. J., Boyd, J. D., and Mossman, H. W.: Human Embryology (Prenatal Development of Form and Function). Baltimore, Williams & Wilkins Company, 1945, 366 pp.

Keibel, F. and Mall, F. P.: Manual of Human Embryology. Vol. 1. Philadelphia, J. B. Lippincott Company, 1910, 548 pp.

Kingsley, J. S.: The Vertebrate Skeleton from the Developmental Standpoint. Philadelphia, P. Blakiston's Son & Co., 1925, p. 337.

McCauley, H. B.: Anatomic Characteristics Important in Radiodontic Interpretation. I. The Maxilla. II. The Mandible. Dent. Radiogr. Photogr. *18:*1–4; 9–12, 1945.

Sweet, A. P. S.: A Statistical Analysis of the Incidence of Nutrient Channels and Foramina in Five Hundred Periapical Full-Mouth Radiodontic Examinations. Am. J. Orthodontics. *28:*427–442 (July) 1942.

Wilder, H. H.: The History of the Human Body. New York, Henry Holt & Company, 1923, 623 pp.

2

ANOMALIES

An anomaly is a deviation from normal. Such deviations may be caused by local conditions. They may arise as inherited dental tendencies, or they may be manifestations of systemic disturbances. Abnormalities that are associated with systemic disease and other developmental disturbances will be dealt with elsewhere.

The most common oral anomalies are those that affect the teeth, and more rarely those that result from faulty development of their supporting structures. Anomalies of the teeth not only affect their form, size, arrangement, number, and time of development but also may affect their histologic structure. An excellent contribution on the subject of dental anomalies is that of Pindborg (1970).

CONGENITALLY MISSING TEETH

As with other serial structures such as digits, vertebrae, and ribs, the teeth have a marked tendency to deviate from the normal number. Congenital absence of teeth is not uncommon, and in many instances it follows a hereditary pattern. Dahlberg (1937) has reported the absence of anterior teeth in the same family over a period of four generations, and Gardner (1927) reported missing teeth in six generations.

Any tooth in the dental arch may fail to develop; however, the order of frequency in which teeth are absent is as follows: third molars, premolars, and maxillary lateral incisors. Absence of one or more of the third molars occurs in approximately 1 of 10 persons, while absence of a canine occurs very rarely. Garn and Lewis (1962) have found that persons with agenesis of one or more of the third molars have an appreciably greater number of other congenitally absent teeth than do those in whom all the third molars are present. Teeth of the permanent series are most frequently absent; however, in some instances the primary tooth, as well as its permanent successor, may be absent. Congenital bilateral absence of teeth is not uncommon. Partial or almost complete anodontia may occur in patients in whom general physical examination gives essentially negative results (Porter and Edwards, 1937). Partial or complete anodontia is almost a constant feature in ectodermal dysplasia. Canines

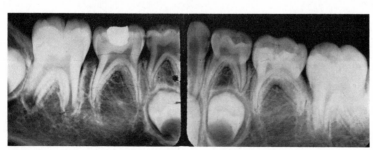

Figure 2–1 Congenital absence of mandibular second premolars in a patient 7 years of age.

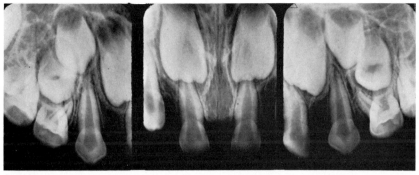

Figure 2–2 Congenital absence of maxillary primary and permanent lateral incisors in a patient 5 years of age.

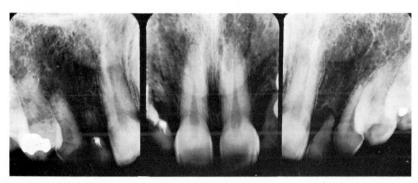

Figure 2–3 Congenital absence of the permanent maxillary lateral incisors and canines. Absence of the canines is a very rare anomaly.

may be absent when several other teeth also have failed to form, but absence of them alone is a very rare occurrence, there being only six cases reported in the literature (Hillam, 1970). A case of bilateral absence of maxillary canines has been reported by Simon and Webster (1970).

Absence of teeth also may be caused by lesions of the jaws that occur in infancy and as a result of irradiation while they are in their early stages of formation. It is of utmost importance to know that teeth are missing and to know this while the child is young, so that planning of proper treatment can be undertaken. Obviously, in the case of missing teeth, it is through roentgenographic examination only that accurate information can be gained (Figs. 2–1, 2–2, 2–3, 2–4, and 2–5).

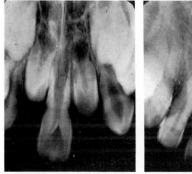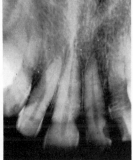

Figure 2–4 Congenital absence of maxillary central incisor. *Left,* Teeth of a boy 9½ years of age. *Right,* Teeth of boy's mother, in whom a maxillary central incisor also failed to develop.

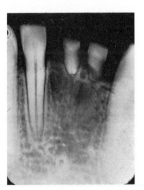

Figure 2–5 Congenital absence of three mandibular incisors.

TOTAL ANODONTIA OF THE PERMANENT DENTITION

An unusual anomaly is one in which the primary dentition is normal, but all teeth of the permanent dentition are congenitally absent. Hutchinson (1953) observed this in a boy 11 years old, and Swallow (1959) in a boy 8 years old. In both cases the skin, hair, and sweat glands were normal, and there were no other ectodermal defects. There was no familial history of a similar anomaly.

The roentgenogram shown in Figure 2–6 was made for a boy 14 years old who had what closely approached a total anodontia of the permanent teeth. Only the maxillary central incisors and right first molar had developed. All of the primary teeth had developed. The maxillary central incisors had undergone normal shedding, and the three missing primary molars had been extracted. All of the primary mandibular teeth were still present. As in the two cases referred to above, there were no other ectodermal defects.

SUPERNUMERARY TEETH

There is a definite tendency for each tooth to duplicate itself, and this tendency in most instances is a familial one. Osborn

(1912) stated, "The paleontological record of the evolution of teeth, which is fairly complete in all mammalian orders, lends no support to the theory of atavism as applied to supernumeraries." Supernumerary teeth are not limited to the permanent dentition but are also present in the primary. The incidence of occurrence is approximately 1 in 100 persons, and the ratio of occurrence in the maxilla to occurrence in the mandible is about 8 to 1 (Stafne, 1932). The ratio of unerupted supernumerary teeth to those that erupt is about 5 to 1; therefore, the majority of them can be demonstrated by means of the roentgenogram only.

As to their form, many supernumerary teeth resemble normal teeth, others have conical crowns, and in some instances they bear no resemblance to any normal tooth form. The form is fairly typical for the region in which they occur; thus, mesiodentes are almost always conical; mandibular incisors, premolars, and mandibular third molars tend to resemble the normal form; and those that occur in the maxillary third molar region may be of either normal or conical shape. In general, supernumerary teeth are smaller; however, mandibular incisors and the premolars are more often equal in size to the normal teeth. The time of development often conforms to that of the normal teeth in the region in which they occur. Any deviation from this is toward retarded develop-

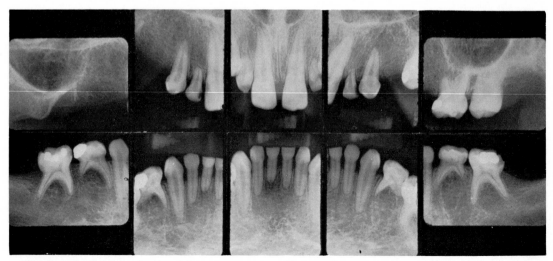

Figure 2–6 Total anodontia of the permanent mandibular teeth and partial anodontia of the permanent maxillary teeth.

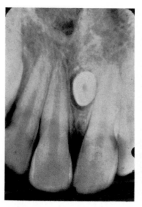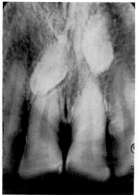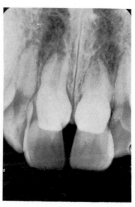

Figure 2–7 Mesiodentes. *Left,* A mesiodens situated directly in the midline, between the roots of the central incisors and in a transverse position. *Center,* Two mesiodentes situated at a higher level. They are asymptomatic and there is no indication for their removal. *Right,* Two mesiodentes with broad incisal edges situated posterior to the normal central incisors. These are partially erupted, and their extraction is indicated.

ment. As with congenitally missing teeth, bilateral occurrence is not uncommon.

The most common complications caused by supernumerary teeth are malposition and noneruption of the normal teeth (Fastlicht, 1943). As with other teeth that remain embedded, there is the possibility of cyst formation (Stafne, 1931). Roentgenologic examination at an early age will reveal their presence and permit removal of those with which complications may be, or may become, associated.

Mesiodentes are situated in the maxilla near the midline, and almost always posterior to the normal central incisors. Many of them, therefore, are bypassed by the permanent incisors which are permitted to erupt into their normal position in the arch (Fig. 2–7). Some of the complications associated with them are shown in Figures 2–8 and 2–9.

Supernumerary teeth that occur in the mandibular incisor region almost always so closely resemble the normal incisors that it is impossible to distinguish between them. Cases in which there have been six mandibular incisors of equal size have been noted. One case in which five incisors were present is shown in Figure 2–10. In some instances supernumerary molars may erupt posterior to, and in alignment with, the third molar. However, most of them do not erupt, and

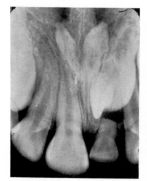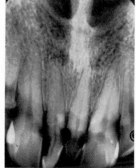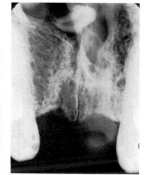

Figure 2–8 Mesiodentes with associated complications. *Left,* Two mesiodentes that have assumed an inverted position and are situated at a high level in the arch. Also there is a third mesiodens situated at a lower level where it has prevented eruption of the permanent right central incisor; removal of the mesiodens at this time will permit normal eruption of the permanent tooth. *Center,* Two fully erupted mesiodentes that have caused marked separation of the permanent incisors. *Right,* A small peg-shaped mesiodens that is erupting into the floor of the nasal fossae.

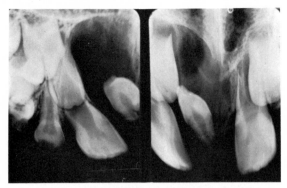

Figure 2–9 Inverted mesiodens from which a dentigerous cyst has developed in a patient 7 years of age.

usually they interfere with eruption of the third molar. Onset of development does not occur until after 7 years of age; therefore, they do not interfere with normal eruption of the second and first molars. In general, their occurrence is of less clinical significance than is the occurrence of supernumerary teeth in the arch anterior to the third molar region. Bilateral occurrence of two supernumerary teeth in both maxillary third molar regions is shown in Figure 2–11. A mandibular fourth molar that is interfering with the eruption of the third molar is shown in Figure 2–12. Obviously, there is not sufficient space for the third molar to achieve

full eruption of the clinical crown; therefore, removal of the third molar would be indicated regardless of the presence of the supernumerary tooth.

Supernumerary premolars occur most frequently in the mandible, and tend to resemble the normal premolars in form and size. There is rarely sufficient space for them to undergo complete eruption, although premature loss of the first molar may afford space for them to do so. The presence of two supernumerary premolars in the right mandible is shown in Figure 2–13. The tendency of supernumerary teeth to undergo development at a time later than that of the normal teeth in the region in which they

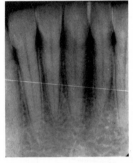

Figure 2–10 Supernumerary mandibular incisor that would be difficult to distinguish from the normal incisors.

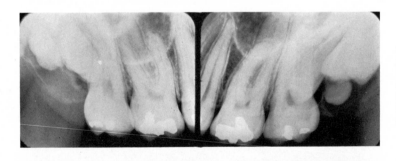

Figure 2–11 Supernumerary maxillary molars. Bilateral occurrence of two in each region. *Left,* Normal third molar is dwarfed. *Right,* The supernumerary teeth are preventing the eruption of a third molar which is of normal size and form.

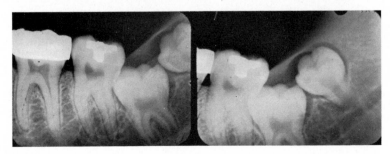

Figure 2–12 Supernumerary mandibular molar which is preventing eruption of the third molar. Such a molar almost always resembles a normal molar in form, but tends to be smaller.

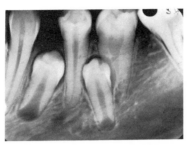

Figure 2–13 Supernumerary mandibular premolars. Both of them are in an earlier stage of development than are the normal premolars.

occur is evidenced by the incomplete formation of their roots as compared with the complete development of the roots of the normal premolars. Morgan et al. (1970) have reported a case in which an additional premolar

appeared later at each site from which three supernumerary mandibular premolars had been removed 5 years previously. The patient, an 11-year-old girl, had been referred by her orthodontist for the removal of the erupted mandibular first premolars and three unerupted supernumerary premolars (Fig. 2–14).

Supernumerary maxillary lateral incisors are not always conical; they often resemble the normal tooth in form, although rarely in size. There is a relatively high incidence of supernumerary lateral incisors associated with cleft palate. They were present in 22 of 60 cases of cleft palate (Millhon and Stafne, 1941). An interesting rarity is the bilateral occurrence of maxillary primary lateral incisors (Fig. 2–15).

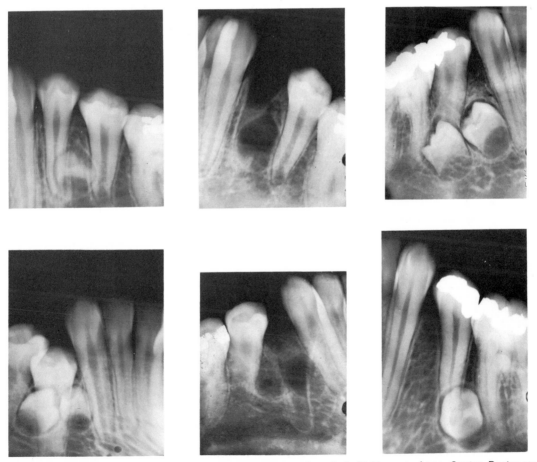

Figure 2–14 Recurring mandibular supernumerary premolars. *Left,* At 11 years of age. *Center,* Postoperatively. *Right,* At 16 years of age, showing recurrence. (Reproduced with permission from Morgan, G. A., Morgan, P. R., and Crouch, S. A.: Recurring Mandibular Supplemental Premolars. Oral Surg., Oral Med. & Oral Path. *30:*501–504 [Oct.] 1970.)

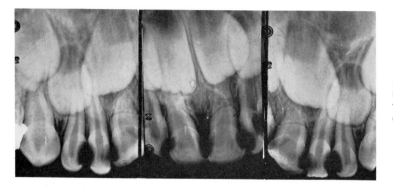

Figure 2–15 Bilateral occurrence of supernumerary primary lateral incisors. Note fracture of the roots of the primary central incisors.

ENAMEL PEARLS (ENAMELOMA)

Enamel pearls are most often attached to the surface of the root of the tooth at or close to the cementoenamel junction. In some instances they are attached to dentin and in others to cementum. Those attached to cementum most likely arise in the periodontium, and become fused to the root of the tooth following complete development of the root. Cavanha (1965) has found pearls that contain enamel only, others that contain enamel and dentin, and some that include a pulp chamber that connects with the central pulp chamber of the tooth.

The number of pearls on a tooth is most often limited to one. However, the occurrence may be multiple, although more than two is considered rare. They are recognized in the roentgenogram by their globular shape and by their radiographic density, which is similar to that of enamel (Fig. 2–16).

MICRODONTIA

The size of the teeth is not necessarily proportionate to the size of the individual,

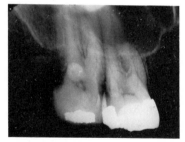

Figure 2–16 Enamel pearl situated near the bifurcation of the roots of a maxillary second molar.

and rarely is their size influenced by a generalized developmental suppression. Small teeth in a person of large stature can most often be attributed to a hereditary tendency. Microdontia of individual teeth also tends to follow a familial pattern, and the teeth involved most frequently are those that are more apt to be congenitally absent, namely the third molars, the maxillary lateral incisors, and more rarely the second premolars (Fig. 2–17). In some instances the entire tooth may be abnormally small; in others, either its crown or root only.

Microdontia is not an uncommon finding in osteogenesis imperfecta and in hemiatrophy of the face in which there is an associated underdevelopment of the jaws. Dwarfing of teeth also may be produced by irradiation used in the treatment of tumors of the jaws and adjacent structures.

FUSION AND CONCRESCENCE

Fusion is a developmental union of two or more teeth in which the dentin and one other dental tissue are united. There may be complete union to form one abnormally large tooth, or union of the crowns, or union of the roots only. A supernumerary tooth is frequently one of the teeth involved. It affects primary teeth as well as permanent ones. Illustrations of fused teeth are shown in Figures 2–18, 2–19, and 2–20.

Concrescence is a condition in which only the cementum of two or more teeth becomes united. The molars are involved most frequently. More often one or both of the united teeth remain unerupted; therefore, in most instances, they are first recog-

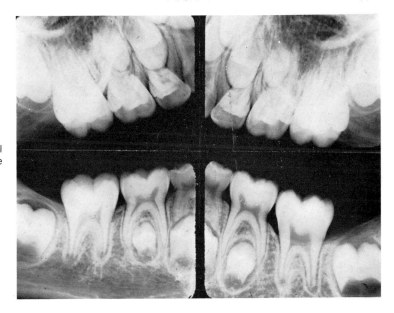

Figure 2–17 Microdontia. All developing second premolars are abnormally small.

nized incidental to a roentgenographic examination (Figs. 2–21 and 2–22). However, it is not always possible by means of the roentgenogram to distinguish between actual concrescence and images of teeth that are in close contact but are merely superimposed, one on the other. Concrescence, if not recognized, presents a hazard in extraction, particularly if undue and indiscriminate force is applied.

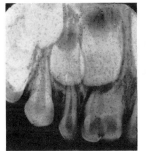
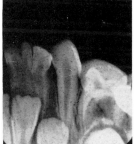

Figure 2–18 Fusion of primary teeth. *Left,* Maxillary incisor and a supernumerary lateral incisor. *Right,* Fusion of the mandibular central and lateral incisors with a small supernumerary tooth between them. The pulp chambers of the three are merged.

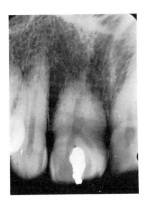
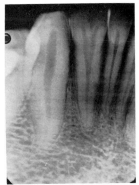

Figure 2–19 Fusion of permanent incisors. *Left,* Maxillary central and lateral incisors. *Right,* Mandibular lateral and supernumerary lateral incisors. There is convergence of the pulp canals to form a single canal and root.

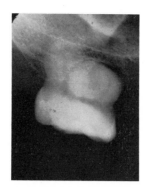

Figure 2–20   Fusion of posterior teeth. Two molars with pulp chambers merged, but with separate root canals.

DENS IN DENTE
(DENS INVAGINATUS)

The so-called dens in dente is an anomaly in development of a tooth wherein there is disarrangement of the enamel organ, producing an invagination within the body of the tooth which becomes lined with enamel. The cavity so formed retains communication with the outside through a small opening on the surface of the crown. The histologic structure of this condition has been described by Kronfeld (1934), Kitchin (1935), and others.

The anomaly occurs most frequently in the anterior teeth, particularly the maxillary lateral incisors. The posterior teeth, especially the molars, are affected to a much lesser degree. Bilateral occurrence is not uncommon (Morgan and Poyton, 1960).

Oehlers (1957) has grouped the invaginations into three types: (1) those confined within the crown of the tooth, (2) those that invade into the root but remain within

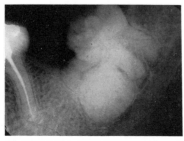

Figure 2–21   Concrescence of mandibular second and third molars. The second molar remains unerupted.

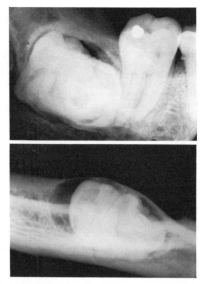

Figure 2–22   Concrescence. Two cases in which mandibular molars are involved. In both instances the teeth have remained embedded. The one in the lower picture shows evidence of early cyst formation.

it as a blind sac, and (3) those that penetrate to the surface of the root to produce a "second foramen." An example of type 3 is shown in Figure 2–23 (*left*).

The condition is recognized roentgenographically as a shadow which depicts the enamel that covers the surface of the cavity or invagination and which may approach the radiographic density of the enamel that covers the surface of the crown (Fig. 2–24).

In instances in which the invagination is extensive, the crowns of the teeth involved are invariably malformed. With the accumulation and retention of fluid and debris within the invagination, the enamel that covers its surface is particularly vulnerable to decay and, as a result, there is a high incidence of infection and degeneration of the pulp (Fig. 2–23).

The roentgenogram often reveals enamel invaginations of lesser extent when there is no clinical evidence of their presence. A common site for these is the lingual surface of maxillary lateral incisors (Fig. 2–25). Because of the high incidence of infected and gangrenous pulps caused by this condition, obliteration of the defect by placing a filling as a prophylactic or preventive measure may be indicated.

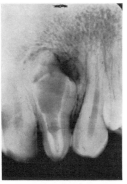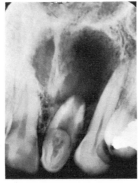

Figure 2–23 Dens in dente with periapical involvement. *Left,* Extensive invagination that involves a large portion of the root adjacent to which there is evidence of bone destruction caused by infection. *Right,* Dens in dente with radicular cyst.

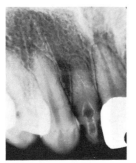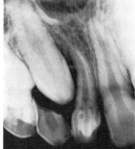

Figure 2–24 Dens in dente. *Left,* Single invagination of enamel extending from the apex of the conically shaped crown well up into the root of the tooth. *Right,* Two invaginations of enamel present in the same tooth. Pulps in both teeth were vital.

TUBERCULATED PREMOLAR (EVAGINATED ODONTOMA)

The tuberculated premolar also has been referred to as Leong's premolar and oriental premolar. The anomaly is one in which a tubercle, or protuberance, is located on the occlusal surface of premolar teeth. The tubercle, which varies in form, may arise from the center of the occlusal surface and obliterate the central groove, or it may arise from the lingual ridge of the buccal cusp. It consists of an outer layer of enamel with a core of dentin into which a horn of the dental pulp extends to varied degrees. The second premolars are involved most frequently and the anomaly is most often bilateral.

It is assumed that this anomaly affects only members of the mongolian race. It has been reported to occur only in Chinese, Japanese, Filipinos, Eskimos, and American Indians. Merrill (1964) examined 650 high-school students in southeastern Alaska, all Eskimos and Indians, and found the anomaly present in 28 of them. The 28 students had a total of 85 anomalous premolars.

The roentgenogram shown in Figure 2–26 was made for an 11-year-old boy of Chinese origin. It is from a case reported by Poyton and Vizcarra (1965) in which conical shaped tubercles are present in three mandibular premolars. The extensions of the pulp into the tubercles are clearly visible in the roentgenogram. The pulp in the left first premolar (shown on the viewer's right) had become exposed and there is evidence of rarefying osteitis near the apex of the root.

The presence of the anomaly obviously presents clinical problems. The tubercles interfere with normal interdigitation of the teeth, and this may lead to occlusal traumatism or malocclusion. As a result of abrasion or fracture of the tubercle, which is not uncommon, the pulp may become infected and thus lead to periapical abscess formation. Perhaps, as a preventive measure, removal of the tubercle and endodontic treatment may be indicated in those patients in whom the roentgenogram reveals that the pulp extends to a point near the surface.

HYPERCEMENTOSIS (CEMENTUM HYPERPLASIA)

Hypercementosis is excessive formation of cementum on the surface of the root

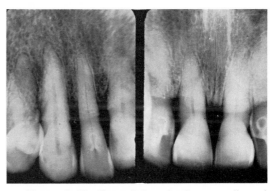

Figure 2–25 Enamel invaginations on lingual surface of both maxillary lateral incisors.

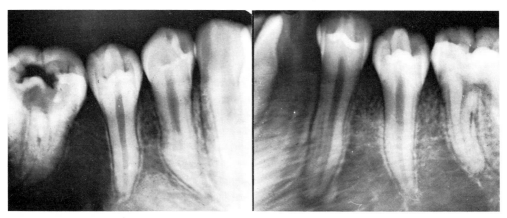

Figure 2–26 Tuberculated premolars in which the dental pulp has extended to a point near the tip of the tubercles. The first premolar on the viewer's right shows a periapical lesion. (Reproduced with permission from Poyton, H. G. and Vizcarra, E. R.: Three Evaginated Odontomes: Case Report, Canad. Dent. A. J. *31*:439–442, 1965.)

of the tooth. It is most often confined to the apical half of the root but, in some instances, may involve the entire root. In a large majority of instances, it affects vital teeth, is not associated with any one particular systemic disease, and therefore might justifiably be regarded as a dental anomaly, as suggested by Zemsky (1931). The premolars are most frequently involved; the incidence in rela-tion to other teeth is approximately 6 to 1 (Gardner and Goldstein, 1931). Next in order of frequency are the first and second molars.

Hypercementosis is seen in the roent-genogram as a bulbous enlargement that has surrounding it a continuous and un-broken periodontal membrane space, and a normal lamina dura (Fig. 2–27). The radio-

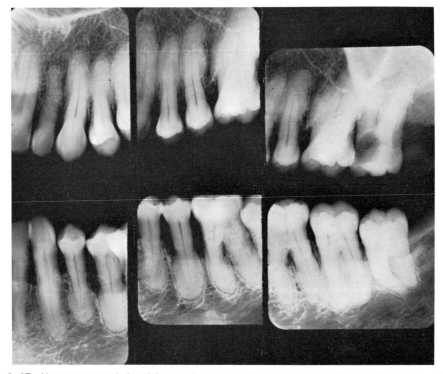

Figure 2–27 Hypercementosis involving canines, premolars, and molars. Teeth affected are vital and free from caries. Teeth on opposite side were similarly affected.

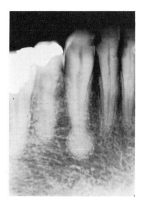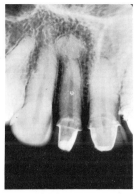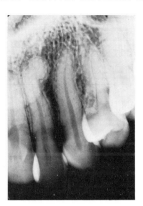

Figure 2–28 Hypercementosis of three anterior teeth, showing spherical mass of cementum situated at apex.

graphic density of hyperplastic cementum is less than that of dentin; therefore, the outline of the limits of the dentin is often discernible. Hypercementosis of anterior teeth often occurs in the form of a spherical mass of cementum situated directly at the apex of the root (Fig. 2–28).

In the case of pulpless teeth, hyperplasia of cementum may be stimulated by chronic inflammation of the periodontal membrane. According to Boyle (1949), the space for formation of the excess cementum is created by the inflammatory destruction of alveolar bone, and the formation is a protective and reparative reaction. This type of hypercementosis is readily recognized in the roentgenogram, for there is a definite break in the continuity of the periodontal membrane space and the lamina dura. Also, usually there is evidence of osseous destruction in the periapical region (Fig. 2–29).

There also is a form of hypercementosis

that is a common feature in Paget's disease (osteitis deformans) that involves the jaws. As seen roentgenographically, there is complete absence of the periodontal membrane space and lamina dura surrounding the hyperplastic cementum; therefore the condition can be readily distinguished from the forms previously discussed.

Nonpathologic hypercementosis, as such, is of very little significance. Many teeth with hypercementosis have in the past been removed on the erroneous assumption that they were the cause of a large variety of systemic conditions. Removal of such teeth with a view of relieving any systemic condition is contraindicated. They do become clinically significant if they must be removed for purely dental reasons, for their extraction obviously presents a difficult problem.

RETARDED DENTAL DEVELOPMENT

Retardation of development that does not exceed much more than 1 year and that involves the entire dentition may be considered as being within normal limits. Such retardation often follows a familial pattern. The most common systemic causes for retardation are hypopituitarism and hypothyroidism. It also may occur in association with another anomaly, namely facial hemiatrophy, in which retarded development may be present on the involved side.

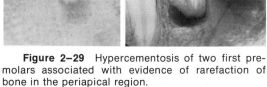

Figure 2–29 Hypercementosis of two first premolars associated with evidence of rarefaction of bone in the periapical region.

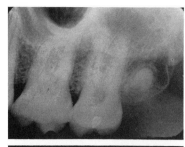

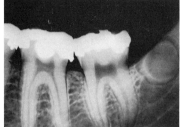

Figure 2–30 Retarded development of third molars. *Above,* Maxillary third molar at 26 years of age. *Below,* Mandibular third molar at 20 years of age.

Retardation also may occur as a distinct dental anomaly involving single teeth only. The teeth involved are those that most often are congenitally missing, particularly the third molars and premolars. Retarded development of third molars is shown in Figure 2–30, and of a premolar in Figure 2–31.

TRANSPOSITION OF TEETH

Exchange of position of teeth most often involves the canine and the teeth

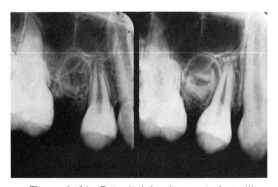

Figure 2–31 Retarded development of maxillary second premolar. *Left,* Tooth bud is shown, with evidence of early stage of calcification of the crown at 14 years of age. *Right,* One year later there is evidence of increased calcification.

adjacent to it. More rarely, transposition of premolars and molars has been noted also. In most instances, the transposed teeth are fully erupted and in normal alignment in the arch. There often is bilateral occurrence, which suggests that the anomaly has its origin in the anlage stage of development and not in a change in position in the course of eruption. Transposition of canines with lateral incisors is shown in Figures 2–32 and 2–33, and of canines with first premolars in Figure 2–34. An extremely rare occurrence is the transposition of a central and a lateral incisor (Fig. 2–35).

DENTINOGENESIS IMPERFECTA (HEREDITARY OPALESCENT DENTIN)

Dentinogenesis imperfecta is a hereditary anomaly of dominant character which can be expected to be passed on to one-half of the children of a parent (Hodge et al., 1939; Roberts, 1949; Skillen, 1937). The primary as well as the permanent teeth are involved. Physical examinations have revealed no disturbance to which it could be attributed, although a similar condition of the teeth does occur in association with osteogenesis imperfecta. The anomaly is characterized by imperfectly formed dentin and a crown that has an opalescent or amber color. The enamel is softer than normal, and the crowns may be worn away rapidly by attrition. This may result in early loss of teeth, if preventive measures are not taken. Small, underdeveloped roots also may be a feature of the anomaly.

Microscopic studies have shown that the histologic appearance of the enamel is normal, but there are pronounced pathologic changes in the dentin. Next to the enamel and cementum there is usually a thin layer of dentin which, while not quite normal, is fairly well developed. Next to this zone the dentinal tubules become fewer, are irregular in their course, and, as the central portion of the tooth is approached, may be absent. Apposition of this dentin of poor quality may continue until most or all of the pulp cavity is obliterated, and usually

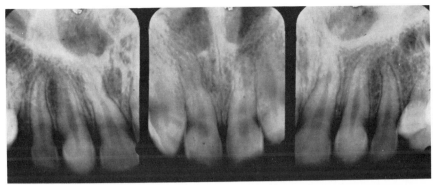

Figure 2–32 Transposition of maxillary canines and lateral incisors. Bilateral occurrence.

this takes place while the tooth is undergoing development.

The roentgenogram reveals the relative size of the crowns and roots of the teeth; where the pulp cavities have been obliterated the entire tooth has an increased opacity. The enamel may be distinguishable from dentin, but the peripheral zone of dentin, which is said to be nearly normal, cannot be distinguished roentgenographically from the dentin of poorer quality that occupies the central portion of the tooth.

The dental roentgenogram in Figure 2–36, made for a patient 3 years of age, demonstrates the early obliteration of the pulp chambers of the primary teeth. The replacement of the pulp chambers by a calcified substance gives the impression that the crowns of the teeth are abnormally dense; however, the density of the dentin actually is less than normal. The dental roentgenograms in Figure 2–37, made for a patient 10 years of age, reveal roots that are small in proportion to the size of the crowns, and obliteration of the pulp chambers almost simultaneously with calcification of the teeth. The incisors and first molars are fully developed and the pulp chambers are absent.

The dental roentgenogram made for a girl 19 years of age is shown in Figure 2–38. It illustrates the rapidity with which the crowns of the teeth may be worn away through attrition. The maxillary teeth had

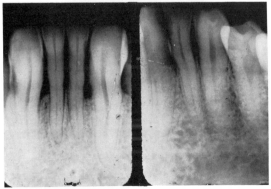

Figure 2–33 Transposition of mandibular canines and lateral incisors. Bilateral occurrence.

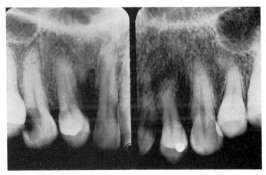

Figure 2–34 Transposition of maxillary canines and first premolars.

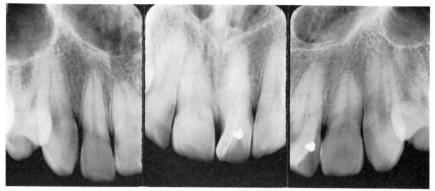

Figure 2–35 Transposition of a maxillary central and lateral incisor.

been extracted 2 years previously. The anomaly was known to be present in four generations. The teeth of two sisters were similarly involved, and two brothers and one sister had normal teeth.

DENTINAL DYSPLASIA

Dentinal dysplasia is a term used by Rushton (1939) to designate a rare anomaly characterized by dentin that contains an enormous number of spherical bodies. It produces partial or complete obliteration of the pulp. The roots are malformed, and there is a marked tendency to abscess and cyst formation. The primary as well as the permanent teeth are involved, and the condition is hereditary. Logan and co-workers (1962) have reported its occurrence in nine children of one family, and in two of four grandchildren. Their report includes excellent roentgenograms and ground sections of some of the teeth that demonstrate the bizarre histogenetic pattern of the dentin. The enamel is apparently normal, and the crowns of the teeth are of normal size. The dentin in the coronal portion of the tooth appears to have a near-normal tubular pattern which ends somewhat abruptly at about the point where the pulp chamber normally would be present. From this juncture on, there is a formation of whorl-like, spherical structures with a variable number of dentinal tubules, which continues apically and terminates at the apex of the root. The size and arrangement of the spherical bodies may vary greatly. Those situated near the coronal portion are in general larger and tend to be laid down in successive layers which are arranged in

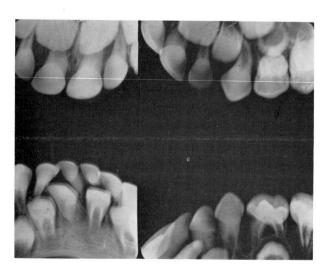

Figure 2–36 Dentinogenesis imperfecta in a patient 3 years of age, showing obliteration of the pulp chambers and root canals of the primary teeth.

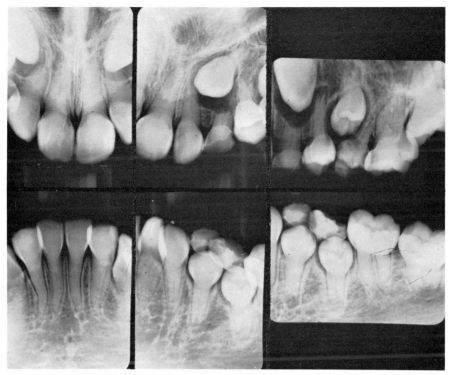

Figure 2–37 Dentinogenesis imperfecta in a patient 10 years of age, showing obliteration of the pulp chambers and root canals of the incisors and first molars; also, small underdeveloped roots are shown.

horizontal rows. As the apex of the root is approached the spherical bodies are smaller and their arrangement is completely disorganized and haphazard.

The roentgenographic examination is important in the identification of the anomaly. It reveals the size and shape of the roots of the teeth. With the possible exception of the canines, the roots are abnormally short; those of the single-rooted teeth are tapered, and those of the molars usually are blunt and stubby. There are no pulp chambers or root canals in evidence. Abscess and cyst formation is seen frequently and often affects teeth that are free from caries. The roentgenogram shown in Figure 2–39 reveals a total of 16 periapical lesions; those on the maxillary right and the mandibular left first molars resemble peridontal cysts. The most characteristic roentgenographic feature, which is peculiar to the anomaly, is the presence of one or more horizontal radio-

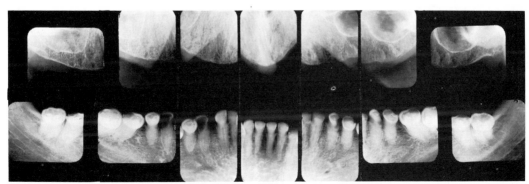

Figure 2–38 Dentinogenesis imperfecta in a patient 19 years of age, showing absence of pulp chambers and root canals, and marked incisal and occlusal wear.

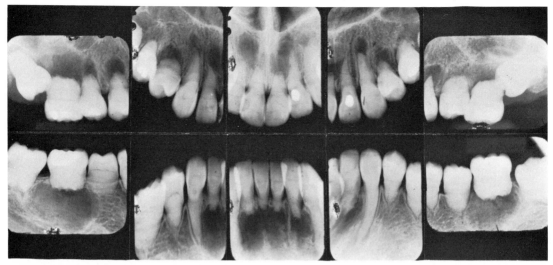

Figure 2–39 Dentinal dysplasia, showing deformities of the roots, absence of normal pulp cavities, horizontal radiolucent lines near the base of the crowns of some of the teeth, and a large number of periapical rarefactions.

lucent lines situated near the base of the crown. These lines correspond to and represent the space between layers of the spherical bodies that are arranged in horizontal rows. This feature is illustrated exceptionally well in Figure 2–40.

That dentinal dysplasia does not necessarily involve all of the teeth in a given case and that there may be variants in morphology of the teeth that it produces are suggested by cases reported by Elzay and Robinson (1967) and Stafne and Gibilisco (1961). In the latter case, the abnormality was confined to the mandibular canines and premolars only (Fig.

2–41). The middle third of the roots are more bulbous, and their diameter almost equals that of the crowns of the teeth. The apical portion of the roots are narrow and spindle-shaped. Hoggins and Marsland (1952) found that the calcified mass within the roots of teeth of similar morphology consisted chiefly of small foci of calcific degeneration and dentinal tubules of irregular pattern running parallel to the long axis of the tooth. The mass was surrounded by a thin layer of normal dentin. In a case reported by Petersson (1972), all of the incisors, canines, and premolars presented a roentgenographic ap-

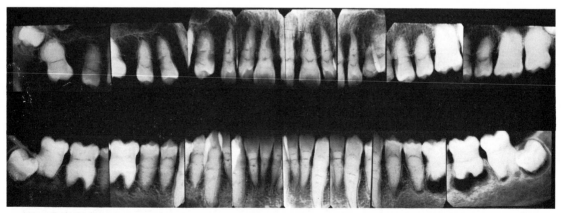

Figure 2–40 Dentinal dysplasia in a 13-year-old boy, demonstrating at various levels one or more of the horizontal radiolucent lines characteristic of the anomaly. (Reproduced with permission from Logan, J., Becks, H., Silverman, S., Jr., and Pindborg, J. J.: Dentinal Dysplasia. Oral. Surg., Oral Med. & Oral Path. *15*:317–333 [Mar.] 1962.)

Figure 2–41 Enlargement and deformity of the roots of the canine and premolars caused by dentinal dysplasia. (Reproduced with permission from Stafne, E. C. and Gibilisco, J. A.: Calcifications of the Dentinal Papilla That May Cause Anomalies of the Roots of Teeth. Oral Surg., Oral Med. & Oral Path, *14*:683–686 [June] 1961.)

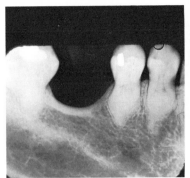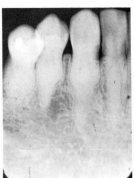

pearance similar to that seen in Figure 2–41, and an anomaly of the molars resembled dentinal dysplasia.

AMELOGENESIS IMPERFECTA (HEREDITARY HYPOPLASIA OF ENAMEL)

Hereditary hypoplasia of the enamel is an anomaly of dominant character. The hypoplasia probably is caused by generalized disturbance of the ameloblasts. The enamel of all the teeth is affected. The dentin, cementum, and pulp are normal. Roentgenographically, such teeth are recognized by the absence of the radiopaque image that depicts the enamel of normal teeth (Fig. 2–42). Because of the thinness or absence of enamel, the crowns have a dark, yellowish color, and are tapered.

The primary as well as the permanent teeth may be affected (Cameron and Bradford, 1957; Chaudhry et al., 1959), and the incidence of caries is low (Toller, 1959).

TURNER'S TEETH

A Turner tooth is one with hypoplasia of enamel that is of local origin. It is usually confined to single teeth, and the mandibular premolars are the teeth most frequently affected. The hypoplasia is caused by periapical infection and inflammation involving a primary tooth that spread to the enamel organ of the underlying tooth germ before development of the enamel is completed. Damage to the ameloblasts leads to the defects of the enamel (Morningstar, 1937). The defect may involve the entire surface, or only a small portion of it. Figure 2–43 shows varied degrees of hypoplasia involving two mandibular premolars.

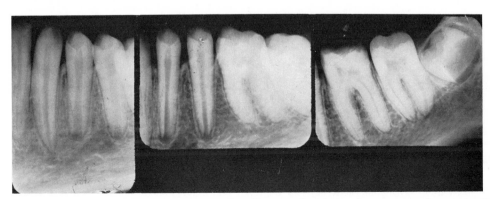

Figure 2–42 Amelogenesis imperfecta in a patient 12 years of age, showing absence of enamel and tapering crowns, including unerupted third molar; all teeth are similarly affected. A sister had a like condition.

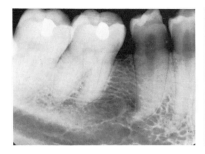

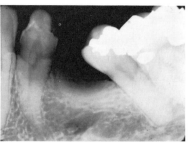

Figure 2–43 Turner's teeth showing enamel hypoplasia of local origin. *Left,* Only a portion of the crown is involved. *Right,* The entire crown is involved.

ODONTODYSPLASIA (ODONTOGENESIS IMPERFECTA)

Odontodysplasia is characterized by a marked hypoplasia and hypocalcification of the enamel and dentin. The cementum may have a normal mineral content but is much thinner than normal. The cause is unknown. Teeth of both dentitions may be affected, and when the primary teeth are involved their permanent successors are prone to present a similar condition. In most instances more than one tooth is affected and these tend to occur in consecutive series in the arch. To our knowledge there have been no instances in which all of the teeth have been affected; however, Chaudhry and colleagues (1961) reported the case of a 7-year-old girl whose mandibular first molars and all teeth anterior to them were involved. Also the left maxillary posterior teeth were involved.

Rushton (1965) studied the distribution on the basis of 18 cases and found that the teeth of the maxilla were affected in 14 cases and the mandible in 4. In both jaws the teeth most frequently affected were the anteriors. In the case of the primary incisors one can assume that the disorder had its onset at about the sixth month of prenatal

life, and that of the permanent incisors prior to the sixth month of postnatal life. The anomaly probably results from a disorderly proliferation of the dental epithelium during the early stage of hard dental-tissue formation followed by premature degeneration of the enamel organ. The histologic aspects of the anomaly have been well established by Bergman and colleagues (1963) and Zegarelli and colleagues (1963). Gardner and Sapp (1973) reviewed the literature and reported the histologic findings in two cases of their own. In one of them, a periapical lesion on one of the affected teeth was found to be an empty cavity, similar to a traumatic bone cyst. Burch et al. (1973) reported a case in which a periapical cyst lined by squamous epithelioma had developed on one of the involved teeth.

Figure 2–44 illustrates the features of odontodysplasia. The patient was a 9-year-old boy. The right mandibular incisors and canine are affected. The central incisor has undergone partial eruption; the lateral incisor and canine remain embedded. There is a hypoplasia of enamel which involves the entire surface of the crowns. The roots of the incisors are almost completely formed, as evidenced by a thin layer of dentin that depicts their outline. Only a very thin layer

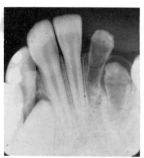

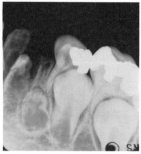

Figure 2–44 Odontogenesis imperfecta involving the right mandibular incisors and canine.

of dentin is present next to the enamel and cementum. The pulp cavities are abnormally large. Since noneruption is not uncommon, teeth that remain embedded may erroneously be mistaken for those that are undergoing resorption.

In the case represented in Figure 2–44, the corresponding primary teeth were said to be discolored and hypoplastic. The anomaly could not be attributed to a systemic disturbance or a familial tendency.

COMPLEX DENTAL ANOMALY

A case reported by Bruce (1954) is unusual in that it presented a composite of several anomalous features that may affect the teeth. These consisted of early maturation, eruption, and exfoliation of the primary teeth and several of the permanent teeth. Also, dentinogenesis imperfecta, cementogenesis imperfecta, microdontia, and a supernumerary tooth were present. The patient was normal otherwise, and the dental condition could not be explained on a hereditary basis.

The primary incisors had erupted and shed and the primary first molars were undergoing eruption at 10½ months of age. At 3 years and 8 months of age (Fig. 2–45)

the mandibular incisor and first molars of the permanent dentition had erupted. Of the primary dentition, only four of the molars remained; a supernumerary tooth was present in the right maxillary incisor region.

Microscopic examination of some of the exfoliated teeth revealed that the enamel was essentially normal. The dentin was abnormal in that the tubules were sparse and widely spaced, and in some areas had a whorled arrangement. There were very few odontoblasts, and the pulp chamber was prematurely reduced in size. Little, if any, cementum was present on the root surfaces. In the absence of cementum, adequate fixation and retention of the tooth are not afforded, and Bruce thought that this may have accounted for the early and rapid sloughing of the teeth.

This anomaly, which is primarily of mesenchymal origin, is of interest in that the disturbance caused cementogenesis imperfecta as well as dentinogenesis imperfecta.

TAURODONTIA

Taurodontia is a descriptive term suggested by Keith (1913) for molar teeth that in

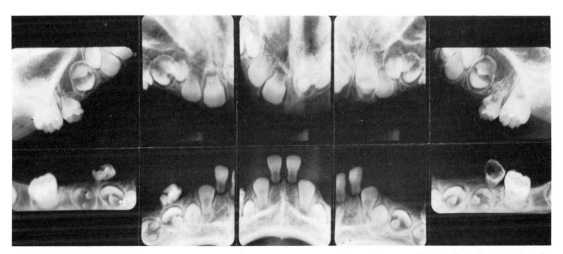

Figure 2–45 Complex dental anomaly. Roentgenogram made at 3 years 8 months of age, showing premature loss of the primary teeth, eruption of the permanent first molars and mandibular central incisors, and obliteration of the pulp chambers of the incisor teeth. (Reproduced with permission from Bruce, K. W.: Dental Anomaly: Early Exfoliation of Deciduous and Permanent Teeth. J. Am. Dent. A. *48*:414–421 [Apr.] 1954.)

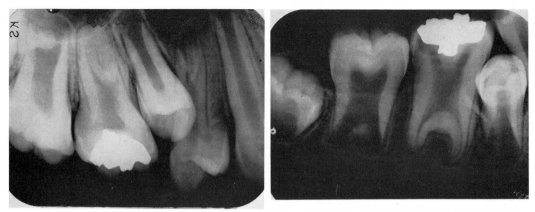

Figure 2–46 Taurodontism. Roentgenograms of maxillary and mandibular first and second molars which have the typical features of the taurodont form of molar. These are abnormally long pulp chambers and short root canals. (Reproduced with permission from Hamner, J. E., III, Witkop, C. J., Jr., and Metro, P. S.: Taurodontism: Report of a Case. Oral Surg., Oral Med. & Oral Path. *18*:409–418 [Sept.] 1964.)

many respects resemble in form those of the ox and some other hoofed mammals. The prominent feature is an extension of the pulp chamber deep into the root portion of the tooth; in some instances the pulp chamber almost reaches the apex. Since the overall length of these teeth is not greater than that of normal teeth, the end result is one of abnormally short root canals. The anomaly occurs in the primary as well as in the permanent molars, and there is a marked tendency to bilateral occurrence.

Hamner and colleagues (1964) have expressed the opinion that taurodontism is caused by failure of Hertwig's sheath to evaginate at the proper horizontal level, and may not do so to form the root cleft until it has reached a point near the apex of the root. Figure 2–46 illustrates the main features of the anomaly in a white girl 13 years of age.

Taurodontism has been of interest to the anthropologist, since it has been found in certain prehistoric men, particularly the Neanderthal man. However, there is evidence that it does occur on occasion in the various races of modern man. As with many other anomalies of dentition, it might be considered as a retrograde or atavistic feature (Album, 1958; Stoy, 1960). The dental roentgenogram often reveals variants of the taurodont form of molars; therefore it cannot be considered rare.

CLEFTS OF THE PALATE AND JAW

Clefts of the alveolar process and palate result from complete or partial failure of the facial processes to fuse. Failure of the palatine processes to fuse results in cleft palate; failure of the globular process and the maxillary bone to fuse results in a cleft of the alveolar process, which most often is situated between the canine and lateral incisor. Disturbance of dental development in the region of the cleft is not uncommon, and this is manifested by the formation of supernumerary teeth, or absence of teeth. Teeth

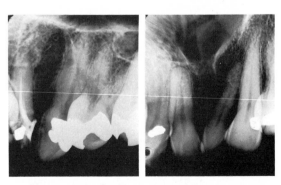

Figure 2–47 Clefts of the jaw. *Left,* Cleft involving jaws only and situated between canine and lateral incisor. Incomplete union of osseous structure is evidenced by radiolucence in interseptal space. *Right,* Incomplete fusion of maxillary bone with premaxilla.

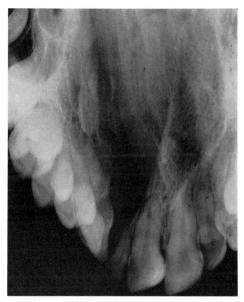

Figure 2–48   Cleft of jaw and palate.

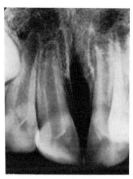

Figure 2–50   Median alveolar cleft of the jaw. True clefts in this region are exceedingly rare.

may remain embedded in bone, or may erupt into the cleft or the nostril. Clefts of the palate and the jaw are often combined with one another, and with cleft lip (harelip) (Chase, 1945). Clefts also may occur bilaterally.

Roentgenographic examination is of value in that it reveals the extent and size of the osseous deformity, and also the position and number of teeth present in the region of the cleft. Use of occlusal as well as intraoral

dental views is necessary. Partial clefts of the jaw that have produced no clinically significant abnormality are shown in Figure 2–47. In Figure 2–48 are views of a combined cleft of the jaw and palate as seen in an occlusal view. In Figure 2–49 is an occlusal view of a bilateral cleft of the jaw and palate. A small median alveolar cleft of the jaw is shown in Figure 2–50. This occurs as a result of nonunion of the two centers of calcification of the globular process.

HYPERTROPHY OF THE TUBEROSITY

Hypertrophy of the tuberosities is almost always bilateral, and overdevelopment may take place in some instances to such an extent that it inteferes with normal closure of the teeth. If artificial dentures must be worn, there may be inadequate space for their insertion, or the presence of the prominence may not permit construction of the artificial denture to the desired occlusal plane. The excess bone can be removed readily and with assurance that there will be no recurrence. The roentgenogram (Fig. 2–51) will reveal the amount by which the prominence safely can be reduced without encroachment on the maxillary sinus.

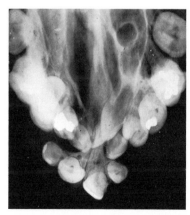

Figure 2–49   Bilateral clefts. The premaxilla contains the incisor teeth, and a supernumerary right lateral incisor is situated in the maxillary bone. A view of the palate reveals a wide cleft. (Reproduced with permission from Millhon, J. A. and Stafne, E. C.: Incidence of Supernumerary and Congenitally Missing Lateral Incisor Teeth in 81 Cases of Harelip and Cleft Palate. Am. J. Orthodontics [Oral Surg. Sect.]. 27:599–604 [Nov.] 1941.)

HYPERTROPHY OF THE ANGLE OF THE MANDIBLE

Hypertrophy of the angle of the mandible may be of genetic origin, or it may be

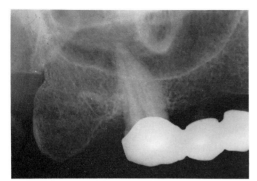

Figure 2–51 Hypertrophy of the tuberosity.

acquired. In the genetic form the prominence is bilateral, and there may or may not be a relative enlargement of the masseter muscle. Acquired hypertrophy of the angle may be bilateral or unilateral, and usually results from excessive function of the masseter muscle. The hypertrophy occurs at the site of insertion of the muscle on the mandible, and there is compensatory hypertrophy of the muscle as well. Among the contributory causes are abnormal masticating habits, bruxism, and habitual clenching of the teeth. The enlargement of bone and muscle in some instances is so extensive that it causes a disproportion in the shape of the face, particularly when there is unilateral involvement. The hypertrophy of the soft tissue may be thought to represent a disturbance of the parotid gland, a lipoma, or

some other tumor. A roentgenogram that demonstrates hypertrophy of bone as well should be of aid in differential diagnosis (Fig. 2–52).

The deformity of the face may be of great concern to the patient. In such cases markedly improved cosmetic results have been obtained by removing a portion of the muscle and reducing the bony prominence (Caldwell and Hughes, 1957; Eubanks, 1957).

HYPERTROPHY OF THE CORONOID PROCESS

Enlargement of the coronoid process most often occurs as a result of tumor formation. However, enlargement of the process also occurs as a result of a hyperplasia of normal bone and may be so extensive that it limits the movement of the mandible in all directions. This limitation of movement is produced by an extension into the infraorbital fossa with infringement upon the posterior aspect of the zygomatic bone and arch.

The onset of the condition is thought to be at about puberty, and in some instances the involvement may be bilateral. The first report of bilateral hyperplasia apparently was made by Van Zile and Johnson (1957). Other reports are those by Shira and Lister (1958) and Allison et al. (1969). The tomo-

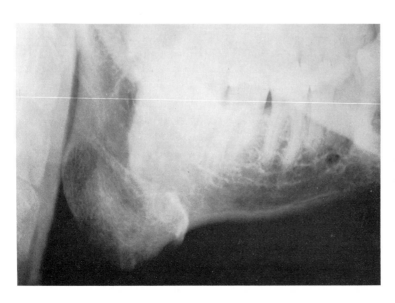

Figure 2–52 Hypertrophy of the angle of the mandible associated with an overdeveloped and enlarged masseter muscle. A similar enlargement was present on the opposite side.

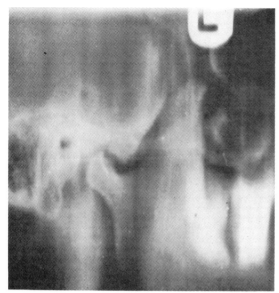

Figure 2–53 Hypertrophy of the coronoid process. (Reproduced with permission from Davidson, J. S. H.: Unilateral Coronoid Hypertrophy Causing Restricted Opening of Mouth. Brit. J. Radiol. 38:478–479 [June] 1965.)

gram of a case of unilateral involvement reported by Davidson (1965) is shown in Figure 2–53.

Excellent results have been obtained by surgical removal of the enlarged portion of the coronoid process, and normal movement and function of the mandible have been restored.

DEVELOPMENTAL DEFECT OF THE MANDIBLE CONTAINING SALIVARY GLAND TISSUE

A defect that occurs in the posterior region of the mandible near the inferior border simulates in some respects the roentgenographic appearance of epithelium-lined cysts, although its borders tend to be more opaque and wide. Selected views of nine of these defects are shown in Figure 2–54, bilateral occurrence is shown in Figure 2–55, and a defect that was revealed by a lateral-oblique view of the mandible is shown in Figure 2–56. In the roentgenogram the defect presents either an elliptical or a round radiolucent image that is most often situated slightly above the inferior border. In some defects the continuity of the inferior border is interrupted and in this region cortical bone

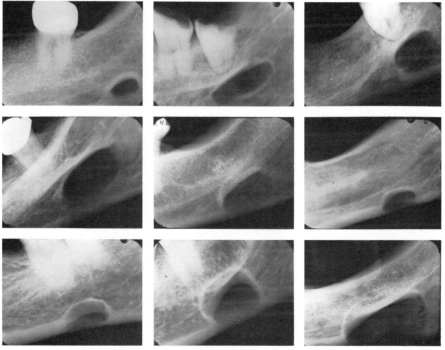

Figure 2–54 Developmental defects of the mandible presumably containing salivary gland tissue. Nine cases are illustrated to show the common location and the typical roentgenographic appearance. (Reproduced with permission from Stafne, E. C.: Bone Cavities Situated Near the Angle of the Mandible. J. Am. Dent. A. 29:1969–1972 [Nov. 1] 1942.)

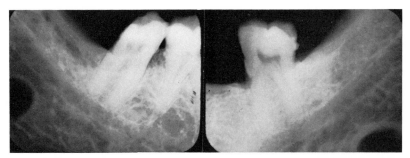

Figure 2-55 Bilateral developmental defects of the mandible.

is absent, which demonstrates that it is not a closed bone cavity (Stafne, 1942).

In almost all cases the defect was first detected incidentally in routine dental roentgenographic examination, when all or a portion of the image of the defect would appear at the lower border of a roentgenogram that had been positioned to include as much of the third molar and retromolar region as possible. In some cases the defect has been observed for several years, and no change in size or alteration in the roentgenographic appearance has been seen. None of the defects was observed in children; however, in children a dental film can rarely be placed downward and posteriorly to a position where it would include such a defect even if it were present.

The consistency of locale and similarity of roentgenographic appearance suggest that the condition is a definite entity.

It is unlikely that such a defect is of odontogenic origin, since it is situated below the mandibular canal. It has been suggested that such defects represent eosinophilic granulomas; however, general physical examination has not revealed polycystic disease, and it is doubtful that all of them could represent solitary eosinophilic granuloma of bone. Their dense and definite borders also differentiate them from eosinophilic granuloma. Furthermore, it is doubtful whether an eosinophilic granuloma involving the mandible ever arises below the mandibular canal.

Rushton (1946) expressed the belief that these defects represent constricted remains of solitary cysts present at an earlier age, and referred to them as "latent bone cysts." That they can be explained on this basis can be questioned, for in no instance was there a history of a previous solitary or traumatic bone cyst in more than 100 cases observed. Neither was there any residual enlargement or deformity of the mandible, which is often present following resolution

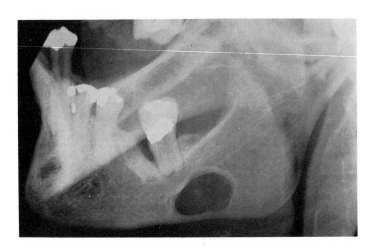

Figure 2-56 Developmental defect of the mandible as viewed in a lateral roentgenogram of the mandible.

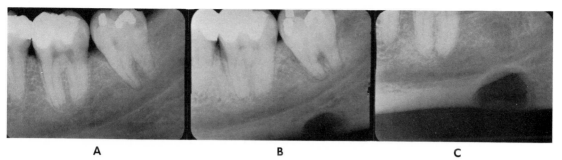

Figure 2–57 Developmental bony defect of the mandible. *A*, Negative (1947). *B*, Early rarefaction of bone (1954). *C*, Typical defect present (1967). (Reproduced with permission from Tolman, D. E. and Stafne, E. C.: Developmental Bone Defects of the Mandible. Oral Surg., Oral Med. & Oral Path. *24*:488–490 [Oct.] 1967.)

of a solitary cyst, many of which reach an appreciable size and expand the cortex.

In recent years several cases have been reported in which microscopic examination has demonstrated that the contents of such defects consisted of normal salivary gland tissue. Among these reports are those of Choukas and Toto (1960), Amaral and Jacobs (1961), and Hayes (1961). More recently, Choukas (1973) reported two cases in which normal salivary gland tissue occupied the defects. Reasonable evidence that the concavity contains a lobule of the submaxillary gland similar to those found at operation is provided by sialograms. Seward (1960) studied two defects by means of the sialogram, and from the occlusal views demonstrated that a branch of the submaxillary gland extended directly into the defect in the mandible. It also has been established that they are not confined to the molar region only, but may be present in the anterior portion of the mandible where they are occupied by sublingual salivary gland tissue (Richard and Ziskind, 1957; Camilleri, 1963; Palladino et al., 1965; Miller and Winnick, 1971).

The consensus has been that the condition is congenital. This has been based on the supposition that a premature growth of the gland had to be accommodated by an abnormally deep submaxillary fossa or even a deeper concavity or defect on the lingual surface of the mandible. This is conceivable since, in the embryo, the differentiation of the gland precedes the development of the mandible. However, Tolman and Stafne (1967) reported two cases in which typical roentgenographic evidence of the defect first had appeared after the patients had reached middle age. A series of dental roentgenograms made for one of them, a man who was 59 years old when typical evidence of the defect appeared, is shown in Figure 2–57; Figure 2–58 shows a roentgenogram made for the same patient in 1973, six years after the one shown in Figure 2–57C. During the six-year period there was no change in the shape or size of the defect. Roentgenograms made for a man who was 58 years of age when the defect first was observed are shown in Figure 2–59. In both cases, the defects had appeared without any symptoms referable to the mandible. Apparently they had developed slowly and progressively, and were not the remains of a larger lesion or cyst of the jaws.

The roentgenographic findings would indicate that these bony defects are not exclusively congenital in origin.

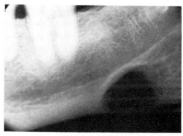

Figure 2–58 Developmental bony defect of the mandible. Roentgenogram made 6 years after the one shown in Figure 2–57C which demonstrates no change in size or shape of the defect.

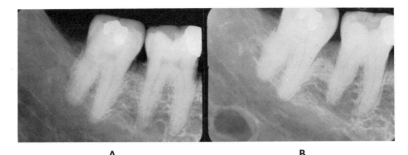

A   **B**

Figure 2–59 Developmental bony defect of the mandible. *A,* Negative (1944). *B,* Bony defect present (1954). (Reproduced with permission from Tolman, D. E. and Stafne, E. C.: Developmental Bone Defects of the Mandible. Oral Surg., Oral Med. & Oral Path. *24:*488–490 [Oct.] 1967.)

REFERENCES

Album, M. M.: Taurodontia in Deciduous First Molars. J. Am. Dent. A. *56:*562 (Apr.) 1958.

Allison, M. L., Wallace, W. R., and Von Wyl, H.: Coronoid Abnormalities Causing Limitation of Mandibular Movement. J. Oral Surg. *27:*229–233 (Mar.) 1969.

Amaral, W. J. and Jacobs, D. S.: Aberrant Salivary Gland Defect in the Mandible: Report of a Case. Oral Surg., Oral Med. & Oral Path. *14:*748–752 (June) 1961.

Bergman, G., Lysell, L., and Pindborg, J. J.: Unilateral Dental Malformation: Report of Two Cases. Oral Surg., Oral Med. & Oral Path. *16:*48–60 (Jan.) 1963.

Boyle, P. E.: Histopathology of the Teeth and Their Supporting Structures. Ed. 3. Philadelphia, Lea & Febiger, 1949, 514 pp.

Bruce, K. W.: Dental Anomaly: Early Exfoliation of Deciduous and Permanent Teeth. J. Am. Dent. A. *48:*414–421 (Apr.) 1954.

Burch, M. S., Besley, K. W., and Samuels, H. S.: Regional Odontodysplasia with Associated Midline Mandibular Cyst: Report of Case. J. Oral Surg. *31:*44–48 (Jan.) 1973.

Caldwell, J. B. and Hughes, K. W.: Hypertrophy of the Masseter Muscles and Mandible: Report of Case. Oral Surg., Oral Med. & Oral Path. *15:*329–333 (Oct.) 1957.

Cameron, I. W. and Bradford, E. W.: Amelogenesis Imperfecta: A Case Report of a Family. Brit. Dent. J. *102:*129–133 (Feb. 19) 1957.

Camilleri, G.: Salivary Gland Inclusion of the Mandible. Brit. Dent. J. *114:*515–516 (June 18) 1963.

Cavanha, A. O.: Enamel Pearls. Oral Surg., Oral Med. & Oral Path. *19:*373–382 (Mar.) 1965.

Chase, S. W.: The Abnormal Development of the Oral Region. In Hill, T. J.: A Textbook of Oral Pathology. Ed. 3. Philadelphia, Lea & Febiger, 1945, 398 pp.

Chaudhry, A. P., Johnson, O. N., Mitchell, D. F., Gorlin, R. J., and Bartholdi, W. L.: Hereditary Enamel Dysplasia. J. Pediat. *54:*776–785 (May) 1959.

Chaudhry, A. P., Wittich, H. C., Stickel, F. R., and Holland, M. R.: Odontogenesis Imperfecta: Report of a Case. Oral Surg., Oral Med. & Oral Path. *14:*1099–1103 (Sept.) 1961.

Choukas, N. C.: Developmental Submandibular Gland Defect of the Mandible: Review of the Literature and Report of Two Cases. J. Oral Surg. *31:*209–211 (Mar.) 1973.

Choukas, N. C. and Toto, P. D.: Etiology of Static Bone Defects of the Mandible. J. Oral Surg. *18:*16–20 (Jan.) 1960.

Dahlberg, A. A.: Inherited Congenital Absence of Six Incisors, Deciduous and Permanent. J. Dent. Res. *16:*59–62 (Feb.) 1937.

Davidson, J. S. H.: Unilateral Coronoid Hypertrophy Causing Restricted Opening of Mouth. Brit. J. Radiol. *38:*478–479 (June) 1965.

Elzay, R. P. and Robinson, C. T.: Dentinal Dysplasia: Report of a Case. Oral Surg., Oral Med. & Oral Path. *23:*338–342 (Mar.) 1967.

Eubanks, R. J.: Surgical Correction of Masseter Muscle Hypertrophy Associated with Unilateral Prognathism: Report of Case. J. Oral Surg. *15:*66–69 (Jan.) 1957.

Fastlicht, S.: Supernumerary Teeth and Malocclusion. Am. J. Orthodontics. *29:*623–637 (Nov.) 1943.

Gardner, B. S. and Goldstein, H.: The Significance of Hypercementosis. Dent. Cosmos. *73:*1065–1069 (Nov.) 1931.

Gardner, D. G. and Sapp, J. P.: Regional Odontodysplasia. Oral Surg., Oral Med. & Oral Path. *35:*351–365 (Mar.) 1973.

Gardner, T. A.: Six Generations of Congenitally Missing Teeth. Dent. Cosmos. *69:*1041–1045 (Oct.) 1927.

Garn, S. M. and Lewis, A. B.: The Relationship Between Third Molar Agenesis and Reduction in Tooth Number. Angle Orthodont. *32:*14–18 (Jan.) 1962.

Hamner, J. E., III, Witkop, C. J., Jr., and Metro, P. S.: Taurodontism: Report of a Case. Oral Surg., Oral Med. & Oral Path. *18:*409–418 (Sept.) 1964.

Hayes, H.: Aberrant Submaxillary Gland Tissue Presenting as a Cyst of the Jaw: Report of a Case. Oral Surg., Oral Med. & Oral Path. *14:*313–316 (Mar.) 1961.

Hillam, D. G.: Congenital Absence of Permanent Maxillary Canines. Dent. Pract. (Bristol). *20:*268–270 (Apr.) 1970.

Hodge, H. C., Finn, S. B., Lose, G. B., Gachet, F. S., and Bassett, S. H.: Hereditary Opalescent Dentin: General and Oral Clinical Studies. J. Am. Dent. A. *26:*1663–1674 (Oct.) 1939.

Hoggins, G. S. and Marsland, E. A.: Developmental Abnormalities of the Dentine and Pulp Associated with Calcinosis. Brit. Dent. J. *92*:305–311 (June 17) 1952.

Hutchinson, A. C. W.: A Case of Total Anodontia of the Permanent Dentition. Brit. Dent. J. *94*:16–17 (Jan. 6) 1953.

Keith, A.: Problems Relating to the Teeth of the Earlier Forms of Prehistoric Man. Proc. Roy. Soc. Med. 6 (part 3):103–124, 1913.

Kitchin, P. C.: Dens in Dente. J. Dent. Res. *15*:117–121 (Apr.) 1935.

Kronfeld, R.: Dens in Dente. J. Dent. Res. *14*:49–66 (Feb.) 1934.

Logan, J., Becks, H., Silverman, S., Jr., and Pindborg, J. J.: Dentinal Dysplasia. Oral Surg., Oral Med. & Oral Path. *15*:317–333 (Mar.) 1962.

Merrill, R. G.: Occlusal Anomalous Tubercles on Premolars of Alaskan Eskimos and Indians. Oral Surg., Oral Med. & Oral Path. *17*:484–496 (Apr.) 1964.

Miller, A. S. and Winnick, M.: Salivary Gland Inclusion in the Anterior Mandible: Report of a Case with a Review of the Literature on Aberrant Salivary Gland Tissue and Neoplasms. Oral Surg., Oral Med. & Oral Path. *31*:790–797 (June) 1971.

Millhon, J. A. and Stafne, E. C.: Incidence of Supernumerary and Congenitally Missing Lateral Incisor Teeth in Eighty-one Cases of Harelip and Cleft Palate. Am. J. Orthodontics (Oral Surg. Sect.) 27:599–604 (Nov.) 1941.

Morgan, G. A., Morgan, P. R., and Crouch, S. A.: Recurring Mandibular Supplemental Premolars. Oral Surg., Oral Med. & Oral Path. *30*:501–504 (Oct.) 1970.

Morgan, G. A. and Poyton, H. G.: Bilateral Dens in Dente. Oral Surg., Oral Med. & Oral Path. *13*: 63–66 (Jan.) 1960.

Morningstar, C. H.: Effect of Infection of Deciduous Molar on the Permanent Tooth Germ. J. Am. Dent. A. *24*:786–791 (May) 1937.

Oehlers, F. A. C.: Dens Invaginatus (Dilated Composite Odontome). I. Variations of the Invagination Process on Associated Anterior Crown Forms. Oral Surg., Oral Med. & Oral Path. *10*:1204–1218 (Nov.) 1957.

Osborn, R. C.: On Supernumerary Teeth in Man and Other Mammals. Dent. Cosmos. *54*:1193–1203 (Nov.) 1912.

Palladino, V. S., Rose, S. A., and Curran, T.: Salivary Gland Tissue in the Mandible and Stafne's Mandibular 'Cysts.' J. Am. Dent. A. *70*:388–393 (Feb.) 1965.

Petersson, A.: A Case of Dentinal Dysplasia and/or Calcification of the Dentinal Papilla. Oral Surg., Oral Med. & Oral Path. 33:1014–1017 (June) 1972.

Pindborg, J. J.: Pathology of the Dental Hard Tissues. Philadelphia, W. B. Saunders Company, 1970, 443 pp.

Porter, C. G. and Edwards, R. W.: Congenital Absence of Twenty-nine Permanent Teeth: Report of Case. J. Am. Dent. A. *24*:1852–1854 (Nov.) 1937.

Poyton, H. G. and Vizcarra, E. R.: Three Evaginated Odontomes: Case Report. Canad. Dent. A. J. *31*: 439–442, 1965.

Richard, E. L. and Ziskind, J.: Aberrant Salivary Gland Tissue in Mandible. Oral Surg., Oral Med. & Oral Path. *10*:1086–1090 (Oct.) 1957.

Roberts, W. R.: Hereditary Dentinogenesis Imperfecta (Opalescent Dentine). Brit. Dent. J. *87*:6–10 (July 1) 1949.

Rushton, M. A.: A Case of Dentinal Dysplasia. Guy's Hosp. Rep. 89:369–373, 1939.

Rushton, M. A.: Solitary Bone Cysts in the Mandible. Brit. Dent. J. *81*:37–49 (July 19) 1946.

Rushton, M. A.: Odontodysplasia: 'Ghost Teeth.' Brit. Dent. J. *119*:109–113 (Aug. 3) 1965.

Seward, G. R.: Salivary Gland Inclusions in the Mandible. Brit. Dent. J. *108*:321–325 (May) 1960.

Shira, R. B. and Lister, R. L.: Limited Mandibular Movements Due to Enlargement of the Coronoid Process. J. Oral Surg. *16*:183–191 (May) 1958.

Simon, J. F., Jr. and Webster, G. M.: Developmental Absence of Maxillary Permanent Cuspids. Oral Surg., Oral Med. & Oral Path. *30*:647–648 (Nov.) 1970.

Skillen, W. G.: Histologic and Clinical Study of Hereditary Opalescent Dentin. J. Am. Dent. A. *24*:1426–1433 (Sept.) 1937.

Stafne, E. C.: Supernumerary Upper Central Incisors. Dent. Cosmos. 73:976–980 (Oct.) 1931.

Stafne, E. C.: Supernumerary Teeth. Dent. Cosmos. 74:653–659 (July) 1932.

Stafne, E. C.: Bone Cavities Situated Near the Angle of the Mandible. J. Am. Dent. A. 29:1969–1972 (Nov. 1) 1942.

Stafne, E. C. and Gibilisco, J. A.: Calcifications of the Dentinal Papilla That May Cause Anomalies of the Roots of Teeth. Oral Surg., Oral Med. & Oral Path. *14*:683–686 (June) 1961.

Stoy, P. J.: Taurodontism Associated with Other Dental Anomalies. Dent. Pract. & Dent. Rec. *10*:202–205 (May) 1960.

Swallow, J. N.: Complete Anodontia of the Permanent Dentition: A Case Report. Brit. Dent. J. *107*: 143–145 (Sept.) 1959.

Toller, P. A.: A Clinical Report on Six Cases of Amelogenesis Imperfecta. Oral Surg., Oral Med. & Oral Path. *12*:325–333 (Mar.) 1959.

Tolman, D. E. and Stafne, E. C.: Developmental Bone Defects of the Mandible. Oral Surg., Oral Med. & Oral Path. *24*:488–490 (Oct.) 1967.

Van Zile, W. N. and Johnson, W. B.: Bilateral Coronoid Process Exostoses Simulating Partial Ankylosis of the Temporo-mandibular Joint: Report of Case. J. Oral Surg. *15*:72–77 (Jan.) 1957.

Zegarelli, E. V., Kutscher, A. H., Applebaum, E., and Archard, H. O.: Odontodysplasia. Oral Surg., Oral Med. & Oral Path. *16*:187–193 (Feb.) 1963.

Zemsky, J. L.: Hypercementosis and Heredity: An Introduction and Plan of Investigation. Dent. Items of Interest. *53*:335–347 (May) 1931.

MALPOSITION OF TEETH

3

A malposed tooth is one that is not in its normal position. Malposed teeth that have erupted are best seen and evaluated by clinical examination, but those that remain unerupted can be detected and evaluated by roentgenographic examination only. Embedded teeth are those that have failed to erupt, and remain completely or partially covered by bone or soft tissue or both. Those that have been obstructed by contact against another erupted or unerupted tooth in the course of their eruption are referred to as impacted teeth.

The causes for noneruption of teeth are numerous. Chiefly, these are lack of space; obstruction by cysts, tumors, supernumerary and primary teeth; infection; trauma; anomalous conditions affecting the jaws and teeth; and systemic conditions.

The most common cause of noneruption is lack of space. Often there is not sufficient space in the jaws to accommodate all of the teeth, and those that erupt first may occupy a portion or all of the space that is intended for those teeth that erupt later, namely the canines and third molars. Insufficient space is created as a result of premature loss of a primary tooth, and this often occurs following loss of a primary second molar, in which instance the permanent first molar may move forward, leaving little if any space into which the second premolar can erupt.

Obstruction by supernumerary teeth, and by primary teeth that are retained beyond their normal time for exfoliation, is not an uncommon cause of noneruption of the teeth of the permanent dentition. A dentigerous cyst that develops on a tooth that is still in its formative stage often prevents eruption of the involved tooth, and if the cyst is not destroyed the tooth remains embedded. Likewise the early formation of odontogenic and other tumors may prevent eruption of one or more teeth in the region in which it occurs.

Infections involving primary teeth may result in the formation of dense sclerotic bone adjacent to the crown of the permanent successor, which will prevent its eruption. In some instances, resorption on the surface of the crown may take place, producing actual ankylosis. Fractures of the jaws sustained at an early age may cause sufficient damage either to the tooth or the surrounding bone to prevent its eruption.

Among the anomalous causes of noneruption of the teeth, abnormal primary displacement of the tooth germ is the most common. In most instances the tooth germ is in its normal location, but it assumes a position in which the developing tooth may have an abnormal version, which may range from an angular version toward the alveolar ridge to complete inversion. In rare instances the tooth germ may develop in a region remote from the normal location. Such cases have been reported by Balendra (1949), Zernov (1949), and others.

One of the abnormalities of the jaws that most often cause noneruption of the teeth is alveolar cleft. In these patients the teeth adjoining the cleft tend to erupt toward the cleft, and most often remain embedded in either bone or soft tissue.

Noneruption of teeth may occur as a definite hereditary anomaly. This is evidenced by a familial tendency for failure of certain teeth to erupt in persons who are otherwise normal and in whom there are no apparent local causes for noneruption.

Teeth that have become fused with one another or have been joined by concrescence often fail to undergo eruption.

Systemic conditions that have an influence upon the eruption of teeth are those that cause underdevelopment of the jaws, structural defects of the teeth, or poor quality of bone. In hypothyroidism (cretinism) the jaws may be so small that they cannot accommodate all of the teeth. In hypoparathyroidism, when the disturbance has its onset early in life, the teeth may become ankylosed as a result of structural defects of enamel. In skeletal developmental disturbances, such as achondroplasia and cleidocranial dysostosis, the quality of bone may be of a character that prevents normal eruption of the teeth. A general physical examination, including a roentgenologic survey, is therefore indicated in patients in whom many of the teeth fail to erupt, to rule out skeletal and other disturbances as a possible cause. However, multiple noneruption of teeth also occurs in patients whose general physical examination gives essentially negative results, as illustrated in Figure 3–1. Here the left maxillary canine and third molar had been removed shortly prior to the time the roentgenogram was made.

The various positions that an embedded tooth assumes in relation to the occlusal plane of the jaws might adequately be described as being vertical when it is in a normal position for eruption, mesioangular, distoangular, horizontal, inverted, or transverse. Those that are in a transverse position may have either a lingual or a buccal version. This description as to position can be applied to all embedded teeth, including unerupted supernumerary teeth.

The teeth of the normal permanent dentition that are more often embedded are, in order of decreasing frequency, the mandibular third molar, maxillary third molar, maxillary canine, mandibular second premolar and maxillary premolar. The other teeth may remain embedded also, but to a lesser degree. With the third molars and maxillary canines there is a marked tendency to bilateral occurrence. Supernumerary teeth account for a large number of embedded teeth. Approximately 75% of them remain embedded, and of the mesiodentes, which represent the largest group of supernumerary teeth, only about 10% undergo eruption.

MANDIBULAR THIRD MOLAR

The most common cause of noneruption of the mandibular third molar is insufficient space. Frequently there is not enough room between the second molar and the anterior border of the ascending ramus, and as a result the third molar becomes impacted against the second molar in its course of eruption. If it does not become impacted and assumes a vertical or nearly vertical position, it may reach the level of occlusion but still have a portion of its crown embedded in bone of the anterior border of the

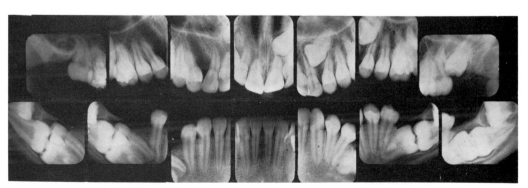

Figure 3–1 Noneruption of 11 teeth in an otherwise normal person.

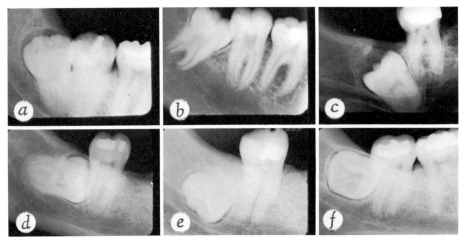

Figure 3–2   Embedded mandibular third molars. *a,* Vertical. *b,* Mesioangular. *c,* Distoangular. *d.* Horizontal. *e.* Inverted. *f.* Transverse.

ascending ramus. Mandibular third molars are often prevented from erupting by dentigerous cysts (so-called eruptive cysts), which arise on them while they are still in the stage of development and prior to the normal time for their eruption.

Because of its frequent occurrence and the high incidence of complications associated with it, noneruption of the mandibular third molar plays an important role from the standpoint of clinical significance. Most nonerupted mandibular third molars are situated in a mesioangular or a vertical position; however, they may assume many varied positions in the arch (Fig. 3–2).

MAXILLARY THIRD MOLAR

As with the mandibular third molar, the cause of noneruption of the maxillary third molar is, in most instances, lack of space. The second molar frequently occupies nearly all of the space near and up to the termination of the alveolar process, leaving very little if any room for the third molar to erupt. If the space is not too greatly reduced it will move downward in a vertical direction, but before eruption is completed it may become impacted against the second molar. Also in its movement downward it may be diverted posteriorly, but rarely will it erupt through the bone on the posterior surface of the tuberosity.

Early formation of dentigerous cysts and obstruction by supernumerary teeth, which is not an uncommon occurrence in this region, are not infrequent causes of noneruption.

Unlike the mandibular third molar, the maxillary third molar does not have as much space in the jaws in which to develop; therefore there is a greater tendency for the tooth germ to be displaced and assume an abnormal position. As a result there is a higher incidence of inversion of the maxillary third molar. Those that are inverted tend to move upward to reach a position that is at some distance from the alveolar crest and in a location where they may not be revealed by the routine dental roentgenographic examination.

Some of the variable positions in which maxillary third molars occur in the jaw are shown in Figure 3–3.

CANINES

While the incidence of embedded maxillary canines is appreciably higher than that of mandibular canines, the causes for noneruption are somewhat similar. In the maxilla there is a high frequency of bilateral occurrence, whereas in the mandible the frequency is much less.

One of the causes of noneruption is in-

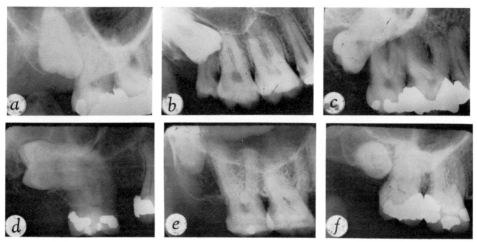

Figure 3–3 Embedded maxillary third molars. *a*, Vertical. *b*, Mesioangular. Eruption obstructed by supernumerary tooth. *c*, Distoangular. *d*, Horizontal. *e*, Inverted. *f*, Transverse.

sufficient space in the jaw to accommodate all of the teeth. The lateral incisor and the first premolar, since they erupt first, may be occupying a part or all of the space intended for the canine, thus preventing its eruption. Also, premature loss of the primary canine permits the first premolar to move forward, thereby reducing the space between it and the lateral incisor to the extent that the permanent canine will become impacted or will erupt into malposition. If the primary canine is retained beyond its normal time for shedding, the permanent canine may be diverted from its normal course and direction for eruption and as a result become impacted. Disorientation of the tooth germ no doubt accounts for some embedded canines, particularly those that are in an inverted position.

Why many maxillary canines fail to erupt is not clearly understood. The crown, following its complete development, may be in a favorable position for normal eruption, but after an appreciable amount of the root has formed, the tooth may begin to deviate anteriorly, even in the absence of any obstruction or lack of alveolar space. Such deviation may be influenced by forces exerted at the root end, where there may be inadequate vertical dimension and space for the root to undergo development.

Almost all of the embedded maxillary canines that are not in a vertical position are located posterior to the roots of the erupted teeth, while many of those in the mandible assume a position that is anterior to the roots of the erupted teeth.

Illustrations of embedded maxillary canines, as seen in routine dental roentgenographic examination, are shown in Figure 3–4, and of embedded mandibular canines in Figure 3–5.

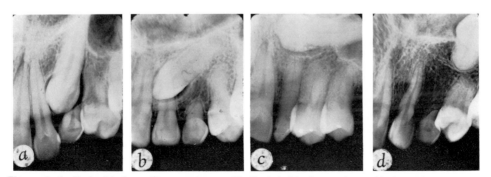

Figure 3–4 Embedded maxillary canines. *a*, Vertical. *b*, Mesioangular. *c*, Horizontal. *d*, Inverted.

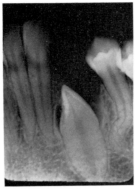
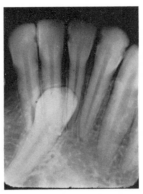
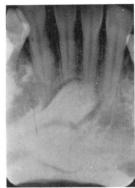

Figure 3–5 Embedded mandibular canines. *Left*, Vertical. *Center*, Mesioangular. *Right*, Bilateral, one of which is in a horizontal position.

PREMOLARS

Embedded premolars are almost always second premolars. Rarely does the first premolar fail to erupt. The causes of noneruption of the maxillary and mandibular premolars are largely similar.

The most common cause for noneruption is the premature loss of the primary second molar. Its loss permits the permanent first molar to move forward into a position where it will obstruct and prevent eruption of the second premolar. Prolonged retention of the primary second molar as a result of ankylosis or failure of its roots to resorb sometimes serves as an obstruction. The direction of the second premolar may be diverted, or if removal of the obstruction is delayed too long, the premolar may fail to erupt even though it has remained in its normal position for eruption. Many premolars may fail to erupt as a result of disorientation of the tooth germ, and this is particularly true of the maxillary second premolar, where complete inversion is not an unusual occurrence.

Most embedded maxillary premolars are situated lingual to the roots of the erupted teeth. Those that are in a horizontal position are most often inclined anteriorly, and complete inversion is not uncommon. Varied positions of embedded maxillary second premolars are shown in Figure 3–6. Embedded mandibular premolars assume more varied positions in relation to the roots of the erupted teeth. Those that are in a horizontal position are invariably inclined posteriorly, and complete inversion is a rarity. Varied positions assumed by embedded mandibular second premolars are shown in Figure 3–7.

SECOND MOLARS

Second molars may fail to erupt as a result of the early formation of cysts and tumors, disorientation of the tooth germ, ankylosis, and an inherent tendency. In

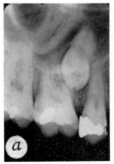
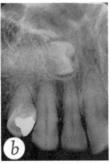
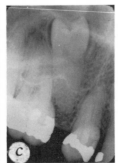
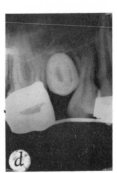

Figure 3–6 Embedded maxillary second premolars. *a*, Vertical. *b*, Horizontal. *c*, Inverted. *d*, Transverse.

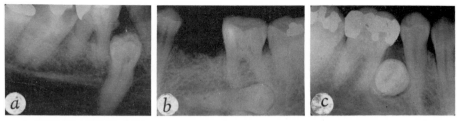

Figure 3–7 Embedded mandibular second premolars. *a*, Vertical. *b*, Horizontal. *c*, Transverse.

most instances, however, the cause of non-eruption is obscure. The tooth may fail to erupt even though it is in a normal vertical position, has had adequate space, has normal surrounding bone, and presents no evidence of having become ankylosed. The third molar, which erupts later, may become impacted or it may have sufficient space to undergo eruption. Sometimes the second molar remains embedded as a result of disorientation of the tooth germ or as a result of ankylosis. Illustrations of unerupted mandibular second molars are shown in Figure 3–8.

INCISORS

Noneruption of the incisors occurs more frequently in the maxilla than in the mandible. Causes of noneruption may be the presence of supernumerary structures, infection, or malformation of the alveolar process. The maxillary central incisor may fail to erupt when the mesiodens obstructs its path (Fig. 3–9), and similarly a compound composite odontoma, which when present almost always occurs in the canine region, may prevent eruption of lateral incisors. Sclerosis or scarring of bone in the incisal region, which results from infection associated with the primary teeth, may also prevent eruption. The crown of the tooth may become ankylosed, in which event the tooth retains its original position and later in life is situated at some distance from the crest of the alveolar ridge (Fig. 3–10). A high incidence of embedded lateral incisors is associated with alveolar clefts.

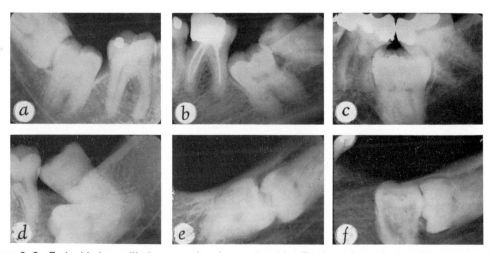

Figure 3–8 Embedded mandibular second molars. *a*, *b*, and *c*, Teeth are in vertical position but they have failed to erupt even though the space was adequate at the time they normally would have undergone eruption. *d*, Horizontal, with mesioversion. *e*, Horizontal with distoversion. *f*, Eruption may have been arrested as a result of idiopathic resorption.

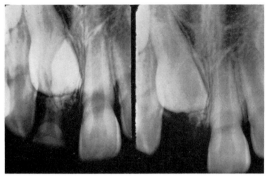

Figure 3–9 Maxillary central incisor which is being prevented from erupting by an inverted mesiodens. The view on the right is a postoperative one.

FIRST MOLARS

As in the case of the second molar, the cause of noneruption of the first molar is often obscure. The tooth may fail to erupt even when it is in a vertical position and has ample space in the arch for normal eruption. In some instances the tooth may become disoriented during the period of development, in which event it may become impacted (Fig. 3–11).

EMBEDDED PRIMARY TEETH

Embedded primary teeth that occur in an otherwise normal jaw are largely confined to the second molars and almost always become embedded as a result of inclusion. In such instances the roots become ankylosed, the primary tooth remains in its original

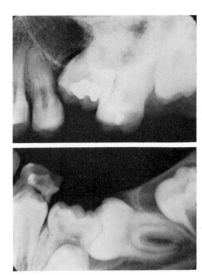

Figure 3–11 Impacted first molars. *Above,* Maxillary. *Below,* Mandibular.

location, and the alveolar bone grows around and over it, so that it may become completely enveloped by bone. The noneruption of a primary tooth is in itself a rarity. Most of the embedded primary teeth undergo early and rapid resorption, since a large portion of the dentin which is very vulnerable to resorption is already exposed (Fig. 3–12).

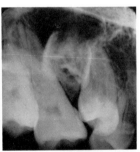

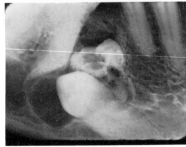

Figure 3–12 Embedded primary teeth. *Above,* Primary maxillary second molar which has become embedded as a result of inclusion. *Below,* Primary mandibular second molar which has prevented eruption of the second premolar; a dentigerous cyst has formed from the premolar.

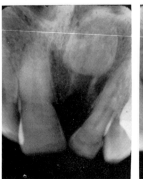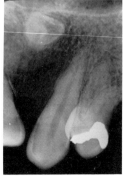

Figure 3–10 Embedded incisors. *Left,* Ankylosed maxillary central incisor. *Right,* Ankylosed maxillary lateral incisor.

MIGRATION OF TEETH

As a result of migration, an unerupted tooth may eventually assume a location that is at some distance from its original site of development. The teeth that are most often involved are the second premolars, canines, and third molars. The movement of the tooth is always in the direction of the crown, and most often the greatest amount of movement takes place prior to complete development of the root of the tooth, or at an early age. However, in rarer instances, an embedded tooth that has shown no tendency to movement for a period of several years may again begin to move.

Embedded maxillary teeth rarely migrate for as great a distance as do embedded mandibular teeth, since their movement is soon obstructed by the roots of the erupted teeth, or by the maxillary sinus. The median suture of the maxilla also serves as an obstruction, and an embedded canine will often reach but never pass through it to reach the opposite side. An exception to the rule that maxillary teeth migrate shorter distances than do mandibular teeth is the maxillary third molar, which when inverted may migrate upward as far as the floor of the orbit, and its presence may first come to light in roentgenograms of the maxillary sinuses or the head.

If a second mandibular premolar migrates, it invariably passes posteriorly through the medullary space and below the roots of the molar teeth, where it tends to meet least resistance and obstruction. A premolar that has migrated to a position near the angle of the mandible is shown in Figure 3–13. That it occupied this position

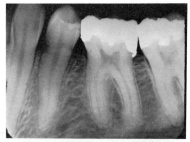

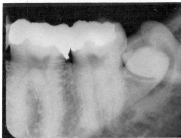

Figure 3–14 Migration of a mandibular premolar into the third molar region.

as a result of a displaced tooth germ is highly improbable, since it is situated below the mandibular canal. A second mandibular premolar that has migrated posteriorly and has attempted to erupt into the third molar space is shown in Figure 3–14.

The direction toward which an unerupted mandibular canine most often deviates is mesially. If it reaches a horizontal position, and if there is no obstruction by the roots of the incisor teeth, it may travel forward toward the midline, cross the symphysis, and assume a position where the entire tooth may be situated on the opposite side of the mandible (Fig. 3–15). Tarsitano et al. (1971) have reported three similar cases and have stated that panoramic views will reveal those which may not be detected otherwise.

Maxillary premolars that have migrated to a point near the midline are shown in Figure 3–16. They are situated palatal to the roots of the incisor teeth, as evidenced by the fact that their image moves posteriorly in relation to the roots of the incisor teeth as the x-ray tube is moved posteriorly. The primary second molars are still in place.

A tooth tends to migrate into an adjacent edentulous space, particularly at the time that it is still undergoing development and eruption. Following the early loss of a first

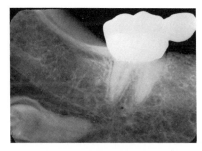

Figure 3–13 Migration of a mandibular premolar to a site near the angle of the mandible.

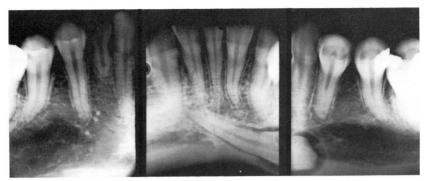

Figure 3-15 Migration of mandibular canine. It has crossed the symphysis to the opposite side of the mandible.

molar it is not unusual for the second molar, which develops and erupts later, to move forward and occupy the first molar space. Likewise, the third molar may move forward into the space formerly occupied by the second molar if the latter is lost early. A mandibular second premolar may migrate in some instances into an edentulous first molar region. The roots of the primary second molar usually keep its successor in proper position, but if the primary second molar and the permanent first molar as well are lost when the second premolar is still in its early formative stage, it may rapidly move posteriorly and assume a position in the permanent second molar space (Fig. 3-17). In the absence of a definite history one should, however, remember that such separation could be accounted for on the basis of transposition of the tooth germs of the second premolar and first molar.

Tumors and cysts that undergo expansion and reach an appreciable size cause malposition of the teeth. Erupted teeth may be forced out of normal alignment in the arch, and unerupted teeth may be forced to a location far remote from their original position. The pressure of the tumor or cyst is sufficient to overcome the eruptive force of the tooth, and the tooth is often moved in a direction that is rootwise (Figs. 3-18, 3-19, and 3-20).

PREOPERATIVE CONSIDERATIONS

For the removal of an embedded tooth the surgeon may require additional roentgenographic views that demonstrate more accurately its exact location, for often the proper surgical approach depends on the information so obtained. The exact location of an embedded mandibular tooth is more readily demonstrated, for an additional occlusal view usually suffices. The occlusal view is essential if, in the lateral view, the image of the embedded tooth is superimposed on the roots of the erupted teeth (Fig. 3-21).

Although the occlusal view is of value preparatory to the removal of a mandibular third molar, a good view of its root is probably more important. The roots of this tooth vary greatly as to number, size, and shape;

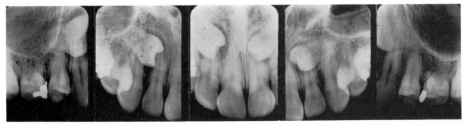

Figure 3-16 Migration of maxillary second premolars to a site near the median line.

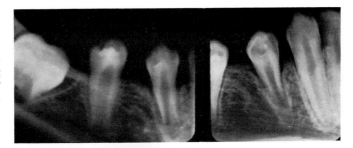

Figure 3-17 Migration of a mandibular second premolar posteriorly as a result of extraction of the permanent first molar and the primary molars at 7 years of age.

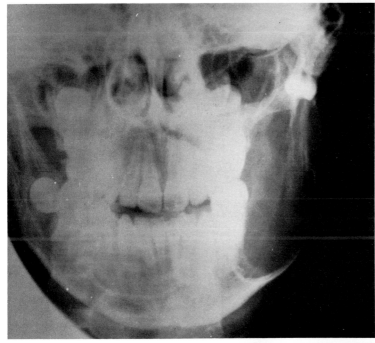

Figure 3-18 Mandibular third molar which has been forced to a site high in the ramus by a dentigerous cyst in a patient 16 years of age. The tooth is not fully developed, and the corresponding tooth on the opposite side is still in its normal position. (Courtesy of Dr. Earl Bettenhausen, Duluth, Minnesota.)

Figure 3-19 Mandibular third molar, the roots of which have been forced into the coronoid notch by a dentigerous cyst which now has undergone partial degeneration.

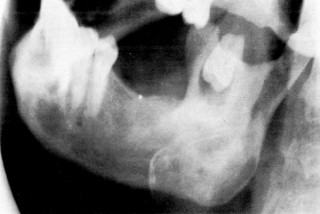

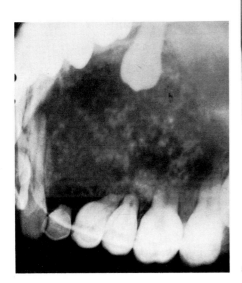

Figure 3-20 Maxillary canine which has been forced far superiorly by an odontogenic adenomatoid tumor.

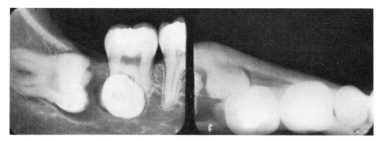

Figure 3–21 *Left,* Lateral view which reveals an embedded cystic third molar and also a supernumerary molar which is superimposed on the roots of the second molar. *Right,* An occlusal view which demonstrates that the supernumerary molar is located on the buccal surface.

many of the roots have a decided curvature, and some may extend below the mandibular canal (Waggener, 1959). Because of the proximity of the roots to the mandibular canal there is the added hazard of causing injury to the inferior dental nerve, which may result in temporary or permanent paresthesia or anesthesia of the lip. If the apex of the root extends below the level of the mandibular canal, there may be a groove present on either the lingual or the buccal surface of the root which a part or all of the contents of the mandibular canal may occupy. Cases have been reported in which the root of the tooth has completely surrounded the mandibular canal (Austin, 1947). Such grooves and canals are not always demonstrable in the roentgenogram; however, when they do appear they are evidenced by a constriction of the root at a point where the image of the mandibular canal is superimposed on it. There also may be a constriction of the mandibular canal, in which event one should suspect that it passes directly through the root (Fig. 3–22).

Figure 3–23 shows three mandibular third molars whose roots demonstrate the relationship they had to the mandibular canal. When the tooth is prevented from continuing its normal movement toward the crest of the alveolar ridge prior to complete development of its root, the root may encroach upon the mandibular canal. As a result of the obstruction of the canal, the root may divide to form a buccal and lingual root. When completely developed, these roots may extend downward below the canal and in some instances converge to surround it completely.

Since the contents of the mandibular canal are fairly strong and elastic, it is sometimes possible to detect that they are attached to the root, before the tooth has been delivered completely from its socket. In this event the root can then be sectioned or divided so as to prevent severance of the inferior dental nerve and mandibular artery.

The location of an embedded maxillary canine can be determined by noting its change in position in relation to the roots of the erupted teeth as the direction of the beam of radiation is changed. If the image

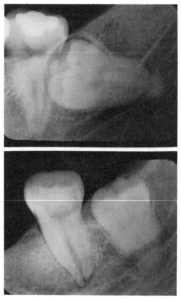

Figure 3–22 Relation of the mandibular canal to the roots of mandibular third molars. *Above,* Constriction of the root, which is evidence of a surface concavity that the contents of the canal may occupy. *Below,* Constriction of the root and of the canal as well, which may be evidence of a canal that passes directly through the root of the tooth.

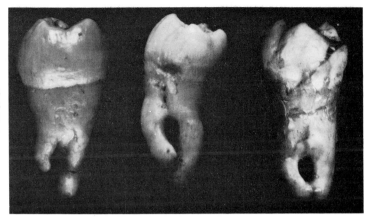

Figure 3-23 Photograph of three mandibular third molars with roots that partially or completely surround the contents of the mandibular canal.

of the canine moves posteriorly as the beam is moved in that direction, it is situated on tha palatal surface (Fig. 3–24). If its image moves forward its location is on the labial surface, and if it remains in the same position it is situated in direct alignment with the roots of the erupted teeth. It is difficult to obtain a view in which the embedded canine is not superimposed on a portion of the roots of the incisor teeth even though it actually may be situated above them.

Determining the exact location of an embedded maxillary premolar prior to operation is essential since there is wide variation in its position, and a decision must be made whether it can be delivered more conveniently from a buccal or palatal approach. Its position can best be demonstrated in an occlusal view. The lateral view of an inverted premolar shown in Figure 3–25 does not provide adequate information as to its version. The occlusal view, however, reveals that the major portion of the tooth is located on the palatal side, and that the logical approach for its removal is from that side.

SIGNIFICANCE OF MALPOSED TEETH

Embedded teeth are often a cause of conditions that are clinically significant. Those that are partially erupted through soft tissue often produce pericoronal infection and periodontal lesions involving the adjacent teeth, particularly in the case of the mandibular third molar. The development of dentigerous cysts from embedded teeth is not an infrequent occurrence, and such teeth also may be a source of odontogenic tumors, namely fibromas, myxomas,

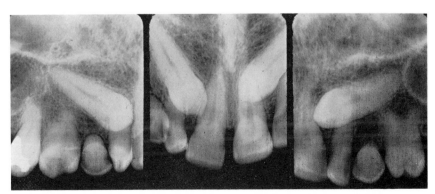

Figure 3-24 Impacted canines which are located on the palatal surface as evidenced by the fact that the images of their crowns move posteriorly in relation to the roots of the incisor teeth as the beam of radiation moves in that direction.

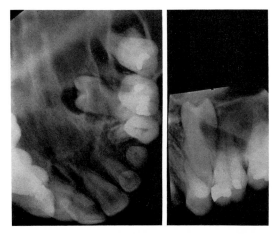

Figure 3–25 Occlusal view which demonstrates that the inverted maxillary second premolar seen in the view on the right is located on the palatal surface.

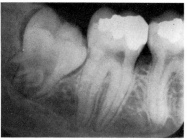

Figure 3–26 Mandibular third molar that is undergoing development and that proved to be the cause of otalgia.

ameloblastomas, and mixed odontogenic tumors. They often cause malposition or pressure resorption of the roots of the adjacent teeth, and in rarer instances they may be a source of referred pain. An instance of such referred pain is that of otalgia that occurs as a result of impaction of a mandibular third molar prior to complete development of its root. Eruption of the molar is then retarded or completely arrested, in which event the formative organ may exert undue pressure on the inferior dental nerve (Fig. 3–26). Removal of such teeth has afforded immediate and complete relief from pain.

Logan (1937) found that there is no evidence of inflammation in the tissue surrounding a tooth that is completely embedded in bone. One therefore should not anticipate any benefit from the removal of such teeth in patients suffering from systemic disease. If there is no roentgenographic evidence of associated infection or other complications, one should consider carefully the age and condition of the patient and the severity of the surgical procedure in determining the indications for removal of teeth that are completely embedded in bone.

REFERENCES

Austin, L. T.: Perforation of Roots of Impacted Lower Third Molars by Contents of Mandibular Canal: Report of a Case. Am. J. Orthodontics (Oral Surg. Sect.). *33*:623–624, 1947.
Balendra, W.: Unerupted Lower Third Molar in the Region of the Condyle. Brit. Dent. J. *86*:229 (May 6) 1949.
Logan, W. H. G.: Are Pulps and Investing Tissues of Completely Embedded Teeth Infected? J. Am. Dent. A. *24*:853–867 (June) 1937.
Tarsitano, J. J., Wooten, J. W., and Burditt, J. T.: Transmigration of Nonerupted Mandibular Canines: Report of Cases. J. Am. Dent. A. *82*:1395–1397 (June) 1971.
Waggener, D. T.: Relationships of Third Molar Roots to the Mandibular Canal. Oral Surg., Oral Med. & Oral Path. *12*:853–856 (July) 1959.
Zernov, M. W.: Misplaced Third Molar in the Region of the Condyle Erupting Through the Cheek. Brit. Dent. J. *87*:295 (Dec. 2) 1949.

PROLONGED RETENTION OF PRIMARY TEETH

4

The retention of a primary tooth beyond the normal time for shedding may occur when the permanent successor or the permanent tooth adjacent to it is congenitally missing, or when the permanent successor fails to assume its normal position for eruption and becomes impacted or remains embedded. In many instances, for reasons unknown, the roots of the primary teeth may fail to undergo resorption and the teeth are retained long beyond the normal time for exfoliation. Prolonged retention of primary teeth is not an uncommon feature in cases of cleidocranial dysostosis and ectodermal dysplasia.

Primary teeth that still may be present in persons beyond 21 years of age are, in order of frequency, the maxillary canine, mandibular second molar, maxillary second molar, mandibular canine, and others very rarely (Austin and Stafne, 1930). Primary second molars have been noted in persons who have reached 80 years of age.

The retention of the primary canine occurs most often when the permanent canine deviates from its normal course for eruption, bypasses the root of the primary tooth, and becomes impacted (Fig. 4–1). It also may be retained when the permanent lateral incisor is congenitally missing and the permanent canine bypasses the primary canine to erupt into the space for the lateral incisor (Figs. 4–2 and 4–3). Congenital absence of the permanent canine is extremely rare; therefore, it rarely accounts for the prolonged retention of its predecessor.

Prolonged retention of the primary second molar most often occurs as a result of congenital absence of the permanent successor (Fig. 4–4, *left*) and more rarely when its permanent successor has been

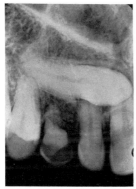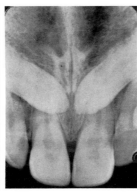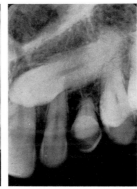

Figure 4–1 Prolonged retention of maxillary primary canines resulting from failure of the permanent successors to erupt into their normal position in the arch.

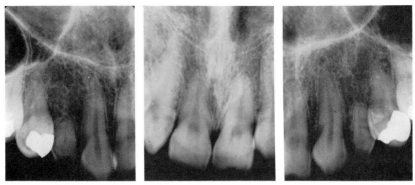

Figure 4–2 Prolonged retention of maxillary primary canines. Their permanent successors have erupted into the space where the lateral incisors are congenitally absent.

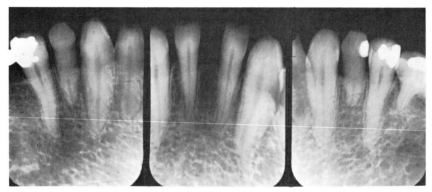

Figure 4–3 Prolonged retention of primary canines resulting from congenital absence of the permanent lateral incisors.

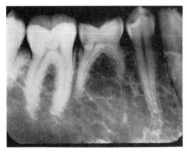 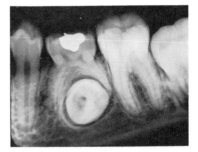

Figure 4–4 Prolonged retention of the primary mandibular second molar where there is congenital absence of its successor *(left),* and where the successor is not in normal position for eruption *(right).*

diverted from its normal course for eruption (Fig. 4–4, *right*). Bilateral occurrence is not infrequent, since congenital absence of second premolars also tends to be bilateral.

An illustration of prolonged retention of all the primary canines and molars, apparently as a result of failure of their roots to undergo normal resorption, is shown in

Figure 4–5*a*. The patient was a normal, healthy girl 16 years of age. The permanent successors were completely formed, and there was evidence of dense sclerotic bone overlying the crowns of many of them. Extraction of the primary teeth and surgical removal of the sclerotic bone were followed by orthodontic treatment, the result of

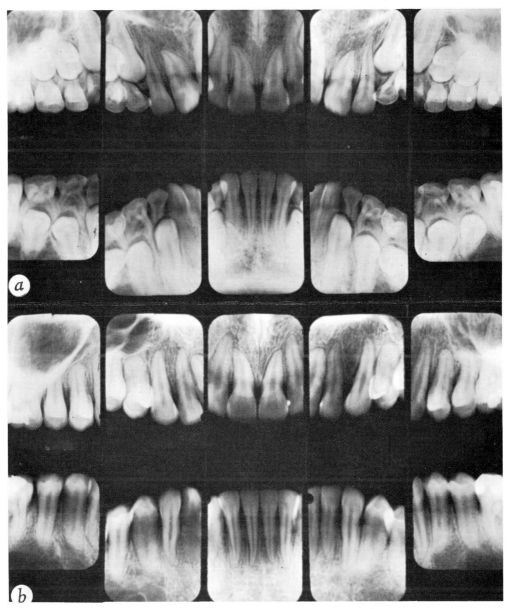

Figure 4–5 *a*, Prolonged retention of all primary canines and molars in a patient 16 years of age. *b*, Appearance following completion of surgical and orthodontic treatment. (Reproduced with permission from Stafne, E. C. and Wentworth, F. L.: Surgical and Orthodontic Treatment in a Case of Noneruption of Twelve Permanent Teeth. Am. J. Orthodontics [Oral Surg. Sect.]. *33*:585–589 [Aug.] 1947.)

which is shown in a roentgenogram made at 21 years of age (Fig. 4–5*b*).

A dental roentgenographic examination is indicated in all instances in which a primary tooth is retained beyond its normal time for exfoliation. It may reveal that the permanent successor has not reached the stage of development at which it is prepared to erupt; however, if it has, the primary tooth should be extracted even though

there may have been very little, if any, resorption of its roots. Its prolonged retention will either prevent eruption of the permanent successor or cause it to erupt into malposition. If the primary tooth is permitted to remain for any great length of time, the bone overlying the crown of the unerupted tooth tends to become sclerotic and, when this occurs, the permanent tooth may fail to erupt even after the primary

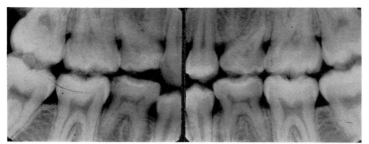

Figure 4–6 Retention of all primary second molars in a patient 38 years of age.

tooth has been extracted. Morgan (1938) has called attention to the ill effects that frequently result from prolonged retention of the primary teeth and has emphasized the importance of extraction as soon as it appears that they may interfere with normal eruption of the permanent teeth.

The roentgenogram may reveal congenital absence of the permanent successor, which is most often the case in prolonged retention of the primary mandibular second molar. If the successor is absent, every effort should be made to retain the primary tooth, at least until the patient has reached an age when it is favorable to replace it with an artificial restoration. Some primary teeth that maintain a normal level of occlusion can be retained indefinitely (Fig. 4–6).

REFERENCES

Austin, L. T. and Stafne, E. C.: Retained Deciduous Teeth. Dent. Cosmos. 72:707–712 (July) 1930.
Morgan, G. E.: Prolonged Retention: When Should Healthy Deciduous Teeth Be Extracted? J. Am. Dent. A. 25:358–363 (Mar.) 1938.

THE PULP CAVITY

5

Fields in which roentgenographic examination is indispensable are operative dentistry and endodontics, if for no other reason than to determine the relative size of the pulp chamber and canals prior to treatment. The pulp cavity may be either very large so that there is an increased hazard of pulp exposure in doing restorative work, or reduced in size by excessive formation of secondary dentin so as to make root-canal therapy more difficult. An excessive amount of pulp calcification also presents a problem in root-canal therapy.

REDUCTION IN SIZE OF PULP CAVITY

Aside from reduction in the size of the pulp cavity which is associated with advanced age, there are some conditions that are known to stimulate prematurely the formation of secondary dentin, thereby reducing the size of the pulp cavity. These are attrition, abrasion, dental caries, dental restorations, injury, and force that is applied by orthodontic appliances. The absence of pulp chambers is seen as a

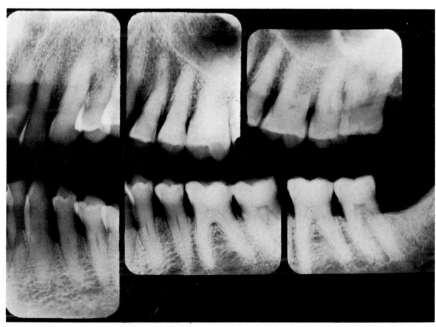

Figure 5-1 Reduction in size of the pulp chambers and canals associated with advanced age. Roentgenogram made at 60 years of age.

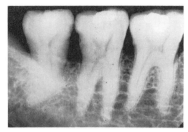

Figure 5–2 The size of the pulp chamber is greatly reduced but the horns of the pulp persist.

characteristic feature of dentinogenesis imperfecta.

Although there is gradual reduction in the size of the pulp chamber and canals with advancing years, there is still wide individual variation in size at any given age. An illustration of reduction in size with advancing age is a roentgenogram made for a person 60 years of age (Fig. 5–1). Here the teeth are free from caries and there is only slight attrition of the occlusal surfaces. There is complete obliteration of the pulp chambers of all the premolars, the chambers of the molars have become reduced to a small size, and the pulp canals of all of them have become very narrow and indistinct. In some instances there may be almost complete obliteration of the pulp

chamber and canals, and yet the horns of the pulp of molar teeth may persist and remain relatively close to the surface of the crown. Such pulp extensions are often discernible in the roentgenogram (Fig. 5–2), or they may be so indistinct that they cannot be recognized. Such pulp extension may account for pulpitis following insertion of a filling that was thought to be placed at some distance from the pulp chamber.

That marked reduction can take place at a relatively early age is illustrated in Figure 5–3, which shows the teeth of a person 31 years of age. The roentgenogram reveals premature reduction in size of the pulp chambers of most of the teeth, including those that are free from caries and do not contain fillings. The pulps have a strong defensive reaction, as evidenced by the formation of secondary dentin beneath restorations that had been placed in the maxillary second premolar and the mandibular first molar.

ATTRITION

Attrition is the loss of tooth structure that results from wear that is produced by opposing teeth coming in contact with one

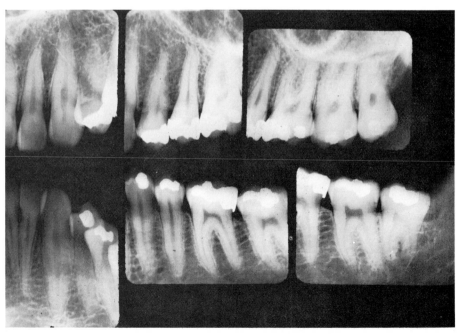

Figure 5–3 Premature reduction in size of the pulp chambers in a person 31 years of age.

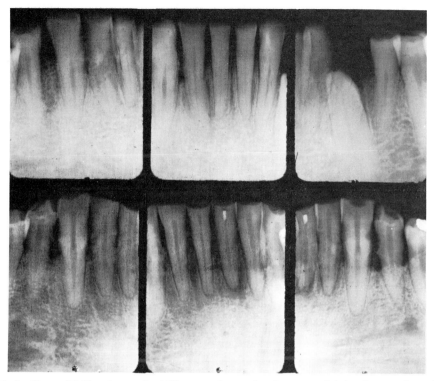

Figure 5–4 *Above,* Attrition in a patient 72 years of age, showing a good defensive reaction of the pulp as evidenced by the formation of secondary dentin. *Below,* Attrition in a patient 69 years of age, showing a poor defensive reaction of the pulp.

another. If all teeth are present in normal alignment and are put to proper use, there is gradual wearing away of the occlusal and incisal surfaces until in older persons the cusps of the teeth are worn away completely and the dentin is exposed; under these conditions the wear is considered to be a normal physiologic change. There also is gradual reduction in the size of the pulp chamber and, where the wear has become extensive, the pulp chamber may be almost completely obliterated. Rarely is the wearing away so rapid that the formation of secondary dentin does not keep pace with it; therefore, pulp exposure is not a common occurrence.

The roentgenograms shown in the upper part of Figure 5–4, made for a patient 72 years of age, exhibit a good defensive reaction of the pulp. In some instances owing to a poor defensive reaction, the formation of secondary dentin does not keep pace with wear and, as a result, the pulp may become exposed. The roentgeno-

grams shown in the lower part of Figure 5–4 are illustrative. Made for a patient 69 years of age, they reveal pulp exposure of the mandibular right central incisor and pulps of other teeth that were on the verge of exposure.

Such predisposing factors as loss of teeth, malocclusion, and habits such as pipe smoking, tobacco chewing, and bruxism may produce attrition that is so rapid that the formation of secondary dentin cannot keep pace with it, and hence pulp exposure occurs at a relatively early age.

ABRASION

Abrasion is the wearing away or loss of tooth structure that is not caused by occlusal or incisal wear. The most common cause of abrasion is incorrect use of the toothbrush. The defect produced by incorrect brushing is situated on the buccal and labial surfaces and is fairly characteristic. It is most often a sharply defined, wedge-shaped, transverse defect which is initially produced at the cementoenamel junction after having forced the gingiva sufficiently far rootward. The extent and size of the defect depend on how long and vigorously the incorrect brushing is continued. The loss of tooth structure is chiefly inward, since the enamel is not readily destroyed by brushing. This type of abrasion invariably stimulates the formation of secondary dentin, and when the defects are extensive it is not unusual to note roentgenographically that the pulp chambers are completely obliterated, and that only the root canal persists. The process of destruction may continue through the secondary dentin, severing the tooth in two and still leaving a vital pulp in the root portion.

The roentgenogram shown in Figure 5–5, of the maxillary anterior teeth, illustrates defects produced by improper brushing. The defects are confined to the labial surface and gingival portion of the teeth, and have reached a depth that is approximately midway through the central incisors. The formation of secondary dentin is evidenced by complete obliteration of the pulp chambers of the incisors. The pulp canals are still present, and the pulps gave a normal response to tests for vitality.

While destruction of normal enamel is not readily accomplished by brushing, it is, in some instances, markedly enhanced by the ingestion of solids and liquids that are highly acid and by the regurgitation or vomiting of acids from the stomach.

DENTAL CARIES

Dental caries stimulates formation of secondary dentin on the surface of the pulpal wall that is directly beneath it. If the carious process progresses slowly, the deposition of secondary dentin may, in a measure, keep pace with its advance and thereby prevent early exposure of the dental pulp. The roentgenogram is of value in that it reveals the extent of secondary dentin formation and the amount and thickness of the dentin that separates the dental pulp from the carious lesion, and often it will be found that a very extensive carious lesion is amenable to treatment without exposure of the dental pulp or the necessity of resort to root-canal therapy.

DENTAL RESTORATIONS

Deposition of secondary dentin to a varied degree continues after insertion of a filling, and roentgenographically this is most often evidenced by obliteration of the horns of the pulps of mandibular molar teeth. This deposition of dentin may take place as a result of the operative procedures necessary for insertion of a restoration in a normal tooth, for it occurs in a noncarious tooth in which an abnormal amount of

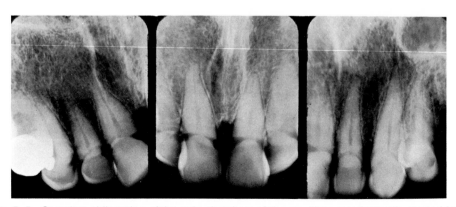

Figure 5–5 Complete obliteration of the pulp chambers of the maxillary anterior teeth, caused by abrasion as a result of incorrect brushing of the teeth.

Figure 5–6 Reduction in size of a pulp cavity following injury. *Left,* After fracture of the crown. *Center,* Complete obliteration of the pulp cavity in a primary incisor. *Right,* Complete obliteration of the pulp cavity in a permanent incisor.

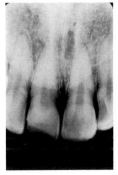 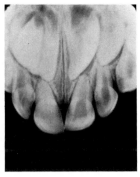 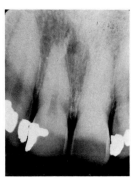

Figure 5–6 Reduction in size of a pulp cavity following injury. *Left,* After fracture of the crown. *Center,* Complete obliteration of the pulp cavity in a primary incisor. *Right,* Complete obliteration of the pulp cavity in a permanent incisor.

secondary dentin was not present prior to its insertion.

INJURY

Alteration and decrease in the size of the pulp chamber and canals often occur as a result of injury. After fractures of the crowns of anterior teeth when the line of fracture is close to the pulp chamber, secondary dentin may form very rapidly. This often can be demonstrated by means of the roentgenogram within a few weeks after injury. A roentgenogram made 1 year after fracture is shown on the left in Figure 5–6. It reveals that a large amount of secondary dentin has formed as a defensive reaction to the injury.

A not uncommon result of injury is complete obliteration of the pulp chamber and root canals. The deposition of calcified substance, which is usually ill-defined secondary dentin, first takes place on the pulpal wall and continues until all the pulp

tissue has been replaced. This phenomenon most often occurs in the early decades of life and in primary (Fig. 5–6, *center*) as well as permanent teeth. Rarely do periapical lesions develop from such pulpless teeth, and these teeth are less susceptible to caries than are the teeth that have normal pulps. A common observation is that such a tooth is caries-free while the adjoining teeth either have active caries or have been treated for caries (Fig. 5–6, *right*). Such a tooth will not respond to tests for vitality and may show no other symptoms. It may be said that it has a most efficient natural root-canal filling.

An unusual sequel of pulp reaction to injury is partial obliteration of the pulp cavity; this is confined to the root canal. When seen in the roentgenogram, only the pulp canal is obliterated, while the chamber retains the size and contour that it presumably had at the time of injury. This picture probably represents varied degrees of degeneration of the pulp following in-

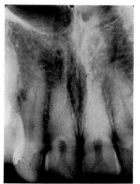 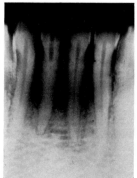 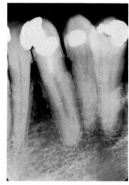

Figure 5–7 Obliteration of the root canals alone as a result of injury or pulpotomy. *Left,* Involvement of the maxillary central incisors. *Center,* Involvement of the mandibular left central incisor. *Right,* Involvement after pulpotomy in a mandibular canine.

jury. The portion that occupied the pulp chamber has undergone complete degeneration, while the portion that occupied the root canal still retains the ability to form secondary dentin. Illustrations of two such cases are shown in Figure 5–7. There was a definite history of injury in both instances. The roentgenogram on the left reveals obliteration of the pulp canals of the maxillary central incisors, large pulp chambers which conform to the size common at about 9 years of age, when the injury was sustained, and a fracture of the incisal edges of the crowns of both teeth. The roentgenogram in the center reveals a similar condition involving the mandibular left central incisor. The lamina dura in the periapical region appeared normal in both cases. Another instance in which the pulp canal alone may be obliterated by the formation of secondary dentin is that in which the pulp chamber is opened and filled prior to complete degeneration of the pulp (Fig. 5–7, *right*).

ORTHODONTIC FORCE

Force applied to a tooth in the course of orthodontic treatment may result in partial or complete obliteration of the pulp cavity (Fig. 5–8). In some instances, pulps that undergo only partial obliteration at the time of completion of treatment may eventually undergo complete obliteration (Fig. 5–9).

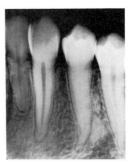

Figure 5–8 Reduction in size of the pulp cavity of a canine and complete obliteration of the pulp cavity in a premolar following orthodontic treatment.

DENTINOGENESIS IMPERFECTA

Absence of the pulp cavity is a characteristic feature of dentinogenesis imperfecta, which occurs either with or without an associated osteogenesis imperfecta. The roentgenogram shown in Figure 5–10, made for a boy 14 years of age who had osteogenesis imperfecta, reveals almost complete absence of pulp cavities.

A tooth in which the size of the pulp chamber has been reduced, whether the reduction is associated with advanced age, injury, or other causes, becomes less sensitive to outside stimuli, particularly if there has been no abnormal loss of structure on the surface of the crown, such as that caused by attrition and abrasion. There may be only slight, and sometimes no, response to tests for vitality. Such tests are then very unreliable, and a correct diagnosis of the condition of the tooth can be

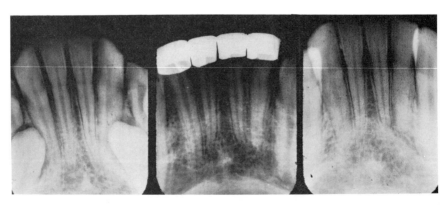

Figure 5–9 Obliteration of the pulp cavity of the mandibular right lateral incisor as a result of force applied incidental to orthodontic treatment. *Left,* Appearance prior to treatment. *Center,* Appearance at completion of treatment, showing partial obliteration. *Right,* Four years after termination of treatment, showing complete obliteration of the pulp cavity.

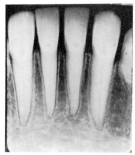

Figure 5–10 Absence of pulp cavities associated with osteogenesis imperfecta in a patient 14 years of age.

made only when the clinical and roentgenographic findings also are considered.

Abnormal reduction in size or complete elimination of the pulp cavity as seen in the roentgenogram may occur with anomalies that are peculiar to the teeth only. Among these are dentinal dysplasia and opalescent dentin (see Chapter 2). Such reductions also may occur as manifestations of progeria, osteopetrosis, and some other syndromes and systemic conditions, as well as of osteogenesis imperfecta.

ABNORMALLY LARGE PULP CAVITIES

Since normally there is gradual reduction in the size of the pulp cavity from the time the tooth is completely formed into old age, a pulp cavity can be considered abnormally large if it does not conform in size to that for a given age, or if it is abnormally large as compared with the pulp cavities of other teeth in the same person. Injury that causes degeneration of the pulp and formation of pulp calcifications at an early age accounts for many abnormally large pulp cavities. In some instances, for reasons unknown, the pulp chambers undergo but very slight reduction in size and remain abnormally large into adult life. Figure 5–11 shows the posterior teeth of a person 29 years of age. The pulp chambers and some of the root canals are still extremely large for a person of that age, and the increased hazard of pulp exposure in the treatment of the carious lesions in such a patient is obvious. There appears to be slight, if any, tendency to the formation of secondary dentin, as evidenced by the fact that a mesio-occlusal metal filling that had been placed in the mandibular first molar 6 years previously had not caused formation of secondary dentin that usually obliterates the horn of the pulp beneath it. Kronfeld (1949) and others have discussed the individual reactions of pulps, and have called attention to the fact that some of them show a weak defensive reaction by a failure to form secondary dentin. The factors that de-

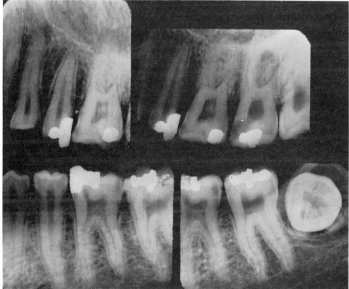

Figure 5–11 Abnormally large pulp chambers in a person 29 years of age.

termine or regulate these individual variations are unknown.

After complete degeneration and liquefaction of the pulp from any cause, there will be no further decrease in the size of the pulp cavity. If the tooth is retained and roentgenograms are made several years later, such a pulp cavity will be noted as being larger in proportion to the pulp cavities of the remaining teeth that have normal pulps. The earlier in life the degeneration takes place, the greater this variation in size will be, and it is often possible from the roentgenographic evidence to determine the approximate age at which degeneration of the pulp occurred. Routine roentgenographic examination often reveals large pulp cavities in teeth in which degeneration of the pulp has been caused by injury. These teeth are associated with a very high incidence of periapical lesions (Fig. 5–12).

Abnormally large pulp cavities may be present as anomalies of the teeth only; among these are taurodontia, regional odontodysplasia, and the "shell teeth" of Rushton (1954). They also may be associated with metabolic diseases such as hypophosphatasia and vitamin D-resistant rickets; in these patients, the horns of the pulp may extend to the dentoenamel junction at the incisal and occlusal surfaces. A comprehensive article dealing with manifestations of genetic diseases in the human pulp is that by Witkop (1971).

CALCIFICATIONS IN THE PULP TISSUE (PULP STONES)

Calcifications in the dental pulp occur in the form of denticles, nodules or stones, and diffuse fibrillar structures. Some denticles consist of irregular dentin; others have a concentric, laminated structure which is produced by deposition of consecutive layers of calcium salts around a central nucleus. The latter are by far the more common. They are often multiple and, as they enlarge, may fuse with one another to form a solid calcified mass. Some that are close to the pulpal wall may become firmly attached to the dentin and, in some instances, become completely surrounded by secondary dentin. Fibrillar calcifications are seen most often in older persons and are one of the manifestations of regressive changes that the pulp undergoes. Calcification may begin in the walls of the blood vessels and in the perineural connective tissue, which provides a nucleus along which additional calcific deposits are made. Fusion of these deposits may form a solid calcified mass.

The presence of calcification in the pulp has been attributed to local irritants of long standing, such as caries, dental restorations, abrasion, erosion, gingival recession, and periodontal disease. That local irritants of long standing are causative factors must be questioned, in view of the large number of calcifications that occur in normal teeth where such irritants are not present. It also has been suggested that their formation is a local manifestation of systemic disturbances. It has been found, however, that there appears to be no relationship between the incidence of pulp calcifications and any one particular systemic disease, with the possible exception of arteriosclerosis, a condition that is most prevalent among older persons and at an age when calcifications of the pulp also are most prevalent (Stafne and Szabo, 1933).

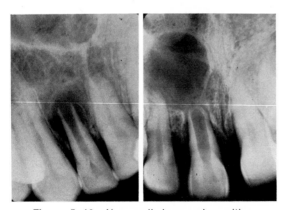

Figure 5–12 Abnormally large pulp cavities, resulting from complete degeneration of the pulp incidental to injury sustained earlier in life and associated with periapical lesions. *Left,* Periapical granuloma. *Right,* Epithelium-lined cyst.

The incidence of calcifications in pulp tissue is relatively high on the basis of microscopic examination. Hill (1934) reported that they occur in 66% of all teeth between the ages of 10 and 20 years, and in 90% of all teeth between the ages of 50 and 70 years. Incidence based on roentgenographic examination would be inaccurate, since so many of the calcifications are not of sufficient size to be discernible in the roentgenogram.

Calcifications of the pulp appear in the roentgenogram as radiopaque structures within the pulp chamber and root canal. They may be round or oval bodies of varied size that may appear singly but more often appear in multiple numbers; others are solid opaque bodies that tend to conform in shape to the outline of the pulp chamber and root canal. A radiolucent line is seen which separates them from the pulpal wall, although when they are present in the molar teeth they may appear to be attached to the floor of the pulp chamber, as, in some instances, they actually may be. The ones that are most readily seen in the roentgenogram and are recognized as pulp calcifications are those that have formed while the pulp chamber is still large. If the calcifications reach appreciable size early in life, they prevent the reduction in size of the pulp chamber that normally takes place with advanced age, and therefore there may be only slight or no alteration in the appearance even many decades later. Diffuse, irregular opacities that probably more often represent fibrillar calcifications are not so readily recognized, particularly when they form later in life, at a time when the pulp cavity has decreased in size and the opacity of the tooth has increased. In general, calcifications of the pulp can be demonstrated more readily by use of the bite-wing film.

A dental roentgenogram of the anterior teeth made for a person 17 years of age is shown in Figure 5–13. It reveals multiple nodules in the pulp chambers, some of which extend into the pulp canals. Such nodules also were present in the pulps of the posterior teeth. The teeth were free from caries and there were no local long-

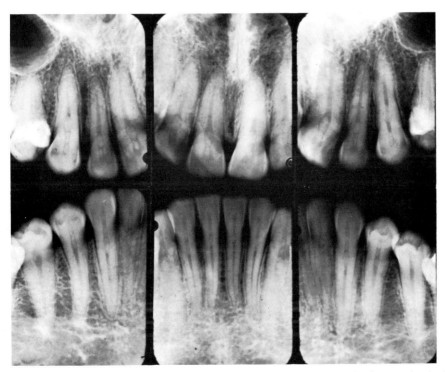

Figure 5–13 Pulp calcifications that appear in the form of multiple nodules in the anterior teeth of a person 17 years of age. Similar nodules were present in the posterior teeth.

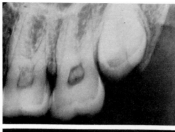
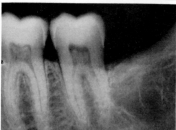

Figure 5–14 Pulp calcifications that involve the molar teeth and that occupy almost all of the pulp chamber.

standing irritants to which the calcifications could be attributed.

Pulp calcifications that occupy almost all the pulp-chamber space of molar teeth that are free from caries are shown in Figure 5–14. The degree of calcification is greater in the first molars, since they had undergone development earlier than the second molars. In the first molars the calcification has come close to the pulpal wall, and there will be no further decrease in the size of the pulp chamber.

The present consensus is that calcifications of the pulp are of no great significance, if one excludes the few instances in which pathologic calcifications occur as a result of inflammation or necrosis of the pulp. According to Kronfeld (1939), pulp calcifications themselves never cause inflammation of the pulp, and therefore they should not be considered a source of dental infection. Calcifications of the pulp present a problem in root-canal therapy and may make such treatment increasingly difficult, particularly when they are extensive or adherent to the pulpal wall.

REFERENCES

Hill, T. J.: Pathology of Dental Pulp. J. Am. Dent. A. *21*:820–844 (May) 1934.

Kronfeld, R.: Histopathology of the Teeth and Their Surrounding Structures. Ed. 2. Philadelphia, Lea & Febiger, 1939, p. 94.

Kronfeld, R.: Histopathology of the Teeth and Their Surrounding Structures. Ed. 3, edited by P. E. Boyle. Philadelphia, Lea & Febiger, 1949, pp. 71–104.

Rushton, M. A.: A New Form of Dentinal Dysplasia: Shell Teeth. Oral Surg., Oral Med. & Oral Path. 7:543–549 (Apr.) 1954.

Stafne, E. C. and Szabo, S. E.: The Significance of Pulp Nodules. Dent. Cosmos. 75:160–164 (Feb.) 1933.

Witkop, C. J., Jr.: Manifestations of Genetic Diseases in the Human Pulp. Oral Surg., Oral Med. & Oral Path. 32:278–316 (Aug.) 1971.

DENTAL CARIES

6

The most important niche that roentgenology has filled as an adjunct to the practice of dentistry has been, and no doubt still is, that of the detection of dental caries and of determining the degree of destruction and penetration of individual carious lesions. The usefulness of the roentgenographic examination lies in the fact that it reveals a high percentage of caries that otherwise would remain undetected. There is some difference of opinion as to the proportion of carious lesions that remain undetected if roentgenographic examination is not used: Cheyne and Horne (1948) expressed the opinion that it is about one-third.

The roentgenographic examination in itself does not adequately provide an efficient examination, for many initial carious lesions of the occlusal surfaces of the posterior teeth, as well as those on the labial, buccal, and lingual surfaces, are not readily visualized roentgenographically. To obtain the greatest efficiency one must, therefore, supplement the roentgenographic with a careful clinical examination. It is the consensus that the highest degree of accuracy in detecting initial caries is attained by clinical examination supplemented by the use of bite-wing films.

An insidious form of caries that frequently is not detected without the aid of a roentgenogram until the pulp has become involved is the form represented in Figure 6–1. Caries on the proximal surface of a mandibular first molar has passed through the enamel by a narrow channel which has become no larger, while the un-

derlying dentin has undergone destruction that has led to exposure of the pulp.

The introduction of the bite-wing film by Raper (1925) not only provided a more efficient method for the early detection of proximal caries but also served to make the periodic dental examination more economical. In recommending the use of the bite-wing film, he stated that no proximal cavity would escape detection. He also emphasized the fact that the interproximal x-ray examination is not a substitute for the periapical x-ray examination.

The method utilizing the bite-wing film, in addition to permitting better visualization of proximal caries (Figs. 6–2 and 6–3), has a decided advantage over the standard dental roentgenographic examination in revealing recurrent caries that occurs under fillings (Fig. 6–4) and near the gingival margins of artificial crowns (Fig. 6–5). The exposure is made at right angles to the long axis of the tooth, and this is most often parallel to the base of the filling, thereby providing a view of more of the tooth struc-

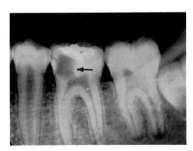

Figure 6–1 Extensive caries of dentin leading to exposure of the pulp. Invasion occurred through a narrow channel in the enamel on the proximal surface of a mandibular first molar.

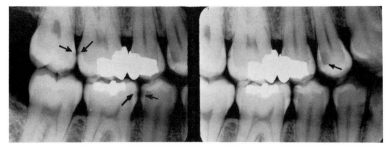

Figure 6–2   Bite-wing roentgenograms that reveal incipient proximal caries of the maxillary first and second molars and canine, and of the mandibular first molar. Caries of the maxillary first and the mandibular second premolars has invaded the dentin.

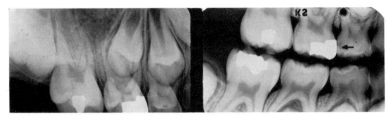

Figure 6–3   Proximal caries in a primary maxillary molar that is not visualized in the standard film *(left)*, but is clearly demonstrated in the bite-wing film *(right)*.

ture beneath it. If a crown is present, there is less superimposition of metal on the cervical and root portion of the tooth when the exposure is made at right angles to the long axis of the tooth.

Sometimes the roentgenogram reveals defects on the proximal surfaces that have been produced by an active carious process that has become completely arrested. These defects invariably involve a small area of the enamel surface and extend directly inward by way of the enamel lamellae, but do not penetrate sufficiently far to reach the dentin. They are most often seen in persons who have a natural or hereditary immunity to dental caries and have few or no filled teeth present, or in persons who have had active caries but have entered a period of immunity. When such a defect is

encountered in an adult patient for whom no previous records are available, one should entertain the thought that it might be arrested caries. Any operative procedure should be postponed until there is roentgenographic evidence of increase in size of the cavity.

Caries that originates in pits and fissures can most often be found on clinical examination but, in some instances, a definite diagnosis cannot be made by means of the exploring tine only. The caries may appear at the bottom of the pit or fissure, extend directly into dentin, and produce extensive destruction in a tooth, the crown of which may still have a normal, healthy clinical appearance at a time when the first symptoms of pulp exposure appear (Fig. 6–6).

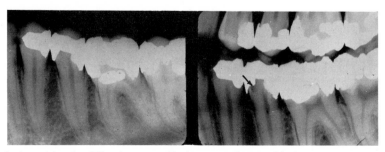

Figure 6–4   Caries under the filling in a mandibular second premolar that was not revealed by the standard technique *(left)*, but was demonstrated in the bite-wing film *(right)*.

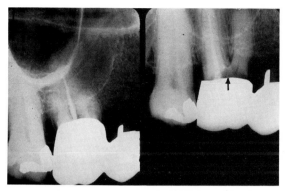

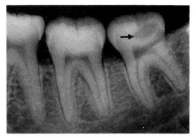

Figure 6–6 Extensive caries of the dentin of the mandibular third molar from invasion through an occlusal fissure. The presence of caries could not be established from clinical examination alone.

Figure 6–5 Caries under a crown, the extent of which was not revealed by the standard technique *(left)* but was visualized in the bite-wing film *(right)*.

Caries that occurs on the distal surface of second molars and is caused by partially erupted impacted third molars often remains undetected without the aid of the roentgenogram. It most often begins at the cementoenamel junction, invades the dentin, but leaves the enamel wall on the distal surface of the tooth intact (Fig. 6–7). The roentgenogram on the right was made for a patient who was referred for removal of the impacted third molar, with a view of relieving a severe pain of 5 days' duration. The nature of the pain, however, was characteristic of pulpitis, and this was verified by roentgenographic examination which revealed extensive caries in the second molar. The roentgenogram on the left, of the same patient, which had been made 6 years previously, shows that a small carious lesion was present at the cementoenamel junction at that time.

The optimal time interval for periodic roentgenographic examination insofar as dental caries is concerned is variable, and is in a large measure dependent upon the age of the patient and the degree of his immunity or susceptibility to caries. Examination should begin at least by 4 years of age, for the onset of most of the carious lesions of the primary teeth occurs at about 4 to 7 years of age. In general, the interval for the bite-wing examination probably should not exceed 6 months until the patient has reached 20 years of age, or until such time that there is definite evidence of decreased susceptibility. While the interval between roentgenographic examinations may be lengthened appreciably after the patient has entered a period of relative immunity, it should not be discontinued. A caries-immune person may, at any time, and particularly in the later decades of life, again become susceptible to caries as a result of change in dietary habits or a decrease in flow of saliva.

REFERENCES

Cheyne, V. D. and Horne, E. V.: Value of Roentgenograph in Detection of Carious Lesions. J. Dent. Res. *27*:58–67 (Feb.) 1948.

Raper, H. R.: Practical Clinical Preventive Dentistry Based Upon Periodic Roentgen-Ray Examinations. J. Am. Dent. A. *12*:1084–1100 (Sept.) 1925.

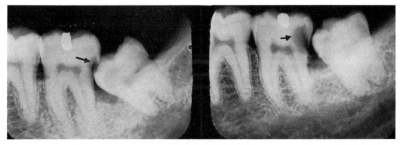

Figure 6–7 Caries near the cementoenamel junction caused by an impacted third molar. The roentgenogram on the left was made 6 years prior to the one on the right.

7

INFECTIONS OF THE JAWS

Infections of the jaws that are of dental origin may be discussed most conveniently under five headings: (1) periapical infection, (2) residual infection, (3) pericoronal infection, (4) periodontal disease, and (5) osteomyelitis. The predisposing causes for such infections are almost always local; however, in some instances, systemic disease and blood-borne infection may be contributing factors. Periodontal infection will be dealt with in the chapter on periodontal disease.

PERIAPICAL INFECTION

Infections that involve the periapical region most often are a result of inflammation and necrosis of the dental pulp. In some instances the source of the infection may be blood-borne, but such cases are rare.

ACUTE PERIAPICAL ABSCESS (DENTOALVEOLAR ABSCESS)

In acute periapical abscess, invasion of the surrounding bone by bacteria produces hyperemia, leukocytic infiltration, and edema, which may extend some distance from the root of the involved tooth. The earliest roentgenographic evidence of acute periapical abscess is widening of the periodontal-membrane space in the periapical region, which results from inflammatory changes in the membrane (Fig. 7–1, *left*). At this stage the involved tooth has

become tender to percussion and, in the majority of cases, the widening of the space is followed by more extensive involvement of the surrounding bone within a relatively short time (Fig. 7–1, *right*). On occasion, acute inflammation may cause widespread demineralization of bone, and roentgenograms made during the acute phase often reveal extensive areas of radiolucence with indefinite borders (Fig. 7–2). Once the acute phase has subsided, a large portion of the bone at the borders returns to normal opacity and trabecular pattern. The end result may be either a chronic periapical abscess or a dental granuloma, either of which is evidenced by periapical radiolucence of smaller size than that exhibited by the acute abscess.

Acute periapical abscess that involves a primary tooth rarely shows roentgenographic evidence of bone involvement

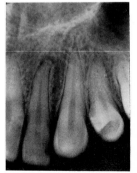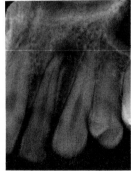

Figure 7–1 Acute periapical abscess. *Left,* Widening of periodontal-membrane space in the periapical region, which often is seen in the early stage. *Right,* Two days later there is extension into surrounding bone.

74

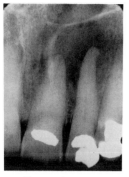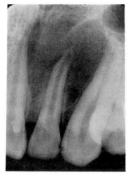

Figure 7–2 Acute periapical abscess. Two illustrations of widespread demineralization of bone that may be present during the acute stage of inflammation and swelling.

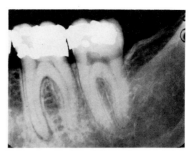

Figure 7–5 Widening of the periodontal-membrane space with condensing osteitis caused by chronic inflammation of a pulp that still gives a positive response to tests for vitality.

beyond the apical region. Destruction of bone invariably extends up into the bifurcation of the roots and presents a very typical picture (Fig. 7–3). Invasion of the cancellous bone of the jaw may occur if the permanent successor is missing or malposed (Fig. 7–4).

Widening of the periodontal-membrane space may be associated with chronic pulpitis even when the pulp still gives a positive response to tests for vitality. This widening may persist for long

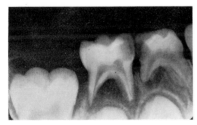

Figure 7–3 Acute periapical abscess involving a primary molar, as evidenced by destruction of the bone within the bifurcation of the roots.

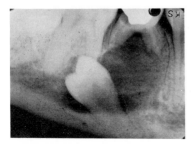

Figure 7–4 Acute periapical abscess of primary molar, which extends into the cancellous bone.

periods, often extending into months, and in most instances there is evidence of condensing osteitis of the surrounding bone (Fig. 7–5). The final outcome in the majority of such patients is either the development of an acute periapical abscess or the formation of a dental granuloma.

CHRONIC PERIAPICAL ABSCESS

A chronic periapical abscess may persist for years, particularly if there is a draining sinus to the surface. Such a sinus through which pus and serum are discharged most often leads from the abscess to the oral cavity, but it may also lead to the surface of the skin. If the latter condition exists, there may be confusion as to the source of the drainage, and such conditions have been treated on the assumption that they were confined to the soft tissues of the face or neck. In such cases dental roentgenograms have revealed abscesses associated either with the roots of pulpless teeth or with a retained dental root. Many of these abscesses are not well circumscribed and the borders may be very irregular.

A roentgenogram made for a woman 23 years of age who had a sinus of the chin that drained intermittently for more than 2 years is shown in Figure 7–6. Surgical incision to establish drainage and plastic operations to correct the scar defect had been done without avail. The roentgenogram revealed an abscess involving the right mandibular central and lateral incisors, which proved to be the source of the infection. The failure to arrive at a correct

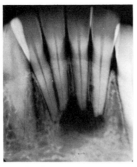

Figure 7–6 Chronic periapical abscess which proved to be the cause of a draining sinus that extended to the chin. There is slight resorption of the root of the right lateral incisor, and there is also reduction in size of the pulp cavity of the left central incisor, suggesting a previous injury to the teeth.

diagnosis earlier is understandable, for, in many such instances, formation of the chronic abscess is not preceded by an acute periapical abscess, and the first symptom referable to it may be localized swelling and redness of the skin. An abscess that is involving a mandibular second molar and that has extended downward and perforated the inferior border of the mandible is shown in Figure 7–7. It had produced a fistula and phlegmon of the neck. Removal of the tooth resulted in a cure. Such cases emphasize the importance of early dental roentgenographic examination to rule out dental infection as a possible source.

A not unusual occurrence is one in which periapical infection associated with maxillary posterior teeth extends upward and into the maxillary sinus to become the source of a chronic sinusitis. The cause of the sinusitis may be obscure until dental roentgenographic evidence is available. More rarely, an extensive periodontal lesion may be the source of a maxillary sinusitis (see Chapter 9). Periapical infection that has extended upward from maxillary incisors and established drainage on the floor of the nares also has been observed.

DENTAL GRANULOMA

A dental granuloma may form as a result of the reparative process that follows resolution of a periapical abscess. It also may form by direct extension from an inflamed periodontal membrane into the periapical bone when it is not preceded by an acute periapical abscess. It is usually round or oval, and is surrounded by a fibrous-tissue capsule which is continuous with the periodontal membrane. It may contain lymphocytic elements and plasma cells, and, according to Hill (1930), epithelium is present in all stages of proliferation, from that of epithelial rests to that of cystic formation. Many granulomas are infected, although microscopic examination as well as cultures has disclosed that many of them are sterile. Once formed, the granuloma may remain symptomless and unchanged indefinitely. The granulomatous process may undergo exacerbation and cause an acute periapical abscess to form, or the

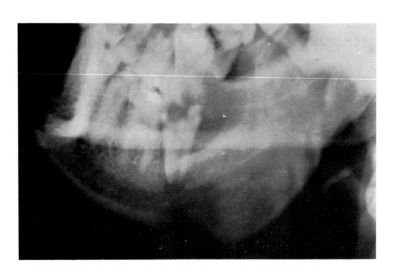

Figure 7–7 Abscess that extends from a lower second molar downward through the lower border of the mandible.

epithelial elements present may proliferate and form a radicular cyst. Priebe and co-workers (1954) demonstrated epithelial tissue in lumen formation in 55% of 101 cases of periapical lesions studied.

Roentgenographically, a granuloma is seen as a round or oval radiolucence that extends away from the apical portion of the root of the tooth. The borders are most often fairly well circumscribed, but in general they are not as definite and well demarcated, nor do they extend as abruptly away from the surface of the root, as is true of the small, fully developed radicular cyst. Frequently, however, a granuloma and a radicular cyst of equal size cannot be distinguished roentgenographically one from the other, but it should be kept in mind that an encapsulated granuloma rarely exceeds 1 cm in diameter. Evidence of resorption of the root or hyperplasia of the cementum may be associated with granulomas of long standing, but such evidence may be associated also with radicular cysts and therefore it is not important to differential diagnosis.

Some of the features of differential diagnosis are exhibited in Figure 7–8. The roentgenogram on the left is that of a granuloma, and the one on the right that of a radicular cyst. They are of equal size and are asymptomatic, and the diagnosis of both was based on microscopic examination. The borders of the granuloma are not as sharply defined and the central portion is slightly more radiopaque than that of the cyst. While the roentgenographic features were suggestive, it must be said that a correct diagnosis could be arrived at only by microscopic examination.

The inability to differentiate roentgenographically between a granuloma and a radicular cyst is of minor importance if the treatment chosen is either extraction of the tooth or complete apicoectomy. In each instance the lesion can be removed in its entirety. Lack of such differentiation does present a problem in root-canal therapy when apicoectomy is not contemplated, for then success of treatment often depends on the nature of the lesion.

In rare instances a dental granuloma may not be manifested roentgenographically. Such a granuloma occurs most often on the maxillary central incisors and first molars and is situated beneath the periosteum, where it is in direct communication with a small portion of the root through a very thin cortical plate. Digital examination reveals a firm, circumscribed swelling which is adherent to the surface of the jaw. There may or may not be a history of previous acute pulpitis, and the involved tooth does not respond to tests for vitality. The roentgenographic appearance of the bone in the periapical region is normal, and the lamina dura surrounding the apical portion of the root may appear to be intact.

RESIDUAL INFECTION

Residual infection is that which remains following extraction of a tooth, and is almost always associated with a retained root. The root may have been infected prior to extraction of the tooth, or it may have become infected as a result of being dislodged from its socket at the time of extraction. More rarely, a chronic periapical abscess that remains after extraction of the tooth may not undergo resolution and disappear, but may persist as a residual infection. In this event it is evidenced by a well-circumscribed radiolucent area which should not be confused with the diffuse radiolucent marrow spaces that some years

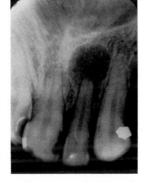

Figure 7–8 Dental granuloma or dental-root cyst? The similarity in roentgenographic appearance of the two conditions is illustrated. The one on the left proved to be a granuloma, the one on the right a cyst.

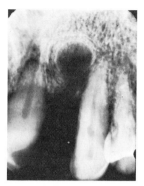

Figure 7–9 Residual infection. The cavity in the bone contained chronic inflammatory tissue. The tooth had been extracted 8 years previously.

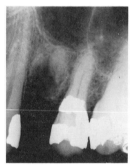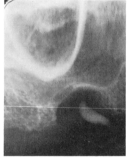

Figure 7–10 Residual infection associated with retained dental roots, as evidenced by areas of radiolucence adjacent to them. *Left,* Adjacent to fractured surface of root. *Right,* Infection surrounding entire root and causing chronic maxillary sinusitis.

ago were often interpreted as representing residual infection. Roentgenographic evidence of chronic inflammatory tissue that was still present 8 years after extraction of a maxillary lateral incisor is shown in Figure 7–9.

Residual infection that is associated with retained roots is recognized by a radiolucence that is adjacent to, or may com-

pletely surround, the root (Fig. 7–10). A root that had been forced through the cortex and had become lodged beneath the periosteum, where several years later it caused a subperiosteal abscess, is shown in Figure 7–11. From the lateral view *(left)* one might well assume that the root was still located within the jaw; however, the occlusal view *(right)* definitely demonstrates its exact location.

RETAINED ROOTS

Fortunately, the majority of retained roots are not infected. Most of these root fragments have not been dislodged from their sockets, and are from teeth that had normal vital pulps or had inflammation of the pulp which was still confined to the pulp chamber at the time of extraction. According to Kronfeld (1949) and others, the pulp in the fragment may remain vital; normal bone forms around it, and the fractured surface often becomes covered by cementum. Such roots may remain in the jaws indefinitely without causing any clinical symptoms.

The roentgenographic examination is a very reliable means of determining whether a retained root is, or is not, infected. If the lamina dura is intact and the bone surrounding it has a normal appearance, the possibility that it is infected is very remote (Fig. 7–12). It should be kept in mind, however, that the bone in an edentulous region is often more radiolucent than bone that is still supporting a tooth, and this should not be confused with reduced radiopacity caused by inflammation and infection.

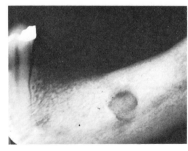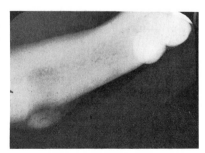

Figure 7–11 Retained dental root situated adjacent to the buccal surface of the mandible, where it caused an acute subperiosteal abscess.

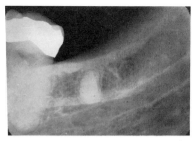

Figure 7-12 Retained dental root, showing intact lamina dura and normal appearance of the bone surrounding it.

The fact that many retained roots are not infected and remain asymptomatic should not encourage one to permit them to remain at the time of extraction, for there is no assurance that a root, even from a vital tooth, will not become infected.

PERICORONAL INFECTION

Pericoronal infection is a frequent occurrence if one includes that which is associated with the eruption of some teeth and subsides when the tooth has erupted. Such infections are of relatively short duration and do not produce any defects in the bone.

Chronic and acute pericoronal abscesses are frequently associated with teeth that remain only partially erupted, and they are not uncommonly associated with teeth that remain embedded. The teeth most frequently involved are the third molars, particularly the mandibular third molars.

Partially erupted mandibular third molars in which an appreciable amount of the occlusal surface remains covered by soft tissue are often associated with chronic pericoronal abscess. On clinical examination the overlying tissue may or may not appear to be healthy, although pressure most often reveals a purulent exudate. The roentgenogram usually shows a crater-like defect of the bone in the retromolar region which contains inflammatory tissue (Fig. 7–13, *left*). This condition not only is a source of focal infection, but also may provide an incubation zone for initiating an ulcerative gingivitis. The chronic abscess also may become acute and lead to cellulitis of the face and neck.

The most common source of pericoronal infection of teeth that are completely embedded either in soft tissue or in bone is the oral flora. The extent of bone destruction it produces may include the entire periphery of the tooth (Fig. 7–13, *center*), and it is not unusual to find that bone supporting the adjacent tooth has been destroyed to the extent that that tooth also must be extracted (Fig. 7–13, *right*). A chronic pericoronal abscess often may go undetected and first come to light only incidental to roentgenographic examination.

OSTEOMYELITIS

Osteomyelitis is a progressive inflammation of bone, usually of infectious origin, which tends to spread and in some instances may involve the entire bone. The extent and character of the changes it pro-

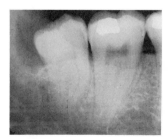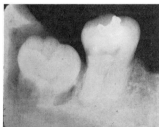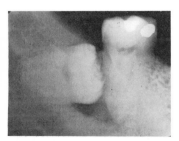

Figure 7-13 Chronic pericoronal abscess. *Left,* Abscess situated posterior to a partially erupted mandibular third molar and evidenced by the saucer-shaped defect in bone. *Center,* Abscess surrounding the major portion of an embedded mandibular third molar. *Right,* Abscess associated with an impacted mandibular third molar and with marked destruction of bone adjacent to the erupted second molar.

duces in bone are dependent on the stage of the disease, the resistance of the host, and the virulence of the infection. It may occur in an acute and a chronic form. The mandible is involved more frequently than the maxilla.

Most cases of osteomyelitis of the jaws result from local causes. These are acute periapical infection, pericoronitis, acute periodontal lesions (Ivy and Cook, 1942), trauma, particularly that associated with fracture, acute infection of the maxillary sinus, and, by direct extension, furunculosis of the face. Osteomyelitis may follow extraction of teeth or superimposed dental infection in bone that is of poor quality, such as irradiated bone, marble bone (osteopetrosis), and other conditions in which the bone is highly vulnerable to infection. It may occur in the metastatic form, in which the original infection is at a site in the skeleton far remote from the jaws. Other causes of osteomyelitis of the jaws may be syphilis, tuberculosis, and actinomycosis. The roentgenographic appearance may be similar, in many respects, and a positive diagnosis is based on the presence of the specific organism.

ACUTE OSTEOMYELITIS

Acute pyogenic osteomyelitis has a sudden onset which is usually associated with severe pain and an elevation in temperature. The infection may spread rapidly, destroy and penetrate the cortical bone and periosteum, and extend into the surrounding soft tissues to produce cellulitis of the face or neck. The course may be very rapid, with pus formation occurring in many instances within 2 to 4 days. Destruction of the blood supply within the bone leads to necrosis and formation of sequestra which are characteristic of the disease.

During the first few days after onset of the infection, there may be no roentgenographic evidence of either alteration of trabecular pattern or destruction of bone. The first change is manifested by indistinct trabeculations and destruction of bone at the site of infection (Fig. 7–14). If osteomyelitis follows extraction of a tooth, first

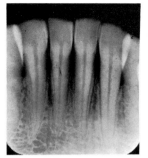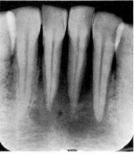

Figure 7–14 Osteomyelitis that had its origin in acute gingivitis. *Left,* Roentgenogram, with negative findings, made 3 days after onset, at a time when severe pain and marked swelling had appeared. *Right,* Roentgenogram made 8 days after onset, which reveals diffuse destruction of bone in the interseptal and periapical regions.

roentgenographic evidence of the nature of the infection is that of destruction and obliteration of the radiopaque lines that depict the walls of the dental root socket (Fig. 7–15). This is a characteristic feature that serves to distinguish it from so-called dry socket, a condition that also may be associated with severe postoperative pain. In acute infection, rapid diffuse destruction of bone may take place which will, within a relatively short time, extend some distance from the original site (Fig. 7–16).

In many instances the destruction of bone follows a linear pattern, and between the channels of destruction there are, at one stage of the disease, areas of bone in which the trabeculae are well preserved—that is, segments of bone that apparently have temporarily resisted destruction (Fig. 7–17). Later the isolated segments of bone may become devitalized and form sequestra. Sequestration occurs in almost all untreated and unsuccessfully treated patients with osteomyelitis, and is pathognomonic of the disease. Such sequestra are well demonstrated by the dental roentgenogram (Fig. 7–18).

The roentgenographic picture of osteomyelitis may be altered by the administration of antibiotics. If they are administered during the early stage of the infection, the osteomyelitis may be aborted to the extent that no evidence of decalcification, bone destruction, and sequestration appears. It is therefore often impossible to make a diag-

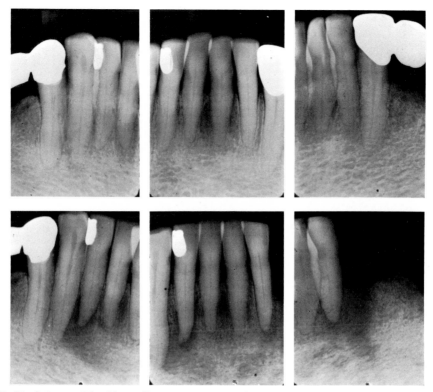

Figure 7–15   Osteomyelitis. *Above,* Roentgenogram made 2 years prior to the one below, showing normal bone pattern. *Below,* Roentgenogram made 2 weeks following extraction of a periapically infected mandibular canine, showing complete destruction of the walls of the dental-root socket and evidence of bone destruction extending away from it and across the symphysis.

nosis by means of the roentgenographic examination alone. If the osteomyelitis is well developed and advanced prior to the administration of antibiotics, the symptoms may be masked, although destruction of bone and sequestration may continue unchecked. In such patients the progress of the disease and its response to treatment should be observed by frequent roentgenographic examinations.

The roentgenographic picture of healed osteomyelitis, particularly if of long standing, is fairly typical. The cortical bone shows an irregular increase in width and density. The medullary cavity is narrowed, and the bone may be abnormally dense. In the jaws it is often possible to make a diagnosis of a previous osteomyelitis on the basis of roentgenographic evidence alone.

A conservative attitude should be

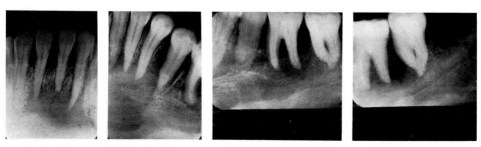

Figure 7–16   Osteomyelitis that had its origin in an acute pericoronal abscess associated with a mandibular third molar. The roentgenogram reveals diffuse destruction of bone that extends as far anteriorly as the midline and that had taken place within a period of 2 weeks.

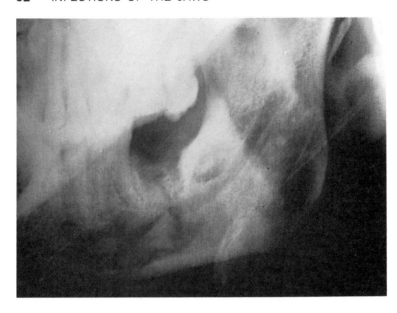

Figure 7-17 Osteomyelitis that followed extraction of an infected mandibular second molar, showing separated segments of bone that still have normal trabecular pattern.

taken toward extraction of teeth during the active phase of the disease, since many of them for which extraction appears to be indicated at the time may prove to be useful teeth after the infection has subsided. Extraction should therefore be limited to those that are certain to undergo sloughing and those that are associated with acute periapical abscesses that might interfere with successful treatment of the osteomyelitis.

In view of the fact that most cases of osteomyelitis of the jaws arise from acute odontogenic infections, a measure that might tend to reduce the incidence may be the early extraction of the offending tooth,

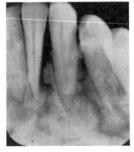

Figure 7-18 Osteomyelitis. Dental roentgenogram illustrating the worm-eaten pattern of bone destruction and the radiopaque islands of bone that represent formation of sequestra.

thereby providing early drainage for the infection present. This applies particularly to pericoronitis. There is still some diversity of opinion as to whether early extraction should be done since, in many instances, the osteomyelitis may continue unabated following the extraction, in which event it might be concluded that it arose as the result of the extraction. However, it would be more logical to assume that in the majority of patients the osteomyelitis was present prior to the surgical procedure.

In cases of known vulnerability to osteomyelitis, as in patients with irradiated bone, teeth should be extracted only when necessary. As an added precaution, antibiotics should be administered prior to and following the surgical procedure.

HEMATOGENOUS OSTEOMYELITIS

Hematogenous osteomyelitis most often occurs in children and adolescents, according to Weinmann and Sicher (1947) and Fabe (1950), and it is usually caused by *Micrococcus (Staphylococcus) pyogenes* var. *aureus.* Its onset may follow measles, scarlet fever, and other childhood diseases, and also injuries and skin infections. Subsequent to the initial infection, several

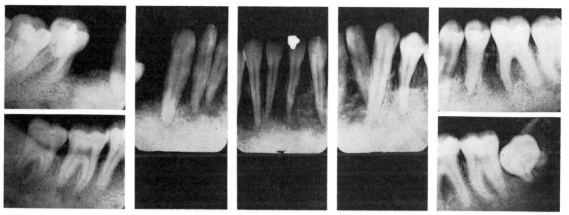

Figure 7–19   Osteomyelitis (hematogenous). Infection in the mandible occurred subsequent to involvement of other bones of the skeleton. Source of the original infection was a blister on the heel.

bones may become involved successively, and often active infection is present in a number of bones simultaneously. The roentgenographic appearance is similar to that seen in osteomyelitis that arises from odontogenic infections and other infectious sources.

A dental roentgenogram made for a boy 16 years of age who had mandibular osteomyelitis of hematogenous origin is shown in Figure 7–19. The right ramus and the entire body of the mandible were involved, and the site of the greatest destruction of bone was in the anterior region. There was no acute periapical infection or recent operation or trauma that could account for it on a local basis. The initial lesion was an infected blister on the heel of the left foot. This was followed in a few days by acute osteitis of the fibula, and within a few weeks the left knee, right scapula, ribs, and mandible had become involved successively.

CHRONIC SCLEROSING OSTEOMYELITIS

Chronic diffuse sclerosing osteomyelitis represents a proliferative reaction of bone to a low-grade infection. It may occur at any age but is seen most often in older persons. The mandible is most frequently involved, sometimes bilaterally.

The roentgenographic appearance of this form of osteomyelitis is fairly typical. There is a partial obliteration of the marrow spaces and a thickening of the cortex that results in a marked roentgenographic density of the bone. The bone may be slightly enlarged, and its surface may be slightly irregular (Fig. 7–20). In some respects the roentgenographic picture may be somewhat similar to that of Paget's disease of bone.

Occasionally there may be intermittent inflammation and swelling of the mucoperiosteum with draining fistulae onto the mucosal surface. This form of osteomyelitis is very resistant to treatment.

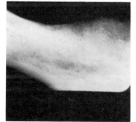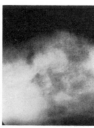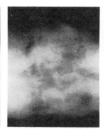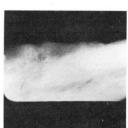

Figure 7–20   Chronic sclerosing osteomyelitis involving the major portion of the mandible and showing generalized increased density of bone and numerous areas of rarefaction.

GARRÉ'S OSTEOMYELITIS
(PERIOSTITIS OSSIFICANS)

According to Bennett (1948), Garré's osteomyelitis is a form of sclerosing osteomyelitis in which the infectious agent localizes in the periosteum and produces an overgrowth of bone on the outer surface of the cortex. If the condition persists, the infection may spread into the interior of the bone. Involvement of the jaws occurs almost always in children or young adults and has a definite predilection for the mandible (Shafer et al., 1974). Suydam and Mikity (1969) reported three cases, in infants less than 2 years of age, in which infection of the soft tissues overlying the bone of the mandible caused periosteal new bone formation without involvement of the underlying bone. Administration of antibiotics resulted in recovery and almost complete disappearance of the periosteal new bone.

A periostitis with bone formation that eventually led to invasion of the medullary portion of the mandible is illustrated in Figure 7–21. A roentgenogram made for a white 17-year-old girl revealed the presence of dense bone overlying the inferior border of the mandible, extending from the premolar region posteriorly onto the ramus. This is typical of periosteal bone formation of long standing. The roentgenogram also showed a path of bone destruction through the periosteal bone formation that extended upward into the medullary spaces of the body and ramus of the mandible. There was a several-year history of intermittent pain and swelling of the overlying soft tissues; this pain and swelling had been relieved by the administration of antibiotics at the time of the exacerbations. In view of this history, surgical treatment was advised. This consisted of extraction of the premolar and first and second molars, removal of dense bone from above the mandibular canal, and decortication of a portion of the buccal plate extending down to the inferior border of the mandible. The roentgenogram made 15 months postoperatively showed partial return of the normal contour of the mandible, and there was no evidence of osteomyelitis. The patient had experienced no pain or other symptoms of osteomyelitis for the last 11 of those 15 months.

When this type of periosteal bone formation occurs during infancy, it may be confused with infantile cortical hyperos-

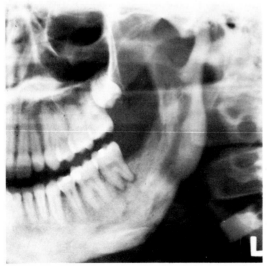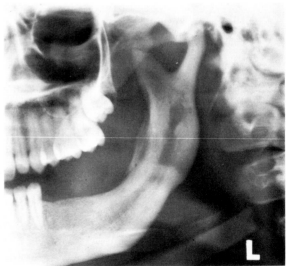

Figure 7–21 Garré's osteomyelitis (periostitis ossificans). *Left,* Roentgenogram made at 17 years of age, showing periosteal bone formation overlying inferior border of mandible, and destruction of bone through it that extends upward into the medullary portion. *Right,* Roentgenogram made 15 months after operation, with no evidence of active osteomyelitis.

tosis (Caffey's syndrome). However, the clavicles, pelvis, and extremities also are involved in Caffey's syndrome. The presence of pain, swelling, and favorable response to antibiotics should rule out fibrous dysplasia.

SERIOUS SEQUELAE RESULTING FROM ORAL INFECTION

Serious complications may arise when the infection perforates the cortical bone of the jaws and invades the adjacent soft tissues and tissue spaces. (The attachment of the muscles may determine the path that the infection will follow, channeling it into the various tissue spaces.) The virulence of the organism and the resistance of the host influence the degree of spread of the infection. Among the severe complications are cellulitis, Ludwig's angina, and cavernous sinus thrombosis.

CELLULITIS (PHLEGMON)

Cellulitis of the face and neck is a diffuse inflammation of the soft tissues that most often occurs as a result of a periapical abscess, osteomyelitis, or pericoronitis involving erupting and partially impacted mandibular third molars. The cellulitis is characterized by painful swelling of the soft tissues, fever, leukocytosis, and lymphadenitis. Early administration of antibiotics and removal of the cause of the infection will in large measure prevent the formation of a draining sinus to the surface of the skin.

LUDWIG'S ANGINA

Ludwig's angina is a severe cellulitis that most often has its onset in the submaxillary space, from which it extends into the sublingual and submental spaces. The source of the infection is most often the mandibular molars, where the thin lingual plate offers the least resistance to perfora-

tion and thereby leads to the direct extension of the infection to the floor of the mouth. There it rapidly produces a firm swelling that does not localize but extends downward to involve the neck. Edema of the glottis may also occur, which carries with it the risk of suffocation. Prior to the advent of antibiotics the mortality rate was very high, but now it has been markedly decreased.

CAVERNOUS SINUS THROMBOSIS

Cavernous sinus thrombosis consists of formation of a thrombus in the cavernous sinus and the branches that communicate with it. Infections of the face and intraoral structures are the common sources of this condition, particularly those that occur above the maxilla. The path of a dental infection is by way of the pterygoid plexus. Death occurs as a result of meningitis or a brain abscess, and prior to the use of antibiotics the condition was invariably fatal.

REFERENCES

Bennett, G. A.: The Bones. In Anderson, W. A. D.: Pathology. St. Louis, The C. V. Mosby Company, 1948, pp. 1263–1326.

Fabe, S. S.: Acute Hematogenous Osteomyelitis of Mandible: Report of Case. Oral Surg., Oral Med. & Oral Path. 3:22–26 (Jan.) 1950.

Hill, T. J.: Epithelium in Dental Granulomata. J. Dent. Res. 10:323–332 (June) 1930.

Ivy, R. H. and Cook, T. J.: Osteomyelitis Arising from Periodontium. Am. J. Orthodontics (Oral Surg. Sect.). 28:86–94 (Feb.) 1942.

Kronfeld, R.: Histopathology of the Teeth and Their Surrounding Structures. Ed. 3, edited by P. E. Boyle. Philadelphia, Lea & Febiger, 1949, p. 351.

Priebe, W. A., Lazansky, J. P., and Wuehrmann, A. H.: Value of Roentgenographic Film in Differential Diagnosis of Periapical Lesions. Oral Surg., Oral Med. & Oral Path. 7:979–983 (Sept.) 1954.

Shafer, W. G., Hine, M. K., and Levy, B. M.: A Textbook of Oral Pathology. Ed. 3. Philadelphia, W. B. Saunders Company, 1974, p. 459.

Suydam, M. J. and Mikity, V. G.: Cellulitis with Underlying Inflammatory Periostitis of the Mandible. Am. J. Roentgenol. 106:133–135 (May) 1969.

Weinmann, J. P. and Sicher, H.: Bone and Bones: Fundamentals of Bone Biology. St. Louis, The C. V. Mosby Company, 1947, p. 321.

8 PERIODONTAL DISEASE

PHILLIP J. SHERIDAN, D.D.S.
CHARLES M. REEVE, D.D.S.

The term "periodontal disease" refers to a group of diseases that affect the investing or supporting structures of the teeth. These structures (the periodontium) comprise the gingiva, periodontal ligament, alveolar bone, and cementum. Exceptions to this definition are the pathologic changes localized in the periapical region and associated with pulpal disease; these are not included in the customary usage of the term.

Periodontal diseases have been classified under the headings "inflammatory" and "dystrophic" (Bernier, 1957). A recent classification (Tobias et al., 1972) substitutes "degenerative" for "dystrophic." However, because the term "degenerative" by definition excludes some entities (for example, gingival hyperplasia), in this chapter the older but more appropriate heading, "dystrophic," will be used. Inflammatory disease includes gingivitis and periodontitis. Dystrophic disease includes recession, disuse atrophy, gingival hyperplasia, and periodontosis. Trauma from occlusion also affects the supporting tissues of the teeth and some authorities include this as a separate pathologic entity (Grant et al., 1972). In addition, periodontal disease will be discussed with respect to its relationship to certain systemic diseases and syndromes.

Dental roentgenographic examination is one of the most valuable adjuncts in the detection of periodontal disease. It also plays an important role in specific diagnosis and in treatment planning. However, it should not be relied on as the sole diagnostic method, because it does not reveal periodontal pockets and it often fails to disclose osseous destruction, particularly that confined to the buccal or lingual surfaces of the teeth (Figs. 8–1 and 8–2). It does not provide information as to the health of the soft tissues, and the condition of the gingiva cannot be predicted from the roentgenographic appearance of the alveolar crest (Massler et al., 1953). Nevertheless, the roentgenogram can supply very important knowledge of the variations in

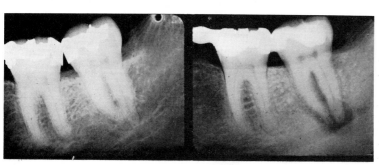

Figure 8–1 Periodontal pocket on buccal aspect of root that extends beyond the apex and resembles a periapical abscess. Roentgenogram on the left was made 2 years prior to the one on the right.

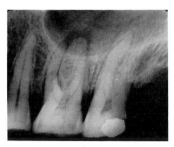

Figure 8–2 Periodontal pocket on palatal aspect of lingual root that extends beyond the apex and resembles a periapical abscess.

contour of the interdental alveolar septa that may exist in the absence of periodontal disease. Ritchey and Orban (1953) demonstrated that the maximal height of any interdental septum is determined by an imaginary straight line connecting the cementoenamel junctions of adjoining teeth; therefore, the configuration of the alveolar crest is oblique when there is a difference in the length of crowns, when there is a variation in the degree of eruption of adjoining teeth, or when there is an inclination in position of the teeth in the jaws. Such deviation in configuration from a horizontal crest might erroneously be interpreted as evidence of early angular bone destruction.

Often the roentgenogram does not demonstrate the characteristic radiopacity of the cortical bone of the interdental alveolar crest, even in the presence of a normal cortex; this is particularly true of the incisor region where, because of the thinness of the alveolar process, the x-ray beam may not encounter sufficient compact

bone to make it visible. Variations in the angulation of the beam may also cause disappearance or appearance of the radiopacity that depicts a normal cortex.

Roentgenograms made by the parallel or right-angle technique will demonstrate more accurately the features of periodontal disease, because this technique provides a better view of bone in the crest and reveals more accurately the actual extent or depth of the periodontal lesion in relation to the root of the tooth (Prichard, 1961). Roentgenograms made by the bisecting-angle technique may show greater destruction of the supporting bone than that actually present, because the central ray is directed obliquely to the long axis of the teeth and jaw, which produces dimensional distortion. Also, with the bisecting-angle technique, subgingival calculus may be superimposed on alveolar bone and thus would not be detected. The bite-wing film will demonstrate deposits of subgingival calculus and defects of the cementum, but it may not cover a sufficient area to demonstrate extensive periodontal lesions adequately.

The panoramic roentgenogram is useful for examination of the maxilla and mandible. In many instances it facilitates the diagnosis of fractures, impacted teeth, bony lesions, and some temporomandibular joint changes (Chapter 19). However, owing to lack of definition and overlapping of teeth, it is of little value in the diagnosis of periodontitis. A detailed examination of the periodontal ligament space and interprox-

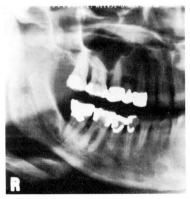
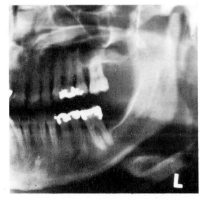

Figure 8–3 Panoramic roentgenogram provides a continuous picture of the bone level, but definition is poor.

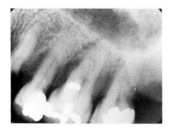 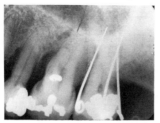

Figure 8–4 Periodontal pocket with bone loss extending beyond apex of palatal root of second molar is not evident on roentgenogram *(left)* because intact buccal bone masks loss of lingual bone. Note result when silver points are inserted into lingual pocket *(right)*.

imal alveolar crest requires the use of intraoral roentgenograms. The panoramic survey does provide a continuous picture of the bone level about the teeth, and thus it might be used in some instances to supplement intraoral roentgenograms in the diagnosis of periodontitis (Fig. 8–3).

The bone loss caused by periodontal disease can be underestimated on the roentgenogram because of the superimposition of all or part of the lesion on tooth structure. Using dried specimens of human jaw with fine wires adapted to the teeth at the base of the infrabony deformities, Theilade (1960) showed that the actual loss of bone was appreciably greater than the loss apparent on the roentgenogram. Goldman and Stallard (1973) made roentgenograms of dried human skulls before and after filling the osseous defects with a radiopaque paste; they found that the buccal and lingual walls of interproximal osseous defects did not register on the roentgenogram. To demonstrate and confirm in vivo the presence of deep osseous defects that are not discernible in the roentgenogram, one can insert gutta-percha or metal points into the pockets and expose the film while they are in place (Fig. 8–4). This method is useful for purposes of teaching and it also may be of practical clinical value.

Roentgenographic examination is important in evaluation of the success or failure of periodontal treatment. Successful treatment is often evidenced by restoration of a cortical plate. From a follow-up of several patients over a period of years, Bell and colleagues (1950) concluded that, if there is no evidence of further resorption and destruction of bone, it must be accepted that the original inflammatory process has been eliminated by treatment

and that no persistent chronic inflammation or infectious process has recurred in the meantime.

SUPRAGINGIVAL AND SUBGINGIVAL CALCULUS

Calculus plays a major part in the production of gingival inflammation. Two types have been referred to by Stones (1951) and others: supragingival and subgingival.

Supragingival calculus tends to be deposited on the lingual surfaces of the mandibular incisors and on the buccal surfaces of the molars, the regions that are near the openings of the ducts of the submaxillary and parotid glands, respectively (Figs. 8–5 and 8–6). This type of calculus is often superimposed on the crowns of the teeth and is not always discernible in the roentgenogram until the deposits have become extensive.

In contrast, the roentgenogram is invaluable in detecting the location and amount of subgingival calculus; the deposits are seen as pointed or irregular radiopaque projections extending from the sur-

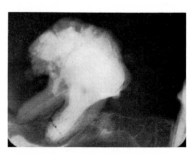

Figure 8–5 Supragingival calculus. Extensive deposits on the molar in the region of opening of the parotid duct.

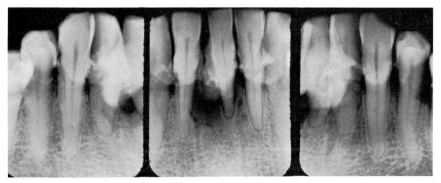

Figure 8–6 Supragingival calculus associated with resorption of the alveolar ridge in the region of the mandibular incisor teeth.

face of the root. The calcareous deposits are best demonstrated on a film that is placed parallel to the long axis of the tooth, with exposure time decreased. The bite-wing film is especially useful for this purpose (Fig. 8–7). Obviously, one should not rely solely on the roentgenogram for detection of the deposits, because some of them may not be opaque enough to be demonstrable.

INFLAMMATORY PERIODONTAL DISEASE

GINGIVITIS

Gingivitis is defined as inflammation of the gingiva. It may be chronic or acute. The primary etiologic factor is the accumulation of bacterial plaque due to inadequate oral hygiene. Local predisposing factors include calculus, malposed teeth, defective restorations, and the presence of prosthodontic and orthodontic appliances. In addition, gingivitis may occur as an oral manifestation of allergy, blood dyscrasia, endocrine or nutritional disturbances, or other systemic conditions. Gingivitis due to local irritation is considered to be the simplest form of inflammatory periodontal disease and as such is a forerunner of periodontitis.

PERIODONTITIS

Periodontitis results from the extension of gingival inflammation to involve the remainder of the periodontium. Initially,

inflammatory destruction of the coronal portion of the periodontal ligament permits apical migration of the epithelial attachment and the formation of a periodontal pocket. If the inflammatory disease is permitted to progress, the crestal portion of the alveolar process begins to resorb. In the roentgenogram this destruction of the cortical layer of the alveolar process often is evidenced by a cup-shaped notch or scalloping of the crest. The resorption may proceed apically on a horizontal level. Beyond this, the lamina dura appears to be normal and there is no widening of the periodontal ligament space. Many of the

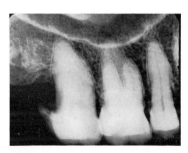

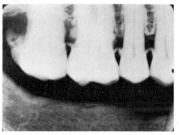

Figure 8–7 Subgingival calculus. *Above,* Roentgenogram made with the bisecting-angle technique does not adequately demonstrate the calculus present. *Below,* Bite-wing film not only demonstrates more clearly the amount and location of the calculus but also provides a better view of the alveolar crest.

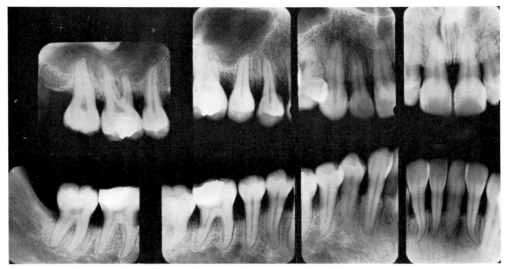

Figure 8–8 Periodontitis with uniform resorption of the alveolar margin on a horizontal level.

teeth remain solid in their sockets (Fig. 8–8). When the loss of bone has reached a level at which support for the teeth is no longer adequate, leverage becomes so unfavorable that the lateral force developed even by normal function cannot be compensated for.

The pattern of bone destruction may progress in a vertical direction along the root to form angular bony defects. In the roentgenogram these usually are evidenced by a vertical or V-shaped flaw, with the root of the tooth forming one side of the defect (Fig. 8–9).

PERIODONTAL ABSCESS

Periodontal abscess is an acute exacerbation of the process occurring in a chronic periodontal pocket; it usually results from partial or complete occlusion of the orifice of the pocket. Although it may occur in a fairly shallow pocket, it most often develops in a deep one (Fig. 8–10); the bifur-

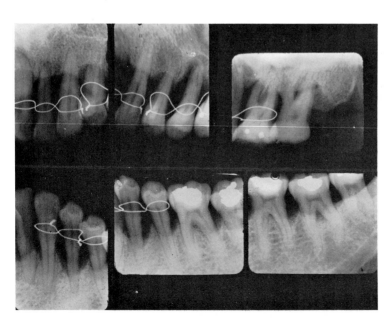

Figure 8–9 Periodontitis with vertical destruction of bone, which extends along the roots toward their apices.

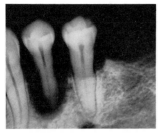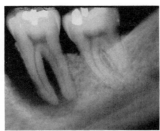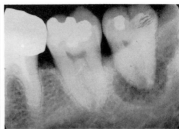

Figure 8–10 Three cases in which acute periodontal abscesses occurred within chronic periodontal pockets extending beyond the root apices. The chronicity of the bone destruction is evidenced by the presence of calculus on the apical one-third of the root (see bicuspid).

cation or trifurcation of the molar teeth is a common site of occurrence. An abscess also may begin in a normal periodontium if a foreign body is forced beyond the epithelial attachment (Fig. 8–11). Like the acute periapical abscess, the acute periodontal abscess may produce rapid and extensive bone destruction. In some instances it will extend beyond the level of the apices of the roots of the teeth.

Multiple acute periodontal abscesses may occur in some cases of advanced generalized periodontitis. Destruction of bone usually is rapid and extensive, and there is a tendency for the formation of draining sinuses that extend into the adjacent mucosa.

DYSTROPHIC PERIODONTAL DISEASE

Prichard (1972) described dystrophic changes as those resulting from atrophic,

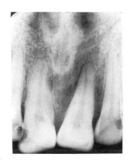

Figure 8–11 Periodontal abscess. A popcorn hull forced beyond the epithelial attachment on the mesiolingual aspect of the central incisor tooth resulted in an acute periodontal abscess that extended apically and then labially, perforating the labial bony plate on the mesial aspect of the root and producing swelling labial to the root apex. The tooth was vital and the pulp remained uninvolved.

hypertrophic, degenerative, or mechanical (traumatic) influences, or from other circumstances leading to interference with the normal physiology of the periodontium.

ATROPHY

In atrophy, the part or its cellular elements are decreased in size after reaching full maturity; this usually is manifested by recession of the gingiva and the crest of the alveolar process and by diminution of the cellular elements of the supporting bone. The recession sometimes occurs early in life, but usually it is associated with senility. The length of the clinical crown may be greatly increased, although this might be accounted for partially on the basis of continuous eruption of the teeth. Atrophy from disuse affects primarily the supporting bone and is manifested by osteoporosis that appears in the roentgenogram as a decrease in the number of the bony trabeculations and narrowing of the cortex. Disuse atrophy most often follows loss of opposing teeth; it also may result from developmental and acquired disabilities that decrease masticating function. The occurrence of such atrophies rarely leads to inflammatory periodontal disease if good oral hygiene is maintained and if the teeth retain their normal positions in the arch.

HYPERPLASIA

The hyperplasia attributed to dystrophic changes is a diffuse fibromatosis that may involve part or all of the gingiva. The gingiva is pale, and there is no inflammation in the original state. The fibromatosis sometimes is idiopathic, although a similar hyperplasia of the gingiva may occur in patients on diphenylhydantoin (Dilantin) therapy. The condition rarely produces any roentgenographic changes. However, defects of alveolar bone caused by pressure of the dense fibrous tissue have been noted in a few instances.

PERIODONTOSIS (DEGENERATION)

Periodontosis is defined as a noninflammatory destruction of the periodontium. According to Frankl et al. (1973), it occurs most frequently in young persons and usually before age 20 years. Degeneration of the principal fibers of the periodontal ligament causes increased mobility and migration of the teeth, which is one of the earliest and most characteristic signs of the disease. Later, localized deep periodontal pockets and angular bony defects become the predominating features. In many patients these degenerative changes appear to be confined to the supporting structures of the incisors and first molars (Fig. 8–12), but in some instances all of the teeth present may be involved. Often, only a few teeth are lost and the remaining ones may become firm and remain with a normally functioning attachment apparatus.

Roentgenograms made during the early stages of the disease reveal widening of the periodontal ligament space, which tends to be uniform in width in its entirety, and an irregular lamina dura. In the later stages, marked resorption of bone is a feature and is evidenced by deep, vertical, osseous defects.

All efforts to relate periodontosis to systemic disease have been futile, with the exception of the rare Papillon-Lefèvre syndrome (see page 95). A number of inves-tigators have observed periodontosis to follow a familial pattern. In spite of the unusual features of the disease, however, there are some who question whether periodontosis can be considered a definite clinical entity separable from juvenile periodontitis.

OCCLUSAL TRAUMATISM

Tissue changes in the periodontium that may result from occlusal traumatism are thrombosis of the blood vessels, necrosis, and hyalinization of the connective tissue of the periodontal ligament. The cementum and bony wall of the alveolus may undergo varied degrees of resorption (Glickman, 1972). The traumatism may be confined to one or a few teeth only, or it may involve all of the teeth present.

Occlusal traumatism is said to be primary or secondary (Orban et al., 1958). "Primary trauma" is that which occurs when excessive force is exerted on a tooth that has normal bone support. "Secondary trauma" occurs when excessive force is exerted on a tooth that has diminished support owing to periodontitis. In advanced periodontitis, even the normal masticatory forces may become excessive and result in secondary occlusal traumatism.

Essential for occlusal traumatism is premature contact between opposing teeth. Such premature contact may result from cuspal interference, drifting and tilting of a tooth after loss of a neighboring tooth, or improper prosthetic appliances or occlusal fillings. Some discomfort is commonly associated with the traumatism. This may range from a dull to a severe pain, the latter occurring most frequently when the tooth is still firm in its socket.

When a tooth is subjected to abnormal

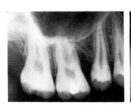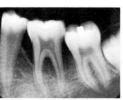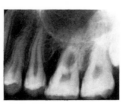

Figure 8–12 Periodontosis in a 14-year-old boy, with deep, vertical, osseous defects involving the first molars. No other defects were present.

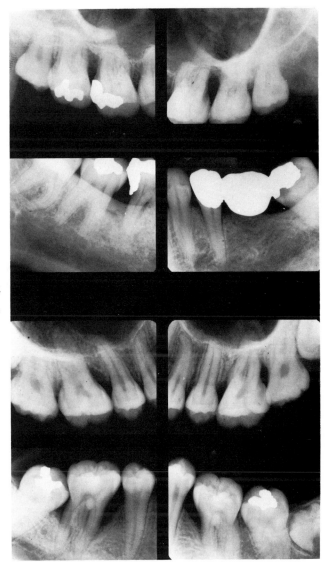

Figure 8–13 Periodontosis in mother, age 54 years *(upper),* and daughter, age 17 years *(lower).* Note similarity of deep, vertical, osseous defects.

or excessive stress, one of two things may result. The structures that support it either are damaged and break down or they become reinforced, thereby making the tooth able to withstand the increased functional demand. It is possible therefore that there is less damage to the supporting structures of some of the teeth that appear to be bearing the most severe occlusal stresses. Here, the direction of the force may be an important factor. Conceivably these teeth are subjected to a lesser degree of lateral stress. It long has been recognized that the supporting structures will tolerate a considerable amount of vertical stress because the force is more evenly distributed over all of the principal fibers of the periodontal ligament.

PARAFUNCTION

Habits of forcible clenching of the teeth and bruxism (gritting the teeth) may produce sufficient trauma to cause pathologic changes in the periodontium. Clenching is usually a tensional manifestation and frequently comes into play during mental concentration and nervous tension. The patient often is unaware of the habit. The degree of injury to the periodontal tissues

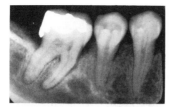

Figure 8–14 Clenching habit apparently has led to widening of periodontal ligament space. Patient had worn a complete maxillary denture for 12 years.

depends largely on the amount of force placed on the tooth, on whether it is constant or intermittent, and how frequently it is applied. Usually, the habit of clenching is not acquired until later in life, and the supporting structures of the molars usually are the first to show its deleterious effects. The destructive changes in the periodontium and the changes in the mobility of the teeth are more extensive than in brusixm, because the frequency, duration, and severity of the occlusal load are often greater in clenching. Early evidence of these changes is seen in the roentgenogram as a widening of the periodontal ligament space, particularly in the crestal and periapical regions (Fig. 8–14).

Bruxism is largely confined to the time of sleep. This habit usually is acquired early in life. Like the habit of clenching, it may be a tensional manifestation, but occlusal imbalance also may be an initiating factor. Continuation of the habit results in abnormal occlusal wear. If the habit is long-standing, the cusps may be worn away, leaving a flat occlusal surface. Flat occlusal surfaces will permit free lateral movement, and in many cases the supporting structures of the teeth will adapt to the forces of bruxism (Fig. 8–15). The chief concern in many cases of bruxism is marked loss of tooth structure. The roentgenogram usually reveals a wide lamina dura and abnormally dense supporting bone. The picture is very similar to that presented by the habitual tobacco chewer.

SYSTEMIC DISEASES AFFECTING THE PERIODONTIUM

Although systemic disease does not initiate the lesions of inflammatory periodontal disease (gingivitis or periodontitis), certain systemic conditions (for example, diabetes) may predispose to or alter the severity of inflammatory periodontal disease. Other systemic disease processes (scleroderma, hyperparathyroidism) or neoplastic processes (eosinophilic granuloma) can cause roentgenographically or clinically observable lesions or changes in the periodontium; however, the existence of these lesions in conjunction with inflammatory periodontal disease is a matter of coincidence. A third group that should be considered here are those systemic conditions (Papillon-Lefèvre syndrome, hypophosphatasia) that apparently can cause some types of dystrophic periodontal disease. Diabetes mellitus (see Chapter 18), a disorder of carbohydrate metabolism, for many years has been considered to be associated with an increased severity of inflammatory periodontal disease. Particularly impressive is the severe periodontitis with advanced bone destruction (Fig. 8–16) often seen in young adult diabetics (Rutledge, 1940; Sheppard, 1936; Swenson, 1954). Recently, electron microscopic studies (Frantzis et al., 1971) have demonstrated

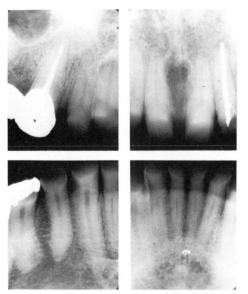

Figure 8–15 Bruxism. The periodontium has adapted well to the forces of bruxism in this 67-year-old man.

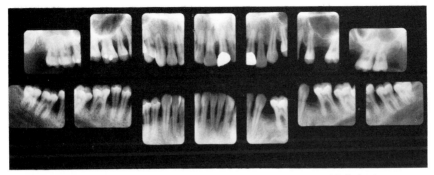

Figure 8–16   Diabetes. Advanced periodontitis in a 24-year-old diabetic man.

significant thickening of the capillary base-ment membrane in the gingival connective tissue of diabetics. Such microangiopathies might well alter the host susceptibility to inflammatory periodontal disease.

Scleroderma is a collagen disease in which a primary feature is enlargement and disorientation of the principal fibers of the periodontal ligament. The changes in the periodontium usually are first noted when roentgenographic examination reveals wid-ening of the periodontal ligament space (Stafne and Austin, 1944) (Figs. 8–17 and 8–18).

Hyperparathyroidism frequently leads to changes in the alveolar bone. The dental roentgenogram may show rarefaction of bone, transformation of trabecular pattern, and absence of lamina dura (Fig. 8–19).

Eosinophilic granuloma of bone, a form of histiocytosis X, has a predilection for alveolar bone (Lichtenstein, 1953). In the adult, the pattern of destruction of al-veolar bone simulates in large measure that of active and advanced periodontitis (Grupe and Orban, 1950). The oral lesions

may be associated with eosinophilic granu-lomas elsewhere in the skeleton, but in some instances they are confined to the jaws (Figs. 8–20 and 8–21).

PAPILLON-LEFÈVRE SYNDROME

The Papillon-Lefèvre syndrome is characterized by hyperkeratosis of the palms and soles and precocious destruction of the supporting structures of the primary and permanent teeth. According to Gorlin and Pindborg (1964), there is evidence that the syndrome is inherited as an autosomal recessive trait, and the onset is usually in the second to fourth years of life. At onset, the palms and soles become red and scaly; later, the skin markings become accentu-ated and assume a parchmentlike quality.

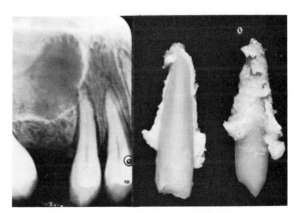

Figure 8–18   Scleroderma. *Left,* Roentgenogram of maxillary second premolar, showing abnormal wi-dening of the periodontal ligament space. *Right,* Longitudinal section through center of tooth, show-ing attached periodontal ligament. (Reproduced with permission from Stafne, E. C. and Austin, L. T.: A Characteristic Dental Finding in Acrosclerosis and Diffuse Scleroderma. Am. J. Orthodontics (Oral Surg. Sect.). *30*:25–29 [Jan.] 1944.)

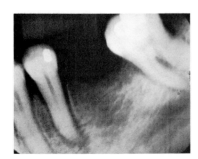

Figure 8–17   Scleroderma. There is uniform wi-dening of the periodontal ligament space, a salient feature of the disease.

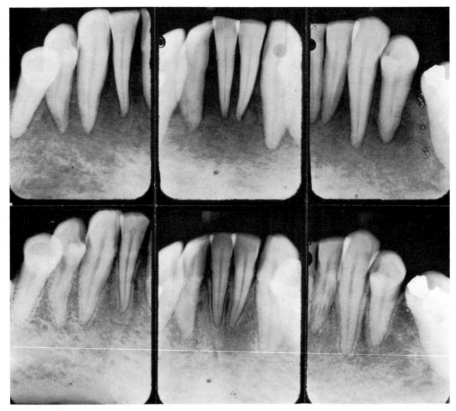

Figure 8–19   Primary hyperparathyroidism. *Above,* Roentgenogram showing marked radiolucence of bone and absence of lamina dura. *Below,* Roentgenogram made 3 years after removal of an adenoma of the parathyroid gland, showing reappearance of the lamina dura and bone of normal density.

The hyperkeratotic plaques also have been noted on the knees, elbows, and other parts of the body.

Development and eruption of the primary and permanent teeth are essentially normal. The onset of periodontal involve-

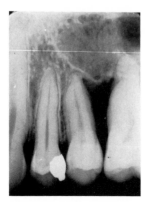

Figure 8–20   Histiocytosis X. Lesion has caused complete destruction of the interdental septum between a maxillary second premolar and first molar.

ment and destruction of alveolar bone occur soon after the eruption of the last primary tooth, and this almost always coincides with the appearance of the palmar and plantar hyperkeratosis.

The first symptom of oral involvement is inflammation and swelling confined to the gingivae. This is followed by destruction of the alveolar bone, which becomes so extensive that all of the primary teeth usually are exfoliated or must be removed prior to 5 years of age. With the loss of the teeth, the inflammation subsides and the tissues overlying the alveolar ridge return to normal. When the permanent dentition erupts, the gingival inflammation and destruction of the alveolar process are repeated in essentially the same manner as in the primary dentition. Again, the destruction of alveolar bone is so extensive that the alveolar process often is completely destroyed, and the permanent dentition, with

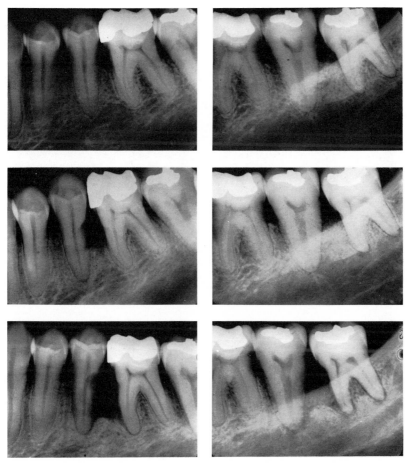

Figure 8–21 Histiocytosis X. *Top,* April 1953. No clinical symptoms of the.lesions were as yet present. *Center,* April 1954. There is destruction of bone between the second premolar and first molar, and early involvement of the crest of the alveolar ridge between the second and third molars. *Bottom,* August 1955. There has been progressive destruction of bone and resorption of the roots of the adjoining teeth.

the exception of the third molars, is lost in the second decade of life (Coccia et al., 1966).

From review of the literature and examination of the roentgenograms of the reported cases, it is apparent that the destruction of the alveolar bone follows a fairly definite pattern. The teeth become involved in about the same order in which they erupt, and the destruction of the alveolar process is initiated at the alveolar crest and progresses on a horizontal plane. Roentgenographic evidence of the formation of deep vertical periodontal pockets is exceptional.

The dental roentgenogram shown in Figure 8–22 was made for a 9-year-old girl who had a palmar-plantar hyperkeratosis. It revealed marked destruction of alveolar bone around the maxillary incisors and the mandibular canines. A rather unusual finding was that the canines, which had erupted prematurely, had also undergone complete maturation at 9 years of age. In this patient, hyperkeratosis of the soles and palms had been present at age 2 years; at age 5 years, similar lesions had appeared on the knees, elbows, and knuckles. The primary teeth had erupted at the normal time and had been exfoliated within 6 months after all of them had erupted. The patient then was clinically edentulous until the permanent teeth began to erupt. The first molars were exfoliated shortly after

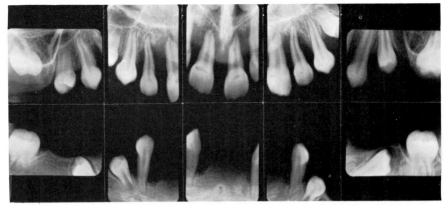

Figure 8–22 Papillon-Lefèvre syndrome. Roentgenogram of a girl 9 years of age, showing extensive destruction of alveolar bone surrounding the anterior teeth and premature maturation and eruption of the canines.

they erupted, and the mandibular incisors became loose and were extracted at age 8 years.

HYPOPHOSPHATASIA

Hypophosphatasia is a familial metabolic disorder in which a salient feature is premature exfoliation of the primary teeth. Baer and colleagues (1964) reported on the dental findings in two cases of hypophosphatasia. On microscopic examination they found definite histologic evidence of hypocementogenesis of the affected teeth. The roentgenogram shown in Figure 8–23 was made of one of their patients, a 2-year-old white girl. It revealed abnormally large pulp chambers, which is a characteristic feature of the condition, and destruction of alveolar bone that becomes apparent when the teeth begin to undergo exfoliation. Un-

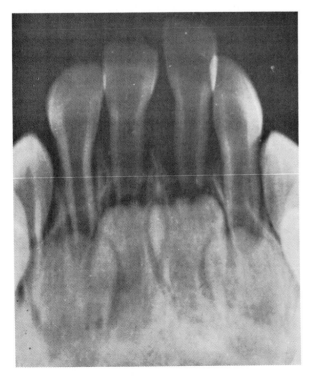

Figure 8–23 Hypophosphatasia. Roentgenogram of a 2-year-old girl, showing abnormally large pulp chambers and loss of alveolar bone in the region of the mandibular incisors. (Reproduced with permission from Baer, P. N., Brown, N. C., and Hamner, J. E., III: Hypophosphatasia: Report of Two Cases with Dental Findings. Periodontics. 2:209–215 [Sept. - Oct.] 1964.)

like the premature loss of teeth that occurs with the Papillon-Lefèvre syndrome, only the primary teeth are affected and gingival inflammation is not a prominent feature.

REFERENCES

Baer, P. N., Brown, N. C., and Hamner, J. E., III: Hypophosphatasia: Report of Two Cases with Dental Findings. Periodontics. 2:209–215 (Sept.-Oct.) 1964.

Bell, D. G., Rule, R. W., Jr., Dienstein, B., and Nuckolls, J.: The Periodontal Lesion. II. A Roentgenographic Evaluation of Treated Periodontal Cases: A Biological Approach. J. Periodont. 21:70–78 (Apr.) 1950.

Bernier, J. L.: Report of Committee of Classification and Nomenclature. J. Periodont. 28:56–58 (Jan.) 1957.

Coccia, C. T., McDonald, R. E.., and Mitchell, D. F.: Papillon-Lefevre Syndrome: Precocious Periodontosis with Palmar-Plantar Hyperkeratosis. J. Periodont. 37:408–414 (Sept.-Oct.) 1966.

Frankl, S. N., Goldman, H. M., and Cohen, D. W.: Periodontal Disease in Children. In Goldman, H. M. and Cohen, D. W.: Periodontal Therapy. Ed. 5. St. Louis, The C. V. Mosby Company, 1973, p. 264.

Frantzis, T. G., Reeve, C. M., and Brown, A. L., Jr.: The Ultrastructure of Capillary Basement Membranes in the Attached Gingiva of Diabetic and Nondiabetic Patients with Periodontal Disease. J. Periodont. 42:406–411 (July) 1971.

Glickman, I.: Clinical Periodontology: Prevention, Diagnosis and Treatment of Periodontal Disease in the Practice of General Dentistry. Ed. 4. Philadelphia, W. B. Saunders Company, 1972, p. 331.

Goldman, H. M. and Stallard, R. E.: Limitations of the Radiograph in the Diagnosis of Osseous Defects in Periodontal Disease. J. Periodont. 44:626–628 (Oct.) 1973.

Gorlin, R. J. and Pindborg, J. J.: Hyperkeratosis Palmoplantaris and Periodontoclasia in Childhood (Papillon-Lefèvre Syndrome, Parodontopathia Acroectodermalis). In Gorlin, R. J. and Pindborg, J. J.: Syndromes of the Head and Neck. New York, McGraw-Hill Book Company, 1964, pp. 287–291.

Grant, D. A., Stern, I. B., and Everett, F. G.: Orban's Periodontics: A Concept – Theory and Practice. Ed. 4. St. Louis, The C. V. Mosby Company, 1972, p. 563.

Grupe, H. E. and Orban, B.: Eosinophilic Granuloma Diagnosed by Gingival Biopsy. J. Periodont. 21:19–23 (Jan.) 1950.

Lichtenstein, L.: Histiocytosis X: Integration of Eosinophilic Granuloma of Bone, "Letterer-Siwe Disease," and "Schüller-Christian Disease" as Related Manifestations of a Single Nosologic Entity. A.M.A. Arch. Path. 56:84–102 (July) 1953.

Massler, M., Muhlemann, H. R., and Schour, I.: Relation of Gingival Inflammation to Alveolar Crest Resorption. (Abstr.) J. Dent. Res. 32:704 (Oct.) 1953.

Orban, B., Wentz, F. M., Everett, F. G., and Grant, D. A.: Periodontics: A Concept – Theory and Practice. St. Louis, The C. V. Mosby Company, 1958, pp. 86–87.

Prichard, J. F.: The Role of the Roentgenogram in the Diagnosis and Prognosis of Periodontal Disease. Oral Surg., Oral Med. & Oral Path. 14:182–196 (Feb.) 1961.

Prichard, J. F.: Advanced Periodontal Disease: Surgical and Prosthetic Management. Ed. 2. Philadelphia, W. B. Saunders Company. 1972, p. 115.

Ritchey, B. and Orban, B.: The Crests of the Interdental Alveolar Septa. J. Periodont. 24:75–87 (Apr.) 1953.

Rutledge, C. E.: Oral and Roentgenographic Aspects of the Teeth and Jaws of Juvenile Diabetics. J. Am. Dent. A. 27:1740–1750 (Nov.) 1940.

Sheppard, I. M.: Alveolar Resorption in Diabetes Mellitus. Dent. Cosmos. 78:1075–1079 (Oct.) 1936.

Stafne, E. C. and Austin, L. T.: A Characteristic Dental Finding in Acrosclerosis and Diffuse Scleroderma. Am. J. Orthodontics. 30:25–29 (Jan.) 1944.

Stones, H. H.: Oral and Dental Diseases: Aetiology, Histopathology, Clinical Features and Treatment; A Textbook for Dental Students and a Reference Book for Dental and Medical Practitioners. Ed. 2. Edinburgh, E. & S. Livingstone, Ltd., 1951, pp. 4, 6, 511.

Swenson, H. M.: Alveolar Bone Resorption Associated with Diabetes. J. Periodont. 25:52–53 (Jan.) 1954.

Theilade, J.: An Evaluation of the Reliability of Radiographs in the Measurement of Bone Loss in Periodontal Disease. J. Periodont. 31:143–153 (Apr.) 1960.

Tobias, J. A., Prichard, J. F., Clark, J. W., and Gilson, C. M. (Eds.): Current Procedural Terminology for Periodontists. Ed. 3. Chicago, American Academy of Periodontology, 1972, p. 9.

9

THE MAXILLARY SINUS

The image of a portion of the maxillary sinus appears almost constantly in the dental roentgenogram, and it so often reveals associated pathologic processes that it appears justifiable to deal with this sinus as a separate entity. The dentist also is often confronted with the problem of differential diagnosis of odontalgia and disturbances of the maxillary sinus, for patients frequently first seek his services, believing that the pain they experience is of dental origin.

ANATOMY

Some knowledge of the anatomy of the maxillary sinus and its variations as to size and form as viewed in the dental roentgenogram is pertinent. Ennis (1937) and Ennis and Batson (1936) made excellent and detailed descriptions of the anatomy of the maxillary sinus as demonstrated by intraoral films. Maxillary sinuses vary greatly in size, some being so small that evidence of them does not appear in the dental roentgenogram. Others are so large that they extend well downward into the interseptal spaces of the posterior maxillary teeth and the region of the tuberosity. The size may also vary from one side to the other in the same person. In general, the larger the maxillary sinus the more radiolucent it is, for there is then less bone surrounding it in proportion to the size of the air cavity.

A dental roentgenogram in which the image of the maxillary sinus does not appear is shown in Figure 9–1. A small maxillary sinus is expected to be situated well upward and posteriorly, and may be obscured by superimposition of the malar process, as in this instance.

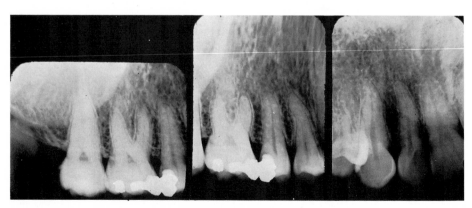

Figure 9–1 Posterior maxillary region in which the image of the maxillary sinus does not appear. (Reproduced with permission from Stafne, E. C.: Roentgenologic Interpretation. In Grossman, L. J.: Lippincott's Handbook of Dental Practice. Ed. 2. Philadelphia, J. B. Lippincott Company, 1952, pp. 63–92.)

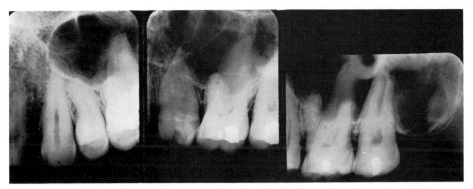

Figure 9–2 Posterior maxillary region, revealing a large maxillary sinus that extends downward between the roots of the molar teeth and also into the region of the tuberosity.

A large maxillary sinus is shown in Figure 9–2. It extends downward and occupies all the space in the trifurcation of the roots of the first molar, and extends into the interseptal space of the first and second molars, the third molar space, and the tuberosity. Knowledge of the relation of the maxillary sinus to the roots of the teeth is of utmost importance when extraction of teeth and other surgical measures are contemplated in that region, and the advantage of preoperative roentgenograms cannot be overemphasized.

Figure 9–3 shows the dental roentgenogram of a maxillary sinus with two septa which appear to separate it into three distinct compartments. These apparent compartments may be confused with epithelium-lined cysts, and in some instances a cyst may produce a similar image when it is superimposed on the maxillary sinus, so that it may require aspiration or injection of a radiopaque fluid before a correct diagnosis can be made.

PNEUMATIZATION OF THE MAXILLARY SINUS

From a slitlike cavity on the lateral wall of the middle meatus, the maxillary sinus proceeds to enlarge by pneumatization in pace with growth of the maxilla and the alveolar process. After adult life has been reached the size remains stationary under normal conditions and function. Downward growth of the alveolar process with downward movement of the posterior teeth following loss of posterior mandibular teeth brings about an increase in its size.

Not infrequently the maxillary sinus, by further pneumatization, resorbs alveolar bone that formerly served to support a missing tooth or teeth and then occupies the edentulous space. A thin cortex remains over the alveolar ridge to maintain a normal contour. An edentulous space into which the maxillary sinus has extended

Figure 9–3 Maxillary sinus, showing septa that appear to divide it into three different and separate compartments.

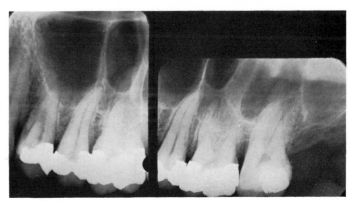

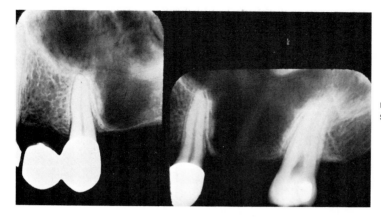

Figure 9–4 Extension of the maxillary sinus into an edentulous space as a result of pneumatization.

after the loss of posterior teeth is shown in Figure 9–4.

Marked increase in the size of the maxillary sinus by pneumatization may take place after extraction of all the maxillary teeth. It is also more likely to occur when the teeth are removed during the earlier decades of life, and when the supporting bone is healthy and normal. Such a case is shown in Figure 9–5. The opposite side presented a similar condition. The vertical dimension of the alveolar process in the anterior region has been maintained, and a thin cortex remains over the alveolar ridge in the posterior regions. Once this has occurred there can be no resorption of the crest of what remains of the alveolar process in the posterior regions. The alveolar ridge should retain its size and contour, which in turn reduces the problems associated with the wearing of artificial dentures.

Following removal of cysts and other pathologic conditions that have reduced the size of the maxillary sinus, there is a marked tendency for the sinus to return to its normal size. This also applies to inflammatory lesions that are associated with the roots of the teeth and that have extended into the sinus and occupied a part of its space. Such a case is shown in Figure 9–6, where an inflammatory lesion associated with a first molar is seen extending upward into the maxillary sinus.

MAXILLARY SINUSITIS

Maxillary sinusitis may be caused by colds and other infectious diseases, trauma, and infection associated with the teeth. The proportion of instances in which sinusitis is of dental origin has been estimated at anywhere from 15 to 75%. It would be difficult to determine the exact incidence; however, the number of those in which dental infection is the cause is appreciably high, but probably would conform more closely to the lower figure.

Dental sources of maxillary sinusitis

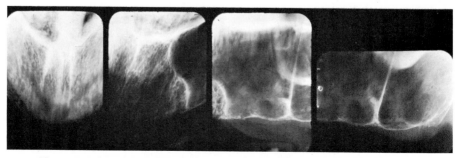

Figure 9–5   Pneumatization of the maxillary sinus in an edentulous maxilla.

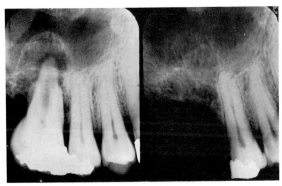

Figure 9–6 *Left,* Inflammatory lesion that is associated with the first molar and that is extending up into the maxillary sinus and replacing a portion of it. *Right,* Maxillary sinus has returned to normal size 7 months after removal of the tooth and lesion.

may be acute periapical abscess, chronic periapical infection, extensive periodontal lesions, or perforation of the antral floor and antral mucosa at the time of dental extraction. Roots and foreign bodies forced into the maxillary sinus at the time of operation also may be a cause.

The onset of acute maxillary sinusitis may often follow an acute periapical abscess of a posterior maxillary tooth. Roentgenograms made for a patient in whom acute sinusitis appeared a few days after the onset of an acute periapical abscess of a right first premolar are shown in Figure 9–7. The acute sinusitis is recognized by the uniform cloudiness or abnormally increased radiopacity of the sinus, particularly as contrasted to that of the maxillary sinus on the opposite side. The increased radiographic density is accounted for by a thickened antral mucosa and the presence of secretions and pus in a cavity that normally contains only air. A similar roentgenographic picture is seen when acute sinusitis is caused by a perforation into the sinus at the time of tooth extraction (Fig. 9–8). The tooth need not necessarily be an infected one at the time it is extracted, for no doubt the infection that is introduced from the oral cavity is responsible for the sinusitis. When it is known that an opening to the sinus has been produced, every effort should be made to effect a closure, to prevent continued passage of fluid and air from the oral cavity into the sinus.

The intraoral roentgenogram offers a reliable means of determining the presence of acute maxillary sinusitis. Austin and Hempstead (1939) studied a series of cases of clinically acute maxillary sinusitis and found that in all instances the intraoral roentgenographic examination served to verify the diagnosis.

Acute sinusitis may clear up completely, leaving little if any damage to the antral mucosa (Stafne, 1957). In such instances, the roentgenographic appearance returns to normal. In the event that chronic sinusitis develops as a result of the acute phase, the roentgenographic appearance changes also. The uniform radiopacity may no longer be present, but in its place are irregular areas of density which are evidence of an uneven sclerosing of the bone of the antral wall, thickened antral mucosa, and perhaps the presence of polyps. The fine radiopaque lines that depict the borders of the maxillary sinus may become wider and irregular. A similar roentgenographic picture is present in chronic sinusitis that is not pre-

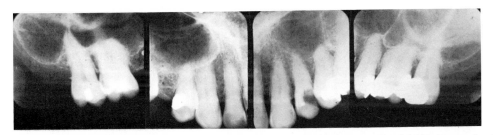

Figure 9–7 Acute maxillary sinusitis caused by an acute periapical abscess of a right first premolar. There is marked radiopacity as compared with the sinus on the left, which is normal. (Reproduced with permission from Stafne, E. C.: Dental Roentgenographic Interpretation Dealing with the Pulp Cavity and the Maxillary Sinus. J. Ohio State Dent. A. *31*:62–73 [Spring] 1957.)

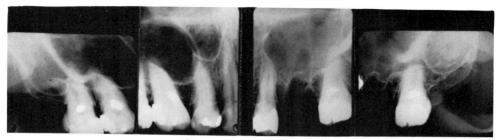

Figure 9–8 Acute maxillary sinusitis following extraction of a right first molar, as evidenced by its marked opacity in contrast to that of the normal sinus on the opposite side.

ceded by the acute phase. Furthermore, once sclerosed changes of the bone of the walls of the sinus have taken place, they may remain in evidence even after the infection has subsided and the patient is free of symptoms.

Dental infection no doubt is the cause of more cases of chronic sinusitis than is generally supposed. Bauer (1943) called attention to the fact that the roentgenogram is not always a reliable indicator in determining maxillary sinusitis of dental origin. He found by microscopic examination that the antral mucosa is often affected in cases of periapical infection that is separated from the maxillary sinus by a relatively thick layer of bone. He also observed local inflammatory reactions of the antral mucosa caused by extensive periodontal lesions.

Maxillary sinusitis that is caused by periapical infection is most often recognized because there usually is a history of pulpitis, the tooth fails to respond to tests for vitality, and the periapical lesion can almost always be demonstrated by roentgenographic examination (Fig. 9–9). Periodontal lesions that cause maxillary sinusitis often go undetected, for there may be no symptoms referable to the involved teeth. These lesions may closely proximate the wall of the sinus as a result of extension into the trifurcation of molar teeth and over

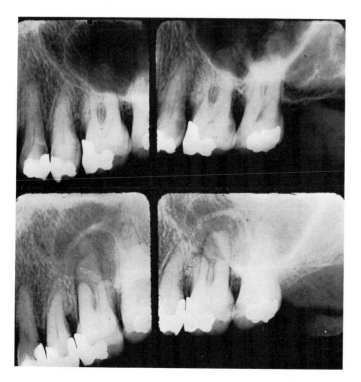

Figure 9–9 Recurrent maxillary sinusitis caused by periapical infection. *Above,* View prior to onset of sinusitis, showing normal-appearing sinus cavity. *Below,* View 1 year after onset of sinusitis. Treatment, including radical operation, had failed to relieve. (Reproduced with permission from Stafne, E. C.: Dental Roentgenographic Interpretation Dealing with the Pulp Cavity and the Maxillary Sinus. J. Ohio State Dent. A. *31*:62–73 [Spring] 1957.)

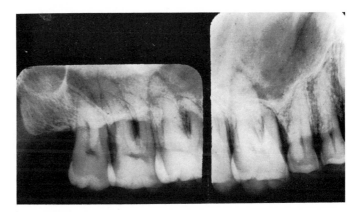

Figure 9–10 Chronic sinusitis caused by extensive periodontal lesions involving the molar teeth.

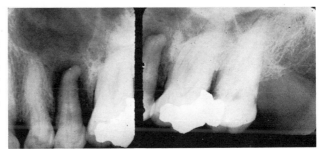

Figure 9–11 Chronic maxillary sinusitis caused by a periodontal lesion associated with a second premolar. (Reproduced with permission from Stafne, E. C.: Dental Roentgenographic Interpretation Dealing with the Pulp Cavity and the Maxillary Sinus. J. Ohio State Dent. A. *31*:62–73 [Spring] 1957.)

the apexes of their palatal roots (Fig. 9–10). Chronic maxillary sinusitis that resulted from perforation of the floor of the sinus by a periodontal lesion involving a vital, caries-free second premolar is shown in Figure 9–11. In some instances, both periodontal and periapical lesions may be contributing factors in causing sinusitis (Fig. 9–12).

Dental infection no doubt is the cause of chronic maxillary sinusitis in a sufficient percentage of cases to warrant a routine dental roentgenographic examination to rule it out as a possible source.

ROOTS AND FOREIGN BODIES IN THE MAXILLARY SINUS

The shadows of roots of teeth that remain after extraction and that are superimposed on the maxillary sinus are often seen in the roentgenogram. Nearly all of these roots are situated in their original position in the dental alveolar socket. Roots that are located within the maxillary sinus are rarely encountered. When they do occur in this location, they are most often recognized by a deviation from their normal vertical position in the arch, and by absence of

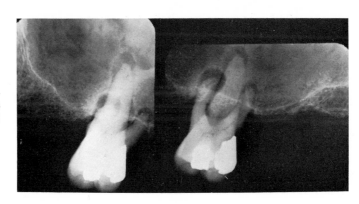

Figure 9–12 Chronic maxillary sinusitis in which periodontal as well as periapical lesions involved the offending tooth.

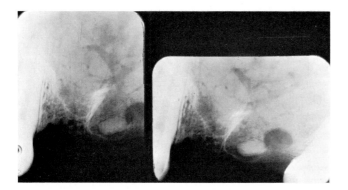

Figure 9–13 Dental root situated between the antral mucosa and the wall of the sinus. There is marked opacity of the sinus cavity.

the lamina dura that normally surrounds them. The entire root may be situated between the antral mucosa and the wall of the maxillary sinus, or a part or all of the root may be situated within the sinus cavity. Some idea as to its location can be gained from the roentgenographic evidence, for roots that lie exposed in the maxillary sinus tend to gather calcific deposits on their surfaces in sufficient amounts to be discernible in the roentgenogram. A root situated under the antral mucosa would not gather such calcific deposits.

If a root becomes lodged between the antral mucosa and the wall of the maxillary sinus, it may become a source of local inflammation or sinusitis (Fig. 9–13).

Two illustrations in which calcific deposits are present on roots in the maxillary sinus are shown in Figure 9–14. In the one on the right the root projected partially into the sinus cavity and it had an appreciable

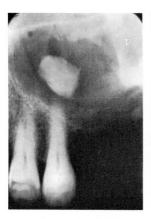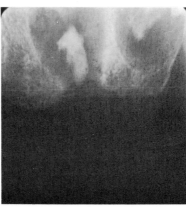

Figure 9–14 Dental roots in the maxillary sinus, on which there are calcific deposits. *Left,* Entire root is within the sinus cavity. *Right,* Apex of root projects into the sinus cavity. (Reproduced with permission from Stafne, E. C.: Dental Roentgenographic Interpretation Dealing with the Pulp Cavity and the Maxillary Sinus. J. Ohio State Dent. A. *31*:62–73 [Spring] 1957.)

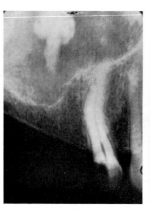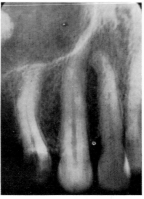

Figure 9–15 Calcific deposits on the apex of a root that projects into the sinus cavity and has formed a bizarre image resembling the shape of a mushroom. (Reproduced with permission from Stafne, E. C.: Roentgeno-oddities. Oral Surg., Oral Med. & Oral Path. *15*:948–949 [Aug.] 1962.)

amount of deposit over the apex. Another example of calcific deposits on the apex of a root which projects into the maxillary sinus is shown in Figure 9–15.

A root fragment that is forced into the maxillary sinus may become a nucleus for the formation of a rhinolith, as shown in Figure 9–16. In this case the roentgenogram revealed a radiopaque object in the left maxillary sinus. It also revealed an absence of bone of the floor of the maxillary sinus in the first molar region, which

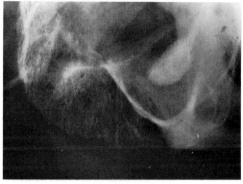

Figure 9–17 Large rhinolith in the sinus of a patient with chronic maxillary sinusitis.

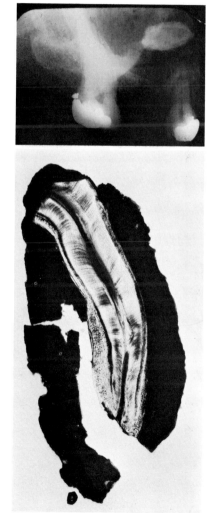

Figure 9–16 Rhinolith in the maxillary sinus. A dental root was the nidus. *Above,* Roentgenogram, and *below,* ground section, showing calcific deposits within which a dental root is present (× 8). (Reproduced with permission from Stafne, E. C.: Dental Roots in Maxillary Sinus. Am. J. Orthodontics. [Oral Surg. Sect.] *33*:582–584 [Aug.] 1947.

suggested that the object might have been introduced into the sinus from the oral cavity. The degree of radiopacity of the periphery of the object suggested that it might be the crown of a tooth. After removal, a ground section was prepared which revealed a dental root covered by a heavy deposit of calculus.

Other small foreign bodies in the maxillary sinus no doubt serve as nidi for the formation of rhinoliths. A case of rhinolith of the sinus was reported by Stafne (1947) in which, upon decalcification, a thread about 1 cm in length was found.

A roentgenogram made for a patient suffering from chronic maxillary sinusitis revealed a rhinolith (Fig. 9–17). Some indication as to the nature of the foreign body might be gained from the fact that a rhinolith is slightly more radiopaque than root structure and less radiopaque than the enamel of a tooth.

Foreign bodies other than tooth structure may be introduced into the maxillary sinus through an antro-oral opening. Ennis and Novak (1943) reported a case in which an appreciable amount of denture relining paste was forced into the sinus when an immediate artificial denture was inserted. Materials used in the postoperative treatment of dental sockets may also be forced into the maxillary sinus. In the event that these materials are radiopaque they are readily seen in the roentgenogram.

The radiopaque body seen in the maxillary sinus in Figure 9–18 proved to be a

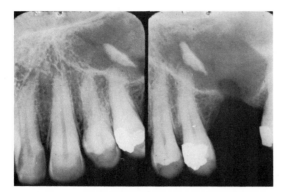

Figure 9–18 Foreign body introduced into the maxillary sinus through the tooth socket.

fragment of radiopaque surgical cement that had been used in treatment of a root socket several years previously. The opening through bone leading from the floor of the sinus to the crest of the alveolar ridge is one that is often seen in cases of antroalveolar fistula of long standing.

Some dental roots, particularly those of small size, that are forced into the maxillary sinus and are not recovered may become incorporated in mucous secretions and may be eliminated through the sinus opening into the nostril. It is therefore important to make preoperative roentgenograms shortly prior to the time removal of the root is contemplated, for there have been some instances in which patients have been referred for removal of dental roots that had recently been forced into the maxillary sinus but in whom the roots were no longer present when the patients came for removal of them. In a review of 50 consecutive cases in which the roots of teeth had been displaced into the maxillary sinus, Killey and Kay (1964) found that spontaneous exfoliation of the roots into the nose occurred in five cases, some of them in the act of sneezing. It was their opinion that the incidence of such an occurrence is presumably greater than heretofore realized.

CYSTS OF THE MAXILLARY SINUS

Dentigerous and radicular cysts, although they do not have their origin in the maxillary sinus, may encroach upon it and partially or in some instances almost entirely obliterate it. An extremely thin layer of bone is retained, separating the cyst and the antral cavity; a layer of connective tissue covered by epithelium lines the cyst wall, and the antral mucosa remains intact on the walls of the maxillary sinus. In a few instances such a cyst may become infected, perforate, and drain into the sinus cavity, or in removal of the cyst the thin antral wall may be destroyed and as a result the maxillary sinus and the cavity produced by the cyst sometimes become a common cavity.

A cyst of dental origin that encroaches upon the maxillary sinus is seen in the roentgenogram as a rounded area of uniform radiolucency, bordered by a thin, well-defined radiopaque margin which displaces the cavity of the maxillary sinus upward or posteriorly, as the case may be. The cyst may have its origin from a pulpless tooth, a retained dental root, or an embedded tooth, or it may be a residual epithelium-lined cyst. It is rarely possible to obtain satisfactory information as to the source of these cysts without the aid of intraoral roentgenographic examination. A case in point is one reported by Hallberg and Stafne (1947). A roentgenogram of the maxillary sinus was made for a man 26 years of age who complained of slight tenderness of the left maxilla. It revealed a large cyst which occupied almost all of the sinus cavity and had expanded to the extent that it had reduced the size of the left nasal chamber (Fig. 9–19). No evidence could be gained from this roentgenogram that the cyst was of dental origin. However, a dental roentgenogram revealed an unerupted premolar of which the crown and distal surface of the root were denuded and completely devoid of bone (Fig. 9–20). A tentative diagnosis of dentigerous cyst was made, which was verified at the time of operation when it was found that the crown of the tooth was situated within the lumen of the cyst and was firmly attached to the wall of the cyst. Microscopic examination revealed that the cyst was lined with stratified squamous epithelium.

The image of mucoid retention cysts

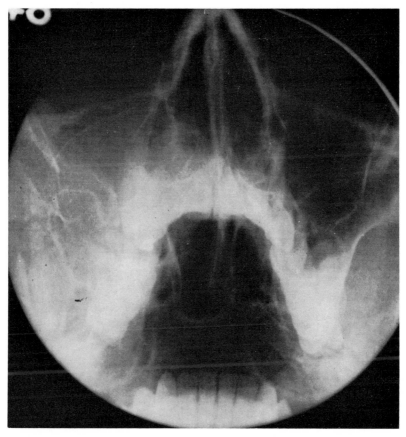

Figure 9–19 Dentigerous cyst that occupies the entire left maxillary sinus. (Reproduced with permission from Hallberg, O. E. and Stafne, E. C.: Treatment of Dentigerous Cysts: Report of a Case. Am. J. Orthodontics [Oral Surg. Sect.] *33*:633–636 [Aug.] 1947.)

that have their origin in the mucosa of the maxillary sinus appears frequently in the dental roentgenogram and often is seen with unusual clarity. Millhon and Brown (1944) have called attention to the high incidence. Skillern (1920) stated that such cysts are characterized by single or multiple, hemispherical, yellow or whitish protuberances on the wall of the antrum, ranging in size from a millet seed to a walnut, and occasionally they may grow to such an extent as to fill the antral cavity completely. Although most of the cysts are asymptomatic, there have been reports of cases in which symptoms were present, such as a sensation of fullness in the orbital and frontal regions or a blockage of the nares caused by extrusion of large cysts into the

Figure 9–20 Same patient as in Figure 9–19, showing an unerupted second premolar from which the dentigerous cyst developed. (Reproduced with permission from Hallberg, O. E. and Stafne, E. C.: Treatment of Dentigerous Cysts: Report of a Case. Am. J. Orthodontics [Oral Surg. Sect.] *33*:633–636 [Aug.] 1947.)

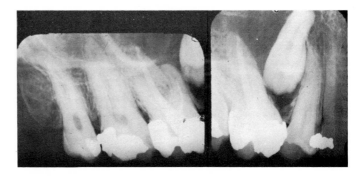

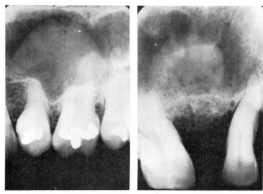

Figure 9–21 Two illustrations of mucoid retention cysts that arose from the floor of the maxillary sinus.

nasal vestibule. Apparently, dental infection is seldom if ever the initiating cause in the formation of these cysts. At any rate, they have been seen to develop in maxillary sinuses when the jaws were edentulous and free from infection.

In the roentgenogram such a cyst is recognized by its radiopaque, dome-shaped or hemispherical form, with the antral wall as its base. The edge of the cyst is smooth and sharply defined, and there is an absence of a peripheral cortical line that is characteristic of odontogenic cysts. Furthermore, unlike the odontogenic cyst, it is

very unlikely to produce an expansion of the bony antral walls as a result of pressure atrophy, even when it occupies the entire maxillary sinus. Two illustrations of such cysts of moderate size are shown in Figure 9–21, both of them arising from the floor of the maxillary sinus.

A case in which two mucoid retention cysts had formed in the maxillary sinus of an edentulous maxilla, after negative x-ray evidence of them 3½ years previously, is shown in Figure 9–22. It has been noted that these cysts may remain stationary in size over a period of many years after they are first observed. Again, they may rupture and disappear completely within a relatively short time. That they may slowly and gradually decrease in size, probably by a slight escape of liquid, is evidenced by the case illustrated in Figure 9–23. In the roentgenogram made in 1940 (above) there was evidence of a cyst that completely occupied the maxillary sinus. A roentgenogram made in 1950 (below) revealed a cyst that had its base on the posterior wall of the sinus and that had become appreciably smaller during the 10-year interval. This change had occurred in the absence of any surgical intervention, and at no time had there been any symptoms referable to the

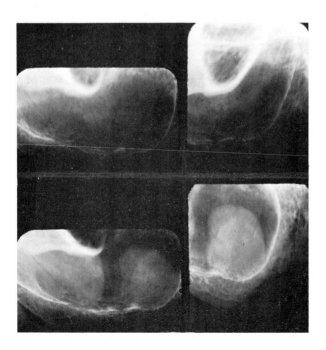

Figure 9–22 Mucoid retention cysts of the maxillary sinus. *Above,* Negative. *Below,* Two cysts are evident in the roentgenograms made 3½ years later.

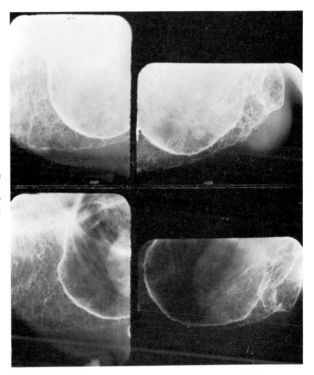

Figure 9–23 Mucoid retention cyst of the maxillary sinus. *Above,* Appearance in 1940, when the cyst occupied the entire antrum. *Below,* View in 1950, showing that the cyst has been reduced appreciably in size.

maxillary sinus. An interesting case is one reported by Sammartino (1965) in which spontaneous rupture of the cyst occurred and all roentgenographic evidence of its presence disappeared within a few days.

From serial roentgenography, it has been noted that some of the cysts will persist without change for a long period, others will gradually increase in size, and some will disappear spontaneously. Those that are of moderate size and asymptomatic can be left untreated. If symptoms are present, the simplest form of treatment is cannulation and drainage; if this is unsuccessful, surgical removal is mandatory (Killey and Kay, 1970).

TUMORS OF THE MAXILLARY SINUS

Tumors, both benign and malignant, may have an origin from within or may secondarily encroach upon and involve the

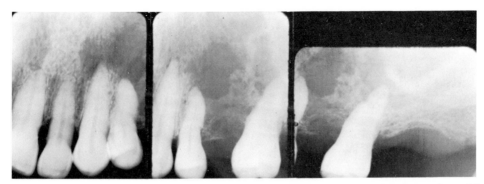

Figure 9–24 Sarcoma that has invaded the maxillary sinus, showing marked destruction of its walls. (Reproduced with permission from Stafne, E. C.: Dental Roentgenographic Interpretation Dealing with the Pulp Cavity and the Maxillary Sinus. J. Ohio State Dent. A. *31*:62–73 [Spring] 1957.)

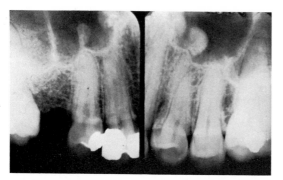

Figure 9–25 Exostoses or osteomas arising from the wall of the maxillary sinus. Bilateral and pedunculated. (Reproduced with permission from Stafne, E. C.: Dental Roentgenographic Interpretation Dealing with the Pulp Cavity and the Maxillary Sinus. J. Ohio State Dent. A. *31*:62–73 [Spring] 1957.)

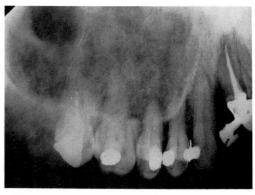

Figure 9–26 Fibrous dysplasia that has encroached upon and obliterated most of the sinus cavity.

maxillary sinus. These would include all of the many tumors that may involve the maxilla. The dental roentgenogram may be a means of early recognition of these lesions, at a time when they are amenable to successful treatment. Any destruction of the antral wall revealed by the roentgenogram should be suspected as being caused by a tumor.

Carcinoma of the maxillary sinus rarely is recognized early, although one of the authors (Stafne) has encountered a few cases in which the dental roentgenogram revealed only slight evidence of destruction of the floor of the sinus wall and which proved to be cases of carcinoma, at a time prior to any swelling of the alveolar process and the palate. Advanced cases of carcinoma are more readily recognized, for the bony walls of the sinus are completely destroyed. A sarcoma that has destroyed the walls and invaded the maxillary sinus is shown in Figure 9–24.

Osteomas rarely arise in the maxillary sinus, but when they do occur the intraoral roentgenogram is invaluable in the differential diagnosis. Exostoses or osteomas similar to those that arise on the wall of the orbit may arise from the walls of the maxillary sinus. These are seen as radiopaque elevations on the walls of the sinus, and they may have either a broad or a narrow base. Bilateral occurrence of osteomas with a narrow base, which presents a mushroom

appearance, is shown in Figure 9–25. Two such pedunculated bony growths are seen in each sinus.

Fibrous dysplasia of the maxilla and zygoma may, as it enlarges, encroach upon and replace the cavity of the maxillary sinus almost completely (Fig. 9–26). The roentgenogram reveals an enlargement of the alveolar process in the molar region, which suggests that the lesion may have had its origin in the jaw. The appearance shown in Figure 9–26 also may, in many respects, be similar to that of fibro-osseous lesions that are resectable. Such a case was reported by Small and Goodman (1973) in which, on removal, the lesion proved to be a cemento-ossifying fibroma. Among the generalized bone diseases that reduce the size or obscure the image of the maxillary sinus are osteopetrosis and Paget's disease of bone. The extreme density of bone in osteopetrosis may obscure the image of the maxillary sinus completely, and in the advanced osteosclerotic stage of Paget's disease, a large part of the sinus may be encroached upon and reduced in size.

REFERENCES

Austin, L. T. and Hempstead, B. E.: Dental Roentgenographic Evidence of Infection of Maxillary Sinus. J. Am. Dent. A. 26:1849–1858 (Nov.) 1939.
Bauer, W. H.: Maxillary Sinusitis of Dental Origin. Am. J. Orthodontics (Oral Surg. Sect.). 29:133–151 (Mar.) 1943.

Ennis, L. M.: Roentgenographic Variations of Maxillary Sinus and Nutrient Canals of Maxilla and Mandible. Internat. J. Orthodontia. 23:173–193 (Feb.) 1937.

Ennis, L. M. and Batson, O. V.: Variations of Maxillary Sinus as Seen in Roentgenogram. J. Am. Dent. A. 23:201–212 (Feb.) 1936.

Ennis, L. M. and Novak, A. J.: Foreign Body (Denture Relining Paste) in Maxillary Sinus: Report of Case. Am. J. Orthodontics (Oral Surg. Sect.). 29:377–379 (July) 1943.

Hallberg, O. E. and Stafne, E. C.: Treatment of Dentigerous Cysts: Report of a Case. Am. J. Orthodontics (Oral Surg. Sect.). 33:633–636 (Aug.) 1947.

Killey, H. C. and Kay, L. W.: Possible Sequelae When A Tooth or Root Is Dislodged into the Maxillary Sinus. Brit. Dent. J. 116:73–77 (Jan. 21) 1964.

Killey, H. C. and Kay, L. W.: Benign Mucosal Cysts of the Maxillary Sinus. Internat. Surg. 53:235–244 (Apr.) 1970.

Millhon, J. A. and Brown, H. A.: Cysts Arising from Mucosa of Maxillary Sinus as Seen in Dental Roentgenogram. Am. J. Orthodontics (Oral Surg. Sect.). 30:12–15 (Jan.) 1944.

Sammartino, F. J.: Radiographic Appearance of a Mucoid Retention Cyst. Oral Surg., Oral Med. & Oral Path. 20:454–455 (Oct.) 1965.

Skillern, R. H.: The Catarrhal and Suppurative Diseases of the Accessory Sinuses of the Nose. Ed. 3. Philadelphia, J. B. Lippincott Company, 1920, p. 130.

Small, I. A. and Goodman, P. A.: Giant Cemento-ossifying Fibroma of the Maxilla: Report of Case and Discussion. J. Oral Surg. 31:113–119 (Feb.) 1973.

Stafne, E. C.: Dental Roots in Maxillary Sinus. Am. J. Orthodontics (Oral Surg. Sect.). 33:582–584 (Aug.) 1947.

Stafne, E. C.: Dental Roentgenographic Interpretation Dealing with the Pulp Cavity and the Maxillary Sinus. J. Ohio State Dent. A. 31:62–73 (Spring) 1957.

10 RESORPTIVE PROCESSES

Evidence of resorptive processes is a very common finding in the roentgenogram, if one includes resorption of the alveolar process as well as that of the dental structures. Resorption of the dental structures is recognized in the roentgenogram by the defects it produces. In general, it might be said that defects that appear in those parts of a tooth that are not exposed to the oral cavity are produced by a resorptive process. In many instances the cause of the resorption is known; in others it may be obscure.

RESORPTION OF ALVEOLAR PROCESS

Following removal of the teeth, there is marked tendency for the bone that formerly supported the teeth to undergo resorption, particularly if periodontal disease has produced partial destruction of the cortical bone prior to extraction of the teeth, or if too much of the buccal and labial bone has been removed at the time of extraction of the teeth. Such resorption of alveolar bone may take place in otherwise normal individuals who have no disturbance of mineral metabolism. Resorption may take place in advance of inflammation of such tissue produced by trauma of a denture. Resorption of the alveolar ridge is much more common in the mandible, where it often presents a major problem in the wearing of dentures. Gradual resorption may continue over a period of many years, requiring frequent refittings of the dentures. The ridge may become thin and narrow, and is painful to pressure. The roentgenogram reveals jagged, thin, spinous projections of the alveolar process which are best demonstrated by a shorter exposure of the dental film than that ordinarily used (Fig. 10–1). If a great deal of pain and inflammation are associated with this condition, surgical removal of the sharp, bony projections may be the treatment of choice.

In some instances the entire alveolar portion of the mandible may undergo resorption, reducing markedly its vertical dimen-

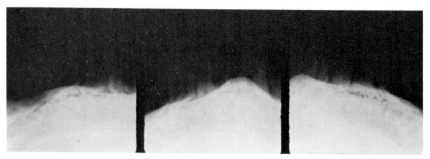

Figure 10–1 Partial resorption of the lower anterior alveolar process, showing thin spinous projections of bone that persist on the crest of the ridge.

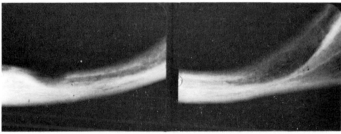

Figure 10–2 Complete resorption of the alveolar process of the mandible, showing reduced vertical dimension of the mandible and situation of the mental foramen on its superior surface.

sion and leaving a flat, broad superior surface. The mental foramen then assumes a position near the superior surface, and the spinous process, which does not undergo resorption, extends well above the level of the ridge (Fig. 10–2). Undue pressure of a denture over the region of the mental foramen in such instances may be a cause of referred pain or paresthesia of the lower lip.

The alveolar process of the maxilla may also undergo resorption to the extent that only a thin layer of bone remains to cover the floor of the maxillary sinus and the floor of the nasal fossae. The roentgenogram in Figure 10–3 was made at a short exposure to show the soft tissue of the ridge that remains.

Rarely alveolar bone becomes separated from the main portion of the jaw and does not undergo complete resorption, but remains in the soft tissue as viable bone. The soft tissue in such instances may or may not be inflamed (Fig. 10–4). Figure 10–5 re-

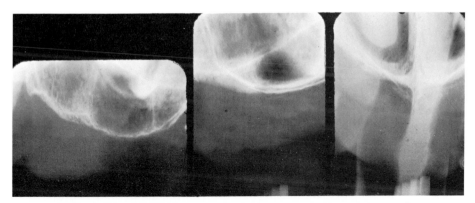

Figure 10–3 Complete resorption of the alveolar process of the maxilla.

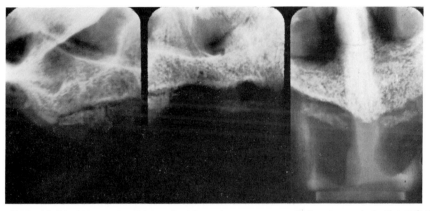

Figure 10–4 Viable fragments of bone that have become separated and remain in the soft tissue.

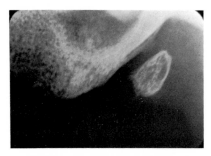

Figure 10–5 Viable fragment of bone situated in the tuberosity region.

veals a fragment of bone situated in the tuberosity region. In this instance the bone may have become separated as a result of fracture during extraction of the third molar; although the fragment may have undergone partial resorption, an appreciable amount of viable bone remains.

RESORPTION OF EMBEDDED TEETH

Teeth that are more prone than others to undergo resorption are those that remain completely embedded and have no communication with the surface of the oral cavity (Stafne and Austin, 1945). The resorptive process originates on the enamel surface or at the cementoenamel junction, and very rarely on the surface of the cementum. It is preceded by degeneration of the enamel epithelium, following which the enamel comes in contact with connective tissue which produces its resorption. The hard dental structures that are destroyed are replaced by bone. The bone is of lesser radiographic density than that of the tooth structure that it replaces; therefore, the defect produced by the resorption is readily discernible in the roentgenogram. The defects when seen in the roentgenogram have been referred to erroneously as caries, decalcification, and evidence of infection. The teeth most frequently involved are the canines and third molars, since they are the teeth that most often remain embedded.

The incidence of resorption of embedded teeth is highest in the later decades of life, although in some instances it may occur early. Resorption of the crown of a maxillary second molar which had its onset prior to the age of 10 is shown in Figure 10–6. The patient was 10 years of age when the upper roentgenogram was made. It revealed a defect in the coronal portion of the tooth. The lower roentgenogram was made at 12 years of age at a time when the tooth was undergoing eruption. Destruction had become more extensive and there was a perforation through to the enamel surface. On microscopic examination it was found that the cavity contained vascular tissue and an appreciable amount of amorphous calcified tissue.

Almost all primary teeth that do not erupt, or become ankylosed and then become embedded as a result of inclusion, undergo marked resorption. In the case of primary teeth, active resorption of the root is already taking place and this continues with progressive destruction of the dentin within the coronal portion of the tooth, in some instances leaving a thin layer of enamel only. An embedded mandibular primary second molar that has undergone

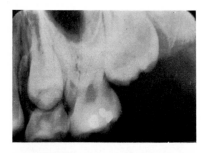

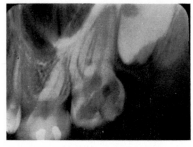

Figure 10–6 Resorption of the crown of a maxillary second molar. *Above,* Appearance at the age of 10 years and prior to eruption. *Below,* Appearance at the age of 12 years, when the tooth was undergoing eruption.

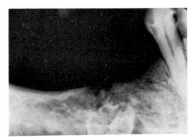

Figure 10–7 Resorption of an embedded primary mandibular second molar of which only remnants of enamel remain.

almost complete resorption is shown in Figure 10–7.

Maxillary anterior teeth that have undergone resorption are shown in Figure 10–8; on the left a central incisor, in the center a lateral incisor, and on the right a canine are involved. The rate of resorption may be very slow, for onset of resorption of the canine in this case had been noted 28 years previously.

Once an appreciable amount of resorption of the coronal portion of an embedded tooth has taken place, it becomes ankylosed and then there is no further movement or migration of the tooth. The presence of resorption in itself is not an indication for the removal of the tooth. If, for other reasons, removal is indicated, it becomes increasingly difficult.

RESORPTION OF ROOTS OF ERUPTED TEETH

Resorption of the roots of primary teeth, which is associated with their shed-

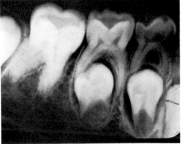

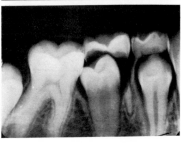

Figure 10–9 Incomplete resorption of the root of a primary mandibular second molar. *Above*, Appearance at 8 years of age. *Below*, Appearance at 11 years of age. The apical portion of the mesial root is unresorbed and remains in the alveolar bone.

ding, is a normal physiologic process. As the permanent tooth develops and moves in an occlusal direction, the roots of the primary tooth are destroyed, until finally only the crown remains. In some instances, however, resorption of the root of the primary tooth is incomplete and a portion of it may remain in the alveolar bone between the roots of the permanent teeth. If the roots of the primary molar are widely bifurcated, the premolar in the course of its eruption may move up into the bifurcation and produce a resorptive process that ex-

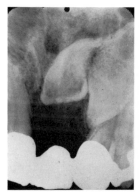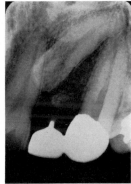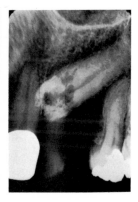

Figure 10–8 Resorption of three maxillary anterior teeth. *Left,* A central incisor. *Center,* A lateral incisor. *Right,* A canine.

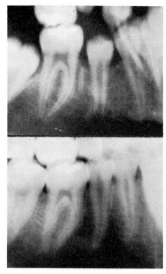

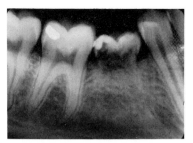

Figure 10–12 Partial resorption of the roots and coronal portion of a primary molar.

Figure 10–10 Retained root of a primary molar that has undergone resorption. *Above,* Root in interseptal bone posterior to the second premolar. *Below,* Three years later, root has been completely resorbed.

tends transversely across the root, leaving the apical portion of it undisturbed. The premolar in the course of eruption also may come in contact with and produce resorption of one root only, in which event the unresorbed root remains (Fig. 10–9). The roots that so remain are almost wholly confined to those of the primary molars, and the incidence is greater in the mandible than in the maxilla, the ratio being approximately 4 to 1. Many of these root fragments undergo complete resorption at some time following shedding of the crown of the primary tooth and complete eruption of its permanent successor (Fig. 10–10). Those roots that do not undergo resorption and

remain into adult life assume varied positions in relation to the crest of the alveolar ridge. Some of them are near the crest of the ridge; others will, as the alveolar process increases in vertical dimension, remain in their original alveolar sockets and finally assume a position at some distance from the alveolar crest (Fig. 10–11). Many of them become covered by thick layers of cellular cementum. They then become rounded or elliptical and approach the size of roots of the permanent teeth. When seen in roentgenograms of edentulous jaws, they may be mistaken for roots of permanent teeth (Austin and Stafne, 1932).

The question arises whether an effort should be made to remove such roots at an early age. Because of the danger of dislodging the unerupted premolar, it may be unwise to attempt removal until the premolar has undergone complete eruption and has become firmly fixed in its socket. If left undisturbed, the root may undergo complete resorption, or it may become encapsulated in cementum. In either event it would have no clinical significance. Re-

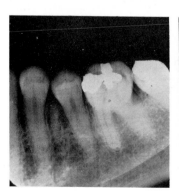 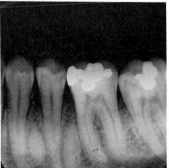 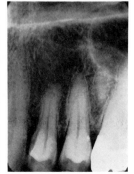

Figure 10–11 Retained roots of primary teeth, showing varied positions they assume in the alveolar process.

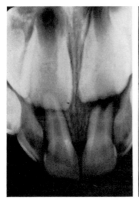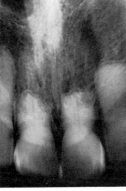

Figure 10–13 Resorption of root ends of teeth as a result of injury. *Left,* Primary right central incisor. *Right,* Permanent central incisors.

moval is indicated for those that project beyond the crest of the alveolar ridge and produce inflammation of the mucoperiosteum and for those that interfere with the movement of teeth in orthodontic treatment.

Roots of an erupted primary tooth may undergo varied degrees of resorption even though the permanent successor is not present. Unlike resorption of the roots of permanent teeth, the resorptive process is most often more extensive and tends to invade the coronal portion of the tooth (Fig.

10–12). Such teeth may become ankylosed and retained for a long time.

The root of a tooth that has been dislodged from the socket and has been reinserted almost always undergoes resorption, which in some instances may be very extensive. The root of a tooth that receives a blow may undergo resorption, even though the tooth may not have been loosened in its socket. Resorption of the root of a primary maxillary central incisor and of permanent maxillary central incisors that has occurred as a result of injury is shown in Figure 10–13.

Resorption that results from force exerted by means of orthodontic appliances is not uncommon and is generally recognized. Becks (1936) has found that resorption is more likely to occur from orthodontic treatment in those patients who have endocrine disturbances. The lateral surface of the root is rarely attacked. Most often the resorption takes place at the apex and, in the event that it continues, the result is a shortened root with a blunt root end (Fig. 10–14).

Resorption also occurs as a result of pressure exerted by impacted teeth, tumors, and osteosclerosis. The eruptive

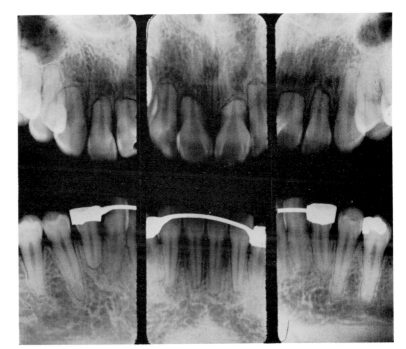

Figure 10–14 Resorption of root ends of teeth caused by force of orthodontic appliance.

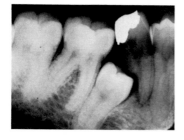

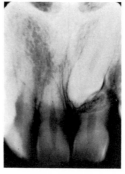

Figure 10–15 Resorption of roots caused by eruptive force of impacted teeth.

force of an impacted tooth is sufficient to produce resorption of the root of the tooth that impedes its eruption. The crown of the impacted tooth does not come in contact with the root during the period of active resorption, but is separated from it by a layer of connective tissue. Two examples of resorption caused by impacted teeth are shown in Figure 10–15. In the one on the left a supernumerary premolar has produced a resorptive defect in the root of a mandibular second premolar. In the one on the right an impacted maxillary canine has caused resorption of most of the root of a central incisor.

Tumors that produce resorption of the roots of teeth are most frequently those in which growth and expansion are not rapid, such as epithelium-lined cysts, ameloblastomas, giant cell tumors, and fibro-osseous tumors. Rapidly growing and malignant tumors produce resorption to a lesser degree. Soft as well as hard tumors are capable of causing resorption. An ameloblastoma of the mandible that has caused marked resorption of the roots of the teeth

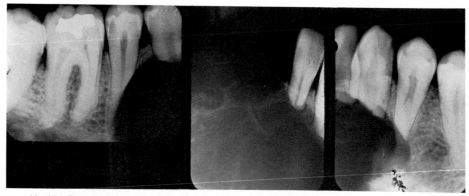

Figure 10–16 Resorption of the root ends of teeth caused by pressure of a tumor (ameloblastoma).

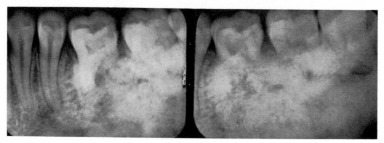

Figure 10–17 Resorption of the roots of mandibular first and second molars caused by pressure of fibrous dysplasia.

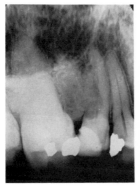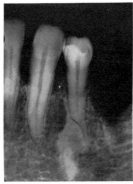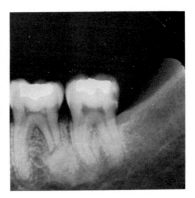

Figure 10–18   Resorption of roots of teeth caused by sclerosis of bone.

on which it has encroached is shown in Figure 10–16. Figure 10–17 illustrates fibrous dysplasia of the mandible that has caused almost complete resorption of the roots of the first and second molars.

Sclerotic bone that expands and increases in size may produce resorption of the root of a tooth upon which it encroaches. The apex of the root is most frequently involved, although osteosclerosis that occurs in the interseptal bone may produce resorption of the lateral surface of the root. Three examples of resorption from osteosclerotic bone are shown in Figure 10–18. On the left is shown osteosclerosis that is confined to the interseptal space and has produced a large defect on the distal surface of a maxillary second premolar; in the center is shown resorption of the root end of a noncarious mandibular first premolar; and on the right is shown resorption of the distal root of a mandibular first molar that contains a normal and vital pulp. Usually teeth so affected are asymptomatic, retain their vitality, and rarely are lost as a result of the resorption.

A fairly high incidence of resorption of the root occurs as a result of inflammation and infection in the periapical region following degeneration and infection of the dental pulp. Such resorption may be slight, but in some cases it is sufficient to produce a defect that is demonstrable in the roentgenogram. A periapical inflammatory lesion that had caused resorption of the root end of a maxillary lateral incisor is shown in Figure 10–19.

Resorption of the apical portion of the root may occur when there is no plausible explanation for it and when the bone adjacent to the root has a normal roentgenographic appearance. Such resorption most frequently involves the incisor teeth and cannot be distinguished from resorption that results from force exerted by orthodontic appliances. It might well be that such resorption is brought about as a result of abnormal stress of occlusion. A roentgenogram that reveals resorption of the root ends of the maxillary incisors is shown in Figure 10–20. The teeth had been forced anteriorly and had become separated as a result of a marked overbite.

Fortunately, resorption of a root in most instances does not result in loss of the tooth involved. The pulp most often remains vital, and usually the resorptive process is arrested or becomes inactive before the entire root is destroyed. Removal

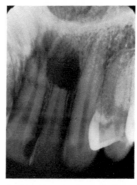

Figure 10–19   Resorption of the root end of a lateral incisor caused by an inflammatory lesion (granuloma).

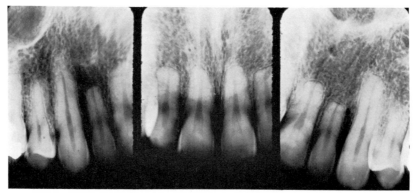

Figure 10–20 Resorption of the root ends of teeth simulating resorption that may be produced by orthodontic force, but in which the cause is obscure.

of unerupted teeth and tumors that caused the resorption, and decreasing or discontinuing orthodontic force, will lead to cessation of the resorptive process. If destruction has not been too extensive, the tooth can be retained as a useful one indefinitely.

IDIOPATHIC RESORPTION OF TEETH

Idiopathic resorption includes some forms of resorption for which the cause is not clearly understood. Authors have referred to this condition by various terms, such as "pink spots" (Mummery, 1920), "internal granuloma," "chronic perforating hyperplasia of the pulp," and "internal resorption of the teeth" (Warner and colleagues, 1947). Numerous investigators have reported cases and discussed this condition, and several theories have been advanced as to the probable causes. Among the suggested causes are inflammatory processes, loss of vitality of cementum, vascular changes in the pulp, accessory root canals, systemic disease, and trauma.

All of these factors may at some time play a part. The tendency to multiple occurrence suggests that systemic disease may be a factor; however, general physical examination of 179 patients who had such resorption of the teeth revealed that it apparently was not associated with any particular systemic disease (Stafne and Slocumb,

1944). Trauma appears to be the most important local factor in the production of resorption. Of 200 teeth that were undergoing resorption, 147 were anterior and 53 were posterior. The anterior teeth are more often subjected to injury and are more often subjected to excessive lateral stress in occluding than are posterior teeth. Henry and Weinmann (1951) noted that resorption of cementum occurs more readily upon surfaces of the root that are facing toward the direction of movement. In lower incisors, onset of resorption invariably occurs on the lingual surface of the root.

There are two types of resorption: central and peripheral. The central type has its origin on the pulpal wall, and the peripheral on the surface of the cementum. The onset of resorption is on the root surface in the majority of instances. Following perforation of the cementum, the resorptive process tends to progress through dentin parallel to the long axis of the tooth. That part of the dentin proximal to the pulp, as well as the cementum adjacent to the perforation, appears to be more resistant to resorption and is destroyed only when resorption has become extensive. Resorption may extend into the coronal portion of the tooth and destroy almost all of the dentin, and yet not produce a perforation into the pulp chamber.

Fortunately, the process of resorption is more often limited in extent and produces only minor defects in the tooth, some of them so slight that they cannot be detected in the roentgenogram. Comparatively few teeth that have undergone resorption are lost because of it. Loss of the tooth may result from complete destruction of its root, from involvement of the pulp, or from perforation through to the dental surface that is exposed to the oral cavity.

Most often, resorption is followed by apposition of a calcified substance (osteodentin). Such apposition may be immediate or delayed, and in most instances the resorbed dental tissue is replaced totally or partially by calcified substance.

The defects produced by resorption are evidenced in the roentgenogram by reduced radiographic density which is most often irregular and diffuse, but which may, in instances of resorption of the central type, show a well-circumscribed enlargement of the pulp chamber or root canal. The calcified substance that is formed is not as radiopaque as the normal dentin that it replaces; therefore, a defect that has been produced by resorption is always visible in the roentgenogram, even when there is no longer any active resorption and even though the resorbed dentin has been completely replaced by the calcified substance.

Resorption may occur in primary teeth, particularly if they are retained beyond the normal time for exfoliation. Such a case is illustrated in Figure 10–21, *left,* as evidenced by marked enlargement of the pulp canal, suggesting that the resorption had its origin from the pulp and could therefore be designated as resorption of the central type. Another case of resorption of the central type is shown in Figure 10–21, *center.*

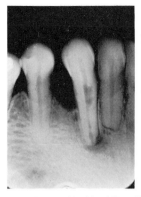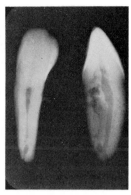

Figure 10–22 Idiopathic resorption of the peripheral type. *Left,* Labiolingual view shows defect superimposed on the pulp canal; defect appears to be in the center of the root. *Right,* Lateral view shows that an opening is present on the surface of the root and that pulp is not involved.

The resorption involves a maxillary permanent lateral incisor and is evidenced by an appreciable enlargement of the root canal. The wall of the cavity produced is regular and smooth, and it does not appear to communicate with the surface. A lateral view of the tooth made following extraction is shown on the right. The dentin surrounding the defect appears to be intact, and microscopic examination did not reveal any communication to the surface of the root.

A resorptive defect that appears on the roentgenogram to be confined to the center of the tooth in a labiolingual and buccolingual view actually may be found situated on, or communicating with, the outer surface of the root. Applebaum (1934) has stressed this fact. The roentgenogram of a mandibular canine shown in Figure 10–22 reveals a defect that is superimposed on

Figure 10–21 Idiopathic resorption of the central type. *Left,* Involvement of a primary canine. *Center,* Involvement of a permanent lateral incisor—appearance prior to extraction. *Right,* Lateral view of extracted tooth, showing that there is no communication with the surface of the root.

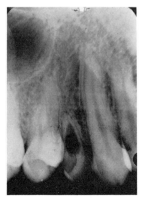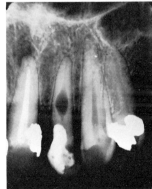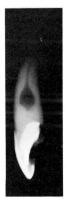

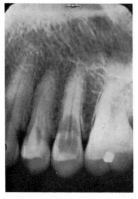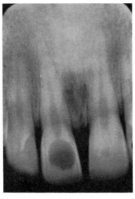

Figure 10–23 *Left,* Extensive idiopathic resorption of dentin in a maxillary second premolar. The radiopaque line that surrounds the pulp chamber is evidence of unresorbed dentin. *Right,* Idiopathic resorption within the crown of a maxillary central incisor ("pink tooth").

the pulp canal and appears to be situated in the center of the tooth. A lateral view (Fig. 10–22, *right*) reveals that the defect extends through the dentin from the cervical to the apical portion of the root. There is evidence of an opening to the lingual surface of the root, but there is no evidence of invasion or perforation into the pulp canal.

The dentin adjacent to the pulp is very resistant to resorption. Careful examination of roentgenograms often reveals evidence of a thin layer of unresorbed dentin; in some instances this dentin produces radiopaque lines that frame the pulp chamber and pulp canal with striking clearness. Such evidence is present in a roentgenogram of a maxillary second premolar that has undergone resorption (Fig. 10–23, *left*). The pulp appears to be completely surrounded by dentin, a finding that leads one to question whether the resorptive process had its origin from the pulpal wall, even though resorption has been confined almost wholly to the coronal portion of the tooth. Clinical examination did not reveal any defect on the exposed surface of the tooth. The enamel presented a pinkish hue, owing to the highly vascular tissue that lay immediately beneath it. There was a normal response to tests for vitality, and the tooth had at no time been painful. A defect in a maxillary central incisor that appears to be more definitely confined to the coronal portion of the tooth may have had its origin from the dental pulp. Such a case is shown in Figure 10–23, *right.* Microscopic examination did not reveal any communication with the surface of the tooth.

The extent and rapidity of the resorptive process that has been initiated are unpredictable. Often the process is very slow and may continue over a period of many years. The roentgenograms of a patient in whom active resorption was in progress for more than 12 years are shown in Figure 10–24. Destruction of tooth structure had extended to the cervical region and had produced an opening that communicated with the oral cavity, with acute pulpitis as a result.

It is not unusual for resorption to occur following injury. Failure to get a history of trauma does not rule out this factor as a possible cause. Two instances of resorption following trauma in which adult patients could offer no information concerning the incident are shown in Figure 10–25. The

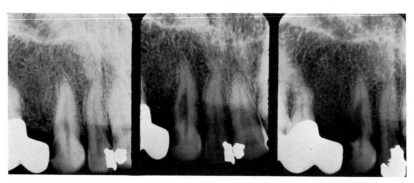

Figure 10–24 Idiopathic resorption of a maxillary canine. *Left,* Negative. *Center,* View 2 years later, showing first evidence of resorptive defect. *Right,* View 12 years later, showing increase in size of defect.

roentgenogram on the left reveals a defect in the middle part of a mandibular lateral incisor. The tooth did not give a response to tests for vitality, and the crown was slightly discolored. The pulp chamber is abnormally large, suggesting that the injury was sustained during childhood. In the roentgenogram on the right there is evidence of resorption of the root of the maxillary central incisor; also there is evidence of a transverse fracture of the root, of which the patient was unaware.

A case of resorption in which there was a definite history of trauma is shown in Figure 10–26. The roentgenogram on the left, made in 1932 shortly after the patient had received a blow that had loosened the mandibular incisor teeth, reveals a transverse fracture of the alveolar bone at the level of the root ends of the incisor teeth. The roentgenogram on the right, made 17 years later, reveals marked resorption of the lateral incisors and, to a lesser degree, of the apex of the root of the left central incisor. The injury had caused degeneration of the pulps, and therefore the size of the pulp chambers and root canals had not been altered.

Unfortunately, in most instances there are no measures that can be taken to arrest the resorptive process. However, if the pulp cavity alone is involved, the tissue within the cavity can be removed and the

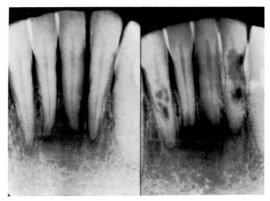

Figure 10–26 Resorption caused by injury. *Left,* View soon after injury, showing fracture of alveolar process. *Right,* View 17 years later reveals resorption of lateral incisors and left central incisor.

root canal treated to preserve the tooth. More rarely, resorption of the peripheral type can be treated if the defect is accessible to filling. Figure 10–27 shows a mandibular second molar in which there is evidence of resorption. On exploration, a painless soft area was detected on the buccal surface and beneath the gingival margin; a silver-alloy filling was inserted, and when the tooth was examined 3 years later its color was still normal and it responded to tests for vitality.

Figure 10–28 demonstrates three types of resorption occurring in the same individual. The cervical portion of the crown of the embedded left canine is undergoing resorption, there is idiopathic resorption of the root of the erupted left central incisor, and most of the root of the erupted right central incisor has been resorbed as a result of pressure by the embedded right canine.

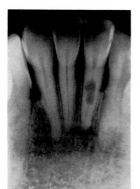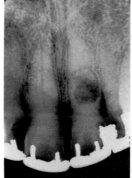

Figure 10–25 Resorption of roots following injury. *Left,* Mandibular central incisor. *Right,* Maxillary central incisor in which there is also a transverse fracture of the root.

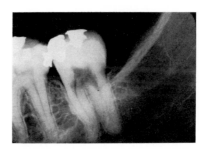

Figure 10–27 Idiopathic resorption involving a mandibular second molar.

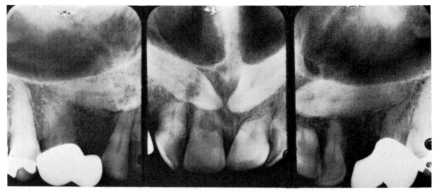

Figure 10–28 Roentgenogram showing three types of resorption: resorption of embedded canine, idiopathic resorption of left central incisor, and resorption of root of right central incisor caused by pressure of an embedded canine.

MULTIPLE IDIOPATHIC ROOT RESORPTION

Multiple idiopathic resorption involving all or nearly all of the teeth in any one patient is a rare occurrence. The resorption is on the external surface and has its origin in the region of the cementoenamel junction. The condition is progressive over a short span of years and nearly all of the teeth may become involved. Kerr et al. (1970) reported two cases. The roentgenograms of one of them are shown in Figure 10–29. This patient was a 30-year-old white woman, and the roentgenograms revealed that all but 1 of the remaining 19 teeth had some degree of cervical resorption. Marginal gingivitis was absent; there was hyperplasia of the papillae. Microscopic examination revealed that the epithelial attachment was at the cementoenamel junction, and the alveolar crest fibers were intact and inserted into the alveolar crest. The tissue occupying the area of resorption was granulation tissue, and the surface of the dentin had Howship's lacunae with multiple multinucleated giant cells in the areas of active resorption. The authors stated that clinical laboratory examinations and histologic study, combined with a

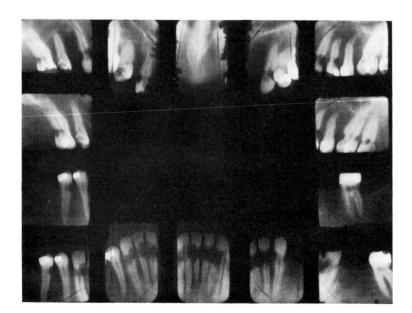

Figure 10–29 Multiple idiopathic root resorption, showing distribution and extent of resorption. (Reproduced with permission from Kerr, D. A., Courtney, R. M., and Burkes, E. J.: Multiple Idiopathic Root Resorption. Oral Surg., Oral Med. & Oral Path. *29*:552–565 [Apr.] 1970.)

search of the literature, failed to reveal or suggest the cause of this pathologic condition.

REFERENCES

Applebaum, E.: Internal Resorption of Teeth. Dent. Cosmos. 76:847–853 (Aug.) 1934.

Austin, L. T. and Stafne, E. C.: Retained Deciduous Roots. J. Am. Dent. A. 19:1320–1323 (Aug.) 1932.

Becks, H.: Root Resorptions and Their Relation to Pathologic Bone Formation. Internat. J. Orthodontia. 22:445–482 (May) 1936.

Henry, J. L. and Weinmann, J. P.: The Pattern of Resorption and Repair of Human Cementum. J. Am. Dent. A. 42:270–290 (Mar.) 1951.

Kerr, D. A., Courtney, R. M., and Burkes, E. J.: Multiple Idiopathic Root Resorption. Oral Surg., Oral Med. & Oral Path. 29:552–565 (Apr.) 1970.

Mummery, J. H.: The Pathology of "Pink Spots" on Teeth. Brit. Dent. J. 41:300–311, 1920.

Stafne, E. C. and Austin, L. T.: Resorption of Embedded Teeth. J. Am. Dent. A. 32:1003–1009 (Aug. 1) 1945.

Stafne, E. C. and Slocumb C. H.: Idiopathic Resorption of Teeth. Am. J. Orthodontics. 30:41–49 (Jan.) 1944.

Warner, G. R., Orban, B., Hine, M. K., and Ritchey, B. T.: Internal Resorption of Teeth: Interpretation of Histologic Findings. J. Am. Dent. A. 34:468–483 (Apr. 1) 1947.

11 CONDENSING OSTEITIS AND OSTEOSCLEROSIS

Localized areas of compact sclerotic bone frequently form within the jaws, and evidence of such bone is often encountered in routine dental roentgenographic examinations. The bone appears in the roentgenogram as an increased radiographic density which may be either diffuse or well defined. If well defined, it does not conform to any particular pattern as to shape, and the borders are most often irregular. The sclerosis is confined to the limits of the bone and does not produce an expansion of the cortex.

The basis for the formation of the sclerotic bone can in many instances be explained; in others it is obscure. The bone may form as a result of a low-grade infection or irritation, or as a reparative process following trauma and acute infections such as osteomyelitis and acute periapical infection. It may occur as a postsurgical sequel, in which event abnormally dense bone may form in a tooth socket or in the space from which a tumor has been removed. It may occur in healed tumors that have not been subjected to surgical intervention, as in giant-cell tumors in successfully treated hyperparathyroidism. There also is reason to believe that root fragments of primary as well as permanent teeth may provide a nidus around which sclerotic bone may form.

CONDENSING OSTEITIS

In the following discussion the term "condensing osteitis" is limited to instances in which sclerotic bone has been formed as a direct result of infection. This type of sclerotic bone is most often seen with periapical and periodontal infection of relatively long standing. When the infection is removed, the radiographic density of the involved bone often returns partially or completely to normal.

Evidence of condensing osteitis may appear in the periapical region prior to complete degeneration of the dental pulp, when the pulp still responds to tests for vitality and when there has as yet been no acute periapical infection with destructive or rarefying osteitis. In such cases, widening of the periodontal-membrane space in the periapical region usually is in evidence (Fig. 11–1).

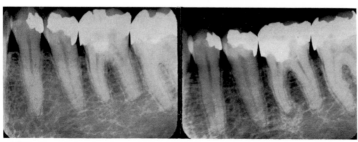

Figure 11–1 Condensing osteitis. *Left,* View taken 3 years prior to the one on the right, showing normal bone in the region of the first molar. *Right,* View revealing sclerotic bone that has formed in the periapical region of the mesial root prior to the onset of acute pulpitis.

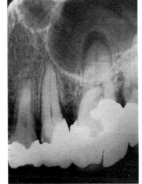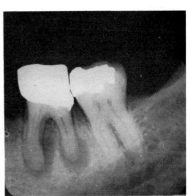

Figure 11–2 Condensing osteitis caused by periapical infection. *Left,* Involvement of maxillary first molar. *Right,* Involvement of mandibular first molar.

The roentgenogram on the left showed bone of normal pattern and density in the periapical region of the first molar. The roentgenogram on the right was made 3 years later to determine the cause of pain of several months' standing which was suggestive of pulpitis. It revealed widening of the periodontal-membrane space and an increase in radiographic density of bone in the periapical region of the mesial root. On thermal test the pulp proved to be hypersensitive. In similar cases in which there is such evidence of condensed bone, the condition may remain asymptomatic for many years following insertion of a large restoration; however, it is predictable that complete degeneration of the pulp followed by acute periapical infection will occur eventually in a high percentage of cases. This type of sclerosis should not be confused with bone of increased density that forms as a result of abnormal occlusal stress.

Examples of condensing osteitis associated with periapical infection of long standing are shown in Figure 11–2. On the left, the bone of the wall of the maxillary sinus surrounding a lesion on the palatal root of a first molar is abnormally dense; on the right, bone of markedly increased density surrounds lesions involving both roots of a mandibular first molar. Widespread condensing osteitis caused by periapical infection involving mandibular incisors is shown in Figure 11–3.

Condensing osteitis similar to that associated with chronic periapical infection often occurs with periodontal lesions of long standing (Fig. 11–4).

The density of bone that has become sclerotic as a result of chronic periapical and periodontal infection tends to return to normal following removal of the infection. As evidenced by roentgenographic examination, this return to normal density may be partial or complete. A case of partial return to normal density is illustrated in Figure 11–5. The roentgenogram on the left shows dense sclerotic bone surrounding

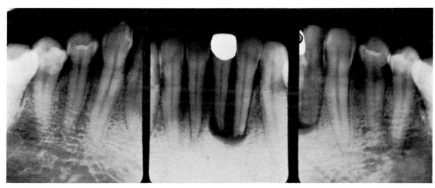

Figure 11–3 Condensing osteitis caused by periapical infection involving mandibular incisors.

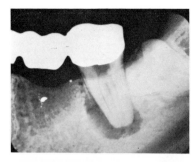

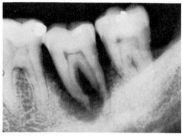

Figure 11–4 Condensing osteitis caused by extensive periodontal lesions involving mandibular molars.

the root of a mandibular molar. The roentgenogram on the right, made 2 years after extraction of the tooth, reveals marked decrease in radiographic density of the involved bone. A case in which the bone has returned to normal radiographic density is shown in Figure 11–6. In the illustration on the left, there is evidence of diffuse and

extensive condensing osteitis associated with an infected mandibular first molar. The illustration on the right, made 1 year after extraction of the tooth, reveals that the roentgenographic appearance of the involved bone has returned to normal.

OSTEOSCLEROSIS

The term "osteosclerosis" refers to certain localized regions of abnormally dense bone that apparently are not a direct result of infection. It includes sclerotic bone that forms as a reparative process, and other kinds for which the cause is obscure.

Representative of abnormally dense bone that may form in the reparative or healing process following an acute destructive infection is that of osteomyelitis. The healed lesion of osteomyelitis presents a fairly typical roentgenographic picture. The bone is abnormally radiopaque, it has a ground-glass appearance, and often numerous, scattered, minute radiolucent spots are present.

Following operation the bone that replaces the space formerly occupied by a dental root, cyst, or tumor does not always have the same density and roentgenographic appearance as the normal surrounding bone. It may vary in that it may be more

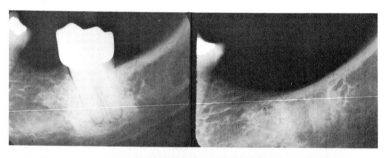

Figure 11–5 Condensing osteitis. *Left,* Appearance prior to extraction of involved mandibular molar. *Right,* View showing reduction in amount and density of sclerotic bone 2 years after extraction.

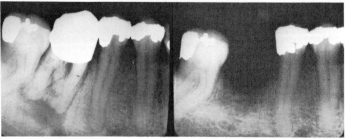

Figure 11–6 Condensing osteitis. The roentgenographic appearance of the bone has returned to normal 1 year after extraction of an infected mandibular first molar.

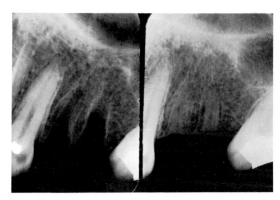

Figure 11–7 Osteosclerosis of a former root socket that resembles a dental root.

radiolucent or more radiopaque, or it may have a normal trabecular pattern.

Sclerotic bone may form within an unresorbed lamina dura after tooth extraction. The lamina dura remains intact, and the bone that is deposited within the wound is of greater density than the adjacent alveolar bone. When this occurs, it is often impossible roentgenographically to distinguish it from the root of a tooth, and the surgeon may be wrongfully accused of having failed to remove the tooth in its entirety. In such instances, routine postoperative roentgenograms prove to be of value. Illustrative of this are those shown in Figure 11–7. The one on the left, made after extraction of the maxillary premolars, shows no root fragments present. The one on the right, made 6 months later, reveals sclerotic bone in both sockets that closely resembles dental roots.

Whether such osteosclerosis is more apt to occur when there is retarded healing of the extraction wound is problematic. In this case, there were no postoperative complications and the patient's general medical examination was negative. Burrell and Goepp (1973) have termed this abnormal repair of the extraction site "socket sclerosis." In a study of dental roentgenograms and hospital charts of patients admitted for treatment at the University of Chicago Hospitals and Clinics, they found that patients with this type of osteosclerosis of the jaws had a significantly higher incidence of gastrointestinal and genitourinary diseases

(especially nephritis and nephrosis) than those without socket sclerosis. Their findings suggest that this form of osteosclerosis is perhaps the result of a disturbance in the osteogenic-osteolytic balance in bone metabolism that is often associated with these diseases.

A common site for the formation of sclerotic bone within the jaws is in the interseptal bone adjoining the premolar teeth. There is some question whether fragments of the roots of primary teeth retained in the interseptal space play a part in the formation of sclerotic bone. These root fragments sometimes become encapsulated by cementum, but most often they undergo complete resorption. However, in some instances at the site of resorption there remain small areas of sclerotic bone which may or may not contain small fragments of dentin. These areas are often seen in the roentgenogram (Fig. 11–8). Apposition of sclerotic bone on such a nidus may account for the frequent occurrence of larger areas of sclerotic bone that extend into the cancellous bone in the region of the premolar teeth. Two illustrations of osteosclerosis occurring adjacent to the roots of vital teeth are shown in Figure 11–9. Osteosclerosis that involves both of the interseptal spaces adjoining a mandibular second premolar and that surrounds the entire root is shown in Figure 11–10; the dense, compact bone contains nutrient canals, which sometimes are discernible in the roentgenogram as in this case.

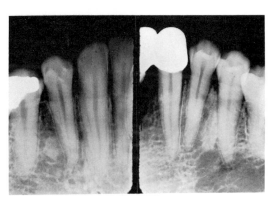

Figure 11–8 Two cases of osteosclerosis that is confined to the interseptal bone adjacent to mandibular premolars.

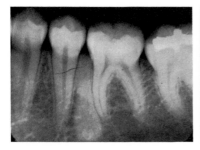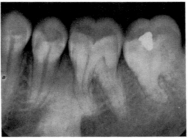

Figure 11–9 Two cases of osteosclerosis that extends from the interseptal space downward into the jaw. The adjacent teeth are normal and free from caries.

In contrast to the bone of condensing osteitis, this form of sclerotic bone does not tend to disappear following extraction of the teeth. If the roots extend into the sclerotic bone, the bone that forms in the socket invariably becomes as dense as the surrounding sclerotic bone (Fig. 11–11). Sclerotic bone seen in edentulous regions is almost always of uniform radiopacity, including the space formerly occupied by the roots of the teeth (Fig. 11–12). Radiopaque osteosclerotic masses of this size have been mistaken for tumors; should there be any question as to their nature, a biopsy could be done, particularly if it will give the patient peace of mind.

A common site of osteosclerosis is the periapical region, most frequently of the posterior teeth. Such sclerosis rarely is of clinical significance, although occasionally it may produce resorption of the root of the tooth. That sclerosis of the walls of nutrient canals leading to the apical foramina may be the forerunner of more extensive sclerosis of bone surrounding them is problematic (Fig. 11–13). Illustrations of more extensive areas of osteosclerosis in the periapical region of vital teeth are shown in Figure 11–14.

Osteosclerosis sometimes occurs in edentulous regions in which it would be difficult to explain on the basis of surgical trauma or retarded healing of the wound, for it may appear several years after operation when there is no roentgenographic evidence of abnormal density. Evidence of small root fragments has been observed in roentgenograms made prior to formation of the sclerotic bone in some of these cases. In Figure 11–15 the roentgenogram on the left, made 2 years after removal of an embedded mandibular third molar, reveals a small root tip and bone of normal density

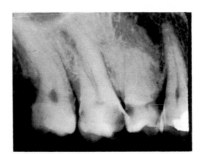

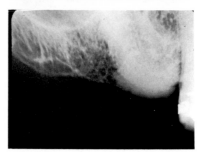

Figure 11–11 *Above,* Osteosclerosis surrounding the root of a maxillary second premolar. *Below,* Appearance several years after extraction. The sclerosis persists and the space formerly occupied by the root also has become filled with sclerotic bone.

Figure 11–10 Osteosclerosis surrounding the root of a normal second premolar. Nutrient canals can be visualized within the sclerosed bone.

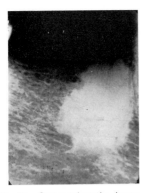

Figure 11–12 Osteosclerotic bone of uniform radiopacity situated in the endentulous mandibular premolar region.

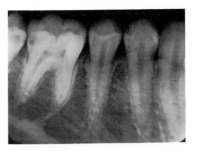

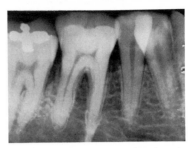

Figure 11–13 Two cases of sclerosis of the walls of nutrient canals that lead to the apical foramina.

and normal trabeculation. The roentgenogram on the right, made several years later, reveals that an appreciable amount of sclerotic bone has formed in this region. A similar case is illustrated in Figure 11–16. In this instance the roentgenogram on the left, made 4 years after removal of a maxillary third molar, shows bone of normal density. The one on the right, made 13 years later, reveals an area of sclerotic bone. Dense bone so formed in an apparently normal edentulous region may be transient, for it also has been observed in rare instances that the density of the bone tends to return to normal.

Hyperostoses that may appear on the crest of the alveolar ridge beneath the pontic of fixed bridges have been noted and one of them is shown in Figure 11–17. The roentgenogram on the left was made shortly after the placement of the bridge, and the one on the right 4 years later. During that interval a dense, compact, bony pro-

Figure 11–14 Osteosclerosis in the periapical region of vital teeth.

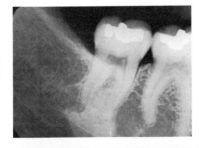

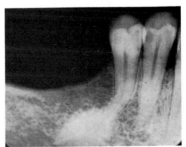

Figure 11–15 Osteosclerosis of obscure origin. *Left,* Roentgenogram made 2 years after removal of a mandibular third molar reveals bone of normal density and a small retained root. *Right,* This view reveals the sclerotic bone that was present several years later.

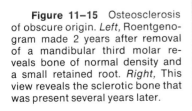

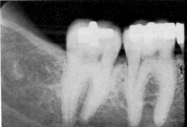

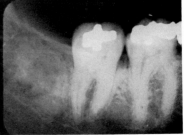

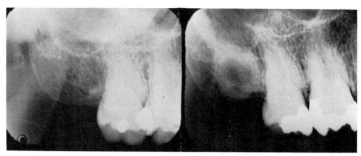

Figure 11–16 Sclerotic bone of obscure origin. *Left,* Four years after removal of the maxillary third molar, bone is of normal density. *Right,* Sclerotic bone is present 13 years later.

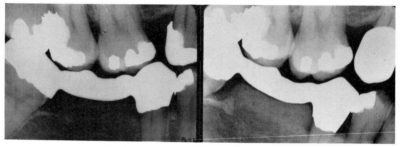

Figure 11–17 Hyperostosis beneath a bridge pontic. The roentgenogram on the left was made 4 years prior to the one on the right. (Courtesy of Dr. J. F. Quinley, Wichita, Kansas.)

tuberance has formed which extends to the lower part of the pontic. It is saucer-shaped and it conforms to the contour of the pontic. In this instance there had been no complaints referable to it. A similar case was reported by Calman et al. (1971). However, cases have been seen in which increased impingement on the pontic had caused inflammation and ulceration of the soft tissues, and it had become necessary to remove the protuberance. What actually causes the condition is problematic. Perhaps a low-grade irritation produced by the pontic initiates a subperiosteal growth of bone.

Fortunately, the localized areas of osteosclerosis within the jaws that are revealed so frequently by routine roentgenographic examination are seldom of clinical significance. There are rare instances in which they may cause resorption of the roots of the teeth or may be the cause of pain. There usually is no indication for surgical intervention. Those that are extensive become firmly fused to both the buccal and the lingual cortex, and surgical removal is a difficult procedure without resort to saucerization, which generally results in needless deformity.

REFERENCES

Burrell, K. H. and Goepp, R. A.: Abnormal Bone Repair in Jaws, Socket Sclerosis: A Sign of Systemic Disease. J. Am. Dent. A. 87:1206–1215 (Nov.) 1973.

Calman, H. I., Eisenberg, M., Grodjesk, J. E., and Szerlip, L.: Interpretation of Radiopacities. Dent. Radiogr. Photogr. 44:3–10, 1971.

PATHOLOGIC CALCIFICATIONS AND OSSIFICATIONS OF THE SOFT TISSUES

12

Deposition of calcium salts occurs normally only in the formation of bone and the teeth. When it occurs elsewhere, including the excretory and secretory passages, it is considered a pathologic process. Anderson (1948) has classified pathologic calcification as (1) dystrophic calcification, (2) metastatic calcification, and (3) calcinosis. Dystrophic calcification is the precipitation of calcium in degenerating and dead tissue and is dependent on a local change in the tissue. Common sites are blood vessels and degenerating tumors. Metastatic calcification is the deposition of calcium salts in previously undamaged tissue as a result of an excess of these salts in the circulating blood. Conditions that tend to produce such calcification are hypervitaminosis D, an excess of parathyroid hormone, and destructive lesions of bone. Common sites of occurrence are the kidneys and blood vessels. Calcinosis is calcification that occurs in or under the skin; one of the conditions with which it may be associated is scleroderma.

According to Anderson (1948), pathologic ossification, unlike simple calcification, forms bone structures. Heteroplastic formation of bone may occur in almost any tissue.

Evidence of many forms of pathologic calcification involving the soft tissues may be seen in regions that are included in the dental and oral roentgenographic examination. Here, calcification in the excretory ducts is represented by salivary calculus (sialolithiasis); dystrophic calcification by phleboliths, calcified lymph nodes, calcification of the larval stage of tapeworm (*Cysticercus*), and calcification of the facial artery; metastatic calcification by calcification of the facial artery in renal osteodystrophy; and pathologic ossification by myositis ossificans and multiple miliary osteomas of the skin.

SALIVARY CALCULUS (SIALOLITHIASIS)

The deposition of calculus in the salivary ducts and glands is not an uncommon occurrence among persons who have reached middle age. It occurs much more frequently in the submaxillary duct (Wharton's) and gland than in the parotid duct (Stensen's) and gland. While most of these calculi arise and are situated in the ducts, there are those that have formed in the gland and have passed on into the duct. They may cause partial or complete obstruction of the duct. The most common and diagnostic symptom of obstruction is increase and decrease in swelling of the

135

gland, particularly at mealtime, swelling that may or may not be associated with pain. Continued obstruction of the duct may lead to inflammation, acute infection, and abscess formation. The calculi may occur as single or multiple stones in the ducts as well as in the glands. They vary in size and may be round, elliptical, or long and cylindrical.

Calculi present in the sublingual and lingual ducts are best demonstrated by use of the intraoral occlusal film, and those situated in the submaxillary gland by occlusal plus extraoral films. Those that are located in the parotid duct can often be demonstrated on a standard dental film that is placed against the inside of the cheek and extended upward into the buccal fold. Calculi in the parotid duct also can be demonstrated on an extraoral film that is placed at a right angle to the surface of the face, with the direction of the tube parallel to the cheek; the exposure is made when the cheek is blown outward and laterally by the patient. Forcing the cheek laterally provides less superimposition of osseous structures.

The calculi are seen in the roentgenogram as radiopaque objects that conform to the size and shape of the particular stone or stones present. The degree of radiopacity varies. Stones that are of long standing and have reached an appreciable size may have a greater radiographic density than normal bone and are readily demonstrated. Others in which the organic content may be relatively high are not sufficiently radiopaque to be seen clearly, and in some instances it may not even be possible to demonstrate roentgenographically calculi that may be causing obstruction of the salivary ducts. Roentgenograms made with a short exposure often reveal calculi that are not clearly discernible otherwise.

It is not unusual for the image of salivary calculi to appear on the roentgenogram incidental to a routine dental roentgenographic examination. Those that occur in the submaxillary duct are most often so disclosed, particularly when roentgenograms of the edentulous mandible are made, for there is then a tendency

to place the films deeper and thereby include a larger portion of the floor of the mouth and its contents (Gardner and Stafne, 1932). When superimposed on the mandible, the image of the calculus may be misinterpreted as a bone whorl, enostosis, or sclerotic bone within the mandible. When such radiopaque images occur it is well to make a digital examination of the floor of the mouth, and to have occlusal roentgenograms of the floor of the mouth made to rule out the possible presence of calculi. An instance in which the image of a calculus of the submaxillary duct was superimposed on the mandible, and in which there were no symptoms referable to it, is shown in Figure 12–1a. Here the dental roentgenograms reveal an elliptical radio-

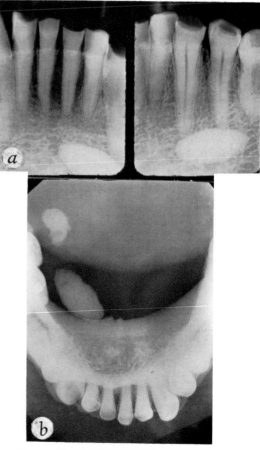

Figure 12–1 Salivary calculi in the duct of the submaxillary gland. *a,* Dental roentgenograms showing image of calculus superimposed on the mandible. *b,* Occlusal view which reveals that there are two distinct calculi in the duct.

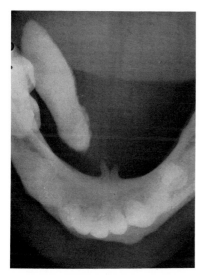

Figure 12-2 Single salivary calculus of large dimension which occupies the greater portion of the duct of the submaxillary gland.

paque object in the anterior region of the mandible. The fact that the position of this object is altered in relation to the roots of the teeth in the two views should lead one to suspect that it is not within the mandible. An occlusal view of the floor of the mouth (Fig. 12-1b) reveals not only one but two separate calculi in the duct of the submaxillary gland.

Calculi that are large and are situated in the anterior portion of the floor of the mouth are readily demonstrated by the occlusal film (Fig. 12-2); however, to be assured that calculi that are situated near or in the submaxillary gland are included, the x-ray tube should be directed forward and upward from a point posterior to the angle and parallel to the lingual surface of the mandible. Figure 12-3 illustrates a case in which the roentgenogram on the left failed to disclose a stone that was present, whereas the one on the right, which was made to include the posterior region of the floor of the mouth, demonstrated the stone clearly. Calculi situated in the submaxillary gland often cannot be demonstrated adequately by the intraoral occlusal film; therefore, it is necessary to supplement it with an extraoral view. One that reveals multiple calculi located in the gland is shown in Figure 12-4.

Illustrations of three cases of calculi of varied size occurring in the duct of the parotid gland are shown in Figure 12-5. They were demonstrated on a standard dental film that is placed inside the cheek and extended upward into the buccal fold. The lower border of the film is moved laterally, forcing the cheek slightly outward. The exposure is made with the x-ray tube directed downward at an angle of

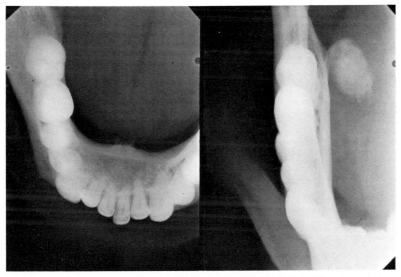

Figure 12-3 Salivary calculus situated near the submaxillary gland. *Left,* View does not include a sufficient area of the floor of the mouth to disclose the stone. *Right,* View is made to include the posterior region and reveals the stone.

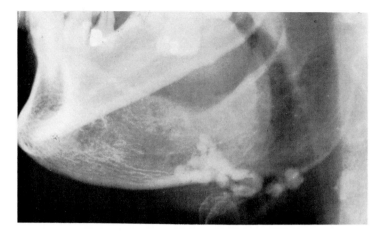

Figure 12–4 Multiple calculi situated in the submaxillary gland.

about 45°, thereby including a larger portion of the cheek above the buccal fold. A calculus in the parotid duct, which is demonstrated by the use of an extraoral film and an exposure made when the cheek is blown outward, is shown in Figure 12–6. Both the intraoral and the extraoral methods should be employed in the search for calculi of the parotid duct.

Some salivary calculi, even though they may have reached an appreciable size, produce no symptoms and are first noted incidental to roentgenographic examination. In view of the complications that may arise as a result of permitting them to remain, the removal of such calculi is justified as a preventive measure.

PHLEBOLITHS AND CERTAIN OTHER DYSTROPHIC CALCIFICATIONS

Phleboliths are calcified thrombi. The ones most often encountered in dental and oral roentgenology are those that occur in cavernous hemangiomas involving the soft tissues adjacent to the jaws. They appear in the roentgenogram as round or oval bodies which are most often uniformly radiopaque, although in some instances they may exhibit the concentric calcific deposits that are characteristic of them. Thoma and co-workers (1948), in describing cross sections of phleboliths, likened them to cross sections of an onion.

Two cases of phlebolithiasis of a hemangioma involving the face are illustrated in Figure 12–7. In the upper illustration there are six radiopaque bodies of varied sizes, four of which are not superimposed on the bone of the maxilla, and therefore must be located in the cheek. In the lower illustration, the phleboliths are superimposed on the mandible and may be mistaken for dental root fragments or small areas of sclerotic bone.

Calcifications in the cheek other than those associated with hemangioma may be encountered incidental to routine

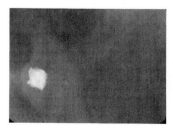
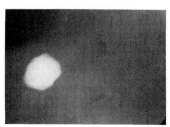
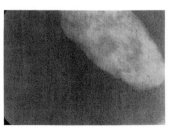

Figure 12–5 Salivary calculi in the duct of the parotid gland. In all three patients the calculus was demonstrated by means of the standard dental film placed on the inside of the cheek.

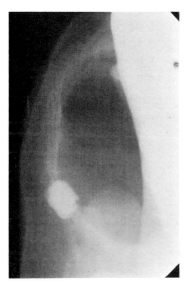

Figure 12–6 Calculus in the duct of the parotid gland demonstrated by means of the extraoral film, with the exposure made while the patient is blowing the cheek outward.

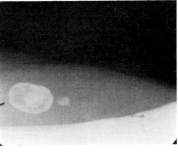

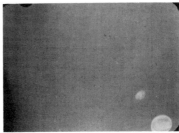

Figure 12–8 Calcifications in the cheek that are of obscure origin.

roentgenographic or digital examination. In some instances the patient may volunteer the information that a firm movable nodule in the cheek has been noted. The calcifications may be single or multiple.

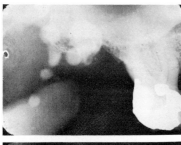

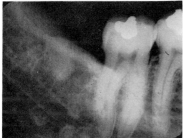

Figure 12–7 Phleboliths in cavernous hemangiomas of the face. *Above,* Multiple phleboliths of varied size, some of which are superimposed on the maxilla and coronoid process. *Below,* Multiple phleboliths superimposed on the mandible; these might be mistaken for roots or bone whorls.

Two cases in which the calcifications were demonstrated with the intraoral film are shown in Figure 12–8; in both instances two calcifications were present. A case in which the calcifications are sufficiently large and dense to be seen when superimposed on the mandible is illustrated in Figure 12–9. The view on the left shows an oval radiopaque mass which resembles a central osteoma. On the right is an occlusal view which reveals that the radiopaque object is not situated within the mandible but in the soft tissues buccal to it, and that it consists of two distinct calcified masses. The larger of the two had three centers of calcification that had coalesced to form a large oval mass around which laminated layers of calcific deposits had been laid down. The patient had been aware of its presence for many years and was under the impression that there had been no increase in size during a period of about 10 years. It is often difficult to determine the source of these calcifications. It is known that they occur in lymph nodes, in epithelial cysts of subcutaneous tissues, in epidermal and sebaceous cysts, and infrequently in cysts of the sweat glands.

Quinn (1965) reported a case in which calcified masses were present in the buccal

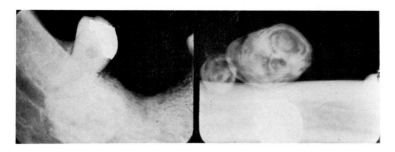

Figure 12–9 Calcifications in the cheek that were said to be calcified lymph nodes. *Left*, Calcifications are superimposed on the mandible and appear to be within the jaw. *Right*, Occlusal view, showing two distinct and separate calcified nodules in the cheek.

soft tissues that were strikingly similar to those shown in Figure 12–9. They first had been noted by the patient 14 years previously, and no information could be gained to account for their presence.

CYSTICERCOSIS

Cysticercus represents the larval stage of the tapeworm. According to Koppisch (1948) it develops in the tissues of man when he ingests ova in water or food contaminated with the excreta of a person who carries the intestinal parasite, or in some instances by autoinfection. Any part of the body may be involved, but in order of frequency are the subcutaneous tissues, brain, orbit, muscles, heart, liver, lungs, and peritoneum.

The cysticerci are round when situated in the viscera, but in the musculature and subcutaneous tissue they are elongated by compression. They vary in diameter from about 2 to 5 mm. When the larvae are alive there is no roentgenographic evidence of their presence; however, after death of the larvae, the cystic spaces they occupy are replaced by fibrous tissue which may undergo calcific degeneration. Those that are situated in muscle or subcutaneous tissue and have undergone calcification are most often seen as radiopaque objects that are elliptical or ovoid in shape. Among other regions, the muscles and skin adjacent to the jaws may be involved, where such calcification may be interpreted as being lithiasis of the salivary ducts and glands (Cheraskin and Langley, 1956). Roentgenograms that demonstrate the varied size and

regular ovoid form of the calcifications are shown in Figure 12–10.

CALCIFICATION OF ARTERIES

Calcific deposits in the walls of the arteries may occur in all forms of arteriosclerosis and secondary to inflammatory conditions involving them. They may occur as extensive deposits within the media or in the fibrous tissue of the intima. According to Fairbairn and colleagues (1972), the latter is a prominent feature in arteriosclerosis obliterans, which is primarily an intimal degenerative process that causes obliteration of the lumen. When seen in the roentgenogram, calcification that accentuates the lateral margins of the artery to produce a tubular configuration almost always means that deposition of calcium has taken place within the medial coat. This type of calcification may occur in persons who may or may not display evidence of occlusive arterial disease (Hays et al., 1966). While the roentgenogram is of distinct value in determining calcification of the aorta and vessels of the extremities, one rarely encounters evidence of calcification of vessels in the dental roentgenogram. Among those who have observed such instances are Ennis and Burket (1942), who reported two cases.

Grossly the vessels vary in thickness; some segments are dilated or contracted, while others are tortuous and may have a pipe-stem appearance. Some of these features are exhibited in the dental roentgenogram shown in Figure 12–11. Another case of calcification of the facial artery is illus-

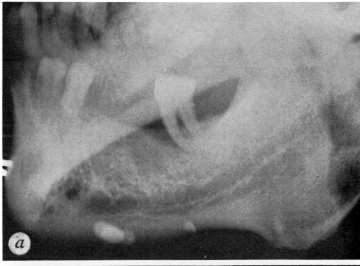

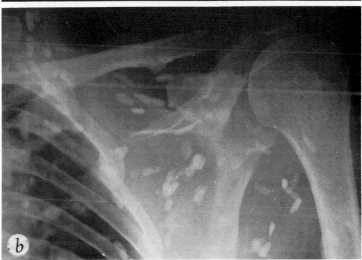

Figure 12–10 Cysticercosis. *a,* View showing four calcified nodules near the inferior border of the mandible, which represent calcific degeneration of the larval stage. *b,* View showing similar ovoid calcifications of the shoulder and thorax. (Reproduced with permission from Cheraskin, E. and Langley, L. L.: Dynamics of Oral Diagnosis. Chicago, Year Book Publishers, 1956, pp. 59–60.)

trated in the roentgenogram shown in Figure 12–12. It was made with a soft-tissue exposure to an occlusal film that had been positioned intraorally against the cheek, and it reveals a much larger segment of the artery than would a dental film of standard size. In both cases the patients suffered from occlusive arterial disease (arteriosclerosis obliterans) of the lower extremities.

Most patients with hyperparathyroid-

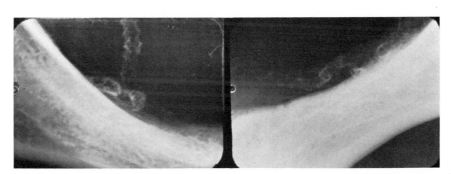

Figure 12–11 Dystrophic calcification of both facial arteries in a patient with arteriosclerosis obliterans.

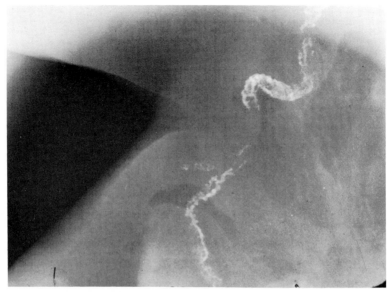

Figure 12–12 Calcification of facial artery demonstrated on occlusal film that has been placed intraorally against the cheek. (Reproduced with permission from Hays, J. B., Gibilisco, J. A., and Juergens, J. L.: Calcification of Vessels in Cheek of Patient with Medial Arteriosclerosis. Oral Surg., Oral Med. & Oral Path. *21*:299–302 [Mar.] 1966.)

ism have some metastatic deposition of calcium salts in the soft tissues, and the kidneys and blood vessels are most frequently involved. Such calcification may be particularly abundant in hyperparathyroidism that is secondary to renal failure and phosphate retention, resulting in high concentration of both calcium and phos-

phorus in the blood. Calcification in the walls of the facial artery in a patient with renal osteodystrophy is shown in Figure 12–13.

The presence of arterial calcification does not necessarily denote a generalized process. However, the possibility of arteriosclerosis in other locations should be

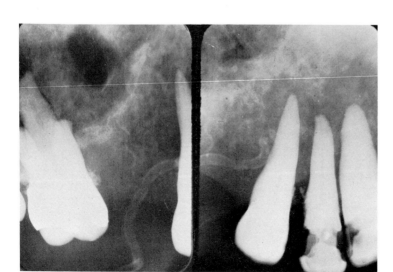

Figure 12–13 Metastatic calcification of the facial artery in a patient with renal osteodystrophy.

suspected whenever localized calcifications are detected.

MYOSITIS OSSIFICANS

Myositis ossificans is characterized by the formation of bony structures, such as lamellae, lacunae, and sometimes marrow, in muscle tissue. It may be present in a progressive widespread form in which there is ossification of muscles, ligaments, fasciae, and tendons, for which the cause is unknown. It may occur in a localized form as a result of single or repeated injury, in which case the ossification is preceded by edema and inflammation of the muscle. The roentgenogram is of aid in determining the character of the lesion, since the calcified substance tends to be quite similar to the trabecular pattern of normal bone.

The muscles of mastication may be involved in some instances. A case of myositis ossificans of the masseter muscle has been reported by Cameron and Stetzer (1945).

The roentgenogram shown in Figure 12–14 was made for a woman 58 years of age who had a hard, diffuse swelling of the soft tissues of the neck on the left side. It reveals strand-like calcifications in the soft

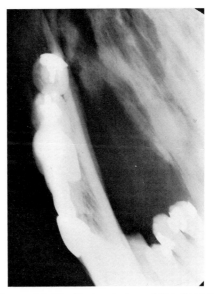

Figure 12–15 Occlusal view of the floor of the mouth, which visualizes more clearly the trabecular pattern of the ossification of the digastric muscle shown in Figure 12–14.

tissues of the neck, particularly of the digastric muscle, where it has a very typical resemblance to bone. An occlusal view (Fig. 12–15) shows more clearly the character of the calcification. There was no history of injury in this instance, and there were no calcifications in muscles elsewhere.

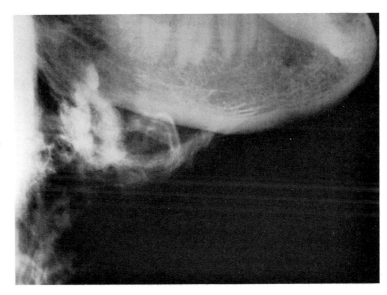

Figure 12–14 Myositis ossificans of the muscles of the neck.

CALCIFIED ACNE LESIONS

A form of dystrophic calcification that may be seen in the dental roentgenogram is that which may occur in degenerated tissue and hypertrophic scarring from lesions of acne. Such calcifications may go unnoticed in routine dental roentgenographic examination, particularly if they are sparse and small. Also, the exposure time customarily used for such examinations may not bring them into view. However, when a reduced soft-tissue exposure is made to a film that is placed in the vestibule of the mouth and directed against the facial tissues, the calcification may become clearly discernible. This has been demonstrated by Ennis (1964), who reported on the roentgenographic features of calcified acne lesions. He stated that since the areas of scarring vary greatly in shape, size, and density, the roentgenographic appearance of the calcific deposits varies similarly. He

referred to them as having somewhat the appearance of snowflakes.

The roentgenographic appearance of calcified acne lesions is illustrated in Figure 12–16. The view on the left was obtained by placing an occlusal film between the teeth and the inside of the cheek, with exposure time altered for soft tissue, in a patient in whom the routine dental roentgenographic examination had given a clue to the presence of calcification. It revealed that calcific deposits were present in large numbers. An enlargement of the view on the left is shown on the right. It demonstrates with clarity the irregular shape of the calcifications.

MULTIPLE MILIARY OSTEOMAS OF THE SKIN

The occurrence of multiple miliary osteomas of the skin is relatively rare. First

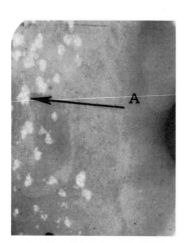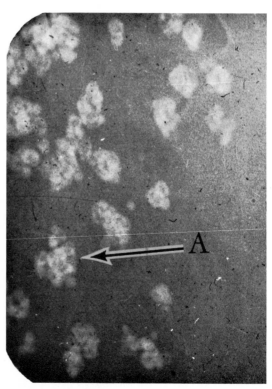

Figure 12–16 Calcified acne lesions. *Left,* Taken with an occlusal film placed in the vestibule of the mouth. *Right,* Enlargement of the view on the left, illustrating the snowflake appearance of the calcific deposits. The arrows point to identical areas. (Reproduced with permission from Ennis, L. M.: Roentgenographic Appearance of Calcified Acne Lesions. J. Am. Dent. A. *68*:351–357 [Mar.] 1964.)

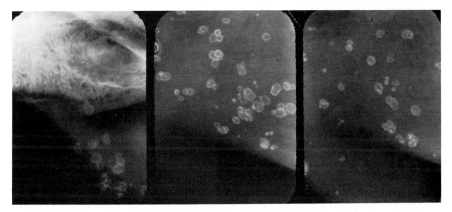

Figure 12–17   Multiple miliary osteomas of the skin of the face, showing the characteristic rounded calcifications with radiolucent centers that give them the appearance of a doughnut. *Left,* As seen in routine dental x-ray examination. *Center,* As seen with dental film placed inside left cheek. *Right,* As seen with dental film placed inside right cheek.

reference to this condition was made by Virchow (1864). The small osteomas, which range from 0.5 to 2.0 mm in diameter, are situated in the cutis and subcutis. Cases in which they have involved the skin of the face, forehead, and chin have been reported (Carney and Radcliffe, 1951; Costello, 1947; Gasner, 1954). The osteomas are round or oval and are surrounded by a capsule of fibrous tissue. They have a smooth surface, and consist of laminated, concentric rings of typical bone with numerous lacunae containing stainable nuclei; they have a central, round, marrow cavity which may contain fat, blood vessels, and a few myeloblastic elements. According to Hopkins (1928) and Leider (1948), they do not necessarily cause any visible change in the skin, although, in most of the cases reported, there has been an associated acne or some other form of dermatosis.

In the roentgenogram they present a very typical picture which conforms to the architecture of the osteoma. Each appears as a small doughnut-shaped shadow with a radiolucent center which represents the central marrow cavity. Such multiple osteomas when present may be seen incidental to routine dental roentgenographic examination. Such a case is shown in Figure 12–17. The roentgenogram on the left reveals several radiopaque nodules in the soft tissue below the alveolar ridge. The roentgenograms in the center and on the right were made by placing a dental film against the inside surface of the cheek, with a reduced time of exposure. This technique demonstrates them more clearly and should be useful in the differential diagnosis of calcifications of the cheeks and lips.

A view made with the tube directed parallel to the surface of the face when the cheek is being blown outward is shown in

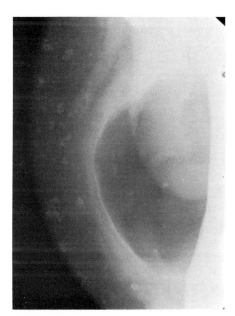

Figure 12–18   Multiple miliary osteomas of the skin of the face. Extraoral view, made when the cheek is blown outward.

Figure 12–18. This technique demonstrates the osteomas less clearly, but it is useful in that it reveals their location in relation to the surface of the skin. It will be noted that in this patient the calcifications appear in proximity to the surface. Calcifications associated with lesions of the oral mucosa would tend to appear on the inner surface of the cheek only.

Theories as to possible pathogenesis have involved (1) metaplastic ossification secondary to chronic inflammatory processes, (2) neoplastic ossification, and (3) embryonal cell rests of osteoblastic elements. Of 11 patients observed roentgenographically by Stafne, in all of whom the osteomas occurred bilaterally, only 1 had any noticeable blemishes on the surface of the skin, and these were nodules from a previous acne. This would tend to support the theory that they are derived from embryonal cell rests, and are not necessarily caused by pre-existing inflammatory processes.

REFERENCES

Anderson, W. A. D.: Pathology: Degenerative Changes and Disturbances of Metabolism. St. Louis, The C. V. Mosby Company, 1948, pp. 67–99.

Cameron, J. R. and Stetzer, J. J., Jr.: Myositis Ossificans of Right Masseter Muscle: Report of Case. J. Oral Surg. 3:170–173 (Apr.) 1945.

Carney, R. G. and Radcliffe, C. E.: Multiple Miliary Osteomas of Skin. Arch. Dermat. & Syph. 64:483–486 (Oct.) 1951.

Cheraskin, E. and Langley, L. L.: Dynamics of Oral Diagnosis. Chicago, Year Book Publishers, 1956, pp. 59–60.

Costello, M. J.: Metaplasia of Bone: Report of Case. Arch. Dermat. & Syph. 56:536–537 (Oct.) 1947.

Ennis, L. M.: Roentgenographic Appearance of Calcified Acne Lesions. J. Am. Dent. A. 68:351–357 (Mar.) 1964.

Ennis, L. M. and Burket, L. W.: Calcified Vessels of Cheeks: Demonstration by Means of Dental Roentgenograms. Ann. Dent. 1:111–113 (Dec.) 1942.

Fairbairn, J. F., II, Juergens, J. L., and Spittell, J. A., Jr.: Peripheral Vascular Diseases. Ed. 4. Philadelphia, W. B. Saunders Company, 1972, pp. 179–190.

Gardner, B. S. and Stafne, E. C.: Misinterpretation of Radiopaque Areas in Dental Roentgenograms. Dent. Cosmos. 74:19–20 (Jan.) 1932.

Gasner, W. G.: Primary Osteoma Cutis: Report of Case. Arch. Dermat. & Syph. 69:101–103 (Jan.) 1954.

Hays, J. B., Gibilisco, J. A., and Juergens, J. L.: Calcification of Vessels in Cheek of Patient with Medial Arteriosclerosis. Oral Surg., Oral Med. & Oral Path. 21:299–302 (Mar.) 1966.

Hopkins, J. G.: Multiple Miliary Osteomas of Skin: Report of Case. Arch. Dermat. & Syph. 18:706–715 (Nov.) 1928.

Koppisch, E.: Protozoal and Helminthic Infections. In Anderson, W. A. D.: Pathology. St. Louis, The C. V. Mosby Company, 1948, pp. 392–446.

Leider, M.: Osteoma Cutis: Report of Case. Arch. Dermat. & Syph. 58:168–176 (Aug.) 1948.

Quinn, J. H.: Calcified Bodies (Idiopathic) in the Buccal Soft Tissues. Oral Surg., Oral Med. & Oral Path. 19:292–294 (Mar.) 1965.

Thoma, K. H., Holland, D. J., Jr., Woodbury, H. W., Burrow, J. G., and Sleeper, E. L.: IV. Contribution to the Oncology of the Jaws: Case 152; Hemangioma of the Cheek with Phlebolithiasis. Oral Surg., Oral Med. & Oral Path. 1:54–57 (Jan.) 1948.

Virchow, R.: Die krankhaften Geschwülste. Berlin, A. Hirschwold, 1864, vol. 2, p. 103.

CYSTS OF THE JAWS

13

Epithelium-lined cysts of the jaws may be divided into two groups: (1) odontogenic and (2) nonodontogenic cysts. They contain fluid or a semisolid material, and they increase in size by their own tension as a result of an osmotic imbalance (James, 1926). The tension from within the cyst exerts an equal pressure in all directions, which accounts for the tendency of the cystic cavity to assume a globular shape. Any variation from the globular form results from variation in resistance to resorption of the structures that the cyst encounters in its growth. The image presented by such a cyst in the roentgenogram is that of a fairly uniform radiolucent cavity in bone which has a well-defined circumscribed border, and the bone adjacent to it appears normal.

A very comprehensive article dealing with the origin and growth of cysts of the jaws and especially with the significance of the odontogenic keratocyst has been published by Toller (1967).

ODONTOGENIC CYSTS

PERIODONTAL CYSTS (RADICULAR, APICAL)

A periodontal cyst is an epithelium-lined sac, usually situated at the apex of the root of the tooth. It is derived from epithelial remnants of the periodontal membrane, and the stimulus that in most instances incites a proliferation of epithelium is probably inflammation. Formation of the cyst is always preceded by degeneration of the pulp of the tooth from which it develops. According to Kronfeld (1939), the cyst can originate in two ways: (1) an abscess cavity in granulation tissue surrounding the root of the tooth may become lined with epithelium because of the inherent tendency for epithelium to cover raw surfaces, or (2) epithelial masses that have formed as a result of proliferation may themselves undergo cystic degeneration and change into cysts. Hill (1930), who examined serial sections of 42 granulomas and found epithelial tissue in all of them, demonstrated epithelium in all stages of proliferation, from that of epithelial rests to that of large cystic regions. Therefore, it appears that all so-called granulomas are potential periodontal cysts.

A periodontal cyst may have its onset at any time during life, and most often is associated with teeth in which there is rampant and untreated caries. In a study of 349 periodontal cysts it was found that such cysts develop more than two and one-half times as often on roots of pulpless teeth with untreated root canals as on roots that have had the root canals treated (Stafne and Millhon, 1945). They occur more frequently in the maxilla than in the mandible, the ratio being approximately 3:2. This difference is accounted for largely by the high incidence of cysts in the incisor-canine region of the maxilla.

Periodontal cysts almost always are lined with squamous epithelium. If any other type of epithelium is present, one must consider the possibility that the cyst originated from some other source.

An epithelium-lined cyst may develop in a periapical lesion that is still relatively small, as evidenced by Figure 13–1. The roentgenogram on the left revealed widening of the periodontal-membrane space in the periapical region of a maxillary second premolar, the pulp of which had undergone degeneration. The roentgenogram on the right was made 2 years later, at which time a round, well-circumscribed radiolucent area had appeared at the apex of the root of this tooth. There had been no symptoms referable to the tooth in the meantime. On microscopic examination the lesion proved to be a cyst lined with stratified squamous epithelium.

How large and extensive a cyst will become or how rapidly it will increase in size is uncertain. Some observed cysts have not increased in size over a period of many years. In others that have undergone enlargement the rate of growth has varied greatly (Figs. 13–2 and 13–3).

Cysts lined with epithelium may develop from epithelium that is associated with roots of primary teeth that remain in the jaws as a result of fracture at the time of extraction, or that remain as a result of incomplete resorption of the root (Stafne, 1937). The majority of such retained roots remain in the premolar regions, particularly in the mandible, and may assume a position ranging from one near the crest of

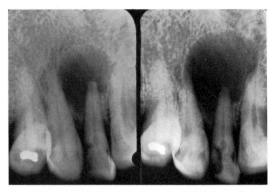

Figure 13–2 Periodontal cyst involving a lateral incisor and showing increase in size over a period of 14 months. (Reproduced with permission from Stafne, E. C. and Millhon, J. A.: Periodontal Cysts. J. Oral Surg. *3*:102–111 [Apr.] 1945.)

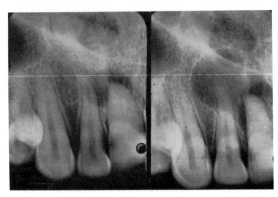

Figure 13–3 Periodontal cyst associated with a central incisor and showing increase in size over a period of about 14 years.

the ridge to one beyond the apex of the roots of the permanent teeth. A cyst that has developed from the retained root of a lower primary second molar is shown in Figure 13–4. The root fragment is situated near the apex of the permanent second premolar. Upon removal of the cyst the root was found to be situated in the wall of the cyst. The cyst was not attached to the roots of the adjoining teeth. A cyst that has developed from the root of a primary tooth which is situated near the crest of the ridge is shown in Figure 13–5.

In most instances such retained roots of primary teeth undergo complete resorption so that they are no longer discernible in the roentgenogram, but leave behind them epithelial rests in the interdental

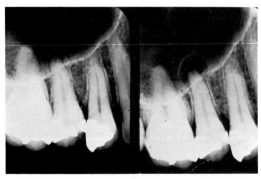

Figure 13–1 Periodontal cyst that has developed from a periodontal lesion of small dimension on a pulpless second premolar. The roentgenogram on the left was made 2 years prior to the one on the right.

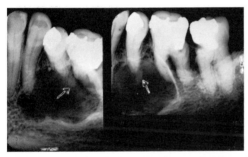

Figure 13–4 Epithelium-lined cyst that has developed from a retained root of a primary tooth. The root is situated near the apex of the root of a vital second premolar. (Reproduced with permission from Stafne, E. C.: Possible Role of Retained Deciduous Roots in Etiology of Cysts of Jaw. *J. Am. Dent. A. 24*:1488–1493 [Sept.] 1937.)

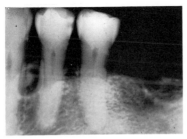

Figure 13–5 Small epithelium-lined cyst that arose from a primary root situated near the crest of the alveolar ridge.

bony septum. These epithelial rests have been mentioned by Orban (1928), who recognized that they were not remainders of the sheath of Hertwig of the permanent teeth and who also called attention to the possibility that such epithelial islands later may develop into epithelial tumors of the jaw. A roentgenogram of a cyst that has developed in the interseptal bone between a

mandibular first and second premolar is shown in Figure 13–6. It developed after the age of 45 years. It was not attached to the roots of either premolar, and it was lined by stratified squamous epithelium. Two cysts in the maxillary premolar region which may have had a similar origin are shown in Figure 13–7. Cysts that are appreciably larger and apparently are not associated with the permanent dentition may in some instances originate from epithelial remnants situated in the interseptal bones of the alveolar process.

DENTIGEROUS CYSTS (FOLLICULAR)

A dentigerous cyst is an epithelium-lined sac that develops from the enamel organ in association with crowns of unerupted teeth. In its early stages it is evidenced in the roentgenogram by widening of the pericoronal space, and a space that has reached 2.5 mm in width represents a cyst with a definite epithelial lining in about 80% of cases (Conklin and Stafne, 1949). The teeth most often involved are, in descending order of frequency of occurrence, the third molars, the canines, and the second premolars. These cysts may occur on any other teeth that remain embedded. Usually a dentigerous cyst begins to develop shortly after complete formation of the crown, by an accumulation of fluid between the enamel surface and the surrounding soft-tissue capsule from which its lining epithelium is derived. Most dentigerous cysts, therefore, have their onset in the early decades of life.

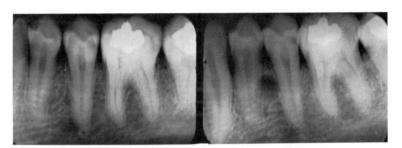

Figure 13–6 *Left*, Roentgenogram shows no abnormality. *Right*, A cyst has developed in the interseptal bone between the premolars. It may have arisen from epithelial remnants once associated with the roots of a primary tooth. (Reproduced with permission from Stafne, E. C.: Possible Role of Retained Deciduous Roots in Etiology of Cysts of Jaw. *J. Am. Dent. A. 24*:1488–1493 [Sept.] 1937.)

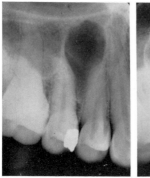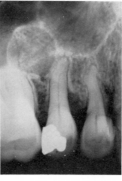

Figure 13–7 Cysts of the maxilla that may have developed from epithelial remnants once associated with the periodontal membrane of primary teeth.

The cyst is given an opportunity to develop and increase in size when the eruption of the tooth on which it occurs is retarded or prevented. Fortunately, in most instances, the eruptive force of the tooth is greater than the pressure of the cyst and, when the crown reaches the surface, the cyst is destroyed. This occurs when the erupting tooth does not encounter any obstruction in the course of eruption. Cysts that have formed and are destroyed as a result of eruption have been referred to as "eruptive cysts." Two of these are illustrated in Figure 13–8. In the one on the left it appears that the tooth will erupt and the cyst will undergo self-destruction as a result of it. In the one on the right, the lower third molar on which the eruptive cyst has developed may become impacted against the erupted second molar and thereby prevented from erupting. If the tooth does not erupt, the cyst may continue to grow and reach an appreciable size. If it is predictable that there is not sufficient space for a third molar to erupt into normal position in the arch, removal of the tooth and cyst is indicated as soon as the condition is detected.

Eruptive cysts involving a maxillary third molar and a maxillary canine are illustrated in Figure 13–9. The third molar shown on the left may not become a useful tooth, and the treatment of choice may be removal of the tooth and cyst. In the case of the canine shown on the right, the cyst is retarding or preventing eruption. In this instance, one should extract the primary canine and destroy the cyst so as to permit normal eruption of the permanent canine.

The rate of growth of a dentigerous cyst and its size vary greatly, although the rate appears to be more rapid at early ages

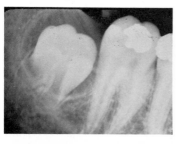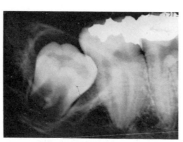

Figure 13–8 Eruptive cysts. Two illustrations showing abnormally wide pericoronal space and roots that are only partially formed.

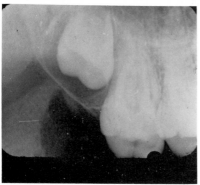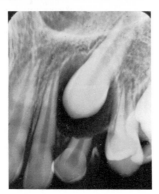

Figure 13–9 Eruptive cysts. *Left,* Maxillary third molar involved. *Right,* Maxillary canine involved.

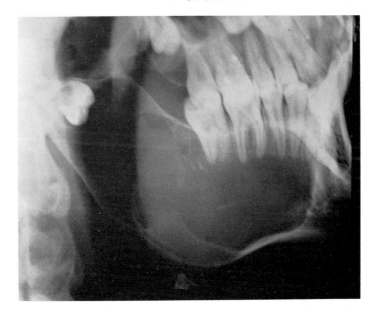

Figure 13-10 Dentigerous cyst in a girl 14 years of age that has undergone rapid growth and reached extensive size. It is associated with a mandibular third molar that has been forced to a location near the condyle.

and in regions of the posterior part of the mandible and ramus where the cyst encounters least resistance to development and also reaches greater size. The lateral x-ray view of the jaw shown in Figure 13-10 is that of an extensive dentigerous cyst that occurred in a girl 14 years of age. It extends from the canine region posteriorly and occupies almost all of the ramus. There is an expansion of the cortex at the inferior border of the mandible, and the cyst has extended upward into the interseptal bone of the premolars and of the first and second molars. The developing third molar from which it originated has been forced by pressure of the cyst from its original position to one in the vicinity of the condyle. This patient also had a similar cyst in the opposite side of the mandible and, in addition, cysts associated with both maxillary upper third molars, and an unerupted maxillary second premolar. The multiple occurrence of dentigerous cysts is not rare, and there also is an hereditary tendency to such cyst formation.

Although in most instances the dentigerous cyst begins to develop prior to complete formation of the tooth with which it is associated, the follicle of a fully embedded tooth does contain viable remnants of epithelium throughout life—epithelium from which a cyst may originate. The roentgenograms shown in Figure 13-11 were made for a patient 35 years of age. The one on the left revealed an embedded mandibular third molar with a pericoronal space of uniform and normal width. The roentgenogram on the right, which was made 4 years later, revealed development of a dentigerous cyst which was forcing the third molar posteriorly.

Dentigerous cysts also may originate

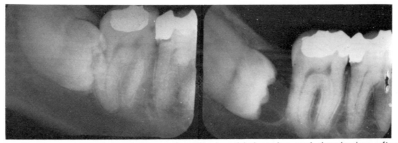

Figure 13-11 Dentigerous cyst involving a mandibular third molar and developing after the age of 35 years. The roentgenogram on the left was made about 4 years prior to the one on the right.

from unerupted supernumerary teeth. In several cases a cyst that developed from an unerupted mesiodens has been noted; one of these is illustrated in Figure 13–12.

The epithelium that is present in an odontoma may proliferate and produce epithelium-lined cysts similar to those that develop from enamel epithelium associated with an embedded tooth, and in this event the cyst is referred to as a cystic odontoma. A patient 42 years of age had swelling and pain in the anterior region of the left maxilla. A roentgenogram (Fig. 13–13) revealed a cyst about 3 cm in diameter and also several radiopaque bodies situated at its lower border. Microscopically, the wall of the cyst was composed of connective tissue of average thickness and it was lined with stratified squamous epithelium. One portion of the wall was markedly thickened, and here epithelium and numerous calcified dental structures were found.

As viewed in the roentgenogram, the crown of the tooth projects into the lumen of the cystic cavity in the majority of cases, and particularly in the early stages of growth. With continuous growth, however, the cyst may alter its position or location in relation to the crown, so that in many instances it remains attached to only a very limited portion of the surface of the enamel and the major portion of the crown is situated outside the cyst wall. This is more prone to occur in those cysts associated with mandibular third molars. Figure 13–

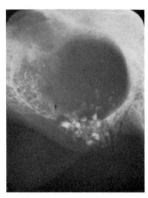

Figure 13–13 Cystic odontoma situated in the canine region of the maxilla.

14 illustrates how this may occur. On the left is an unerupted third molar in a vertical position, on which there is a slightly widened pericoronal space. In most instances such a space is evidence of the early stage of development of a dentigerous cyst. The roentgenogram on the right, made 4 years later, reveals that the third molar has undergone slight eruption only, and that a cystic cavity has developed which extends posteriorly into the retromolar space. This cyst can continue to grow and extend up into the ramus, even though the tooth from which it developed undergoes further eruption. One that is attached to the mesial surface of an unerupted lower third molar is shown in Figure 13–15. It had extended downward in the cancellous portion of the body of the mandible, where least resistance was encountered for its development and growth.

Cysts that are attached to and situated at the side of the crown of an unerupted tooth, as those illustrated, have been referred to as "lateral cysts." This term probably should be referable to their location and position only, and not to their origin. Invariably on removal it is found that enamel of the crown of the tooth is exposed to and fills a part of the lumen of the cyst. Two views of a gross specimen of such a cyst are shown in Figure 13–16. The cyst has been opened to give a view of the inner surface of the wall of the cyst, and, as in many others that have been examined, a portion of the enamel crown of the tooth

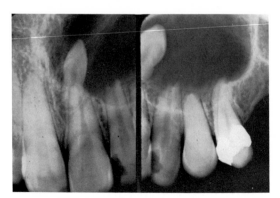

Figure 13–12 Dentigerous cyst that has developed in association with a mesiodens.

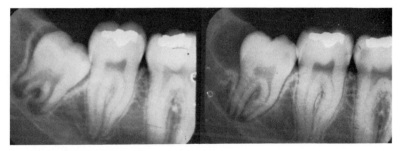

Figure 13–14 *Right,* Dentigerous cyst (lateral type) situated on the distal surface of an unerupted mandibular third molar. *Left,* Appearance 4 years earlier.

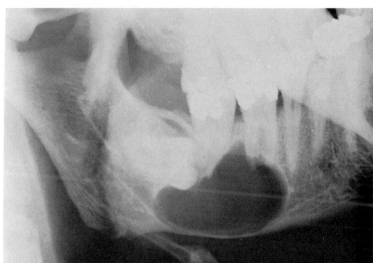

Figure 13–15 Dentigerous cyst (lateral type) situated on the mesial surface of an unerupted mandibular third molar.

fills a part of the lumen of the cavity. This suggests that the lateral cyst most often has an origin similar to that in which the entire crown of the tooth remains situated within the lumen of the cyst. However, Gillette and Weinmann (1958) have reported cases of extrafollicular development of dentigerous cysts.

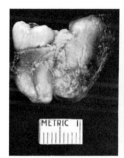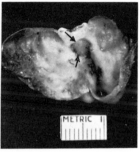

Figure 13–16 Two views of gross specimen of a dentigerous cyst that is attached to the distal surface of a molar. The photograph on the right is the interior view of the cyst wall, showing that the enamel of the tooth fills a portion of the lumen of the cyst.

PRIMORDIAL CYSTS

According to Robinson (1945), a primordial cyst is one of dental origin that develops from the tooth sac while it is still in the embryonal stage, before any calcified structures have been laid down. These cysts are extremely rare and, when they do occur, a definite diagnosis can be made only with difficulty. This would be a situation in which the cyst still is limited as to size, and apparently does not originate from teeth that are present in the region in which it occurs. A cyst that is situated posterior to a third molar and that is not attached to that tooth might justifiably be diagnosed as a primordial cyst. Such a cyst is illustrated in Figure 13–17. It has a circular cavity and does not come in contact with the crown or apex of the root of the tooth. The cyst wall was not attached to the lateral surface of the root of the third molar. Another possible primordial cyst is shown in Figure 13–18. It occurred in a pa-

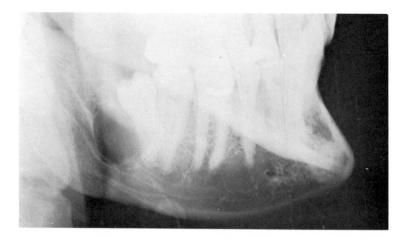

Figure 13-17 Primordial cyst situated posterior to the mandibular third molar, but not attached to the tooth.

tient 13 years of age. It was situated between a mandibular canine and a first premolar and had caused separation of the two teeth. The teeth were vital and, other than bulging of the buccal plate of the mandible and malposition of the teeth, there were no symptoms. The normal number of permanent teeth were present, but since supernumerary premolars are not unusual, it is conceivable that the cyst could have arisen from a supernumerary tooth bud. The cyst was lined with epithelium.

Dentigerous (follicular) cysts are most often lined with a fairly even, uniform layer of squamous epithelium. In rare instances they may be lined with ciliated columnar epithelium (Marsland and Browne, 1965). Gorlin (1957) made a microscopic study of the lining and walls of 200 mandibular dentigerous cysts and from his findings called attention to the potentialities of oral epithelium in such cysts. Since Cahn (1933) reported a case of ame-

loblastoma that had its origin from a dentigerous cyst, many similar cases have been reported.

CALCIFYING ODONTOGENIC CYST

The calcifying odontogenic cyst is one in which the walls are calcified. Most of them are situated within bone, and a few may occur as a cystic mass within the gingiva. They occur more frequently in the mandile than in the maxilla, and they seem to have no significant predilection for either sex. The ages of the patients have ranged from 8 to 74 years. According to Gorlin and colleagues (1962), the basal cells of the cyst become columnar and have the appearance of enamel epithelium. The epithelial layer becomes progressively thicker, and the mural cells develop into large ghost cells. Granulation tissue originating from the connective tissue capsule

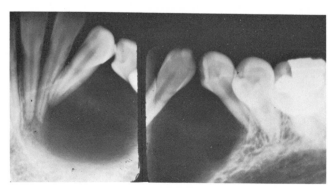

Figure 13-18 Epithelium-lined cyst of the mandible that might be a primordial cyst.

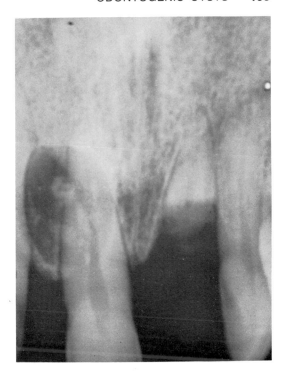

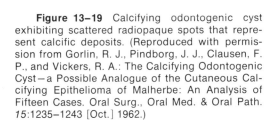

Figure 13–19 Calcifying odontogenic cyst exhibiting scattered radiopaque spots that represent calcific deposits. (Reproduced with permission from Gorlin, R. J., Pindborg, J. J., Clausen, F. P., and Vickers, R. A.: The Calcifying Odontogenic Cyst—a Possible Analogue of the Cutaneous Calcifying Epithelioma of Malherbe: An Analysis of Fifteen Cases. Oral Surg., Oral Med. & Oral Path. *15*:1235–1243 [Oct.] 1962.)

grows up between the ghost cells, and in this tissue a dentin-like material may form. The ghost cells have an affinity for calcium salts, which are deposited when the cells become more homogeneous.

The cyst is seen in the roentgenogram as a unilocular cystic space. In some patients the space may be uniformly radiolucent, like that of a cyst lined by simple stratified squamous epithelium. However, where an appreciable amount of calcific deposition has occurred, scattered radiopaque spots are present at the borders and also within the radiolucent space (Fig. 13–19).

The cystic walls are relatively thick and the cysts are readily enucleated (Gold, 1963). In 1 of the 15 cases reported by Gorlin and colleagues (1962), the cyst recurred 2 years after removal; therefore, one cannot have complete assurance that it will not recur.

MULTILOCULAR CYSTS

Odontogenic cysts are rarely multilocular. When two or more of them are seen adjacent to one another with thin septa separating them, it is likely that they have originated from separate sites and that as they have enlarged they have encroached upon one another. However, many of them cannot be explained on this basis. When multilocular cysts are encountered in the edentulous jaw it is uncertain whether they are of periodontal or follicular origin. A multilocular cyst involving the ramus and a portion of the body of the mandible and containing several separate compartments, all of them lined with stratified squamous epithelium, is shown in Figure 13–20.

It is not uncommon for a single cyst to produce varied degrees of destruction and invasion of the cortex, and to give roentgenographically the impression that distinct and separate compartments are present. A lateral view of a mandible that contained a monocystic epithelium-lined cyst is shown in Figure 13–21 *(above)*. From this view it appears that two separate cysts are present. However, the anteroposterior view *(below)* reveals that it is a single cavity. The illusion that there are two cysts is created because the cortex of the

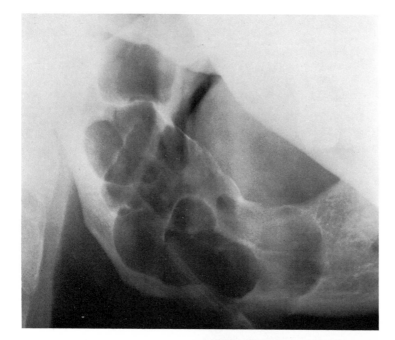

Figure 13–20 Multilocular cyst of the mandible showing several separate compartments, each of which was lined with stratified squamous epithelium.

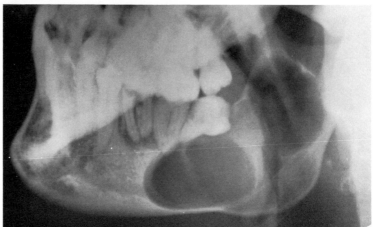

Figure 13–21 Unilocular cyst. *Above,* Lateral view gives the illusion of two separate compartments. *Below,* Anteroposterior view reveals that the cyst contains one compartment only.

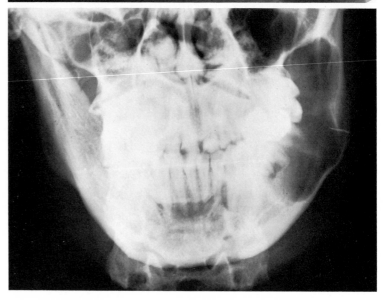

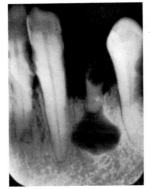
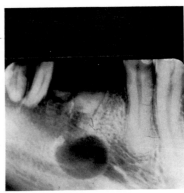

Figure 13–22 *Left*, Periodontal cyst that may persist when the premolar root to which it is attached has exfoliated. *Right*, Periodontal cyst that has become separated from a root which has moved upward and away from it in the process of exfoliation.

buccal plate has undergone less resorption at a point about midway between the anterior and posterior limits of the cyst.

RESIDUAL CYSTS

A residual cyst may be defined as a cyst that still remains in the jaw after the tooth from which it originated is no longer present. This tooth may have exfoliated or it may have been removed surgically. Nearly all residual cysts are periodontal, although on rare occasions a dentigerous cyst may persist after removal of an unerupted tooth.

The incidence of cyst formation with teeth that have extensive untreated caries is relatively high and, as the caries extends rootward, the roots tend to exfoliate. If a periodontal cyst is present it may be left behind when the root sloughs from its socket. The root may become separated from the cyst prior to the time the root is exfoliated completely (Fig. 13–22).

Any cyst may be retained if it is not completely enucleated or if other measures are not taken to destroy it at the time of extraction of the tooth from which it arose. In the absence of preoperative roentgenograms, this could readily occur. Cysts that have a pedunculated form with a constriction near the apex of the root of the tooth would be most prone to be unaffected or undestroyed by extraction of the tooth (Fig. 13–23). The possibility of continued growth of the cyst may be unaltered after loss of the tooth.

The typical roentgenographic appear-

ance of residual epithelium-lined cysts of the maxilla is illustrated in Figure 13–24, and a similar residual cyst of the mandible is shown in Figure 13–25.

Cysts have been observed which are lined with ciliated columnar epithelium and are located near the maxillary sinus, but do not communicate with it. Gregory and Shafer (1958) reported three such cases, all of them in patients who had had previous Caldwell-Luc operations. They concluded that the epithelial lining was derived from cells of the antral mucosa that had been trapped in the wound during closure of the incision and had subsequently proliferated to form the cyst.

It is also possible that such cysts may result from entrapment of a portion of the antral mucosa in a root socket during extraction of a tooth (Royer and Stafne, 1964).

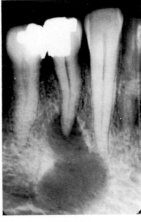

Figure 13–23 Pedunculated periodontal cyst.

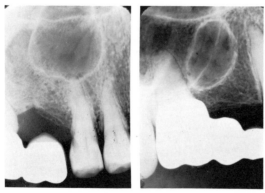

Figure 13–24 Residual epithelium-lined cysts of the maxilla.

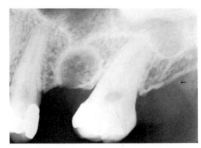

Figure 13–26 Cyst lined with epithelium derived from the antral mucosa. (Reproduced with permission from Royer, R. Q. and Stafne, E. C.: Cyst of Jaw Lined with Ciliated Epithelium. Oral Surg., Oral Med. & Oral Path. *18*:14–15 [July] 1964.)

On delivery of a tooth that is in very close contact with the maxillary sinus, it is not unusual to find a portion of the wall of the sinus and fragments of the antral mucosa attached to its root. A cyst that was lined with ciliated columnar epithelium and that no doubt had its source from epithelium of the antral mucosa is illustrated in Figure 13–26. It is situated in an edentulous first molar space. Roentgenographically there is a suggestion of a small tract leading to the sinus, but when the cyst was removed it was found that the cavity it occupied did not communicate with the maxillary sinus. In this case, a Caldwell-Luc operation had not been performed. The first molar had been extracted 5 years previously.

In some instances a cyst that may have become infected prior to or following extraction of the tooth may establish a draining sinus to the oral cavity and slowly undergo degeneration. When this occurs, the typical roentgenographic appearance of an epithelium-lined cyst disappears. The fine radiopaque line that depicted the border of the cyst tends to vanish, and evidence of new bone formation may be present at the periphery of the cystic cavity (Fig. 13–27); epithelial remnants of the former lining of the cyst may or may not be present in the tissue that then occupies the cavity.

In rare instances a cyst may disappear completely when there is no demonstrable drainage or communication between it and the oral cavity, although it is conceivable that the drainage may be so slight that it cannot be detected. Such a case is illustrated in Figure 13–28. The upper roentgenograms were made for a woman 55 years of age. They revealed a cyst that no doubt arose from the missing second premolar. The lower roentgenograms, made 10 years later, revealed that the cavity formerly occupied by the cyst had been replaced completely by bone. No surgical measures had been taken either to drain or to remove the cyst. Portions of the new bone are sclerotic and of greater radiographic density than normal bone, a not unusual characteristic of bone that replaces cavities in bone that has previously contained cysts or other lesions.

Spontaneous degeneration of a cyst occurs so rarely as compared with continuation of growth that postponement of surgical measures to eradicate such a cyst is not justified.

The rate of growth of odontogenic cysts varies greatly, and it appears that once the cyst develops, the growth most often is continuous until it has reached a

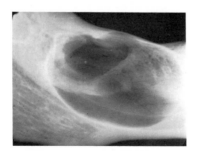

Figure 13–25 Residual epithelium-lined cyst of the mandible.

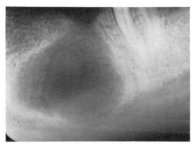

Figure 13–27 Residual cyst with patent sinus leading to the surface of the alveolar ridge. The cystic cavity is being replaced with new bone.

given size. Its size, in some instances, reaches a maximum only when the cyst has perforated the cortical plate and drainage to the outside has been established. A few cysts have been observed in which there has been no increase in size over periods as long as 18 years. In rare instances a cyst may disappear completely for reasons that are obscure. Of the cysts of the jaw, the odontogenic ones present the most difficulty from a clinical standpoint. They may develop at any time during life, and a large

portion of them grow extensively. Therefore, it is well to destroy them when they are first observed.

ODONTOGENIC KERATOCYSTS

Odontogenic keratocysts are those cysts that occur in the jaws and exhibit keratinization of their epithelial lining. The basal cell layer is composed of either columnar or cuboidal cells. There also may be a budding-like hyperplasia of the basal cell layer and microcysts in the wall of the cyst, particularly in those associated with the multiple basal cell nevus syndrome (with which the incidence of occurrence is very high).

Payne (1972) examined 1313 odontogenic cysts and, of these, 103 fulfilled the histologic criteria for odontogenic keratocysts, an incidence of 7.8%. Of the various types of clinical cysts, the keratocysts were found to be most frequently associated with unerupted teeth and were not associated with edentulous areas. Among 659

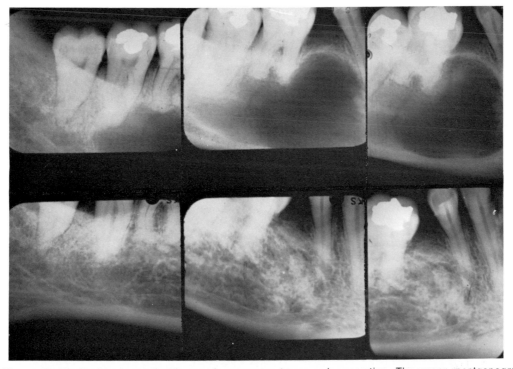

Figure 13–28 Residual cyst that has undergone spontaneous degeneration. The upper roentgenograms were made 10 years prior to those shown below. (Reproduced with permission from Stafne, E. C. and Millhon, J. A.: Periodontal Cysts. J. Oral Surg. 3:102–111 [Apr.] 1945.)

radicular cysts examined, the incidence of keratinization was less than 1%.

The significance of odontogenic keratocysts is the great potential for recurrence after their removal. Among the results of follow-up studies one may find Rud and Pindborg's (1969) recurrence rate of 33% and Payne's (1972) rate of 45%; in one patient, the keratocyst recurred 18 years after the original operation.

There is no specific roentgenographic feature that distinguishes the odontogenic keratocyst from the nonkeratinized odontogenic cyst. Keratocysts may be monolocular or multilocular. That keratinization is most often associated with follicular, residual, or primordial cysts and rarely with radicular cysts probably should be kept in mind.

NONODONTOGENIC EPITHELIUM-LINED CYSTS

CYSTS OF THE INCISIVE CANAL (NASOPALATINE CYSTS)

Of the cysts of the jaw, those that arise from epithelial remnants in the incisive canal are probably the most common. Burket (1937) found microscopic evidence of cyst formation in this region in approximately two-thirds of a series of cases; therefore, it seems quite possible that a cyst of sufficient size to be seen in the roentgenogram can occur in this region.

There are several types of epithelium that may line a cyst of the incisive canal. The type found in a given case probably depends on where it originated in the canal (Stafne et al., 1936). Cysts that arise in the upper portion of the canal may be lined with pseudostratified columnar or columnar epithelium, most often ciliated; those that develop in the middle portion may be lined with primitive or cuboidal epithelium; and those that develop in the lower portion of the canal may be lined with squamous epithelium. Those that are lined with stratified squamous epithelium occur most frequently. However, in a cyst of appreciable size, it may not be possible to determine from what portion of the canal it had its origin, since in some instances the lining of the same cyst may contain two or more types of epithelium.

The wall of the cyst may contain glandular structures, and most often nasopalatine vessels and nerves are present. Abrams and colleagues (1963) have expressed the opinion that the microscopic identification of nerves and blood vessels close to the cystic lumen is the most reliable indication of the presence of a cyst of the incisive canal.

Meyer (1931) was among the first to discuss the anatomic features of the canal, and to describe the typical roentgenographic appearance of these cysts. The anterior palatine system of canals consists of four canals: two minor canals (Scarpa) which are situated in the median line, and two major ones (Stenson) which are lateral canals. The four canals may extend down-

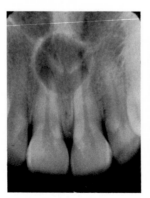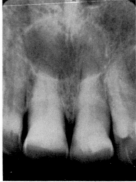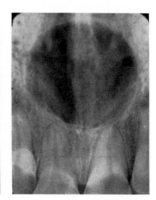

Figure 13–29 Cysts of the incisive canal situated in the median line and extending laterally to both sides.

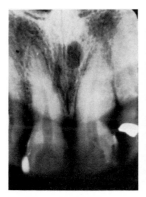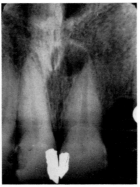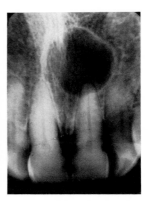

Figure 13–30 Cysts of the incisive canal that have developed in a major lateral canal and extend laterally to one side only.

ward separately to their termination at the anterior palatine foramen, or they may fuse to form a common canal before the foramen has been reached. This anatomic variation may account for the variable location that a cyst of the incisive canal assumes in relation to the median line. In most cases it is situated in the midline and extends laterally to both sides (Fig. 13–29). In some instances it may develop in either the left or the right major lateral canal (Stenson). In this event it extends laterally to one side only. Three such cysts of varied sizes are shown in Figure 13–30. In rare instances cysts may develop independently of one another in both the right and left Stenson canals and form a heart-shaped image in the roentgenogram, as in the three roentgenograms in Figure 13–31. In occlusal film views, the superimposition of the nasal spine may give the impression that there are two cysts present when there is actually only one. In general, the roentgenographic appearance of cysts of the incisive canal is similar to that of odontogenic cysts, although there is a tendency for more of them to be globular.

Cysts of the incisive canal usually are limited as to size. The bone cavity that such a cyst occupies is not closed but communicates directly with the oral and nasal cavities, and drainage of the contents of the cyst to the surfaces may take place to inhibit continued growth. This drainage may be constant or intermittent, and so scant that it cannot be detected grossly. With the aid of a small probe the opening of a small tract leading to the cystic cavity sometimes may be found adjacent to the anterior palatine papilla. On occasion there is continued

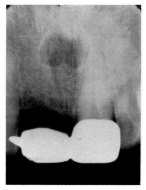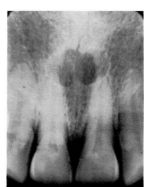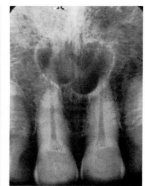

Figure 13–31 Cysts of the incisive canal that have developed independently of one another in each of the two major lateral canals.

growth, and almost always the greatest expansion of the cyst takes place upward and posteriorly in the palate.

A cyst of the incisive canal that has reached an appreciable size by extension upward and posteriorly into the palate is shown in Figure 13–32. Such a cyst, because of its location, might be referred to as a median cyst; however, in the removal of such a cyst and those of intermediate size as well, it will be found that the incisive canal, as such, has been obliterated, and that the contents of the canal are situated within the wall of the cyst; therefore, it is most plausible to infer that these cysts arise in the incisive canal. The dental roentgenogram of one that involves almost the entire palate is shown in Figure 13–33. All the teeth present are vital, and the only clinical evidence of its presence is a slight bulging of the palate. The radiopaque line that follows the median line in the roentgenogram and gives one the impression that two cysts are present is produced by the base of the nasal septum. On removal, the cyst proved to be unilocular, with the contents of the incisive canal attached to the wall of the cyst.

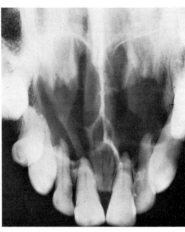

Figure 13–33 Cyst of the incisive canal involving the entire hard palate. This cyst proved to be unilocular. (Reproduced with permission from Stafne, E. C. and Austin, L. T.: Further Observations on Median Anterior Maxillary Cysts. J. Am. Dent. A. *24*:957–963 [June] 1937.)

A few of these cysts have been observed for a period of several years, and those that have increased in size have done so relatively slowly. The roentgenograms of such a cyst are shown in Figure 13–34. The roentgenogram on the left was made 8 years prior to the one on the right, and the increase in size over that period is not great.

Infrequently concrements or stones form within the lumen of cysts of the in-

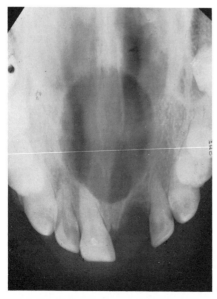

Figure 13–32 Cyst of the incisive canal that has extended posteriorly to involve an appreciable portion of the hard palate. (Courtesy of Dr. O. E. Ranfranz, Houston, Texas.)

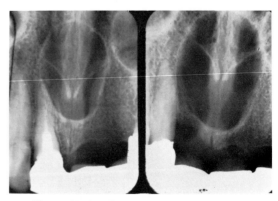

Figure 13–34 Cyst of the incisive canal in which growth is demonstrated. The roentgenogram on the left was made 8 years prior to the one on the right. (Reproduced with permission from Stafne, E. C., Austin, L. T., and Gardner, B. S.: Median Anterior Maxillary Cysts. J. Am. Dent. A. *23*:801–809 [May] 1936.)

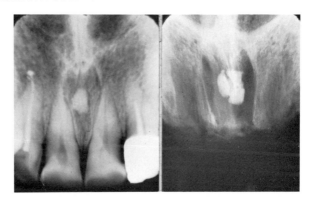

Figure 13–35 Cysts of the incisive canal with concrements. *Left,* Cyst containing one stone. *Right,* Cyst containing two stones. (Reproduced with permission from Lovestedt, S. A. and Bruce, K. W.: Cysts of the Incisive Canal with Concrements. J. Oral Surg. *12*:48–53 [Jan.] 1954.)

cisive canal (Lovestedt and Bruce, 1954). If the cyst becomes infected, tissue debris that is sloughed into the lumen is a potential nidus on which cholesterol or calcium salts can be deposited. Usually in such cases a patent duct of varied size extends from the cyst to the surface of the palate, and spontaneous sloughing of stones through such a duct has been observed. The stones are dense and homogeneous, and have no laminations. In the roentgenogram they are seen as radiopaque bodies situated in the midline, and they are more readily recognized in the customary views made with the intraoral dental film (Fig. 13–35). In the occlusal views they may be obscured by superimposition of the anterior nasal spine and by the junction of the hard palate and the nasal septum.

Cysts of the incisive canal most often remain limited as to size and are asymptomatic. Some of them, however, become infected or show a tendency to grow exten-

sively. When this occurs, surgical intervention is indicated. This may consist of drainage or surgical removal of the cyst. In either event, the approach should be palatal, since this affords better access and provides the lowest point of drainage. Delayed healing and possible devitalization of the incisor teeth usually follow when the labial approach is used. The roentgenogram of a patient in whom the labial approach was employed is shown in Figure 13–36. The left lateral and both central incisors had been rendered pulpless, and there was a purulent discharge from the wound 9 months after operation.

CYSTS OF THE PAPILLA PALATINA

A cyst may arise from the contents of the incisive canal at the site of emergence

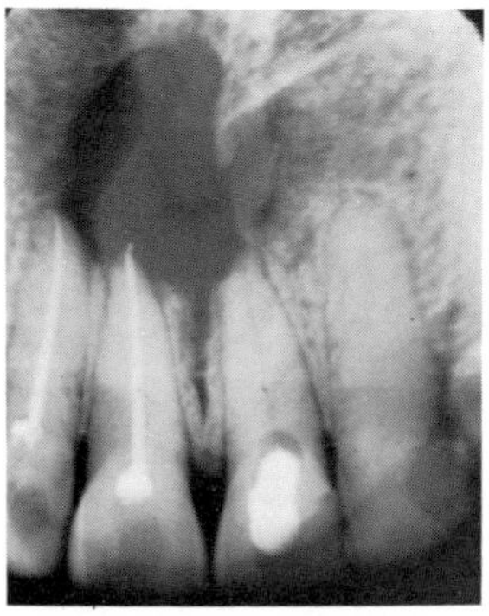

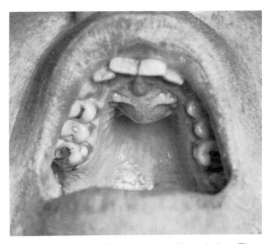

Figure 13–36 Devitalization of the pulps of three incisor teeth following removal of a cyst of the incisive canal from a labial approach.

Figure 13–37 Cyst of the papilla palatina. There was no roentgenographic evidence of its presence.

from the anterior palatine canal. A cyst in this region has been referred to by Thoma (1954) as a cyst of the papilla palatina. It appears as a round soft swelling that extends posteriorly along the midline of the palate, and the anterior palatine papilla is somewhat elevated by the underlying cyst (Fig. 13–37). Such a cyst produces little if any pressure resorption of bone; therefore, there usually is no roentgenographic evidence of its presence.

GLOBULOMAXILLARY CYSTS

The so-called globulomaxillary cyst is situated between the lateral incisor and the canine tooth at the site that corresponds to the incisive suture. It usually extends well down toward the crest of the alveolar ridge, and as it increases in size it may produce a divergence of the roots of the adjoining teeth and assume a pear-shaped appearance (Fig. 13–38). It may extend over the apex of the root of one or both of the adjacent teeth, in which event it is important to determine the vitality of the tooth in question in order to differentiate it from a radicular cyst.

The statement that the globulomaxillary cyst forms at the fusion of the globular and maxillary processes disregards embryologic findings (Ferenczy, 1958; Sicher, 1962). The globular process and the maxillary process are from the beginning united and both take part in the formation of the premaxilla. Therefore, the point of fusion of the globular and maxillary processes cannot correspond to the junction of the premaxilla and maxilla where the incisive suture is found, namely, between the lateral incisor and the canine tooth.

While the term "globulomaxillary" is no doubt incorrect, the origin of the cyst is as yet not clear. There is even considerable doubt that it is a fissural cyst. Similar cysts lined with squamous epithelium have occurred in all interdental spaces anterior to the first molar, and whether these as well as the cyst that is situated between the lateral incisor and the canine have a common origin is problematic. Microscopically, three cases reported by Christ (1970) suggested odontogenic keratocysts, a finding that would support the contention that the cysts are odontogenic in origin.

CONDITIONS THAT SIMULATE EPITHELIUM-LINED CYSTS

SOLITARY BONE CYSTS OF THE MANDIBLE (TRAUMATIC)

A solitary bone cyst of the mandible, which also is referred to as a traumatic, hemorrhagic, or extravasation cyst, is a closed compartment that has a connective-tissue lining of varied thickness. In some instances the lining may be so thin that it cannot be removed intact. The cyst may contain blood, serosanguineous fluid, debris composed chiefly of blood clot, and an occasional giant cell; or it may be completely devoid of solid material. It occurs most frequently in younger persons. While there may be no single common cause for the occurrence of these cysts, it is most generally believed that they result from injury (Ivy and Curtis, 1937; Olech et al., 1951; and Waldron, 1954). An injury sustained by a younger person at a time when the bone is resilient does not easily produce a fracture; however, it may cause an intramedullary hematoma which may undergo disintegration and, as a result, produce a cyst within the bone. A cyst so formed may continue to increase in size until it has become exten-

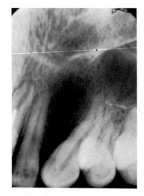

Figure 13–38 Globulomaxillary cyst. (Reproduced with permission from Stafne, E. C.: Globulomaxillary Cyst: Report of a Case. Am. J. Orthodontics [Oral Surg. Sec.] *33*:595–596 [Aug.] 1947.)

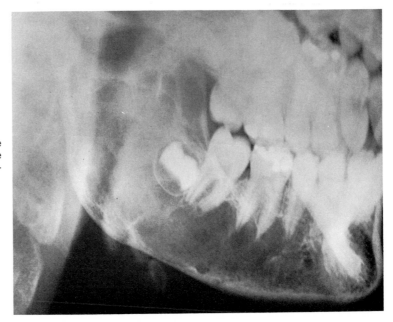

Figure 13–39 Solitary bone cyst involving the body of the mandible and the ramus in a patient 12 years of age.

sive or, in some instances, it may regress spontaneously. In some cases it is difficult to elicit a history of injury, particularly if the presence of the cyst does not come to light for several years after the injury was sustained. It also is believed that some of these cysts represent giant cell lesions that have undergone spontaneous degeneration and cure. A case in which such a cyst of the mandible seemed to be related to a previously existing giant cell reparative granuloma has been reported by Huebner and Turlington (1971). The most common location is the mandibular marrow space that extends posteriorly from the premolar region. More rarely these cysts occur in the incisor region.

The roentgenographic appearance is somewhat dependent on the size and location of the cyst. In general, the borders are not as well defined as, and are more irregular than, those of epithelium-lined cysts. One that occurs in the posterior region is seen as a fairly well-defined area of radio-

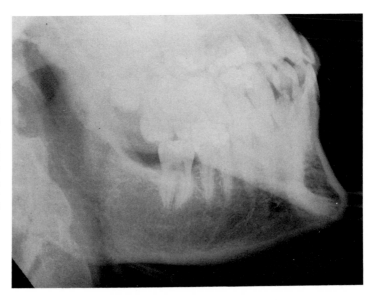

Figure 13–40 Postoperative roentgenogram made 11 months after conservative treatment of the cyst illustrated in Figure 13–39. It revealed that the space formerly occupied by the cyst had become filled with bone, and that the normal cortex had reappeared at the inferior border of the mandible.

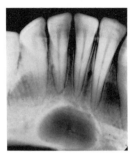

Figure 13-41 Solitary bone cyst in the region of the symphysis.

lucence that tends to conform in shape to the marrow space. When of larger size, it extends upward into the interdental space and also into the ramus, where it may occupy a portion or all of it, and there also may be thinning and expansion of the cortex (Fig. 13-39). The postoperative roentgenogram is shown in Figure 13-40. A mandibular bone cyst that occurs in the anterior region is most often round or oval (Fig. 13-41), a picture that may be very similar to those representing salivary gland inclusions or the rare occurrence of a fissural cyst in this region.

On the basis of roentgenograms made for young persons, there is reason to be-lieve that a solitary cyst may regress spontaneously. Such an instance in a patient 18 years of age is shown in Figure 13-42. Since no biopsy was done, it may be presumptuous to assume that the radiolucent area in the roentgenogram (*above*) represents an extravasation cyst; however, the appearance is strikingly similar to one. A roentgenogram made 5 years later (*below*) revealed that bone had assumed normal radiographic density and trabecular pattern. Szerlip (1966) reported the case of a 15-year-old girl in whom similar cystic spaces in the mandible had been replaced by normal bone within a period of 4½ years, and without surgical intervention. It should be kept in mind, however, that roentgenograms made for patients in the teen age sometimes reveal marrow spaces in the posterior regions of the mandible that appear to be abnormally radiolucent, but these do not present well-defined borders.

Since there may be no symptoms referable to these cysts, many of them are first noted only incidental to routine roentgenographic examination. While a diagnosis based on roentgenographic evidence alone is suggestive, it is not suffi-

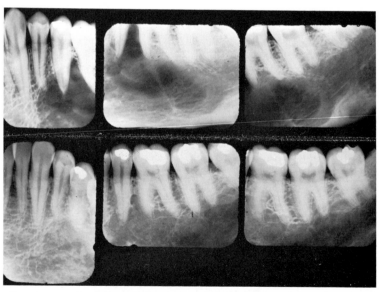

Figure 13-42 Spontaneous healing of what may have been a solitary bone cyst. *Above,* View at 18 years of age. *Below,* View at 23 years of age. (Reproduced with permission from Stafne, E. C.: Value of Roentgenograms in Diagnosis of Tumors of the Jaws. Oral Surg., Oral Med. & Oral Path. 6:82–92 [Jan.] 1953.)

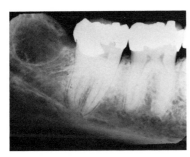

Figure 13-43 Bone cavity that contained petrolatum.

ciently reliable, for the lesion may be of a more serious nature. If it is a solitary bone cyst, there is no way of knowing whether it is static or is increasing in size. Surgical intervention, therefore, is indicated, a measure that invariably leads to successful elimination of the cyst and also serves to arrive at a correct diagnosis.

BONE CAVITY CONTAINING PETROLATUM

A bone cavity that is identical to that presented by a residual epithelium-lined cyst is shown in Figure 13-43. It is globular and is situated in the third molar region. The patient stated that an impacted third molar had been removed 5 years previously. At the current operation it was found that the cavity contained petrolatum. The cavity was lined with fibrous tissue, but there was no epithelium present. The petrolatum no doubt had been used as a vehicle for introducing sulfonamides or other drugs into the socket after removal of the tooth. Although inclusion of petrolatum occurs only rarely when so used, it is well to use a readily absorbed vehicle.

REFERENCES

Abrams, A. M., Howell, F. V., and Bullock, W. K.: Nasopalatine Cysts. Oral Surg., Oral Med. & Oral Path. *16*:306–332 (Mar.) 1963.

Burket, L. W.: Nasopalatine Duct Structures and Peculiar Bone Pattern Observed in Anterior Maxillary Region. Arch. Path. *23*:793–800 (June) 1937.

Cahn, L. R.: The Dentigerous Cyst as a Potential Adamantinoma. Dent. Cosmos. 75:889–893 (Sept.) 1933.

Christ, T. F.: The Globulomaxillary Cyst: An Embryologic Misconception. Oral Surg., Oral Med. & Oral Path. *30*:515–526 (Oct.) 1970.

Conklin, W. W. and Stafne, E. C.: A Study of Odontogenic Epithelium in the Dental Follicle. J. Am. Dent. A. *39*:143–148 (Aug.) 1949.

Ferenczy, K.: The Relationship of Globulomaxillary Cysts to the Fusion of Embryonal Processes and to Cleft Palates. Oral Surg., Oral Med. & Oral Path. *11*:1388–1393 (Dec.) 1958.

Gillette, R., and Weinmann, J. P.: Extrafollicular Stages in Dentigerous Cyst Development. Oral Surg., Oral Med. & Oral Path. *11*:638–645 (June) 1958.

Gold, L.: The Keratinizing and Calcifying Odontogenic Cyst. Oral Surg., Oral Med. & Oral Path. *16*:1414–1424 (Dec.) 1963.

Gorlin, R. J.: Potentialities of Oral Epithelium Manifest by Mandibular Dentigerous Cysts. Oral Surg., Oral Med. & Oral Path. *10*:271–284 (Mar.) 1957.

Gorlin, R. J., Pindborg, J. J., Clausen, F. P., and Vickers, R. A.: The Calcifying Odontogenic Cyst—A Possible Analogue of the Cutaneous Calcifying Epithelioma of Malherbe: An Analysis of Fifteen Cases. Oral Surg., Oral Med. & Oral Path. *15*:1235–1243 (Oct.) 1962.

Gregory, G. T. and Shafer, W. G.: Surgical Ciliated Cysts of the Maxilla: Report of Cases. J. Oral Surg. *16*:251–253 (May) 1958.

Hill, T. J.: Epithelium in Dental Granulomata. J. Dent. Res. *10*:323–332 (June) 1930.

Huebner, G. R. and Turlington, E. G.: So-called Traumatic (Hemorrhagic) Bone Cysts of the Jaws: Review of the Literature and Report of Two Unusual Cases. Oral Surg., Oral Med. & Oral Path. *31*:354–365 (Mar.) 1971.

Ivy, R. H. and Curtis, L.: Hemorrhagic or Traumatic Cysts of Mandible. Surg., Gynec. & Obst. 65:640–643 (Nov.) 1937.

James, W. W.: Do Epithelial Odontomes Increase in Size by Their Own Tension? Proc. Roy. Soc. Med. (Section of Odontology). *19*(pt. 3):73–76 (Apr. 26) 1926.

Kronfeld, R.: Histopathology of the Teeth and Their Surrounding Structures. Ed. 2. Philadelphia, Lea & Febiger, 1939, pp. 195–199.

Lovestedt, S. A. and Bruce, K. W.: Cysts of the Incisive Canal with Concrements. J. Oral Surg. *12*:48–53 (Jan.) 1954.

Marsland, E. A. and Browne, R. M.: Two Odontogenic Cysts, Partially Lined with Ciliated Columnar Epithelium. Oral Surg., Oral Med. & Oral Path. *19*:502–507 (Apr.) 1965.

Meyer, A. W.: Median Anterior Maxillary Cysts. J. Am. Dent. A. *18*:1851–1877 (Oct.) 1931.

Olech, E., Sicher, H., and Weinmann, J. P.: Traumatic Mandibular Bone Cysts. Oral Surg., Oral Med. & Oral Path. *4*:1160–1172 (Sept.) 1951.

Orban, B.: Epithelial Rests in Teeth and Their Supporting Structures. Proc. Am. A. Dent. Schools. 5:121–134, 1928.

Payne, T. F.: An Analysis of the Clinical and Histopathologic Parameters of the Odontogenic Keratocyst. Oral Surg., Oral Med. & Oral Path. *33*:538–546 (Apr.) 1972.

Robinson, H. B. G.: Classification of Cysts of Jaws.

Am. J. Orthodontics (Oral Surg. Sect.). *31*:370–375 (June) 1945.

Royer, R. Q. and Stafne, E. C.: Cyst of Jaw Lined with Ciliated Epithelium. Oral Surg., Oral Med. & Oral Path. *18*:14–15 (July) 1964.

Rud, J. and Pindborg, J. J.: Odontogenic Keratocysts: A Follow-up Study of 21 Cases. J. Oral Surg. *27*:323–330 (May) 1969.

Sicher, H.: Anatomy and Oral Pathology. Oral Surg., Oral Med. & Oral Path. *15*:1264–1269 (Oct.) 1962.

Stafne, E. C.: Possible Role of Retained Deciduous Roots in Etiology of Cysts of Jaw. J. Am. Dent. A. *24*:1488–1493 (Sept.) 1937.

Stafne, E. C., Austin, L. T., and Gardner, B. S.: Median Anterior Maxillary Cysts. J. Am. Dent. A. *23*:801–809 (May) 1936.

Stafne, E. C. and Millhon, J. A.: Periodontal Cysts. J. Oral Surg. *3*:102–111 (Apr.) 1945.

Szerlip, L.: Traumatic Bone Cysts: Resolution Without Surgery. Oral Surg., Oral Med. & Oral Path. *21*:201–204 (Feb.) 1966.

Thoma, K. H.: Oral Pathology: A Histological, Roentgenological, and Clinical Study of the Diseases of the Teeth, Jaws, and Mouth. Ed. 4. St. Louis, The C. V. Mosby Company, 1954, pp. 834–835.

Toller, P.: Origin and Growth of Cysts of the Jaws. Ann. Roy. Coll. Surg. Engl. *40*:306–336 (May) 1967.

Waldron, C. A.: Solitary (Hemorrhagic) Cyst of Mandible. Oral Surg., Oral Med. & Oral Path. *7*:88–95 (Jan.) 1954.

ODONTOGENIC TUMORS

14

Odontogenic tumors result from abnormal proliferation of cells and tissues that are involved in odontogenesis. A classification of benign odontogenic tumors (Pindborg, 1970) has divided them into epithelial and mesodermal tumors. The epithelial tumors have been further subdivided according to whether or not inductive changes are present in the connective tissue (Table 1). The tumors dealt with in this chapter do not include all those listed, but in general this classification has been adhered to.

The roentgenographic appearance of odontogenic tumors varies, depending on their nature, location, and stage of development. Ameloblastomas, odontogenic myxomas, and ameloblastic fibromas that occur in the coronal region may resemble dentigerous cysts. Cementifying fibromas (cementomas) may, in their early stage of development, resemble periodontal (radicular) cysts or dental granulomas. Those in which evidence of calcification is present, notably mixed odontogenic tumors and cementomas, can be diagnosed fairly reliably from the roentgenographic appearance alone. A characteristic of calcified odontogenic tumors is that they do not fuse with the normal surrounding bone, but remain encapsulated by connective tissue; this feature is evidenced roentgenographically by a radiolucent line or area that separates the tumor from the bone.

Table 1. Classification of Benign Odontogenic Tumors*

Epithelial odontogenic tumors
  Without inductive changes in connective tissue
    Ameloblastoma
    Calcifying epithelial odontogenic tumor
  With inductive changes in connective tissue
    Adenomatoid odontogenic tumor
    Ameloblastic fibroma
    Dentinoma
    Calcifying odontogenic cyst
    Odontoameloblastoma
    Odontomas
      Ameloblastic fibro-odontoma
      Complex odontoma
      Compound odontoma

Mesodermal odontogenic tumors
  Odontogenic fibroma
  Odontogenic myxoma
  Cementomas
    Periapical cemental dysplasia
    Cementifying fibroma
    Benign cementoblastoma
    Gigantiform cementoma

---

*Reproduced with permission from Pindborg, J. J.: Pathology of the Dental Hard Tissues. Philadelphia, W. B. Saunders Company, 1970, p. 368.

EPITHELIAL ODONTOGENIC TUMORS WITHOUT INDUCED CHANGES

AMELOBLASTOMA

The ameloblastoma contains ameloblasts which have differentiated from ectodermal epithelium, and it may develop from epithelial cells that occur in the enamel organ, follicle, periodontal membrane, epithelium that lines dentigerous cysts, and marrow spaces of the jaws. In

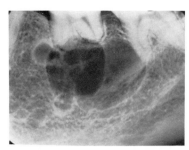

Figure 14–1 Ameloblastoma, showing round cystic spaces of varied size and creating a bubble-like appearance. (Reproduced with permission from Stafne, E. C.: Value of Roentgenograms in Diagnosis of Tumors of Jaws. Oral Surg., Oral Med. & Oral Path. 6:82–92 [Jan.] 1953.)

rare instances it may arise from the surface epithelium, although this would be difficult to determine, for an ameloblastoma that is central in origin often perforates the cortex and invades soft tissue, and becomes contiguous with the surface epithelium.

An ameloblastoma produces more extensive resorption of the roots of the teeth on which it encroaches than do most of the other lesions (Stafne, 1953). If the lesion occupies a single or monocystic cavity only, the roentgenographic diagnosis becomes increasingly difficult because of the striking resemblance to dentigerous cyst and to residual epithelium-lined cyst of the jaw. The tissue of the tumor is more radiopaque than the fluid in an epithelium-lined cyst, but in most instances the difference is so slight that it is not of diagnostic value.

The compartments in bone are rounded and are separated by distinct septa, but there usually is not the fibrillar network that is in evidence in giant cell tumor and fibromyxoma. The compartments vary in size. If there are numerous small compartments, the picture presents a honeycombed appearance. If the compartments are somewhat larger and vary in size, the cyst may have the so-called bubble-like appearance. Those in which the compartments are large and few in number may resemble multilocular epithelium-lined cysts.

An ameloblastoma that is still limited in size and that presents a bubble-like appearance is shown in Figure 14–1. There are two fairly large, round, and distinct compartments, and directly adjacent to one of them are two small round cystic spaces, one at its anterior and the other at its inferior border. The projection of small round compartments into the adjoining bone is very suggestive of ameloblastoma, as is the resorption of the roots of the molar on which it is encroaching.

With growth and expansion of the tumor there may be coalescence and fusion of the compartments, and as a result there is transformation from a multilocular to a monolocular cystic space. Later the lesion that occupies this monolocular space may proliferate into adjacent marrow spaces and form small rounded accessory cysts (Fig. 14–2). Here again the formation of smaller round accessory cysts in the adjoining bone is seen and this appears to be peculiar to ameloblastoma. In evidence also is the resorption of the roots of teeth with which the tumor is in contact.

As the lesion increases in size there is expansion and destruction of the cortex,

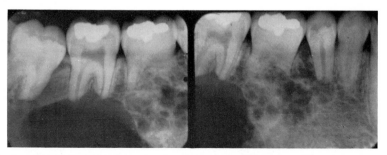

Figure 14–2 Ameloblastoma, showing monolocular lesion with small multilocular spaces adjacent and anterior to it. (Reproduced with permission from Stafne, E. C.: Value of Roentgenograms in Diagnosis of Tumors of Jaws. Oral Surg., Oral Med. & Oral Path. 6:82–92 [Jan.] 1953.)

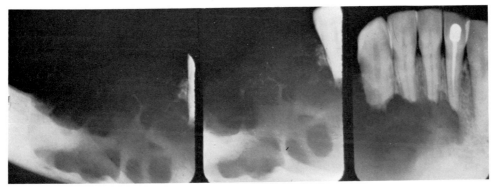

Figure 14–3 Ameloblastoma that has destroyed the cortex and invaded soft tissue.

followed by invasion of the soft tissue. In this respect ameloblastoma differs from fibrous and fibro-osseous lesions, which expand but tend to retain a thin cortex. A roentgenogram of an ameloblastoma of the mandible which reveals destruction of the cortex is shown in Figure 14–3. There are multiple compartments in bone suggestive of ameloblastoma, and there is resorption of the roots of the teeth on which the tumor is encroaching.

An ameloblastoma that resembles closely a multilocular epithelium-lined cyst is shown in Figure 14–4. There are two distinct cystic spaces with well-defined and circumscribed borders situated posterior to the mandibular second molar region. The presence of the mandibular third molar, which has been forced anteriorly, suggests a dentigerous cyst; however, the crown of this tooth is not within the cystic space, and the pericoronal space is intact.

Ameloblastomas that roentgenographically resemble dentigerous cysts have been reported by Cahn (1933), Bailey (1951), and others. A cystic cavity of the mandible into which the crown of an unerupted second molar extends is shown in Figure 14–5. The round shape of the cavity, its even, regular borders, and its position in relation

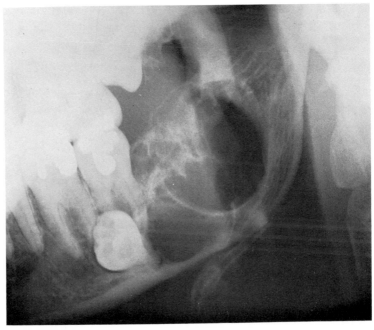

Figure 14–4 Ameloblastoma that roentgenographically resembles a multilocular epithelium-lined cyst.

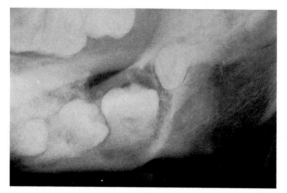

Figure 14-5 Ameloblastoma that roentgenographically resembles a dentigerous cyst.

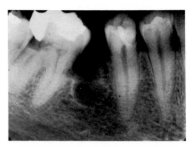

Figure 14-7 Ameloblastoma that occurred in a mandibular first molar edentulous space.

to the unerupted tooth are very suggestive of a dentigerous cyst, but on microscopic examination the contents of the cavity proved it to be ameloblastoma. There is some question whether such an ameloblastoma had its origin from a dentigerous cyst or from epithelium in an enlarged follicle.

An ameloblastoma that roentgenographically resembles a residual epithelium-lined cyst is shown in Figure 14-6. It is round and has a regular, well-defined border. On the left is a roentgenogram made in 1943, 4 years after removal of an embedded third molar. A small defect in the bone was present near the crest of the alveolar ridge, giving a radiolucence that might well be interpreted as a defect following operation. The roentgenogram on the right, made in 1947, revealed a single, circular cavity about 1 cm in diameter. The contents of the cavity proved the tumor to be ameloblastoma. Cahn (1933) has called attention to the possibility that an ameloblastoma may be derived from the follicle, which is not completely removed at the time of removal of an unerupted tooth, and

it is possible that the ameloblastoma present in this instance may have been derived from this source.

The occurrence of ameloblastomas in edentulous spaces from which fully erupted teeth have been extracted some time previously suggests that they might in some instances be derived from epithelial remnants of the periodontal membrane that remain after extraction. The roentgenogram shown in Figure 14-7 reveals a cystic space in an edentulous mandibular first molar region which resembles a residual epithelium-lined cyst, but which on microscopic examination proved to be an ameloblastoma. The molar had been extracted 7 years previously. There was no cortex on the crest of the alveolar ridge, and the lesion was contiguous with the mucous membrane; therefore it also might be contended that it arose from the surface epithelium.

While several variants in the roentgenographic appearance of ameloblastoma have been illustrated, the majority conform to a typical picture in which numerous loculations are present. In a study of 30 cases, Sherman and Caumartin (1955) found that the roentgenographic picture

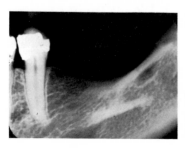
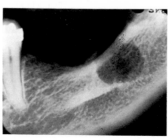

Figure 14-6 Ameloblastoma that roentgenographically resembles a residual epithelium-lined cyst. (Reproduced with permission from Stafne, E. C.: Value of Roentgenograms in Diagnosis of Tumors of Jaws. Oral Surg., Oral Med. & Oral Path. 6:82-92 [Jan.] 1953.)

was characteristic in 24 and stated that a reliable roentgenographic diagnosis in the atypical group appears impossible. A comprehensive article dealing with ameloblastoma has been contributed by Small and Waldron (1955).

ODONTOGENIC ADENOMATOID TUMOR (ADENOAMELOBLASTOMA)

The odontogenic adenomatoid tumor is an epithelial lesion of the jaws that has been recognized as a distinct entity in fairly recent years (Stafne, 1948). It is most frequently associated with unerupted teeth where the epithelial proliferation is confined within a connective-tissue capsule that is attached to the tooth in a manner similar to the attachment of a dentigerous cyst. The tumor also may occur independently of an unerupted tooth, in which instance it also is encapsulated. Most of these tumors are brought to light during the second decade of life, either incidental to routine dental roentgenographic examination or in examinations made to learn the cause for the noneruption of a tooth or to determine the nature of swellings of the jaws that they may produce. Their onset and growth appear to coincide with the time of development of the permanent teeth and most of the odontogenic tumors or hamartomas.

The main cell which forms the bulk of the mass appears to be a regular polyhedral epithelial type of cell with a prominent nucleus and a minimum of cytoplasm. A morphodifferentiation of the basic cells, which is a feature peculiar to the tumor, has been described by Spouge (1967); he has divided the differentiation into three main stages, of which the final one is that of the characteristic spherical duct-like structures lined by ameloblast-like epithelium. However, serial sections have not revealed the presence of ducts; therefore the formation is not that of a conventional gland. There is a variable amount of calcification scattered throughout the lesion. These calcifications appear as rounded, usually structureless, globules which have

some degree of resemblance to cementicles that are associated with remnants of the epithelial root sheath of Hertwig. They tend to occur in grape-like clusters or masses. Such calcifications may be present in sufficient numbers to produce a radiopacity in the roentgenogram.

Giansanti et al. (1970) reviewed 108 cases from the literature and reported 3 additional cases of their own. They found that adenoameloblastoma is predominantly a tumor of young persons; of the 105 cases in which the age was stated, the mean age was 17.8 years. In the 106 cases in which the location was noted, 65% of the tumors occurred in the maxilla and 35% in the mandible. Seventy-six per cent of the lesions occurred in the anterior regions of the jaws, and 74% were definitely associated with unerupted teeth, most often a canine. Roentgenograms that were satisfactory for interpretation invariably revealed that the lesions were monolocular. There was displacement or separation of adjacent roots in 26 cases. Sixty-five per cent of the roentgenograms revealed detectable radiopaque foci representing calcifications that the authors believed might have been odontogenic in origin.

The roentgenogram represented in Figure 14–8, made for a boy 15 years of age, shows a tumor that is associated with

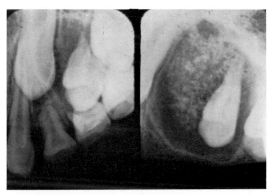

Figure 14–8 Odontogenic adenomatoid tumor associated with an unerupted maxillary first premolar and, on the right, showing roentgenographic evidence of calcification within the tumor. (Reproduced with permission from Stafne, E. C.: Epithelial Tumors Associated with Developmental Cysts of Maxilla: Report of 3 Cases. Oral Surg., Oral Med. & Oral Path. 1:887–894 [Oct.] 1948.)

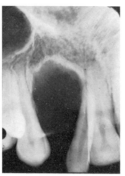

Figure 14–9 Odontogenic adenomatoid tumor located between maxillary canine and lateral incisor. The amount of calcification within the tumor is not sufficient to produce opacity. (Reproduced with permission from Stafne, E. C.: Epithelial Tumors Associated with Developmental Cysts of Maxilla: Report of 3 Cases. Oral Surg., Oral Med. & Oral Path. *1*:887–894 [Oct.] 1948.)

an unerupted tooth and that also contains sufficient calcification to produce a radiopacity. This radiopacity and its association with an unerupted tooth produce a picture which in large measure simulates that of a mixed odontogenic tumor. The tumor had prevented eruption of the first premolar from which it developed and also eruption of the two adjoining teeth.

The roentgenogram represented in

Figure 14–9, made for a girl 14 years of age, shows a tumor in the canine region of the maxilla that was not associated with an unerupted tooth and did not contain sufficient calcification to produce a radiopacity. One could not arrive at a tentative diagnosis on the basis of its roentgenographic appearance, because of the simulation of numerous lesions and cysts that may occur in the jaws.

The tumor may become quite expansive, but unlike the ameloblastoma it is not locally invasive. It is readily removed by simple enucleation or excision, with almost complete assurance that it will not recur. Cina and colleagues (1963) emphasized the importance of correct histologic interpretation and differentiation from ameloblastoma. They reported four cases in which a correct diagnosis had not been made, and in three of them the treatment had been unnecessarily mutilating.

CALCIFYING EPITHELIAL ODONTOGENIC TUMOR (PINDBORG TUMOR)

The calcifying epithelial odontogenic tumor has a predilection for the premolar-

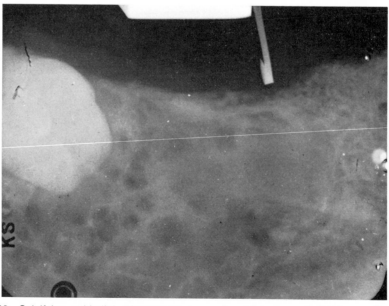

Figure 14–10 Calcifying epithelial odontogenic tumor involving an embedded mandibular third molar. (Reproduced with permission from Shafer, W. G., Hine, M. K., and Levy, B. M.: A Textbook of Oral Pathology. Ed. 2. Philadelphia, W. B. Saunders Company, 1963.)

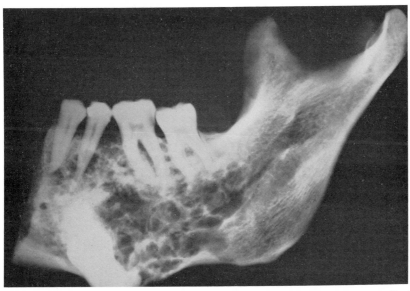

Figure 14–11 Calcifying epithelial odontogenic tumor involving an embedded mandibular first molar, showing extensive invasion and destruction of bone. It has a multilocular, honeycomb appearance. (Reproduced with permission from Pindborg, J. J.: A Calcifying Epithelial Odontogenic Tumor. Cancer, *11*:838–843 [July-Aug.] 1958.)

molar regions, and it occurs in the mandible about twice as often as in the maxilla. The tumor most often grows slowly and is usually first manifested by a painless swelling over the involved region. In a study of 37 cases reported in the literature and an additional 6 cases of their own, Vap et al. (1970) found that 40 of them were intraosseous and 3 of them were located in the overlying soft tissue adjacent to the bone of the jaws. Approximately half are associated with unerupted teeth, and frequently these teeth are those that rarely fail to erupt— namely, first premolars, first molars, and second molars. This suggests that very early onset of the tumor may prevent eruption.

According to Pindborg (1958), the tumor has a peculiar epithelial pattern. There is extensive intracellular degeneration and the degenerated cytoplasm has a great affinity for mineral salts, which are deposited as rings. In some parts of the tumor the calcified cells converge to form masses that appear in the roentgenogram as radiopaque areas. Unlike the ameloblastoma, there are no columnar ameloblast-like cells or central cells similar to stellate reticulum.

The roentgenographic picture is in many respects similar to that exhibited by most ameloblastomas in that it is multiloculated and has a honeycomb appearance. However, the entire lesion is, in general, more radiopaque. The borders are irregular and ill-defined, and this is suggestive of a locally invasive lesion (Figs. 14–10 and 14–11).

The tumor is locally invasive and tends to recur. Clinically, it behaves very much like an ameloblastoma and should be treated accordingly (Shafer et al., 1974).

EPITHELIAL ODONTOGENIC TUMORS WITH INDUCTION (MIXED ODONTOGENIC TUMORS)

The mixed odontogenic tumor results from a proliferation of both elements that play a part in odontogenesis, namely ectoderm and mesoderm. Microscopically, these tumors could be placed in three categories: (1) ameloblastic fibroma (soft mixed odontoma), which consists of epithelial and mesenchymal elements only; (2) ameloblastic odontoma, which contains hard dental structures and a soft-tissue component of odontogenic epithelium and embryonic connective tissue; and (3) complex odontoma, which consists of mature elements of all dental structures, but does not contain the ameloblastic cellular component. The first two categories probably represent varied stages in the development of the complex odontoma. However, a complete stage of induction of the complex odontoma may not always be reached.

AMELOBLASTIC FIBROMA (SOFT MIXED ODONTOMA)

The ameloblastic fibroma develops from the dental follicle usually after the onset of calcification of the tooth. In some instances it may develop in a tooth bud prior to the onset of calcification, in which event formation of the normal tooth is aborted. The tumor results as a proliferation of both epithelial and mesenchymal elements (Shafer, 1955).

The tumor contains strands and buds of epithelium in a connective-tissue stroma, which bears a strong resemblance to the embryonal connective tissue of the dental pulp. The strands resemble dental lamina. Stellate reticulum develops within the larger buds, and the peripheral cells assume a tall columnar appearance similar to that of the inner enamel epithelium of a developing tooth bud. Hard tooth structure is generally absent, although occasional foci of dentin and enamel may be encountered if enough sections are examined (Cina et al., 1961).

The tumor usually occurs within the first two decades of life and with much greater frequency in the mandible than in the maxilla.

The ameloblastic fibroma is seen in the roentgenogram as an area of uniform radiolucency that has a smooth and well-defined border. The appearance of those situated in the pericoronal region of unerupted teeth is similar to that of a dentigerous cyst.

An ameloblastic fibroma that occurred in the pericoronal region is shown in Figure 14–12. A boy, 10 years of age, had a solid swelling over the buccal aspect of the mandible in the region of an unerupted second premolar tooth. The roentgenogram

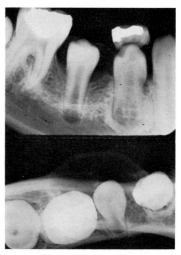

Figure 14–12 Ameloblastic fibroma associated with an unerupted mandibular second premolar. *Above,* Lateral view. *Below,* Occlusal view at reduced exposure to demonstrate the bulge on the buccal surface.

(*upper part*) revealed a well-circumscribed cavity in bone, surrounding the entire crown of the tooth and extending slightly below the cervical margin—a picture very similar to that of a dentigerous cyst. An occlusal view (*lower part* of Figure 14–12) showed expansion of the buccal cortex.

A larger ameloblastic fibroma that occurred in a patient 7 years of age is shown in Figure 14–13. It has formed in association with a developing second molar. The lesion involves the body of the mandible, extends well up into the ramus, and is almost spherical. The crown, which is as yet not fully formed, has been forced downward to the inferior border of the mandible. Although the picture is similar to that of a dentigerous cyst, it should be borne in mind that a dentigerous cyst does not begin to develop and hence never reaches an appreciable size prior to complete formation of the crown and a portion of the root of the tooth. Therefore, in this instance, one should suspect from the roentgenographic appearance a condition other than dentigerous cyst.

The tumor is encapsulated and it is readily removed by simple curettage; however, according to Trodahl (1972) there is a definite potential for recurrence.

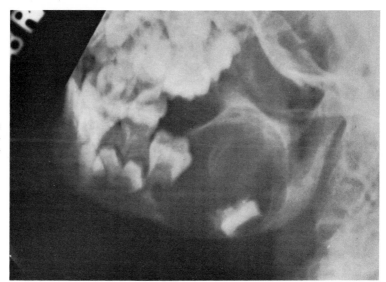

Figure 14–13 Ameloblastic fibroma that has formed in association with a developing mandibular second molar.

AMELOBLASTIC SARCOMA

The ameloblastic sarcoma is a rare form of odontogenic tumor. According to Pindborg (1960), it represents the malignant counterpart of an ameloblastic fibroma. The tumor is composed of benign odontogenic epithelium and a mesodermal component or connective-tissue element that has the histologic features of a sarcoma. Cina and colleagues (1962) state that it differs sharply from the ameloblastoma, in which the connective-tissue element is benign and the epithelial component is neoplastic. In most of the cases reported, the tumor occurred in the mandible and usually was associated with a history of rapid swelling and pain. The ages of the patients in reported cases have varied from 13 to 78 years.

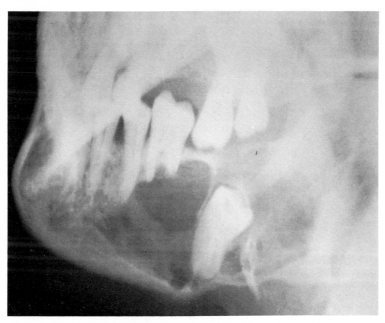

Figure 14–14 Ameloblastic sarcoma, showing destructive process involving the mandible. (Reproduced with permission from Cina, M. T., Dahlin, D. C., and Gores, R. J.: Ameloblastic Sarcoma: Report of Two Cases. Oral Surg., Oral Med. & Oral Path. *15*:696–700 [June] 1962.)

The roentgenographic appearance is not characteristic. However, unlike the ameloblastic fibroma, which tends to be rounded, well circumscribed, and uniformly radiolucent, the ameloblastic sarcoma may have irregular borders and may, in some instances, be traversed by septa to give it a multicystic pattern. A rapidly growing and active lesion such as that in Pindborg's (1960) case may be characterized by diffuse destruction of bone with indistinct borders, similar to that produced by many other malignant tumors involving bone.

The roentgenogram represented in Figure 14–14 was made for a man 39 years of age who had had swelling and pain in the region of the angle of the right mandible for approximately 2 months. It shows bone destruction that extends from the premolar region posteriorly into the ascending ramus. It also reveals an unerupted molar, and anterior to it there is evidence of perforation of the cortical bone. The roentgenographic appearance would not be too helpful in arriving at a correct diagnosis, but it does stress the point that one should never rule out the possibility of malignancy.

The fact that such an ameloblastic tumor can be sarcomatous is significant, and it emphasizes the need for adequate histologic study, especially if the lesion has been symptomatic. Follow-up information was obtained in five of the six cases reported by Leider et al. (1972), and there were recurrences in four (two were multiple recurrences).

AMELOBLASTIC ODONTOMA

The ameloblastic odontoma develops from the dental follicle; when associated with an unerupted tooth it is situated in the pericoronal region. Rarely it may develop early from a tooth bud and replace a normal tooth that would otherwise be present.

The tumor contains hard dental structures arranged in a haphazard fashion, and a soft-tissue component consisting of odontogenic epithelium and embryonic connective tissue similar to that seen in ameloblastic fibroma.

The tumor occurs early in life, most often during the first decade. The premolar-molar region is the most frequent site for occurrence.

In the roentgenogram the lesion is seen as a well-circumscribed cavity in bone; the cavity has a uniformly smooth and even border. Within the cavity are varied amounts of radiopaque material, which represents the hard dental structures present; areas that are not radiopaque represent the soft-tissue or ameloblastic component. The calcified content of the lesion does not fuse with the surrounding bone, as evidenced by a radiolucent line which separates them. A roentgenogram that illustrates these features is shown in Figure 14–15, made for a patient 7 years of age. It shows a large oral cavity in the mandible within which calcified material has been laid down in a radial pattern. The posterior portion of the mass is less opaque and consists largely of the soft-tissue component. The first molar, which has been prevented from erupting, appears to have an intact follicle. Possibly this tumor originated from a second molar tooth bud, particularly since the normal second molar is absent. Whether this tumor, if permitted to remain, would have become completely solid is problematic.

COMPLEX ODONTOMA

The origin of the complex odontoma is similar to that of the ameloblastic odontoma. The tumor contains all mature elements of dental structure: dentin, dentinoid, enamel, enamel matrix, pulp tissue, and cementum. These are laid down in a bizarre and haphazard fashion, and there is no semblance of normal tooth arrangement. The mass of hard dental structure is surrounded by a connective-tissue capsule which could be likened to the periodontal membrane of an unerupted tooth.

The majority of these tumors first are brought to light during the second and third decades of life. They occur with greatest frequency in the mandible, and most of them are situated in the premolar-molar regions.

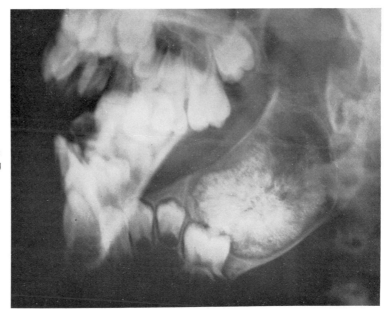

Figure 14-15 Ameloblastic odontoma that is still undergoing active calcification.

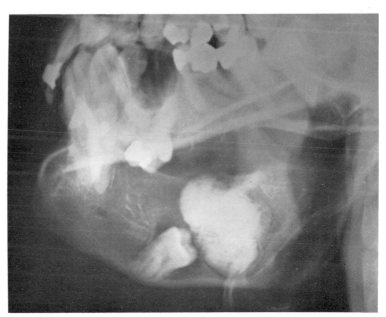

Figure 14-16 Complex odontoma that has undergone complete calcification. (Courtesy of Dr. Edward C. Thompson, Urbana, Illinois.)

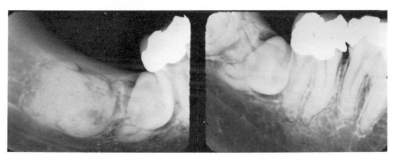

Figure 14-17 Complex odontoma situated posterior to a mandibular third molar, and probably developed from a supernumerary tooth bud.

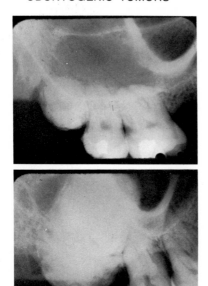

Figure 14–18 Complex odontomas in the maxillary third molar regions. *Above,* No normal third molar is present. *Below,* Lesion is situated adjacent to the crown of an unerupted third molar.

A roentgenogram that illustrates a complex odontoma is shown in Figure 14–16. It reveals a uniformly opaque mass situated adjacent to the crown of an unerupted molar. A radiolucent line of uniform width surrounds the mass, separating it from the normal adjacent bone.

A complex odontoma that probably arose from a supernumerary tooth bud is shown in Figure 14–17. It is situated in the region posterior to a mandibular third molar. The tumor was composed of dentin, cementum, pulp tissue, and a small amount of enamel. Complex odontomas that occurred in the maxillary third molar region are shown in Figure 14–18.

COMPOUND ODONTOMA

The compound odontoma originates from accessory proliferations of odontogenic epithelium that arise directly from the dental lamina, or from whorls that persist as remnants of an epithelial cord that has failed to resorb after closure of the follicle of a normal tooth. The whorls become active enamel-producing organs that form abnormally small teeth. Most of the teeth are conical and usually have single roots. They develop and reach maturity approximately at the same time as do teeth of the permanent dentition. In contrast to complex odontoma, they do not develop from the follicle of normal teeth in the region in which they occur, but develop independently of them. The normal number of permanent teeth is invariably present in the region.

The compound odontoma consists of a bundle of dwarfed, often misshapen teeth which have a normal enamel-dentin-cementum relationship. Foci of ameloblastic proliferation are not present. The number of teeth may vary from a few to several hundred. In general, the larger the number of teeth present the smaller they are.

The lesion occurs most commonly in or near the canine region. Since a supernumerary canine is exceedingly rare, it has been suggested that the odontoma may be a typical form of supernumerary structure associated with the canine tooth (Stafne, 1931). However, on rare occasions it has been seen in the premolar and third molar regions. It occurs with about equal frequency in the mandible and the maxilla, and one in the maxilla contains on the average a greater number of small teeth than does one in the mandible.

In the roentgenogram the compound odontoma is seen as a radiopaque, usually irregular mass within which teeth are recognizable. If only a few teeth are present, a periodontal and pericoronal space characteristic of unerupted teeth may be discernible on each individual tooth (Fig. 14–19, *left*). If a large number of teeth are present, the radiopaque mass is surrounded by a radiolucent line which represents the pericoronal space of the unerupted teeth.

Many of the compound odontomas are first revealed in routine dental roentgenographic examination of adults in whom the normal teeth are fully erupted. In such instances there may be no symptoms or complications attributable to the odontoma (Fig. 14–19). However, as with all embedded teeth, there is a possibility that cysts

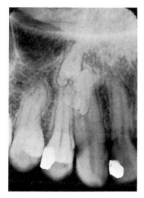
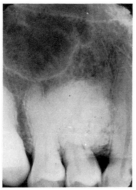
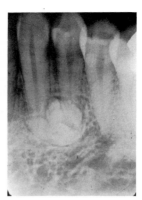

Figure 14–19 Compound odontomas. Three cases in which the normal teeth present have erupted and are in normal alignment. Many of the small teeth of which the odontomas consist are roentgenographically recognizable.

may develop from them; therefore, periodic roentgenographic examination is indicated. In many instances the odontoma is the cause of malposition of normal teeth and often prevents their eruption (Fig. 14–20). Eruption of the normal teeth may follow if the tumor is recognized and removed early in life.

DENTINOMA

The dentinoma is a relatively rare odontogenic tumor composed chiefly of dentin and small amounts of soft tissue and cementum. The cementum is cellular in type and is deposited around the periphery of the tumor. There is no enamel present. Dentinomas are most often associated with the coronal portion of unerupted permanent posterior teeth and, in a few instances, with those of the primary dentition (Manning and Browne, 1970). There also is an amelofibroblastic or immature form of the tumor in which the soft-tissue component predominates.

The roentgenographic appearance of the mature dentinoma is that of a radiopaque mass in close proximity to the crown of an unerupted tooth (Stafne, 1943) (Fig. 14–21). Its location and appearance are similar to those of a complex odontoma.

MESODERMAL ODONTOGENIC TUMORS

ODONTOGENIC MYXOMA (FIBROMYXOMA)

A myxoma is composed of mucous connective tissue that is similar to embryonic mesenchyme and Wharton's jelly. The ori-

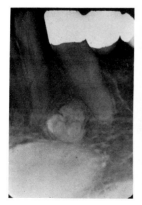
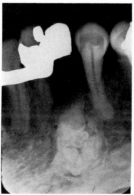
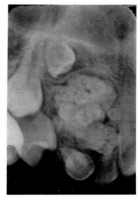

Figure 14–20 Compound odontomas. Three cases in which the odontomas have been the cause of noneruption of permanent teeth.

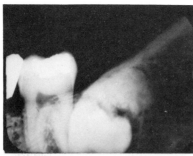

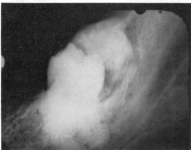

Figure 14–21 Dentinomas. Two cases showing relationship to the crowns of unerupted teeth. (Reproduced with permission from Stafne, E. C.: Dentinoma: Report of Two Cases. Am. J. Orthodontics *29*:156–159 [Mar.] 1943.)

gin of fibromyxoma of the jaws is uncertain. It has been suggested that it may arise from retained islands of undifferentiated embryonic tissue, or from the mesenchymal portion of the tooth germ. That the tumor is odontogenic seems quite plausible, since apparently it is not found in bones outside the facial skeleton (Dahlin, 1957; Lichtenstein, 1952); it occurs almost exclusively in the tooth-bearing regions of the jaws

(Thoma and Goldman, 1947), and the myxomatous tissue histologically resembles the stellate reticulum found in developing teeth. On occasion, fragments of odontogenic epithelium have been encountered within the tumor. In a study of enlarged follicles of unerupted teeth, Conklin and Stafne (1949) found that many of them contained a loose myxomatous type of connective tissue which closely resembled that of a myxoma histologically. The maxilla and mandible are involved with about equal frequency.

In the roentgenogram, fibromyxoma most often presents as a fairly well-circumscribed radiolucent area in which there are multilocular compartments. In this respect, it may resemble ameloblastoma, giant-cell reparative granuloma, and fibrous dysplasia. However, the compartments often differ in that they tend to be angular. They may be separated by straight septa that form square, rectangular, or triangular spaces. The central portion is transversed by fine gracile trabeculations. Sonesson (1950) has an excellent description of the roentgenographic appearance of fibromyxoma of the jaws. Large lesions produce thinning and expansion of the cortex (Fig. 14–22). The dental roentgenogram provides a better view of the interior structure of the lesion (Fig. 14–23).

In some instances the lesion may be unilocular, particularly one that may arise from that part of the follicle which persists

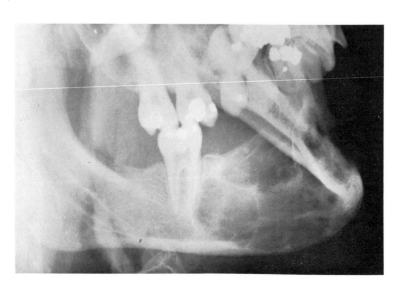

Figure 14–22 Fibromyxoma of the mandible, showing thinning and expansion of the cortex.

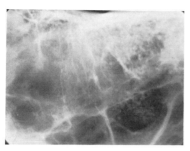

Figure 14–23 Fibromyxoma. The angular compartments are demonstrated.

in the pericoronal region of an unerupted tooth (Millhon and Parkhill, 1946). A myxomatous tumor that had the roentgenographic appearance of a dentigerous cyst is shown in Figure 14–24. The mandibular third molar with which it was associated had assumed a transverse position, and the contents of the cavity directly below it proved to be myxomatous tissue.

Basically, myxomatous tumors are clinically benign (Zimmerman and Dahlin, 1958). They are locally invasive and some of them become large. Treatment consists of enucleation and curettage, or radical excision of the tumor. In view of a high incidence of recurrence, eradication must be thorough. Since they are not radiosensitive, radiation has no place in the treatment.

CEMENTIFYING FIBROMA (CEMENTOMA)

Cementoma is of mesenchymal origin and is almost always derived from the

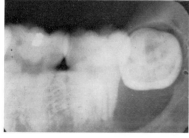

Figure 14–24 Odontogenic myxoma that arose from the follicle of an unerupted mandibular third molar. (Reproduced with permission from Stafne, E. C. and Parkhill, E. M.: Myxomatous Tumor Associated with an Unerupted Tooth: Report of a Case. Am. J. Orthodontics [Oral Surg. Sect.] *33*:597–598 [Aug.] 1947.)

periodontal membrane of fully developed and erupted teeth. Because of its definite course in development, clinical behavior, and roentgenographic appearance, it can be considered a definite pathologic entity (Stafne, 1934). Thoma (1937) has called the early stage of cementoma "cementoblastoma." Other terms have been applied to cementoma, such as ossifying fibroma, enostosis, and periapical osseous dysplasia. Bernier and Thompson (1946) have discussed the histogenesis, and Scannel (1949) and Zegarelli and colleagues (1964) have reported on the findings in a fairly large number of cases.

Cementomas occur more frequently in the mandible than in the maxilla (Chaudhry et al., 1958), the ratio being about 15:1, and there is a decided tendency to multiple occurrence. The lesion results from proliferation of the connective tissue of the periodontal membrane, to form a mass of fibrous tissue of varied size which remains continuous with the periodontal membrane and attached to the root end of the tooth. At this stage there are deposited in that portion of the fibrous mass which more closely proximates the root a sparse number of round or ovoid calcified bodies that resemble cementicles which may be found on occasion in a periodontal membrane of normal thickness. At the peripheral portion of it there is a sparse distribution of normal spicules of bone. Further development may follow one of three courses: (1) the lesion may remain as a periapical fibroma or cementoblastoma for an indefinite period, (2) most of the fibrous mass may be converted to a calcified substance which more closely resembles cementum than normal bone, or (3) in rare instances the mass may be replaced by normal bone.

The roentgenographic appearance depends upon the stage and course of development. In the first stage (Fig. 14–25, *center*), when the lesion consists chiefly of connective tissue, there is a fairly well-circumscribed radiolucent area in the periapical region which is somewhat similar to that produced by a granuloma or epithelium-lined cyst. It is this picture that

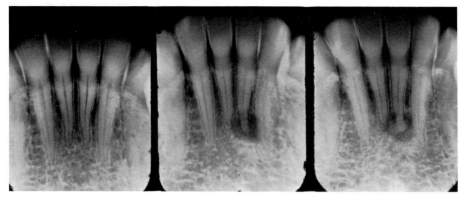

Figure 14–25   Cementoma of mandibular incisor, showing first and second stages of development. *Left,* View in 1941 showing no lesion. *Center,* View in 1948 showing first or early stage. *Right,* View in 1952 showing second stage with calcification within the fibrous mass, and associated hypercementosis of the root of the involved tooth.

causes most confusion in diagnosis, and from which most misinterpretations arise. If the tooth is of normal color and responds normally to tests for vitality, one can arrive at a fairly reliable diagnosis of the early stage of cementoma or cementoblastoma on the basis of the roentgenographic evidence only, and particularly is this so in the absence of a history of pulpitis or trauma.

The second stage, in which the roentgenographic appearance is typical of cementoma, is that seen when a sufficient amount of calcified substance has formed in the central zone to produce a radiopaque

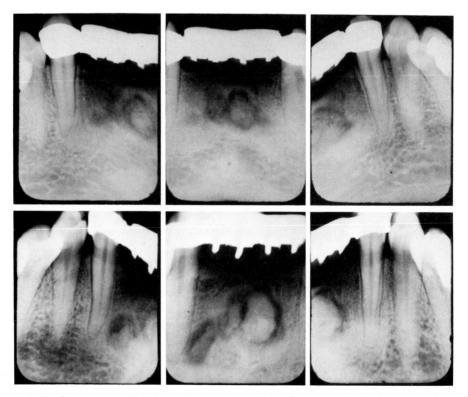

Figure 14–26   Cementomas that have increased in size after removal of the involved teeth. Upper roentgenogram was made 7 years before lower one.

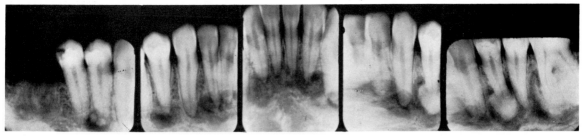

Figure 14–27 Cementoma. Multiple occurrence involving eight mandibular teeth. Most of the lesions are in the early or cementoblastic stage. In the views on the reader's right, an appreciable amount of calcified substance is present in the periapical regions of the first premolar and first molar. (Courtesy of Dr. D. F. Lynch, Washington, D.C.)

image within the original radiolucent area. Once deposition of the calcified substance is discernible in the roentgenogram, it is only in rare instances that the fibrous mass will become more extensive than the limits of the area of radiolucency. Exceptions to this are in cases in which the involved teeth have been extracted or other surgical measures instituted presumably with incomplete removal of the lesion. At this stage there also may become evident a deposition of cementum on the surface of the root, producing hypercementosis (Fig. 14–25, *right*). In no instance is there resorption of the root of the tooth, such as that which is sometimes caused by sclerosis of bone and some of the benign tumors that occur in the jaws.

In Figure 14–26 the first roentgenogram was made for a patient who stated that the lower incisors had been removed because they were infected; it revealed a small radiopaque mass in the right central incisor area and a radiolucence in the space that the two left incisors had occupied. The roentgenogram made 7 years later revealed

that calcification had occurred in all three of the spaces and that the one in the right central incisor area had increased appreciably in size. To what extent they might continue to enlarge is problematic.

A case of multiple occurrence in which eight mandibular teeth are involved is shown in Figure 14–27. Of these lesions, six are in the early stage, and those involving the first premolar and first molar in the views on the right have undergone an appreciable amount of calcification.

The third typical picture is that seen when the lesion has undergone almost complete calcification, as in Figure 14–28. In this case of multiple occurrence, six mandibular teeth are involved, and an additional lesion is present in the edentulous first molar region seen in the view on the extreme left, a lesion that presumably arose from the molar prior to its extraction.

If the involved tooth is extracted and the calcifying mass is permitted to remain, the space formerly occupied by the root will become filled with a similar calcified substance. The result is a round or ovoid

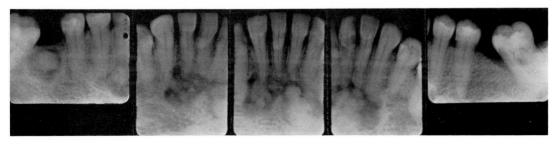

Figure 14–28 Cementomas involving the mandibular canines, incisors, and a first molar edentulous space. These have all reached a highly calcified stage.

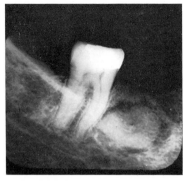
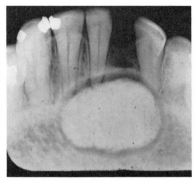

Figure 14-29 Cementomas situated in edentulous spaces—in the molar region in the view on the left, and in the incisor region in the view on the right. Both are surrounded by a radiolucent margin, which represents the connective tissue that separates them from the normal surrounding bone. (Reproduced with permission from Stafne, E. C.: Periapical Osteofibrosis with Formation of Cementoma. J. Am. Dent. A. *21*:1822–1829 [Oct.] 1934.)

radiopaque mass surrounded by a radiolucent space (Fig. 14–29). The significant roentgenographic finding is the radiolucent space which separates the calcified mass from the surrounding normal bone. It is this feature that distinguishes cementomas from osteosclerosis, condensing osteitis, endostosis, and other conditions in which the lesion fuses directly with and is continuous with the adjoining bone.

In rare instances the periapical fibrous lesion may again be converted to normal bone and, in this event, the roentgenographic picture returns to normal, showing no evidence of what has occurred (Fig. 14–30). An unusual case in which the typical roentgenographic evidence of the lesion disappeared after it had undergone an appreciable amount of calcification is shown in Figure 14–31. The change took place within a period of 6 years, and the radiopaque mass was replaced by bone which has a fine ground-glass appearance.

While the so-called cementoma is included under odontogenic tumors of mesenchymal origin, the cause still is obscure. Traumatic occlusion and injury have been mentioned as possible causes, but many cementomas involve mandibular incisors that have never been in occlusion; and maxillary incisors, which are the teeth most often subjected to injury, are rarely involved. Serum calcium, phosphorus, and alkaline phosphatase have been deter-

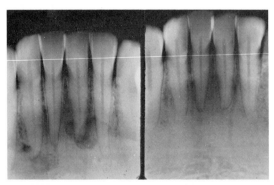

Figure 14-30 Periapical fibromas (cementoblastomas) that involved two incisors and that apparently were converted to bone. *Left,* View showing periapical radiolucent areas. *Right,* View 3 years later showing normal roentgenographic appearance.

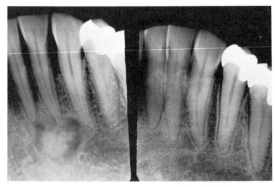

Figure 14-31 Cementoma. *Left,* Appearance in 1950. *Right,* View in 1956, which reveals that the lesion has been replaced by bone that has a fine ground-glass appearance. This change is extremely rare.

mined in several cases in which there has been multiple occurrence, but the values have proved to be within normal limits. The fact that most of these lesions occur in females may some day prove to be significant.

Usually cementomas do not reach an appreciable size, and surgical intervention rarely is indicated, particularly if it will lead to the loss of useful teeth.

REFERENCES

Bailey, J. W.: Dentigerous Cyst with Ameloblastoma: Report of Case. Oral Surg., Oral Med. & Oral Path. 4:1122–1126 (Sept.) 1951.

Bernier, J. L. and Thompson, H. C.: Histogenesis of Cementoma: Report of 15 Cases. Am. J. Orthodontics (Oral Surg. Sect.). 32:543–555 (Sept.) 1946.

Cahn, L. R.: The Dentigerous Cyst Is a Potential Adamantinoma. Dent. Cosmos. 75:889–893 (Sept.) 1933.

Chaudhry, A. P., Spink, J. H., and Gorlin, R. J.: Periapical Fibrous Dysplasia (Cementoma). J. Oral Surg. 16:483–488 (Nov.) 1958.

Cina, M. T., Dahlin, D. C., and Gores, R. J.: Odontogenic Mixed Tumors: A Review of the Mayo Clinic Series. Proc. Staff Meet., Mayo Clin. 36:664–678 (Dec. 6) 1961.

Cina, M. T., Dahlin, D. C., and Gores, R. J.: Ameloblastic Sarcoma: Report of Two Cases. Oral Surg., Oral Med. & Oral Path. 15:696–700 (June) 1962.

Cina, M. T., Dahlin, D. C., and Gores, R. J.: Ameloblastic Adenomatoid Tumors: A Report of Four New Cases. Am. J. Clin. Path. 39:59–65 (Jan.) 1963.

Conklin, W. W. and Stafne, E. C.: A Study of Odontogenic Epithelium in the Dental Follicle. J. Am. Dent. A. 39:143–148 (Aug.) 1949.

Dahlin, D. C.: Bone Tumors: General Aspects and an Analysis of 2276 Cases. Springfield, Illinois, Charles C Thomas, Publisher, 1957, p. 5.

Giansanti, J. S., Someren, A., and Waldron, C. A.: Odontogenic Adenomatoid Tumor (Adenoameloblastoma): Survey of 3 Cases. Oral Surg., Oral Med. & Oral Path. 30:69–88 (July) 1970.

Leider, A. S., Nelson, J. F., and Trodahl, J. N.: Ameloblastic Fibrosarcoma of the Jaws. Oral Surg., Oral Med. & Oral Path. 33:559–569 (Apr.) 1972.

Lichtenstein, L.: Bone Tumors. St. Louis, The C. V. Mosby Company, 1952, p. 20.

Manning, G. L. and Browne, R. M.: Dentinoma. Brit. Dent. J. 128:178–181 (Feb. 17) 1970.

Millhon, J. A. and Parkhill, E. M.: Myxomatous Tumor Simulating Dentigerous Cyst. J. Oral Surg. 4:129–132 (Apr.) 1946.

Pindborg, J. J.: A Calcifying Epithelial Odontogenic Tumor. Cancer. 11:838–843 (July–Aug.) 1958.

Pindborg, J. J.: Ameloblastic Sarcoma in the Maxilla: Report of a Case. Cancer. 13:917–920 (Sept.–Oct.) 1960.

Pindborg, J. J.: Pathology of the Dental Hard Tissues. Philadelphia, W. B. Saunders Company, 1970, p. 368.

Scannell, J. M., Jr.: Cementoma. Oral Surg., Oral Med. & Oral Path. 2:1169–1180 (Sept.) 1949.

Shafer, W. G.: Ameloblastic Fibroma. J. Oral Surg. 13:317–321 (Oct.) 1955.

Shafer, W. G., Hine, M. K., and Levy, B. M.: A Textbook of Oral Pathology. Ed. 3. Philadelphia, W. B. Saunders Company, 1974, p. 260.

Sherman, R. S. and Caumartin, H.: The Roentgen Appearance of Adamantinoma of the Mandible. Radiology. 65:361–366 (Sept.) 1955.

Small, I. A. and Waldron, C. A.: Ameloblastomas of Jaws. Oral Surg., Oral Med. & Oral Path. 8:281–297 (Mar.) 1955.

Sonesson, A.: Odontogenic Cysts and Cystic Tumours of the Jaws: A Roentgen-Diagnostic and Patho-Anatomic Study. Acta Radiol. Suppl. 81, 1950, pp. 104–114.

Spouge, J. D.: The Adenoameloblastoma. Oral Surg., Oral Med. & Oral Path. 23:470–482 (Apr.) 1967.

Stafne, E. C.: Denticles, Supernumerary Cuspids and Compound Composite Odontomes. Dent. Cosmos. 73:796–798 (Aug.) 1931.

Stafne, E. C.: Periapical Osteofibrosis with Formation of Cementoma. J. Am. Dent. A. 21:1822–1829 (Oct.) 1934.

Stafne, E. C.: Dentinoma: Report of Two Cases. Am. J. Orthodontics. 29:156–159 (Mar.) 1943.

Stafne, E. C.: Epithelial Tumors Associated with Developmental Cysts of Maxilla: Report of 3 Cases. Oral Surg., Oral Med. & Oral Path. 1:887–894 (Oct.) 1948.

Stafne, E. C.: Value of Roentgenograms in Diagnosis of Tumors of the Jaws. Oral Surg., Oral Med. & Oral Path. 6:82–92 (Jan.) 1953.

Thoma, K. H.: Cementoblastoma. Internat. J. Orthodontia. 23:1127–1137 (Nov.) 1937.

Thoma, K. H. and Goldman, H. M.: Central Myxoma of Jaw. Am. J. Orthodontics (Oral Surg. Sect.). 33:532–540 (July) 1947.

Trodahl, J. N.: Ameloblastic Fibroma: A Survey of Cases from the Armed Forces Institute of Pathology. Oral Surg., Oral Med. & Oral Path. 33:547–558 (Apr.) 1972.

Vap, D. R., Dahlin, D. C., and Turlington, E. G.: Pindborg Tumor: The So-called Calcifying Epithelial Odontogenic Tumor. Cancer. 25:629–636 (Mar.) 1970.

Zegarelli, E. V., Kutscher, A. H., Napoli, N., Iurono, F., and Hoffman, P.: The Cementoma: A Study of 230 Patients with 435 Cementomas. Oral Surg., Oral Med. & Oral Path. 17:219–224 (Feb.) 1964.

Zimmerman, D. C. and Dahlin, D. C.: Myxomatous Tumors of the Jaws. Oral Surg., Oral Med. & Oral Path. 11:1069–1080 (Oct.) 1958.

15 NONODONTOGENIC TUMORS OF THE JAWBONES

BRUCE A. LUND, D.D.S.

Nonodontogenic tumors of the maxilla and mandible comprise a wide assortment of lesions. By one definition, a tumor is simply an independent overgrowth of tissue that does not serve a useful purpose. This chapter thus will include conditions that are pathologically insignificant as well as primary or metastatic malignant lesions that have serious prognostic implications. It has been stated that there is no such thing as roentgenographic diagnosis, implying that the "findings" observed on a roentgenogram need to be correlated with the clinical evaluation as well as with those findings obtained by other diagnostic aids. The majority of lesions discussed in this chapter do not produce pathognomonic roentgenographic features that will allow one to use the roentgenogram as the sole basis for making a diagnosis. On the other hand, roentgenographic examination is indispensable in revealing the presence (or absence) of lesions in bone, and many times the nature of a tumor can be ascertained from its roentgenographic appearance.

If one carefully analyzes the roentgenogram, certain features may be noted that often will distinguish the benign from the malignant lesion. In the benign tumor, for example, the cortex tends to remain intact even though it may be thinned and expanded; the malignant tumor, on the other hand, frequently produces destruction of the cortex or elevation of the periosteum from the underlying cortex. The margins of the benign lesion are usually well-defined, with a definite demarcation from the surrounding bone. In contrast, the malignant tumor has irregular margins that tend to be less distinct and to blend imperceptibly into the adjacent bone.

The effects on the teeth on which it encroaches may give some information as to the nature of a lesion. These effects are often manifested as resorption of the roots, forcing of the entire tooth away from its normal or original position, or exfoliation of the tooth. Benign tumors that tend to develop and expand slowly, such as the lesions of fibrous dysplasia, central osteoma, giant-cell reparative granuloma, and ameloblastoma, commonly cause resorption of the roots. Tilting of erupted teeth and forcing of unerupted teeth to a location far remote from their original position are common results of pressure by cysts and tumors of odontogenic origin, although these findings occur with giant-cell reparative granuloma and fibro-osseous tumors also. Sloughing of teeth, especially if rapid, is highly suggestive of a malignant tumor.

If the roentgenogram reveals agenesis and noneruption of teeth in the region of a lesion, it generally can be assumed that the lesion had its onset prior to the normal time for development and eruption of these teeth. The approximate duration of the tumor, therefore, often can be arrived at on the basis of this information, even though the tumor may come to light several years later.

Although the entities discussed in this chapter comprise only a small percentage of the pathologic conditions found in the jaws, they are of utmost importance. As emphasized earlier, however, the final diagnosis for any bone lesion must be based on the combined clinical, roentgenographic, and microscopic observations.

BENIGN TUMORS

Benign tumors are usually solitary, although in some instances they may be multiple. They do not produce metastatic lesions in their original state. They grow moderately fast and enlarge by expansion. They generally resemble the mother tissue and usually are classified by the tissue of which they are chiefly composed.

EXOSTOSES AND TORI

Exostoses are localized overgrowths of bone, variable in size and appearing as flat, nodular, or pedunculated protuberances on the surface of the bone. They occur not uncommonly on the surface of the facial bones. The term "tori" often has been used to designate exostoses that occur in the midline of the palate and on the lingual surface of the mandible. The cause of exostosis of the jaws is unknown. The not infrequent history of familial occurrence suggests a genetic basis.

Suzuki and Sakai (1960) studied the genetic aspects of palatal and mandibular tori. They found that, when both parents had either palatal or mandibular tori, the prevalence of those same tori in the children was 63.9% and 58.6%, respectively.

In the roentgenogram, exostosis is seen as an area of increased roentgenographic density that conforms in shape to the outline and form of the particular overgrowth. Exostoses that are composed of compact bone are of uniform radiopacity, whereas some of large size that contain a marrow space have trabeculations. Many exostoses are difficult to demonstrate roentgenographically, particularly those of small size and those that are superimposed on the image of the teeth.

Exostoses that appear on the alveolar process tend to be bilateral and multiple and often produce a nodular protuberance. When multiple, they may coalesce to form an irregular, linear, horizontal elevation. They are almost always limited to the region posterior to the canines, and most of them occur on the buccal surface. In some instances they may occur also on the palatal surface. Figure 15–1 illustrates bilateral exostoses on the palatal surface of the alveolar process in the maxillary molar regions.

Torus Palatinus. Torus palatinus is an exostosis that arises at the margins of the palatal processes at the median suture of the palate. The borders of both sides of the suture line are almost always involved, and in this respect the lesions are bilateral. Invariably, the exostosis from one side will coalesce with the one from the other to form a single protuberance, although often a median groove is present over the protuberance

Figure 15–1 Exostoses (bilateral) situated on the palatal surface of the maxilla in the molar region.

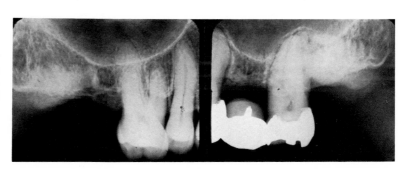

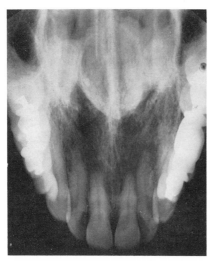

Figure 15–2 Torus palatinus located in the midline and posterior half of the palate. Also an exostosis is present on the palatal surface of each tuberosity.

and tends to divide it into right and left portions.

Kolas and co-workers (1953) categorized palatine tori as flat, spindle-shaped, nodular, or lobular. They found that 20.9% of 2478 patients had torus palatinus as compared with 7.75% who had torus mandibularis; 3.03% of the entire group had both mandibular and palatine tori.

Palatine tori vary greatly in size, from those that are detectable only on palpation to those that occupy almost all of the space of the palate and interfere with function and speech. Their location on the palate also varies. Although most of them are situated in the middle portion of the midline, others are confined to the anterior or posterior region. In some instances the entire midline may be involved, from the anterior

palatine fossa posteriorly to the termination of the hard palate.

Roentgenographically, a palatine torus can be best demonstrated with the occlusal film. One that involved the posterior portion, including the termination of the hard palate, is shown in Figure 15–2. It is evidenced by the oval-shaped opacity situated in the midline. The borders that are more radiopaque represent a cortex, and medullary bone with a normal trabecular pattern can be seen in the inner portion. This case is interesting in that it also illustrates bilateral exostoses arising on the palatal surface in the region of the tuberosities. The two exostoses have similar roentgenographic features in that they exhibit a cortex and medullary bone. Both have reached such a size that they come in contact with the torus in the midline but are separated from it by the overlying mucous membrane.

The image of a portion of a palatine torus may appear in the dental roentgenogram, particularly when the torus is situated in the anterior portion of the palate. The presence of a torus of appreciable size often presents a problem in making a satisfactory roentgenographic examination of the maxillary teeth. When superimposed on the dental roentgenogram, one that is situated in the posterior part of the palate may be mistaken for the zygoma. Dental roentgenograms made for a patient who had a torus of the middle and anterior portions of the palate are shown in Figure 15–3. The torus is evidenced by the marked opacity at the upper border of the roentgenograms. In the roentgenogram of the incisors it is apparent that it extends anteriorly as far as the anterior palatine fossa.

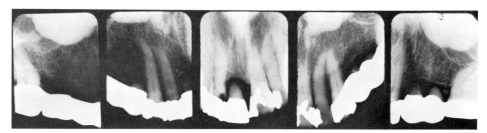

Figure 15–3 Torus palatinus as seen in a dental roentgenogram and evidenced by the marked opacities at the upper border of the films.

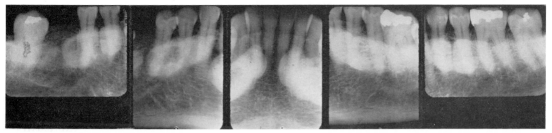

Figure 15–4 Torus mandibularis as viewed in the dental roentgenogram. In this instance the lesions are multiple and bilateral.

Torus Mandibularis. Torus mandibularis occurs on the lingual surface of the mandible, most often in the premolar regions. It may occur singly; however, there is a marked tendency to multiple and bilateral occurrence, and the lesion is not necessarily confined to the premolar region. These tori arise above the mylohyoid ridge. Their size varies, some reaching such size that tori from opposite sides come in contact with each other and occupy a large portion of the floor of the mouth.

Unlike palatine tori, mandibular tori are more readily demonstrated roentgenographically by the standard dental as well as by the occlusal film. The latter has the advantage of revealing the extent, site, and size of the bony projections. A dental roentgenogram that illustrates multiple bilateral tori is shown in Figure 15–4. Such tori may obscure the periapical region, and it is often necessary to make several views in order to visualize the root ends of the teeth. Figure 15–5, an occlusal view of the same case as that shown in Figure 15–4, reveals bilateral occurrence; multiple tori that have coalesced extend from the canine to the third molar regions on both sides. This roentgenogram also illustrates certain features that are to a large extent characteristic of mandibular tori—namely, that they tend to be symmetric in form, number, and size.

Comment. Exostoses and tori are of no pathologic significance, and rarely are they of clinical significance while the normal teeth are still present. If they become so large that they interfere with normal speech and other functions, or if the overlying mucous membrane becomes inflamed or ulcerated from trauma, surgical excision is indicated. Such surgical treatment should be carefully performed, particularly if the exostosis involves the crest of the alveolar ridge, because there is then the added hazard of denuding the root surfaces of useful teeth. After loss of the natural teeth, all exostoses and tori of sufficient prominence to interfere with the wearing of artificial dentures should be removed. It should be kept in mind that exostoses that are present on the alveolar process become increasingly prominent after extraction of the teeth because they are not resorbed, whereas the normal alveolar process adjacent to them invariably does undergo some degree of resorption and atrophy.

Etiologically, it is tempting to associate function with presence of these bony overgrowths. In contrast to this theory, however, Moorrees (1951) found that the anomaly

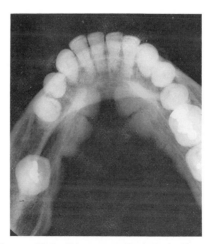

Figure 15–5 Torus mandibularis in the patient shown in Figure 15–4, seen in the occlusal view. The tori are multiple and extend from the canine to the third molar regions on both sides.

had a lower incidence in Eskimo women than in Eskimo men, despite the fact that jaw function was greater among the women as a result of their chewing sealskin pelts.

ENOSTOSIS

Enostosis of the jaws is spoken of as a counterpart of exostosis. The growth is said to arise on the inner surface of the cortex and to extend into medullary space. From the standpoint of the roentgenologist, it is a most confusing entity to recognize. Perhaps some of the opacities within the jaws that are diagnosed as osteosclerosis actually represent enostoses. From observation of roentgenograms of the jaws, at any rate, there appears to be no exact counterpart of exostosis in that there is no similar tendency for multiple and bilateral occurrence.

OSTEOMAS

Osteomas are benign tumors composed of bone. Histologic study often fails to distinguish simple hyperplastic growth of bone from true osteoma, although noninflammatory origin, active participation of osteoblasts, and derivation from cartilage are features that are more prominent in true osteoma. According to Ewing (1928), the gross and clinical features seem to form the best criteria by which to separate osteoma from simple hyperostosis. The bones of the face in particular are subject to a variety of bony overgrowths that are difficult to classify.

Osteomas vary greatly in size, some of them reaching such size as to produce marked disfiguration. In some instances they may be attached to the cortex of the bone by a pedicle; in others they may grow from a wide base. The pedunculated type occurs more frequently in the mandible,

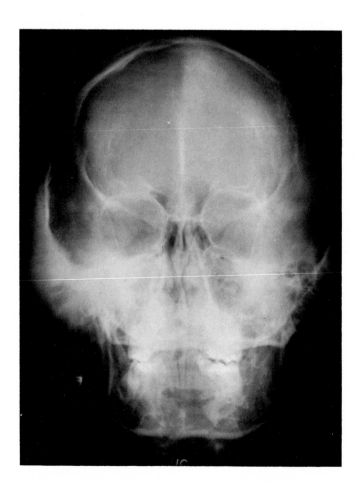

Figure 15–6 Large osteoma attached to the lateral aspect of the skull of a 15-year-old girl.

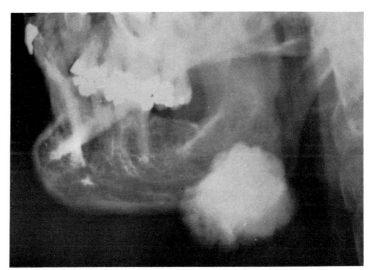

Figure 15–7 Round osteoma attached to the buccal aspect of the mandible, near the inferior border.

where it may appear on any surface and not infrequently arises at the inferior border.

The skull is the most common site for the development of an osteoma, with the calvarium and frontal sinus areas being affected most frequently. The roentgenogram in Figure 15–6 reveals a large osteoma of the skull in a 15-year-old girl. These lesions can be sizable enough to be cosmetic problems and to require surgical removal.

The roentgenogram provides information concerning the shape and size of the tumor and its relationship and attachment to the bone. If the tumor consists chiefly of dense, laminated bone with a few haversian canals, the roentgenographic density is

much greater than that of a tumor containing spongy bone and abundant marrow space. The latter often exhibits normal trabeculation of bone.

A solid, pedunculated osteoma of the mandible is shown in Figure 15–7. It is situated on the buccal aspect, near the inferior border and angle of the mandible. It is round and the border is slightly irregular, suggesting active growth. It is very radiopaque and is characteristic of the dense, eburnated type of osteoma. The one shown in Figure 15–8 is also situated near the inferior border of the mandible and has a bizarre form with projections radiating in all directions. An occlusal view, which is

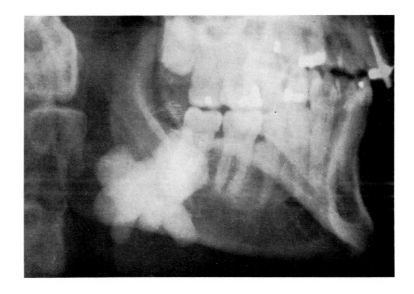

Figure 15–8 Osteoma of the mandible, attached by a pedicle and irregular in shape.

not available for illustration, revealed that it was attached to the buccal surface by a pedicle.

Osteomas tend to be multiple. Multiple osteomas of the jaws may be associated with osteomas in other parts of the skeleton. The first evidence of tumor formation in the body may appear in the jaws, as illustrated by the following case. The dental roentgenograms shown in Figure 15–9 were made for a woman 22 years of age and demonstrate dense, radiopaque bone in the posterior regions of both the maxilla and the mandible. There was some enlargement of both jaws that first had been noted at 11 years of age. From the roentgenographic evidence it is apparent that the medullary bone was involved as well, and failure of the premolar teeth to erupt suggested that the onset of the tumors occurred prior to the normal time for eruption

of these teeth. A roentgenographic survey revealed multiple osteomas of the skull but no evidence of abnormality of the long bones, spinal column, or pelvis. When the patient was seen again at age 30 years, the osteomas of the maxilla and mandible had increased greatly in size to produce a pronounced deformity and a grotesque appearance. An anteroposterior view of the head showing the extent and multiple character of the tumors is presented in Figure 15–10. At this time a skeletal roentgenographic survey also revealed osteomas of the right humerus, radius, and ulna, the left fibula, tibia, and ilium, and four ribs.

It is important to recognize that multiple osteomas may be associated with other lesions. Gardner and Richards (1953) reported a syndrome of multiple osteomas, multiple cutaneous and subcutaneous tumors, multiple polyposis of the large

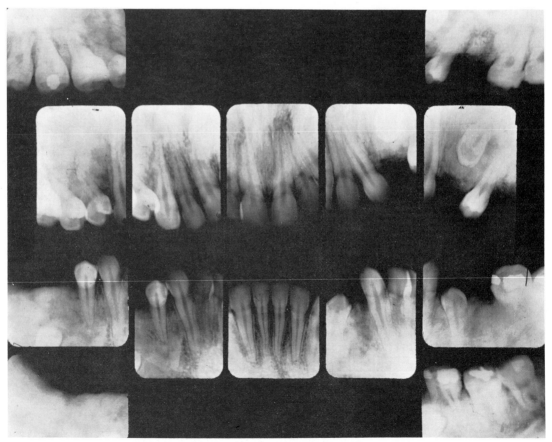

Figure 15–9 Multiple osteomas. Dental roentgenograms made for a patient 22 years of age, showing multiple osteomas of the jaws at a time when they had produced only slight jaw deformity.

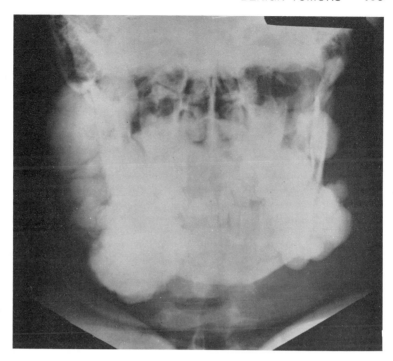

Figure 15–10 Multiple osteomas. Anteroposterior view made at 30 years of age for the patient presented in Figure 15–9, and showing the extent and multiple character of the tumors.

bowel, and desmoid tumor. The patient shown in Figure 15–10 had a desmoid tumor of the left cervical region.

The osteomas that occur in Gardner's syndrome (multiple osteomatosis-polyposis) have a predilection for the frontal bone, maxilla, and mandible, although they may be observed in any of the bones of the cranium or facial skeleton. They generally appear early in the second decade of life and usually are asymptomatic. Compound odontomas and hypercementosis have been reported (Fader et al., 1962) to develop in patients with Gardner's syndrome. Impacted supernumerary and permanent teeth are frequently noted.

It is essential that the dentist be aware of this syndrome in that the multiple osteomas often precede the onset of colonic polyps. Because malignant change occurs in a significant percentage of these polyps and because the syndrome is transmitted as an autosomal dominant trait, relatives of patients with the disease should be investigated (Duncan et al., 1968). Gardner's syndrome is discussed further in the chapter on systemic disease.

Osteoid Osteoma. Osteoid osteoma of the jaws occurs relatively rarely, if inci-

dence can be judged from the paucity of reports. It first was described as a distinct entity and a variation of osteoma by Jaffe (1935). Rushton (1951), Spitzer (1954), and Foss and co-workers (1955) are among those who have reported such lesions of the jaws.

Osteoid osteoma has been defined (Lichenstein, 1965) as a "...small, oval or roundish tumorlike nidus which is composed of osteoid and trabeculae of newly formed bone deposited within a substratum of highly vascularized osteogenic connective tissue." The tumor occurs in or near the cortex, and it may be extremely painful. The lesions are highly unusual in patients over 30 years of age. Either the maxilla or the mandible may be involved (Greene et al., 1968). Frequently, it is noted that salicylates relieve the pain, which otherwise may interrupt sleep. The roentgenographic appearance is fairly typical. There is a radiopaque nidus surrounded by a diffuse and irregular radiolucence, surrounded in turn by bone of increased roentgenographic density.

An osteoid osteoma in the cortex of the inferior border of the mandible directly below the first and second molars is shown

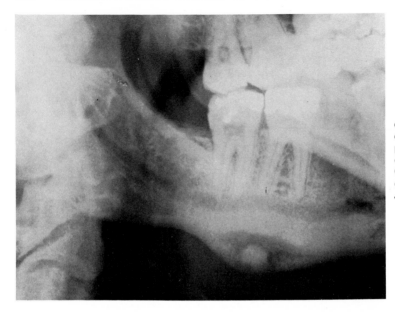

Figure 15-11 Osteoid osteoma situated at the inferior border of the mandible. (Reproduced with permission from Foss, E. L., Dockerty, M. B., and Good, C. A.: Osteoid Osteoma of the Mandible: Report of a Case. Cancer. *8*:592–594 [May-June] 1955.)

in Figure 15–11. The patient had complained of a painful swelling in that region. The roentgenographic appearance was similar to that described for the osteoid osteoma that occurs elsewhere in the skeleton. A tentative diagnosis of osteoid osteoma was made on the basis of the roentgenographic evidence, and this diagnosis was proved to be correct on microscopic examination.

Benign Osteoblastoma. Benign osteoblastoma was described by Dahlin and Johnson in 1954 under the name "giant osteoid osteoma." It was reported in the maxilla by Borello and Sedano (1967) and in the mandible by Kramer (1967). In the Mayo Clinic series (Dahlin, 1967), 28 benign osteoblastomas were reported, with 2 of these occurring in the mandible. Several features distinguish the lesion from an apparently close relative, the osteoid osteoma. The benign osteoblastoma has the potential for becoming moderately large, whereas the osteoid osteoma usually is 1 cm or less in diameter. Symptomatically, the osteoid osteoma is described as being consistently more painful.

CHONDROMA

A chondroma, by definition, is a benign tumor composed of cartilage. On oc-

casion, the chondroma may become partially ossified and is then more appropriately called an osteochondroma. Theoretically, complete replacement of the cartilage by bone could occur—producing an osteoma. On the other hand, these tumors should be carefully evaluated, because any cartilaginous lesion of the jaws must be treated as potentially malignant. There is a possibility of chondrosarcomas arising from pre-existing chondromatous tumors, and therefore the benign chondroma should be completely excised whenever possible.

Chondromas are exceedingly rare in the jaws. The most common sites of occurrence are the toes, fingers, sternum, and ribs. Although these tumors have been separated, by location, into ecchondromas (periosteal chondromas develop on surface of bone) or enchondromas (central chondromas develop deep within bone), this differentiation is not important in the jaws.

A chondroma that involved the cortical portion of the mandible is shown in Figure 15–12. It appears as a raised radiolucent mass in which there are scattered and irregular areas of calcification. Beneath it is a saucer-shaped concavity of the alveolar process that probably was produced by pressure erosion. The base of the concavity is sclerotic, which suggests the benign na-

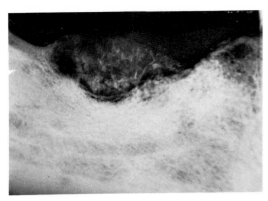

Figure 15-12 Chondroma involving the mandible.

ture of the lesion. However, propensity for these lesions to become malignant has been noted (Chaudhry et al., 1961), and adequate surgical en bloc removal is advised.

NEUROGENIC TUMORS (NEURILEMMOMA, NEUROFIBROMA)

Benign neurogenic tumors are occasionally found centrally within the jaws. Eversole (1969) reviewed the literature and described the findings in 18 cases of neurilemmoma and 11 cases of solitary neurofibroma. At the Mayo Clinic, in a series of nearly 4000 bone tumors, only 4 benign neurogenic tumors were found in the mandible (Dahlin, 1967). Neurilemmoma and neurofibroma can be distinguished microscopically.

The neurilemmoma (schwannoma) is classically described as being composed of two distinct histologic components, Antoni type A tissue and Antoni type B tissue. In addition, there are areas that present an organoid appearance (acellular, hyalinized, eosinophilic mass) and are called Verocay bodies. The lesion is usually encapsulated.

Although the neurofibroma is also a schwannian tumor, it differs from the preceding description in that neurites are found that traverse the tumor. It is not encapsulated. Neurofibromas may occur as solitary nodules (Prescott and White, 1970; Singer et al., 1973), or they may be associated with von Recklinghausen's disease, in which there are multiple cutaneous and subcutaneous tumors, café-au-lait spots of melanin pigmentation, and occasional skeletal deformities.

Benign neurogenic tumors of the jaws may occur at any age, and there appears to be little, if any, significant sex predilection. The great majority of these lesions occur in the mandible. The lesions are relatively slow growing, and pain or paresthesia may be associated symptoms.

The roentgenographic findings vary considerably. The lesion may present as a solitary radiolucency associated with the inferior alveolar canal, or as a cystic multilocular radiolucency that has produced extensive bone damage, cortical expansion, and even perforation.

A neurilemmoma of the inferior dental nerve that is still confined to the interior portion of the mandible is seen as an elongated bulbous enlargement of the mandibular canal in Figure 15-13. Discomfort, pain, or paresthesia may be clinical manifestations of the neurofibroma in this area. On occasion, the intraosseous tumor may perforate the cortex of the jawbone and extend into the overlying soft tissues (Fig. 15-14). This roentgenographic picture is not pathognomonic, and biopsy is necessary to make the diagnosis. A neurofibroma that is adjacent to bone may produce a saucer-shaped erosive defect on the surface of the bone that is similar in appearance to the defects caused by peripheral fibroma,

Figure 15-13 Neurofibroma of the inferior dental nerve, showing bulbous enlargement of the mandibular canal and increased growth. The roentgenogram on the left was made 10 years prior to the one on the right.

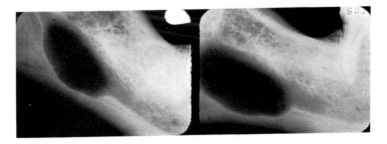

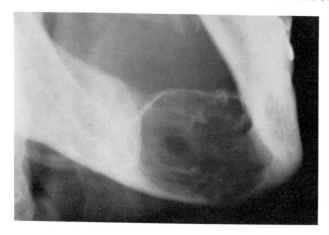

Figure 15–14 Neurofibroma of the mandible. The anterior portion of the tumor has perforated the cortex.

giant-cell reparative granuloma, and some other benign tumors. A case of neurofibroma of the alveolar ridge reported by Bruce (1954) exhibited this roentgenographic feature.

Malignant transformation of pre-existing neurofibromas has been described (DeVore and Waldron, 1961). Malignant peripheral nerve tumors may be difficult to distinguish microscopically because there is a close resemblance between the malignant peripheral nerve tumors (malignant schwannoma) and mesenchymal sarcoma.

TRAUMATIC NEUROMA (AMPUTATION NEUROMA)

A traumatic neuroma is initiated by trauma to a nerve trunk, most commonly amputation (amputation neuroma). In the jaws it may result from fractures, resection, or unavoidable interference with the nerve at the time of surgical removal of a cyst or tumor. It also may follow avulsion of a nerve performed for relief of neuralgia. The tumor appears on the torn or cut end of the nerve, where it forms a ball or swelling, varying in size, on the proximal termination of the nerve fiber. This nodule is formed by neurites seeking the distal portion of the nerve fiber through proliferative tracts of neurilemma cells. The result is a haphazard mixture of axis cylinders, connective tissue elements, and Schwann cells (Eversole, 1969).

A tumor within bone produces a radiolucent defect of varied shape, but it has well-defined borders. The roentgenogram shown in Figure 15–15 was made for a patient who gave a history of having had a large cyst excised from the mandible 5 years previously. A portion of the inferior dental nerve was unavoidably removed, resulting in numbness of the lip on the in-

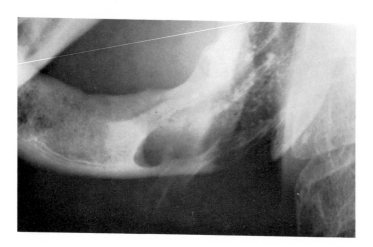

Figure 15–15 Traumatic neuroma (amputation neuroma) of the mandible resulting from injury to the inferior dental nerve.

volved side. At the time of admission the patient was experiencing severe pain. The roentgenogram reveals an elliptic cavity that extends anteriorly and downward from the posterior portion of the mandibular canal; the canal still appears normal and intact. The mandibular canal anterior to the tumor is completely obliterated, presumably by bone that replaced the cavity formerly occupied by the original cyst. This bone cavity might well be mistaken for a residual cyst; however, its direct communication with the mandibular canal and obliteration of the mandibular canal in the region anterior to it should suggest the diagnosis of traumatic neuroma. It is surprising, considering the number of fractures and surgical procedures that insult the inferior alveolar nerve, that this lesion does not occur more frequently.

For a neuroma with associated pain, the treatment is surgical excision.

CALCIFIED PERIPHERAL FIBROMA

A peripheral fibroma arising from the fibrous connective tissue of the periodontium may demonstrate the odontogenic potential of that tissue. It may arise from the gingival crevice on the buccal, labial, or lingual surface; it rarely reaches a diameter of more than 2 cm. Calcified substances form in many of these tumors and may be bone, cementum, amorphous and nonspecific calcifications, or a combination of these. From microscopic examination of 376 peripheral fibromas, Bhaskar and Jacoway (1966) found that almost 50% of them contained foci of bone or other calcified material. Those in which extensive calcification has taken place may become sufficiently radiopaque to permit visualization in the roentgenogram. Such a calcified fibroma previously reported by Stafne (1951) is shown in Figure 15–16. It was attached by a broad pedicle and was covered by an unbroken mucous membrane. The roentgenogram revealed a radiopaque mass that was separate from the alveolar process and therefore apparently was confined to the fibrous growth. On microscopic exami-

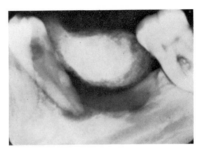

Figure 15–16 Calcified peripheral fibroma. (Reproduced with permission from Stafne, E. C.: Peripheral Fibroma [Epulis] That Contains a Cementum-like Substance. Oral Surg., Oral Med. & Oral Path. *4:* 463–465 [Apr.] 1951.)

nation the calcified substance resembled cementum more closely than normal bone. Because this lesion was situated in an edentulous space, it is uncertain whether it had arisen from the missing first molar or from one of the adjoining teeth.

Because these fibrous growths are rooted in the periodontal membrane, they may recur after simple excision. In some instances, therefore, it may be necessary to remove the teeth from which they arise.

GIANT-CELL GRANULOMA (BENIGN GIANT-CELL TUMOR, GIANT-CELL REPARATIVE GRANULOMA)

The etiology, nomenclature, and classification of giant-cell granulomas of the maxilla and mandible have generated considerable diversity of opinion. Some investigators object to the term "granuloma" while others indicate that the "tumor" aspect is misleading. There has been an attempt to associate trauma or tissue insult with the cause of these lesions; thus the term "reparative" is often used. Two of the questions regarding classification are: (1) Are the peripheral lesion and the central lesion of the jaws first cousins, or is the difference only in location? (2) Are the jaw lesions the same as those found in other bones, or is the separation based on pathogenesis?

Dahlin (1967) maintained that this lesion is peculiar to the jaws and that true giant-cell tumors are rarely, if ever, found in either the maxilla or the mandible. He pointed out that complete removal of giant-cell lesions of the jaws almost always effects a cure, whereas true giant-cell tumors recur in 50% of cases and 10% of them become malignant. However, Shafer et al. (1974) questioned the idea of a "true" giant-cell tumor as a totally separate entity. They subscribed to the view that the benign giant cell tumor of bone is the same as the central giant cell granuloma of the jaws, whereas the malignant lesion represents a form of osteogenic sarcoma whose individual lesions vary in their degree of malignancy.

Giant cell granulomas may be designated as peripheral or central in origin. Microscopic differentiation usually is impossible. The peripheral lesions occur equally in the maxilla or mandible and are located on the gingiva or alveolar process. Although they have a predilection for edentulous areas, they may be located in areas in which teeth are present. The lesions are often pedunculated but may be sessile. They are consistently deep red to blue. In a review of 720 cases, Giansanti and Waldron (1969) found a female-to-male ratio of 2 to 1. The age range in their study was 3 to 77 years (median, 31 years). The peripheral giant-cell granuloma is a benign lesion and responds favorably to simple surgical treatment. Although recurrence is possible, its incidence is extremely low.

Roentgenographically, the peripheral lesion may or may not involve the underlying bone. On occasion, a clearly discernible defect may be noted when the lesion produces a superficial erosion or saucer-shaped concavity on the alveolar ridge. The surface of this bony defect will usually be dense and sclerotic, indicating that invasive bone destruction has not occurred. This feature can be appreciated only with the intraoral dental films. A defect produced by a peripheral giant-cell granuloma that was situated in an edentulous molar region is shown in Figure 15–17. Obviously, this roentgenographic picture cannot be considered pathognomonic for peripheral giant-cell granulomas.

The central giant-cell granuloma occurs more often in children and young adults. Females are affected more than males, and the mandible is involved twice as frequently as the maxilla. The majority of these lesions occur in the region formerly occupied by deciduous teeth—that is, anterior to the molars. Frequently they cross the midline (Waldron and Shafer, 1966). Swelling may be the only presenting symptom and the lesion may be noted as an incidental finding during routine roentgenographic screening. Of 64 giant-cell granulomas reported from the Mayo Clinic (Austin et al., 1959), approximately half were central in origin. Although that paper also discussed two "genuine giant cell tumors," these have subsequently been reclassified as giant-cell granulomas.

The majority of central giant-cell granulomas respond favorably to surgical curettage, but a few resist conservative treatment and have recurred after fairly radical en bloc resection. Radiation therapy is not indicated.

Roentgenographically, the central tumor demonstrates two variations or types. One is a homogeneous, osteolytic, monolocular lesion in which evidence of bone trabeculations is absent from the affected site and in which the cortex may be partially or completely destroyed. The other

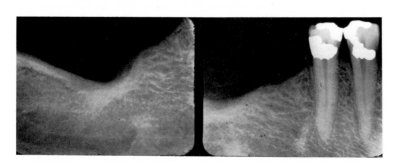

Figure 15–17 Giant-cell reparative granuloma that has produced a defect of the alveolar crest of the mandible from pressure erosion.

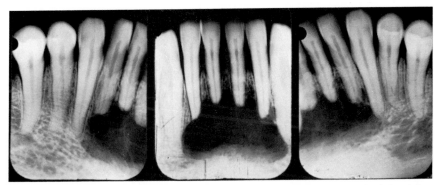

Figure 15–18 Giant-cell reparative granuloma at the symphysis of the mandible. It is of the monolocular type and presents no evidence of bone trabeculations within the lesion. (Reproduced with permission from Stafne, E. C.: Central Giant-Cell Tumor: Report of Case. J. Oral. Surg. 4:224–226 [July] 1946.)

type exhibits multiple osteolytic foci and evidence of the presence of bone trabeculations within the tumor; it may produce thinning and expansion of the cortex but causes perforation only when it has become very extensive. In both types, malposition of teeth and resorption of the roots of the teeth upon which the lesion encroaches are not unusual findings.

The roentgenogram shown in Figure 15–18, made for a woman 29 years of age, illustrates a monolocular type of lesion at the symphysis of the mandible. The tumor is circumscribed, but the margins are not as well-defined as those of an epithelium-lined cyst. No bone trabeculations are in evidence in the central portion of the lesion, and it has caused resorption of the roots of the incisor teeth.

A tumor of the multilocular type that occurred in the premolar region of the mandible is illustrated in Figure 15–19. The dental roentgenogram provided better detail of the interior portions of the tumor than did the extraoral lateral view of the mandible. The tumor extends from the midline to the second molar region and has caused a marked tilting of the premolars and resorption of the roots of the second premolar and first molar. The loculi are irregular in shape and vary in size. A few of them are circular, and in this respect they simulate other multilocular lesions that occur in the jaws, particularly ameloblastoma. Therefore, a diagnosis cannot be made on the basis of the roentgenographic appearance alone. A lateral view of the jaw of a boy 15 years of age that illustrates a multilocular tumor situated at the symphysis is shown in Figure 15–20. The tumor extends posteriorly to the premolar region of both sides. The greatest amount

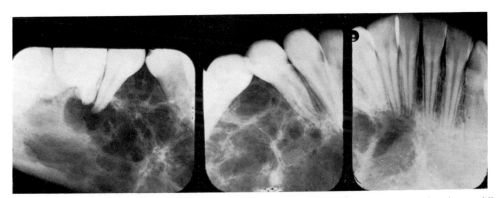

Figure 15–19 Giant-cell reparative granuloma of the mandible. Dental roentgenogram showing multilocular form of lesion. (Reproduced with permission from Stafne, E. C.: Value of Roentgenograms in Diagnosis of Tumors of the Jaws. Oral Surg., Oral Med. & Oral Path. 6:82–92 [Jan.] 1953.)

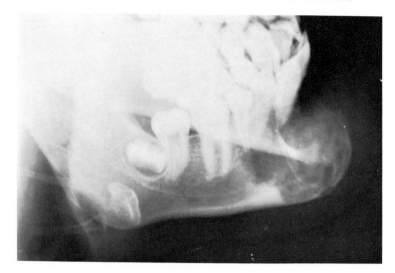

Figure 15–20 Giant-cell reparative granuloma of the multilocular type at the symphysis of the mandible in a boy 15 years of age. It has produced marked deformity of the chin.

of growth had taken place on the labial aspect of the mandible, producing marked deformity of the chin.

On the roentgenogram, these lesions may simulate a variety of pathologic entities. Figure 15–21 illustrates a giant-cell granuloma that easily could be classified as a cyst of the maxilla.

An interesting case of a giant-cell granuloma was reported by Huebner and Turlington (1971). An 11-year-old girl was seen because of left mandibular pain that had been present for about 1 week. About 1 month prior to examination, the child had paresthesia of the left lower lip. Roentgenograms revealed an indistinct lytic area of the left mandible extending from the lower left first molar to the angle. The cortical outline of the mandibular canal was destroyed, and the left inferior cortical border was indistinct (Fig. 15–22). This lesion proved to be a giant-cell granuloma, and it was removed by curettage. One year later, roentgenograms revealed recurrence. At the time of the second surgical procedure, a bony cavity was encountered that was devoid of any tissue or tissue lining and thus was compatible with the so-called traumatic bone cyst. Follow-up roentgenograms 1 year later revealed complete healing of the bone.

Roentgenographic findings that are associated with hormonal imbalance related to hyperparathyroidism are considered in detail in the chapter on systemic disease. It is appropriate, however, that some reference should be made to them here. Certainly, not every patient with hyperparathyroidism will exhibit osseous changes in the jaws and, of course, not all giant-cell lesions are associated with this condition. It is important, however, to suspect parathyroid abnormality whenever a patient develops giant-cell lesions of the jaws, particularly if they are multiple or bilateral. If the endocrine disturbance is treated successfully, the lesion disappears and the bone regains its normal appearance. Hyperparathyroidism is now being recognized in earlier stages, and thus the incidence of

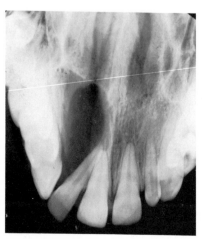

Figure 15–21 Giant-cell reparative granuloma that simulates the roentgenographic appearance of a cyst.

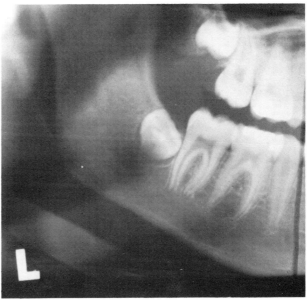

Figure 15–22 Lytic area of the mandible in the developing third molar area. Note that the cortical outline of the mandibular canal is destroyed. This lesion proved histologically to be a giant-cell granuloma. (Reproduced with permission from Huebner, G. R. and Turlington, E. G.: So-called Traumatic (Hemorrhagic) Bone Cysts of the Jaws: Review of the Literature and Report of Two Unusual Cases. Oral Surg., Oral Med. & Oral Path. *31*:354–365 [Mar.] 1971.)

giant-cell lesions (which indicate long-standing disease) is appreciably decreased. The roentgenogram of a patient with advanced hyperparathyroidism is shown in Figure 15–23. In general these lesions do not produce the marked expansion of the cortex with deformity that is often seen in the central giant-cell granuloma. In addition, the location in this particular example would have to be considered as weighing against central giant-cell granuloma.

CENTRAL HEMANGIOMA OF BONE

Hemangiomas are relatively uncommon lesions in the maxilla or mandible. They are composed of blood channels of

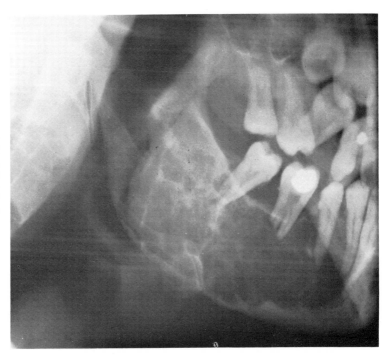

Figure 15–23 Giant-cell tumor of the mandible in a case of advanced hyperparathyroidism. (Reproduced with permission from Stafne, E. C.: Value of Roentgenograms in Diagnosis of Tumors of the Jaws. Oral Surg., Oral Med. & Oral Path. *6*:82–92 [Jan.] 1953.)

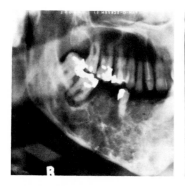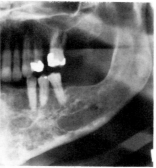

Figure 15–24 Hemangioma involving the entire body of the mandible in a 67-year-old woman.

varied patterns that can be classified histologically as cavernous, capillary, or mixed. The cavernous hemangioma consists of large thin-walled vessels and endothelium-lined sinuses that contain blood and are often interspersed among bony trabeculae. The capillary type is composed of small vessels and capillaries that tend to spread through a variable amount of connective tissue stroma.

In many instances there are no symptoms referable to the hemangioma, and it may be recognized incidentally in a roentgenographic examination that reveals the cystic changes produced by the tumor. In other patients, the presenting symptom is a hard, nontender swelling that has slowly enlarged over several months or years. The swelling may be rather small, or the face may have become noticeably asymmetric because of the bulging of the tumor. Hemorrhaging around the necks of the teeth in the involved region or severe

bleeding after extraction may give a clue to the nature of the lesion; however, spontaneous bleeding is not consistently present. Other clinical findings frequently encountered are mobility of the teeth, hyperthermia of the affected side, bruit, and, less frequently, pain and paresthesia.

The duration of known symptoms varies considerably. A roentgenogram of an extensive hemangioma of the mandible is shown in Figure 15–24. This lesion extends from angle to angle, involving the entire body of the mandible. The patient was a 67-year-old woman who had been aware of her "blood vessel tumor" for 30 years.

Lund and Dahlin (1964) reported that hemangiomas occur twice as frequently in females as in males and that the majority of patients with this lesion are less than 20 years old. It is of interest that hemangiomas are found in the mandible much more frequently than in the maxilla.

Hemangiomas of the maxilla or mandi-

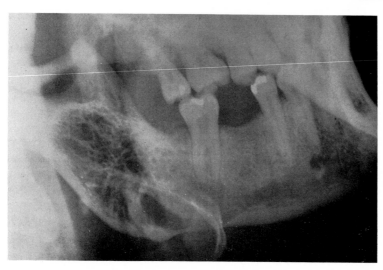

Figure 15–25 Cavernous hemangioma of the ramus of the mandible, showing coarse bone trabeculae radiating from the center toward the periphery of the lesion. (Reproduced with permission from Stafne, E. C.: Value of Roentgenograms in Diagnosis of Tumors of the Jaws. Oral Surg., Oral Med. & Oral Path. 6:82–92 [Jan.] 1953.)

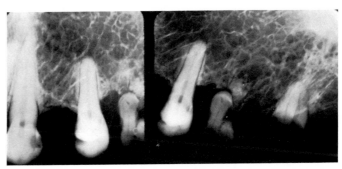

Figure 15–26 Cavernous hemangioma of the maxilla. Bone spicules extending at right angles to the bone and into the lesion can be seen at the anterior border of the lesion.

ble do not demonstrate the classic roentgenographic findings that are often characteristic of this lesion when it is in the skull or long bones. Large lesions in the mandible, however, often consistently reveal cystic spaces interspaced with trabecular patterns and thinned, expanded, eroded cortices.

Hemangiomas may occur in any region of the mandible. A roentgenogram of a lesion involving the ramus is shown in Figure 15–25. The trabeculae extend from the center toward the periphery of the lesion.

Hemangiomas of the maxilla are less likely to have specific roentgenographic patterns, primarily because the bony architecture interferes with a clear roentgenographic evaluation. A roentgenogram of a cavernous hemangioma of the maxilla is shown in Figure 15–26. The dental roentgenogram is presented because it better visualizes the trabecular pattern. In the region between the canine and second premolar where the surrounding bone is still

intact, bone spicules can be seen extending at right angles from the bone into the lesion, a feature that is pathognomonic of hemangioma. When observable, this feature serves to differentiate hemangiomas from ameloblastomas and other lesions that may have a honeycomb appearance. Unfortunately, it is not a consistent finding, as evidenced by Figure 15–27, which shows the roentgenograms of a hemangioma involving most of the maxilla.

When hemangiomas are small, they present no clinical characteristic or radiographic evidence of a vascular lesion. Figure 15–28 shows a well-circumscribed cavity in bone with sclerotic borders.

These vascular lesions are not routinely considered in the differential diagnosis of lytic lesions of the jaws because of their relatively infrequent occurrence. Since profuse, unexpected bleeding may be difficult to control, needle aspiration prior to incisal biopsy procedures should be used in evaluating lytic lesions of the jaws.

Figure 15–27 Hemangioma of the maxilla.

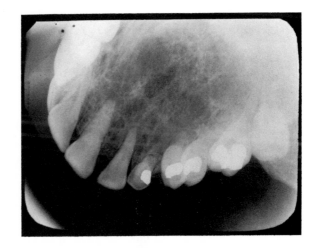

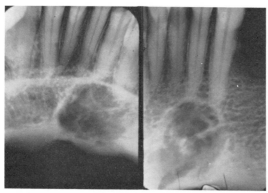

Figure 15–28 Capillary hemangioma of the mandible. Well-circumscribed cavity in bone with sclerotic borders. Within the lesion there is evidence of bone trabeculations that do not have a regular arrangement. (Reproduced with permission from Erich, J. B.: Central Hemangioma of the Mandible: Report of a Case. Am. J. Orthodontics [Oral Surg. Sect.]. *33*:611–613 [Aug.] 1947.)

ARTERIOVENOUS FISTULA

An arteriovenous fistula is a direct communication between an artery and a vein, through which the blood bypasses the capillary circulation. It is a normal feature of the microcirculation; however, by virtue of its size or location, it may be pathologic. Arteries leading into the fistula become dilated and undergo marked degenerative changes. The muscular layers atrophy and the walls become thin and lose their elasticity. The thin-walled arteries and veins tend to rupture and cause progressive formation of new fistulas.

Arteriovenous fistulas may be congenital or acquired. Congenital arteriovenous fistulas result from failure of differentiation of the common embryologic *Anlage* into artery and vein. In the neck and face these congenital fistulas are usually formed by multiple and extensive communications between arteries and veins. Significant local deformity may result, but adverse hemodynamic effects, such as cardiac hypertrophy or decompensation, are absent (Gomes and Bernatz, 1970). Acquired arteriovenous fistulas are most commonly a result of trauma, particularly penetrating wounds such as stab or gunshot wounds.

Indications for surgery may be cosmetic, although bleeding or potential hemorrhage could be compelling.

Early diagnosis and proper treatment of an arteriovenous fistula of the jaws are important to the dentist because a simple extraction of a tooth could cause uncontrollable and fatal hemorrhage (Broderick and Round, 1933). Clinical examination plays an important part in arriving at a correct diagnosis. Enlargement and abnormal warmth of the part, a palpable thrill, and an audible bruit are salient features. Also, there may be loosening of teeth at the site of the fistula and spontaneous hemorrhage from the mouth (Brodsky, 1931).

The roentgenogram shown in Figure

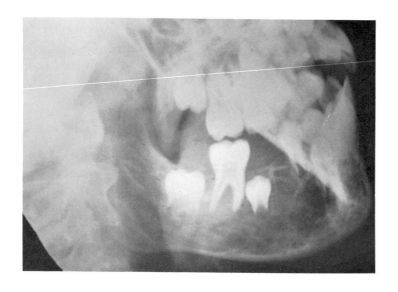

Figure 15–29 Congenital arteriovenous fistula that has caused marked destruction of bone of the body of the mandible. (Reproduced with permission from Devine, K. D., Beahrs, O. H., Lovestedt, S. A., and Erich, J. B.: Congenital Arteriovenous Fistulas of the Face and Neck. Plast. & Reconstruct. Surg. *23*:273–282 [Mar.] 1959.)

15–29 is from a case reported by Devine and colleagues (1959). It was made for a girl 9 years of age who 1½ years previously had had the first of several episodes of severe bleeding from the mouth. A loose deciduous second molar appeared to be the source of the hemorrhage, and it was extracted by her dentist several days after the first episode. This was followed by a profuse hemorrhage that required transfusions. The roentgenogram previously referred to revealed extensive destruction of bone, extending from the canine region posterior to the ramus of the left mandible. The first molar was loose and extruded as a result of loss of its supporting bone. The roentgenographic appearance is not diagnostic, however, because similar marked destruction of bone and sloughing of teeth are characteristic of many malignant tumors. Therefore, one must rely largely on the clinical signs. The treatment in this case was hemimandibulectomy.

Clay and Blalock (1950) stated that, if marked destruction of bone is present, preparation for mandibular resection must be made because this may be the only way to control bleeding successfully and to eradicate the fistula.

ANEURYSMAL BONE CYSTS

Aneurysmal bone cysts occur most frequently in the spinal column and long bones but may be found in almost any part of the skeleton. They are relatively uncommon in the mandible and maxilla, fewer than 20 cases having been reported in the literature.

Jaffe and Lichtenstein (1942) suggested the name "aneurysmal bone cyst" to differentiate these lesions from other solitary cystic lesions of bone. The word "aneurysmal" depicts the distention or ballooning of the bone contour.

These lesions are often noticed in patients during the first and second decades. There does not appear to be any marked sex predilection, but they do occur more frequently in the lower jaw. The presenting symptom is often a progressive swelling of the jaws that may be associated with pain or tenderness. Teeth adjacent to the lesion may be deflected but still vital.

Microscopically, the characteristic feature of aneurysmal bone cyst is the large number of cavernous spaces that vary in size and that lack the usual elastic lamina and muscular layers of blood vessels. The walls and septa consist of fibrous tissue containing variable amounts of fibroblasts, benign giant cells, and long osteoid trabeculae. Solid zones, when present, may have a pronounced resemblance to a giant-cell reparative granuloma. According to Gruskin and Dahlin (1968), a small biopsy specimen may be inadequate for differentiation of these two lesions, and diagnosis may depend solely on the finding of blood-filled spaces in the aneurysmal bone cyst.

Bernier and Bhaskar (1958) have expressed the opinion that aneurysmal bone cyst may result from an overzealous attempt to replace a hematoma in bone marrow. Other theories have been proposed; however, the cause of the cyst remains obscure. Whether it occurs as a primary lesion or develops secondarily in a pre-existing lesion that has been altered by hemorrhage, cystic degeneration, or some other pathologic process is not known (Oliver, 1973).

The roentgenogram often shows a well-circumscribed unilocular cystic lesion. As the lesion increases in size, there may be a marked expansion and thinning of the cortex, resulting in a ballooning or "blow-out" appearance that noticeably distends from the jaw. A roentgenogram that exhibits these features is shown in Figure 15–30. Made for a girl 8 years of age, it reveals marked destruction of the bone extending from the first molar region into the ramus and perforation of the thin cortex at the inferior border of the lesion. If the lesion involves the region of the teeth, root resorption may be seen. A definite diagnosis is not possible roentgenographically, however, and the differential diagnosis would have to include central myxoma, giant-cell lesions, and odontogenic cysts or tumors.

Aneurysmal bone cyst is essentially a benign condition that generally responds

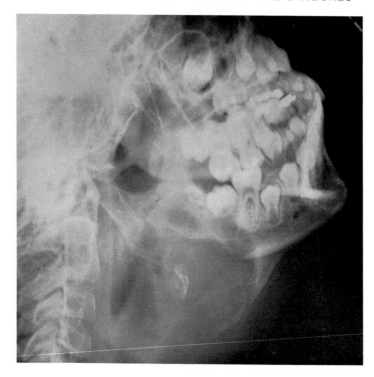

Figure 15–30 Aneurysmal bone cyst of the mandible in an 8-year-old girl, showing marked expansion and thinning of the cortex.

favorably to conservative surgical curettage. The amount of hemorrhage encountered at operation is variable but should be readily controlled. It is important to distinguish between this lesion and arteriovenous fistula, which presents a much greater surgical hazard.

DERMOID CYSTS

Dermoid cysts have this name because they contain elements of dermis, such as epidermal tissue, hair, nails, and sebaceous and sweat glands. They are benign, congenital tumors that may occur in the region near the pituitary gland, in the submaxillary region, and, not uncommonly, in the sex glands, particularly the ovary. Many contain teeth, which permits a fairly reliable diagnosis to be made from the roentgenologic examination alone. Glass and Rosenthal (1937) studied 91 dermoid cysts and found teeth in 18 and teeth and bone in 8. Primary as well as permanent teeth may be present, and all anatomic forms may be found (incisors, canines, premolars, and molars). Jawbones may be represented by a small rudimentary fragment

or may reach appreciable size and development. Heron (1941) reported a dermoid cyst that contained half of a well-formed mandible with a partially formed ramus. Lyon (1942), who made a study of the teeth present in 37 dermoid cysts, found them to be of all forms but, in general, smaller than normal teeth. The roots were smaller, particularly those that were not attached to bone. The periodontal membrane was similar to that of unerupted teeth in that the

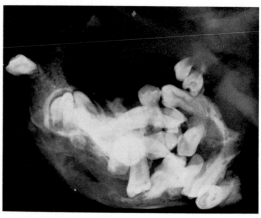

Figure 15–31 Dermoid cyst removed from the ovary. It contained a portion of a mandible and 25 teeth.

fibers ran parallel to the surface of the root. The cementum was thin and of the primary or acellular type, and there was a high incidence of resorption of the roots.

A roentgenogram of the gross specimen of a dermoid cyst removed from the ovary is shown in Figure 15–31. It contained a large portion of the mandible, including one of the rami and 25 teeth. The teeth were in all stages of development; a few were lying free in the soft tissue. A dentigerous cyst had developed from one of the embedded teeth.

MALIGNANT TUMORS

A malignant tumor is one that grows rapidly and invades adjacent tissue. Malignant cells from it may enter blood vessels and lymph channels to be spread from the site of origin and set up secondary foci of malignancy. The primary or original tumor may occur in the oral cavity and jaws, or the tumor in the oral region may result from metastasis of a tumor that arises in another part of the body. The two main types of malignant tumor are carcinoma and sarcoma.

No attempt has been made here to illustrate roentgenographically all forms of malignant tumors that occur in the jaws, either primary or metastatic. Enough are shown, however, to demonstrate the destructive and invasive nature of these tumors, which in general differentiates them from benign tumors. The jaws, more than any other region of the body, are subject to acute infections that produce widespread destruction of bone, and, when seen in the roentgenogram, this tends to simulate the destruction produced by malignant tumors. Therefore, the oral roentgenologist often is confronted with the problem of differentiating between inflammatory and malignant lesions, and the possibility of malignancy should be kept constantly in mind.

CARCINOMA

A carcinoma is a malignant tumor of epithelial origin. It may arise in any organ in which there is epithelial tissue and is the most common of the malignant tumors. There are several types of carcinoma, including basal-cell carcinoma, adenocarcinoma, transitional-cell carcinoma, melanocarcinoma, and squamous-cell (epidermoid) carcinoma. Squamous-cell carcinoma is the one that occurs most frequently in the oral cavity, and the sites of origin may be the lip, tongue, floor of the mouth, palate, buccal surfaces, and gingivae. In rare instances the tumor may arise within the jaws from cell rests remaining from the enamel organ and sheath of Hertwig (Thomas, 1954).

In the early detection of primary squamous-cell carcinoma of the oral cavity, roentgenographic examination is of doubtful value because involvement and invasion of bone may be a late feature in the development of the tumor. When bone is invaded secondarily, erosion of the surface may be sufficient to be readily discernible in the roentgenogram. Later, the lesion may invade the cortex and cause widespread destruction of the bone. The roentgenographic appearance in the advanced stages is one of radiolucency with irregular and ill-defined borders. Expansion of the cortex, characteristic of benign tumor, is seen rarely. In appearance, it most closely simulates infection and an inflammatory process.

A dental roentgenogram made for a patient who had a grade 4 squamous-cell carcinoma of the gingivae that had extended to the floor of the mouth and also involved the cervical lymph nodes is shown in Fig-

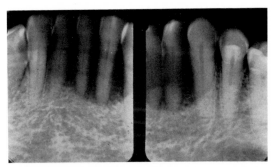

Figure 15–32 Squamous-cell carcinoma of the labial fold and the floor of the mouth, which has destroyed alveolar bone in a manner much like that of periodontal lesions.

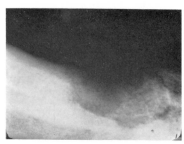

Figure 15–33 Squamous-cell carcinoma of the mucosa of the alveolar ridge of the mandible, showing invasion and diffuse destruction of bone.

ure 15–32. The alveolar process in the region of the incisors has been destroyed and two of the teeth have been loosened, but the destruction is not great in view of the extensive involvement by the tumor. Based on roentgenographic evidence alone, this well could be destruction of bone produced by periodontal disease.

The roentgenogram shown in Figure 15–33 was made for a patient who had an ulcerated lesion on the crest of the alveolar ridge of the mandible. It reveals bone destruction with what appears to be sequestration; therefore, it closely resembles osteomyelitis. However, any ulcerated growth of the soft tissue beneath which there is roentgenographic evidence of destruction of bone should be suspected of being malignant.

Figure 15–34 is a lateral roentgenogram of the jaw made for a patient who had an adenocarcinoma that originated in the lower buccal fold. The lesion has perforated the cortex and entered the cancellous bone of the mandible, where it has produced marked destruction in the region of the premolar and molar teeth.

Carcinomas that occur in the jaws as a result of metastasis from lesions elsewhere most often arise in the central portion of the jaws, because red bone marrow appears to be the most frequent site of metastasis to bone. The first evidence of metastasis may be roentgenographic signs of an osteolytic lesion in a jaw that, on clinical examination, appears to be normal. The lesions that occur in the mandible commonly cause numbness of the lip and chin; when this symptom is present, one should suspect that the lesion is malignant. When the patient is questioned, a history of diagnosis and treatment of the primary lesion may be elicited. However, the presence of the primary lesion may not be known at the time of the oral examination. Aisenberg and Inman (1956) stated that, in two of five cases of metastasis to the jaws, the presence of the primary lesion was known beforehand, whereas in three the primary lesions were discovered after biopsy of the lesions of the jaw.

In a study of 25 cases of malignant tumors metastatic to the jaws, Meyer and Shklar (1965) observed that 5 of them led to the discovery of the primary lesion; in a study of 97 cases, Clausen and Poulsen (1963) found that in 33 the oral metastasis

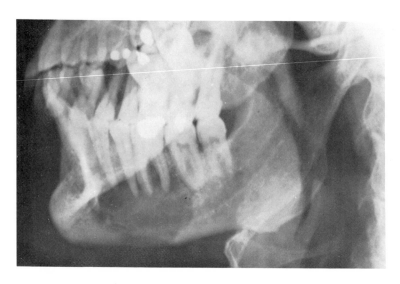

Figure 15–34 Adenocarcinoma of the lower buccal fold, which has perforated the cortex and entered the cancellous portion of the mandible where it has caused marked destruction of bone.

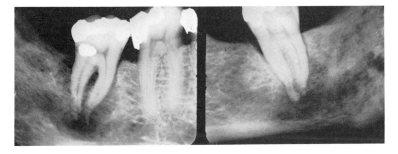

Figure 15–35 Metastatic carcinoma of the mandible in which the primary lesion was a carcinoma of the breast. The dental roentgenogram shows bilateral involvement, as evidenced by osteolytic lesions in the molar regions.

was discovered before the primary lesion. A search for a possible primary lesion always is indicated when a cancer involving the bone of the jaws is first detected, particularly for those that are not the result of direct extension from the oral soft tissues. The mandible is by far the most frequent site of tumors metastatic to the jaws. Although metastasis from the breast is frequently observed, metastasis from any location is possible.

The roentgenogram shown in Figure 15–35 is of interest because it demonstrates bilateral occurrence of carcinoma of the mandible from a primary lesion in the breast. The symptom that led to examination was numbness of the entire lower lip. The roentgenogram revealed osteolytic le-

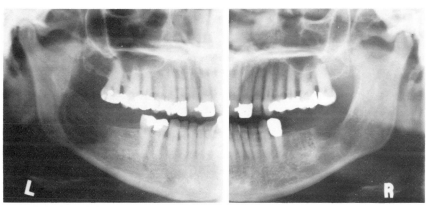

Figure 15–36 Bilateral metastatic carcinoma (same patient as in Figure 15–35), showing unusual symmetric lesions in the third molar areas.

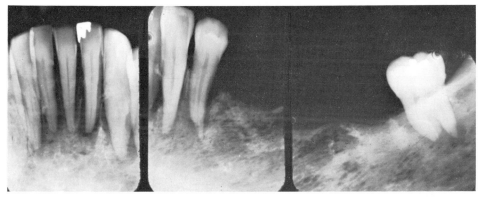

Figure 15–37 Metastatic carcinoma of the mandible, showing diffuse and widespread destruction of bone which resembles that seen in acute osteomyelitis.

sions surrounding the roots and extending posteriorly from both of the mandibular second molars. Figure 15–36 shows bilateral metastatic lesions as they appeared on the panoramic roentgenograms.

A metastatic carcinoma of the mandible that produced more diffuse and widespread destruction of bone is shown in Figure 15–37. It involved the entire right side of the mandible and included the symphysis. There was numbness of the lip on the involved side and also pain and some swelling in the posterior region. The roentgenographic appearance is similar to that seen in acute osteomyelitis, for which carcinoma may be mistaken.

MUCOEPIDERMOID CARCINOMA

Mucoepidermoid carcinomas arise most frequently in the major salivary glands and less frequently in the minor salivary glands. The tumor may be found as a central lesion within the jaws. Nine cases were reported from the Mayo Clinic by Smith et al. (1968). Their findings indicated that either the maxilla or the mandible may be involved but that the molar-premolar area is the usual site. Central lesions appear twice as frequently in women as in men, and the average age at diagnosis is 46 years. The most common roentgenographic finding is a multilocular radiolucency that is similar to ameloblastoma; however, wide variations occur. The presenting symptom is usually a slowly enlarging mass with or without pain.

Figure 15–38 shows the roentgenographic appearance of a lesion in an edentulous patient that proved histologically to be a mucoepidermoid carcinoma. Figure 15–39 shows a lesion of the mandible that mimics a dentigerous cyst. Complete surgical excision of these tumors is the preferred treatment, with radiation therapy used to manage recurrent or inoperable lesions.

SARCOMA

A sarcoma is a malignant tumor of connective tissue origin. It may originate in fibrous tissue, cartilage, bone, muscle, fat, or endothelial tissue. In general, sarcomas differ from malignant epithelial tumors in that they occur in a younger age group. They have a greater propensity to metastasize via the bloodstream rather than the lymphatics; thus, distant sites of secondary tumor are observed more frequently. The roentgenographic examination is important in the early detection of sarcoma that is primary in the jaws, because this type of tumor invariably produces changes in bone in the early stage of development. The roentgenographic evidence of sarcoma may be irregular and diffuse destruction of bone and a patchy appearance, and there may be no line of demarcation from the normal surrounding bone. In some types, excessive cartilage or bone formation within the bone

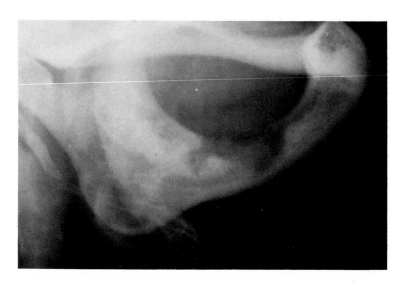

Figure 15–38 Diffuse lytic destruction of the mandible by mucoepidermoid carcinoma. (Reproduced with permission from Smith, R. L., Dahlin, D. C., and Waite, D. E.: Mucoepidermoid Carcinoma of the Jawbones. J. Oral Surg. 26:387–393 [June] 1968.)

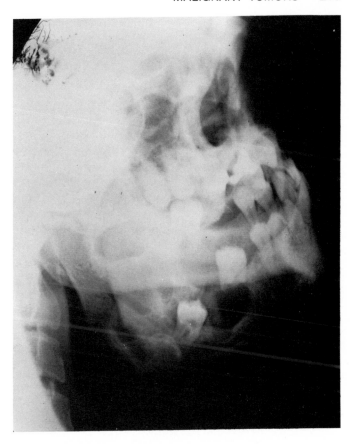

Figure 15-39 Cystic lesion of the mandible that resembles dentigerous cyst but proved histologically to be mucoepidermoid carcinoma. (Reproduced with permission from Smith, R. L., Dahlin, D. C., and Waite, D. E.: Mucoepidermoid Carcinomas of the Jawbones. J. Oral Surg. *26*:387–393 [June] 1968.)

or on its surface (or both) is evidenced by increased opacity.

Fibrosarcoma. Fibrosarcoma may arise in the jaws and is defined as a malignant tumor of spindle-shaped cells that produce no osteoid material in the primary lesion or in secondary deposits. The incidence of fibrosarcoma is less than that of osteosarcoma. These lesions occur equally in both sexes but, in contrast to osteosarcoma, they are found uniformly in both young and older age groups (Dahlin, 1967).

A dental roentgenogram that reveals localized destruction of the alveolar ridge beneath a moderate swelling of 2 months'

duration, which proved to be a fibrosarcoma, is shown in Figure 15–40.

Osteosarcoma (Osteogenic Sarcoma). The osteosarcomas may present a wide range of microscopic and roentgenographic findings. Dahlin (1967) divided this group into osteoblastic, chondroblastic, and fibroblastic tumors, depending on the dominating element.

As pointed out by Dahlin (1967) and by Garrington et al. (1967), there are several aspects of osteosarcomas as they occur in the jaws that deserve comment. The mean age at the time of the first-noted symptom related to the tumor is signifi-

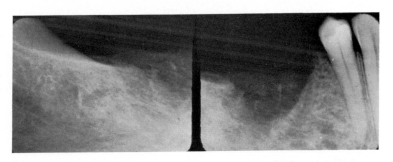

Figure 15-40 Fibrosarcoma of the mandible, showing the osteolytic character of the lesion.

cantly greater (about a decade) than for osteosarcoma of other bones. There appears to be a lesser degree of anaplasia in jaw tumors, with mandibular osteosarcomas having a better prognosis than maxillary tumors. In addition, hematogenous metastasis is less frequently observed.

The presenting symptom is often a swelling of the involved area, with or without associated pain. Paresthesia, loose teeth, and bleeding have been encountered (Kragh et al., 1960). Nasal obstruction may be noted with maxillary lesions.

The osteosarcomas do not produce a typical roentgenographic appearance. The lesion may exhibit a unicentric bony destructive lesion with indistinct borders, it may appear sclerotic or lytic, or there may be a combination of these findings.

Garrington et al. (1967) pointed out that, in some patients, an early osteosarcoma of the jaws may manifest a symmetrically widened periodontal membrane space associated with one or more teeth. This feature, of course, is apparent only on an intraoral periapical roentgenogram.

Figure 15–41, the lateral view of the jaw of a man 58 years of age, illustrates osteolytic osteogenic sarcoma. There is irregular destruction of bone in the posterior half of the ramus and extending to the angle of the mandible. There is no increased radiopacity to suggest any appreciable bone formation.

The roentgenographic features of an osteoblastic or sclerosing osteogenic sarcoma may be seen in the roentgenogram of an excised mandible from a boy 17 years of age (Fig. 15–42); these tumors occur most frequently in the earlier decades of life. The roentgenogram reveals destruction of bone and evidence of new bone formation within the body of the mandible; the shaft of the bone is almost intact. Extending downward from the lower border is evidence of periosteal bone formation that appears as spicules or lamellae situated at right angles to the surface of the bone (this produces a radiating appearance in many instances but is not peculiar to this condition alone). Microscopic examination in this case showed that the pulps of the molar teeth had been invaded by the tumor.

MALIGNANT LYMPHOMA

The malignant lymphomas are a group of neoplasms that are derived from lymphocytes and reticulum cells in any of their developmental stages. Numerous classifications have been suggested, but none is entirely satisfactory because the groups are not histologically exclusive or sharply defined. The term "reticulum-cell sarcoma" commonly is used for this tumor; however, as pointed out by Dahlin (1967), it is a misnomer because relatively few tumors are composed solely of this type of cell.

Malignant lymphomas may appear as primary lesions in bone. The tumor has a predilection for the humerus, femur, and

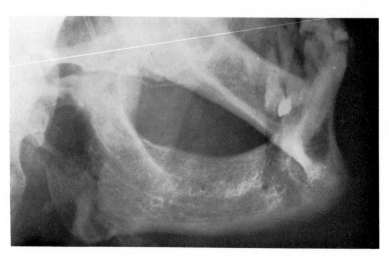

Figure 15–41 Osteogenic sarcoma of the osteolytic type involving the ramus of the mandible.

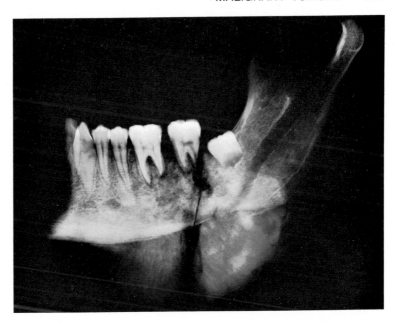

Figure 15–42 Osteogenic sarcoma of the osteoblastic or sclerosing type. Roentgenogram made of a resected mandible showing at its inferior border periosteal bone formation that produces a characteristic sunray or fan appearance.

tibia; however, in a Mayo Clinic series, 13 of 59 solitary lesions involved the mandible (Ivins and Dahlin, 1963). The maxilla is frequently affected, but it is more difficult to ascertain whether the tumors begin in the osseous structures or in the contiguous soft tissue. Steg and associates (1959) reviewed 47 cases of malignant lymphoma in the maxilla and mandible. They noted that the majority of these patients presented with swelling and pain of the involved area. Paresthesia was a frequent finding.

These authors emphasized the necessity of suspecting possible malignant bone tumors when destructive lesions of the jaws produce swelling and pain. In their series, misinterpretation of roentgenographic and clinical evidence resulted in extractions, antral operations, antral treatments, or incision and drainage as the original therapy for some patients with these lesions.

The mainstay in management of malignant lymphoma is irradiation, and this has produced good results. There is no signifi-

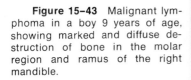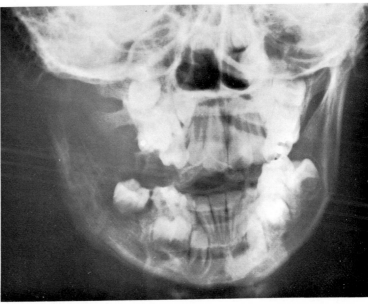

Figure 15–43 Malignant lymphoma in a boy 9 years of age, showing marked and diffuse destruction of bone in the molar region and ramus of the right mandible.

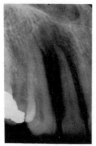 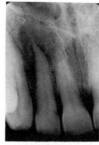

Figure 15-44 Bone loss surrounding maxillary lateral incisor. Film at right was taken 1 month prior to film at left. This was a malignant lymphoma, reticulum-cell type.

cant sex predilection, and all age groups are involved.

An anteroposterior roentgenographic view made for a boy 9 years of age who had a malignant lymphoma is shown in Figure 15–43. An extensive lesion has destroyed a portion of the mandible and the entire ramus. The lesion has caused sloughing of the first and second molars; the partially formed molar that remains but is undergoing exfoliation is probably a third molar.

The lesion represented in Figure 15–44 appears roentgenographically as a periodontal abscess. This patient was a 55-year-old man who had developed a painless swelling in the lateral incisor area. The lateral incisor was removed; the tissue submitted for histopathologic examination was initially described as nonmalignant. The patient was subsequently seen because of continued mobility of the anterior teeth. This time, tissue removed from the area was identified as reticulum-cell sarcoma.

CHONDROSARCOMA

Chondrosarcomas accounted for 11% of all malignant bone tumors in the Mayo Clinic series (Dahlin, 1967). Although these tumors are extremely rare in the jaws, Shafer et al. (1974) reported that they are more prevalent than benign cartilaginous tumors. It has been pointed out that they differ from osteosarcomas in clinical, therapeutic, and prognostic features.

When one considers all skeletal chon-

drosarcomas, there is a predilection for adulthood and older age groups. The tumor apparently may be present for some time before a clinically evident manifestation is observed. Metastasis is a late and often relatively infrequent problem, which contributes to a more favorable prognosis when removal has been adequate (Henderson and Dahlin, 1963).

Mesenchymal Chondrosarcoma. This is a comparatively rare neoplasm of bone, as indicated by the fact that, while there are more than 370 skeletal chondrosarcomas of ordinary type in the Mayo Clinic files, there are only 10 mesenchymal chondrosarcomas arising in bone. Salvador et al. (1971) recently reported their observations on this tumor. They pointed out that the ribs and jaws are the most common sites of involvement and that these tumors are relatively rare in tubular bones. There may be a slight predilection for females in the second and third decades of life.

Swelling is the most frequently recorded symptom. Pain and paresthesia may be associated with the swelling or occasionally may be the presenting complaint. It is conceivable that the lesion may be an incidental roentgenographic finding in the jaws, as it has been in other bones.

The majority of these bony lesions show some degree of calcification on the roentgenogram. Although the roentgenographic findings are suggestive of malignancy, there appear to be no characteristic features that allow differentiation from ordinary chondrosarcomas.

The roentgenogram for a 16-year-old girl is shown in Figure 15–45. This patient's presenting complaint was an enlarging mass in the left jaw that had been noted for about 4 months. The panoramic roentgenogram suggested a slowly growing lesion that had caused resorption of the roots of the second premolar and molars; the third molar was displaced up the ramus. The partial sclerotic border and position of the third molar may indicate a benign nature for this lesion. Figure 15–46 is a posteroanterior view that shows perforation of the lateral cortical plate along with a radiolucent area in the ramus.

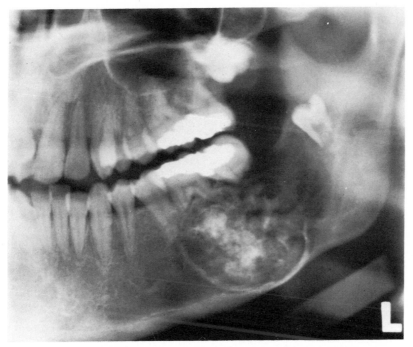

Figure 15–45 Mesenchymal chondrosarcoma of the mandible in a 16-year-old girl. There appears to be a partial well-defined border. Note resorption of the roots of the molar teeth as well as displacement of the third molar.

MULTIPLE MYELOMA

Myeloma is a tumor of bone that arises from bone marrow constituents resembling plasma cells. These neoplasms are almost always multiple and may be widely distributed throughout the skeleton, particularly in the ribs, sternum, skull, clavicles, and spinal column. Involvement of the jaws is not uncommon. Bruce and Royer (1953) studied the roentgenograms of the jaws of 59 patients with myeloma and found evidence of lesions of the jaws in 17

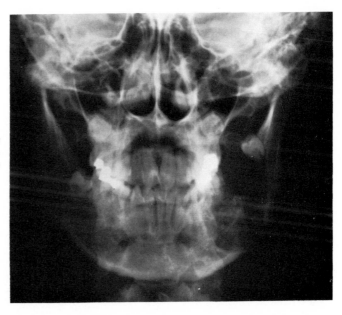

Figure 15–46 Posteroanterior view shows the medial extension of the mesenchymal chondrosarcoma shown in Figure 15–45.

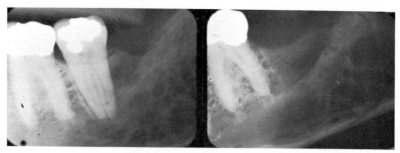

Figure 15–47 Multiple myeloma. *Left,* Dental roentgenogram showing many small, rounded, radiolucent foci that give it a honeycomb appearance. *Right,* Six weeks later, showing increased destruction of bone and coalescence of the multiple foci. (Courtesy of Dr. J. A. Millhon, Springfield, Illinois.)

(29%). The majority of these lesions occurred in the mandible. In seven of the patients the symptoms of myeloma were observed initially in the jaws. These signs and symptoms include swelling, pain, expansion, paresthesia, and looseness of the teeth. The disease occurs most frequently in the fourth to seventh decades of life, and it is fatal. Cataldo and Meyer (1966) reviewed a series of 44 cases of multiple myeloma in which 70% of the patients who had jaw roentgenograms taken had maxillary or mandibular lesions. In the Mayo Clinic series (Dahlin, 1967), in the 242 cases of multiple myeloma from which surgical material was available, 24 lesions were found in the jaws.

In the early stage, small radiolucent regions are confined to the bone marrow. When these become numerous, they coalesce and are manifested as large, irregularly defined regions of radiolucency. The

cortex is secondarily involved by direct extension and, in some instances, an entire bone may be destroyed.

In the jaws there may be a spotty distribution of lesions throughout both the maxilla and the mandible, but in most instances the mandible alone is affected. Here the initial lesions tend to appear in the posterior regions, where the marrow spaces are largest, and extend forward along and below the mandibular canal. There is also a tendency for them to extend up into the marrow spaces of edentulous regions and into the ramus.

The relationship between solitary plasma-cell tumors and multiple myeloma has been discussed by Cataldo and Meyer (1966). Occasionally, a solitary lesion is observed that is not associated with the abnormal laboratory findings so characteristic of multiple myeloma. These patients may develop multiple myeloma, but there

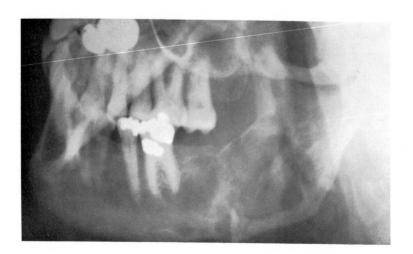

Figure 15–48 Multiple myeloma. Lateral view of the mandible of the patient represented in Figure 15–47, showing widespread destruction but no expansion and deformity of the bone.

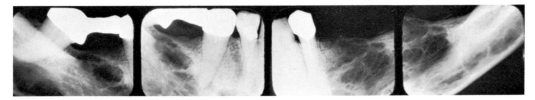

Figure 15–49 Multiple myeloma. Bilateral involvement of the mandible.

may be a latent period of many years. The lesions of multiple myeloma and of solitary plasma-cell tumors are usually histologically similar.

The primary lesion of multiple myeloma may occur in the jaws. Such cases were reported by Meloy and co-workers (1945) and by Wolff and Nolan (1944). The dental roentgenograms shown in Figure 15–47 were made for a woman 56 years of age who had a solitary myeloma of the mandible but no evidence of lesions elsewhere in the skeleton at the time the roentgenogram on the left was made. The one on the right, made 6 weeks later, shows multiple, punched-out, osteolytic foci typical of the first stage of tumor formation (in this later stage, the numerous small radiolucent areas have coalesced to form a large and more uniform radiolucent space). The second molar, evident in the first roentgenogram, had become loose. Biopsy at the time the tooth was extracted led to the correct diagnosis. A lateral view (Fig. 15–48) revealed widespread involvement of that side of the mandible. There is no evidence of osteoblastic activity and, while the lesion has become extensive, there is not the expansion of the cortex with deformity that is often present in ameloblastoma, giant-cell tumor, fibrous dysplasia, and some other conditions in which there may be similarly extensive involvement. In the case shown, similar lesions later appeared in other parts of the skeleton, and death occurred within 2 years after the onset of the lesion in the mandible.

When the jaws are involved, the lesions tend to be multiple. A dental roentgenogram made for a woman 57 years of age who had widespread multiple myeloma that followed a rapidly fatal course is shown in Figure 15–49. It revealed bilateral destruction of bone of the mandible and suggested generalized skeletal involvement. Surgical procedures had been carried out on the assumption that the lesions were benign tumors of the jaw.

The diagnosis of multiple myeloma is often aided by certain laboratory procedures. Many patients exhibit a hyperglobulinemia that is manifested by a reversal of the serum albumin-globulin ratio and an increase in total serum protein. It is well known that Bence Jones protein is noted in the urine in more than half of patients with multiple myeloma. Its absence does not rule out the disease, however.

REFERENCES

Aisenberg, M. S. and Inman, C. L., Sr.: Tumors That Have Metastasized to the Jaws. Oral Surg., Oral Med. & Oral Path. 9:1210–1217 (Nov.) 1956.

Austin, L. T., Dahlin, D. C., and Royer, R. Q.: Giant-Cell Reparative Granuloma and Related Conditions Affecting the Jawbones. Oral Surg., Oral Med. & Oral Path. 12:1285–1295 (Nov.) 1959.

Bernier, J. L. and Bhaskar, S. N.: Aneurysmal Bone Cysts of the Mandible. Oral Surg., Oral Med. & Oral Path. 11:1018–1028 (Sept.) 1958.

Bhaskar, S. N. and Jacoway, J. R.: Peripheral Fibroma and Peripheral Fibroma with Calcification: Report of 376 Cases. J. Am. Dent. A. 73:1312–1320 (Dec.) 1966.

Borello, E. D. and Sedano, H. O.: Giant Osteoid Osteoma of the Maxilla: Report of a Case. Oral Surg., Oral Med. & Oral Path. 23:563–566 (May) 1967.

Broderick, R. A. and Round, H.: Cavernous Angioma of Maxilla: Fatal Haemorrhage After Teeth Extraction, with Notes of Similar Non-fatal Case. Lancet. 2:13–15 (July 1) 1933.

Brodsky, R. H.: Cavernous Hemangioma of the Right Side of the Mandible. Dent. Cosmos. 73:1076–1081 (Nov.) 1931.

Bruce, K. W.: Solitary Neurofibroma (Neurilemmoma, Schwannoma) of Oral Cavity. Oral Surg., Oral Med. & Oral Path. 7:1150–1159 (Nov.) 1954.

Bruce, K. W. and Royer, R. Q.: Multiple Myeloma Occurring in Jaws: Study of 17 Cases. Oral Surg., Oral Med. & Oral Path. 6:729–744 (June) 1953.

Cataldo, E. and Meyer, I.: Solitary and Multiple Plasma-Cell Tumors of the Jaws and Oral Cavity. Oral Surg., Oral Med. & Oral Path. 22:628–639 (Nov.) 1966.

Chaudhry, A. P., Robinovitch, M. R., Mitchell, D. F., and Vickers, R. A.: Chondrogenic Tumors of the Jaws. Am. J. Surg. 102:403–411 (Sept.) 1961.

Clausen, F. and Poulsen, H.: Metastatic Carcinoma to the Jaws. Acta path. et microbiol. scandinav. 57:361–374, 1963.

Clay, R. C. and Blalock, A.: Congenital Arteriovenous Fistulas in the Mandible. Surg., Gynec. & Obst. 90:543–546 (May) 1950.

Dahlin, D. C.: Bone Tumors: General Aspects and Data on 3,987 Cases. Ed. 2. Springfield, Illinois, Charles C Thomas, Publisher, 1967, 285 pp.

Dahlin, D. C. and Johnson, E. W., Jr.: Giant Osteoid Osteoma. J. Bone & Joint Surg. (Am.). 36:559–572 (June) 1954.

Devine, K. D., Beahrs, O. H., Lovestedt, S. A., and Erich, J. B.: Congenital Arteriovenous Fistulas of the Face and Neck. Plast. & Reconstruct. Surg. 23:273–282 (Mar.) 1959.

DeVore, D. T. and Waldron, C. A.: Malignant Peripheral Nerve Tumors of the Oral Cavity: Review of the Literature and Report of a Case. Oral Surg., Oral Med. & Oral Path. 14:56–68 (Jan.) 1961.

Duncan, B. R., Dohner, V. A., and Priest, J. H.: The Gardner Syndrome: Need for Early Diagnosis. J. Pediat. 72:497–505 (Apr.) 1968.

Eversole, L. R.: Central Benign and Malignant Neural Neoplasms of the Jaws: A Review. J. Oral Surg. 27:716–721 (Sept.) 1969.

Ewing, J.: Neoplastic Diseases: A Treatise on Tumors. Ed. 3. Philadelphia, W. B. Saunders Company, 1928, p. 213.

Fader, M., Kline, S. N., Spatz, S. S., and Zubrow, H. J.: Gardner's Syndrome (Intestinal Polyposis, Osteomas, Sebaceous Cysts) and a New Dental Discovery. Oral Surg., Oral Med. & Oral Path. 15:153–172 (Feb.) 1962.

Foss, E. L., Dockerty, M. B., and Good, C. A.: Osteoid Osteoma of the Mandible: Report of a Case. Cancer. 8:592–594 (May-June) 1955.

Gardner, E. J. and Richards, R. C.: Multiple Cutaneous and Subcutaneous Lesions Occurring Simultaneously with Hereditary Polyposis and Osteomatosis. Am. J. Human Genet. 5:139–147 (June) 1953.

Garrington, G. E., Scofield, H. H., Cornyn, J., and Hooker, S. P.: Osteosarcoma of the Jaws: Analysis of 56 Cases. Cancer. 20:377–391 (Mar.) 1967.

Giansanti, J. S. and Waldron, C. A.: Peripheral Giant Cell Granuloma: Review of 720 Cases. J. Oral Surg. 27:787–791 (Oct.) 1969.

Glass, M. and Rosenthal, A. H.: Study of Dermoid Cysts with Suggestion as to Use of X-ray in Diagnosis. Am. J. Obst. & Gynec. 33:813–820 (May) 1937.

Gomes, M. M. R. and Bernatz, P. E.: Arteriovenous Fistulas: A Review and Ten-Year Experience at the Mayo Clinic. Mayo Clin. Proc. 45:81–102 (Feb.) 1970.

Greene, G. W., Jr., Natiella, J. R., and Spring, P. N., Jr.: Osteoid Osteoma of the Jaws: Report of a Case. Oral Surg., Oral Med. & Oral Path. 26:342–351 (Sept.) 1968.

Gruskin, S. E. and Dahlin, D. C.: Aneurysmal Bone Cysts of the Jaws. J. Oral Surg. 26:523–528 (Aug.) 1968.

Henderson, E. D. and Dahlin, D. C.: Chondrosarcoma of Bone: A Study of Two Hundred and Eighty-eight Cases. J. Bone & Joint Surg. (Am.). 45:1450–1458 (Oct.) 1963.

Heron, D. F.: Dentigerous Dermoid Cyst of Ovary Containing Portion of Mandible. J. Am. Dent. A. 28:1624–1626 (Oct.) 1941.

Huebner, G. R. and Turlington, E. G.: So-Called Traumatic (Hemorrhagic) Bone Cysts of the Jaws: Review of the Literature and Report of Two Unusual Cases. Oral Surg., Oral Med. & Oral Path. 31:354–365 (Mar.) 1971.

Ivins, J. C. and Dahlin, D. C.: Malignant Lymphoma (Reticulum Cell Sarcoma) of Bone. Mayo Clin. Proc. 38:375–385 (Aug. 28) 1963.

Jaffe, H. L.: "Osteoid-Osteoma": Benign Osteoblastic Tumor Composed of Osteoid and Atypical Bone. Arch. Surg. 31:709–728 (Nov.) 1935.

Jaffe, H. L. and Lichtenstein, L.: Solitary Unicameral Bone Cyst: With Emphasis on the Roentgen Picture, the Pathologic Appearance and the Pathogenesis. Arch. Surg. 44:1004–1025 (June) 1942.

Kolas, S., Halperin, V., Jefferis, K., Huddleston, S., and Robinson, H. B. G.: The Occurrence of Torus Palatinus and Torus Mandibularis in 2,478 Dental Patients. Oral Surg., Oral Med. & Oral Path. 6:1134–1141 (Sept.) 1953.

Kragh, L. V., Dahlin, D. C., and Erich, J. B.: Cartilaginous Tumors of the Jaws and Facial Regions. Am. J. Surg. 99:852–856 (June) 1960.

Kramer, H. S.: Benign Osteoblastoma of the Mandible: Report of a Case. Oral Surg., Oral Med. & Oral Path. 24:842–851 (Dec.) 1967.

Lichtenstein, L.: Bone Tumors. Ed. 3. St. Louis, The C. V. Mosby Company, 1965, 411 pp.

Lund, B. A. and Dahlin, D. C.: Hemangiomas of the Mandible and Maxilla. J. Oral Surg. 22:234–242 (May) 1964.

Lyon, E. D.: A Morphologic and Histopathologic Study of the Teeth Found in Dermoid Cysts and Teratomata of the Ovaries. Thesis, Mayo Graduate School of Medicine (University of Minnesota), Rochester, 1942.

Meloy, T. M., Jr., Gunter, J. H., and Sampson, D. A.: Mandibular Lesion as First Evidence of Multiple Myeloma. Am. J. Orthodontics (Oral Surg. Sect.). 31:685–689 (Nov.) 1945.

Meyer, I. and Shklar, G.: Malignant Tumors Metastatic to Mouth and Jaws. Oral Surg., Oral Med. & Oral Path. 20:350–362 (Sept.) 1965.

Moorrees, C. F. A.: The Dentition as a Criterion of Race with Special Reference to the Aleut. J. Dent. Res. 30:815–821 (Dec.) 1951.

Oliver, L. P.: Aneurysmal Bone Cyst: Report of a Case. Oral Surg., Oral Med. & Oral Path. 35:67–76 (Jan.) 1973.

Prescott, G. H. and White, R. E.: Solitary, Central Neurofibroma of the Mandible: Report of Case and Review of the Literature. J. Oral Surg. 28:305–309 (Apr.) 1970.

Rushton, M. A.: An Osteoid-Osteoma of the Mandibular Alveolus. Oral Surg., Oral Med. & Oral Path. 4:86–88 (Jan.) 1951.

Salvador, A. H., Beabout, J. W., and Dahlin, D. C.: Mesenchymal Chondrosarcoma: Observations on 30 New Cases. Cancer. 28:605–615 (Sept.) 1971.

Shafer, W. G., Hine, M. K., and Levy, B. M.: A Textbook of Oral Pathology. Ed. 3. Philadelphia, W. B. Saunders Company, 1974, p. 135.

Singer, C. F., Jr., Gienger, G. L., and Kullbom, T. L.: Solitary Intraosseous Neurofibroma Involving the Mandibular Canal: Report of Case. J. Oral Surg. 31:127–129 (Feb.) 1973.

Smith, R. L., Dahlin, D. C., and Waite, D. E.: Mucoepidermoid Carcinomas of the Jawbones. J. Oral Surg. 26:387–393 (June) 1968.

Spitzer, R.: A Case of an Intraosseous Osteoma of the Mandible. Oral Surg., Oral Med. & Oral Path. 7:471–473 (May) 1954.

Stafne, E. C.: Peripheral Fibroma (Epulis) That Contains a Cementum-like Substance. Oral Surg., Oral Med. & Oral Path. 4:463–465 (Apr.) 1951.

Steg, R. F., Dahlin, D. C., and Gores, R. J.: Malignant Lymphoma of the Mandible and Maxillary Region. Oral Surg., Oral Med. & Oral Path. 12:128–141 (Feb.) 1959.

Suzuki, M. and Sakai, T.: A Familial Study of Torus Palatinus and Torus Mandibularis. Am. J. Phys. Anthropol. n.s. 18:263–272 (Dec.) 1960.

Thoma, K. H.: Oral Pathology: A Histological, Roentgenological, and Clinical Study of the Diseases of the Teeth, Jaws, and Mouth. Ed. 4. St. Louis, The C. V. Mosby Company, 1954, p. 1333.

Waldron, C. A. and Shafer, W. G.: The Central Giant Cell Reparative Granuloma of the Jaws: An Analysis of 38 Cases. Am. J. Clin. Path. 45:437–447 (Apr.) 1966.

Wolff, E. and Nolan, L. E.: Multiple Myeloma First Discovered in Mandible. Radiology. 42:76–78 (Jan.) 1944.

16

FIBRO-OSSEOUS LESIONS

Fibro-osseous lesions are characterized by the formation of fibrous connective tissue in the spongiosa of bone—connective tissue that histologically exhibits active osseous metaplasia. Lesions of the jaws that exhibit this histologic feature are not uncommon and, on the basis of clinical features, there are among them several conditions that are considered separate clinical entities. These are fibrous dysplasia, ossifying fibroma (fibro-osteoma), leontiasis ossea, familial intraosseous swellings of the jaws (cherubism), and cementoma. Jaffe (1953), Schlumberger (1946), and Bernier (1959) have expressed the opinion that ossifying fibroma of the jaws should be regarded as a variant of fibrous dysplasia; Pugh (1945) and Cahn (1953) are among those who suggest that hyperostosis and deformity of the facial bones and skull known as "leontiasis ossea" probably represent in some instances fibrous dysplasia of the bone.

FIBROUS DYSPLASIA

Fibrous dysplasia is manifested as a benign fibro-osseous lesion of debatable pathogenesis. Jaffe (1953) has suggested that these lesions may be tumor-like malformations resulting from flaws of development and characterized by defects of tissue combination.

The present concept is that fibrous dysplasia occurs in three forms: (1) monostotic or solitary, (2) polyostotic, in which the multiple lesions tend to have a unilateral distribution, and (3) Albright's syndrome (1937), which is considered a more severe form and in which there is an associated pigmentation of the skin, and precocious puberty and skeletal development in females. Gorlin and Chaudhry (1957) have observed oral melanotic pigmentation in Albright's syndrome. In all three forms the lesions present a similar microscopic appearance.

The tumor is most commonly manifested in patients from 10 to 30 years of age. It often appears in childhood, grows slowly during the general growth period, and sometimes becomes static after general growth has ceased. In some instances deformities of the jaw may not be present, or they may be so slight that the condition first is recognized incidental to a roentgenographic examination only. The incidence is appreciably higher in females than in males.

Fibrous dysplasia occurs more frequently in the maxilla than in the mandible, is most often unilateral, and usually arises in the posterior regions of the jaws. The symptoms are usually swelling, facial asymmetry or distortion of facial contour, malocclusion, and, in a few instances, mild pain.

The roentgenographic appearance varies, depending on the relative amount of fibrous and osseous tissue present in the lesion and on whether it is circumscribed and sharply delineated or fades imperceptibly into normal surrounding bone.

Those tumors in which fibrous tissue is preponderant are cystic in appearance, and may be either monocystic or multilocular. In the latter instance they may in some respects resemble ameloblastoma; however, they differ in that a fibrillary network of fine bony trabeculae and evidence of scattered calcified areas are present within the tumor. This feature can be more clearly demonstrated by the dental roentgenogram. Lesions that appear cystic are most often seen in younger patients, or they have been present for only a short time.

Lesions in which an appreciable amount of osseous tissue has formed show coarser trabeculae and larger masses of dense calcified material that give them a mottled appearance.

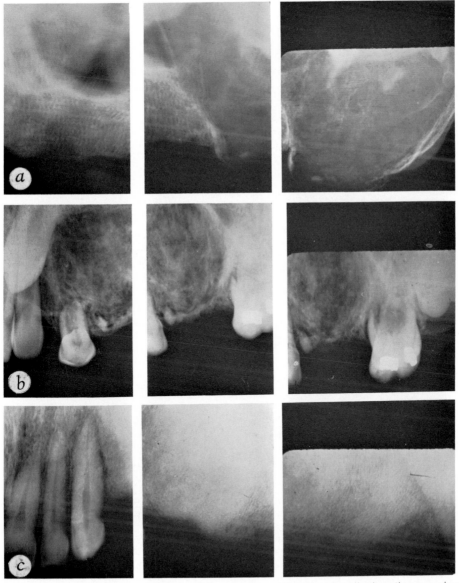

Figure 16–1 Monostotic fibrous dysplasia of the maxilla. *a,* Well-circumscribed cystic-appearing lesion in which there is only slight evidence of calcification. *b,* Well-circumscribed lesion in which there is evidence of scattered masses of highly calcified tissue, giving it a mottled appearance. *c,* Lesion of abnormal radiographic density which fuses imperceptibly with the surrounding bone. (Reproduced with permission from Zimmerman, D. C., Dahlin, D. C., and Stafne, E. C.: Fibrous Dysplasia of the Maxilla and Mandible. Oral Surg., Oral Med. & Oral Path. *11*:55–68 [Jan.] 1958.)

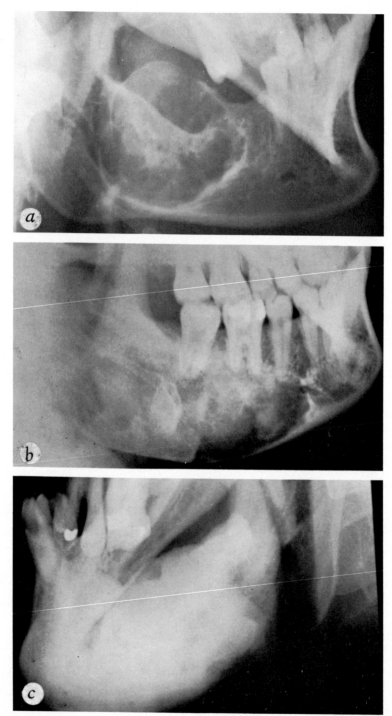

Figure 16–2 Monostotic fibrous dysplasia of the mandible. *a*, Circumscribed with cystic appearance. *b*, Circumscribed with mottled appearance. *c*, Lesion in which the bone is abnormally dense. All these lesions show expansion of the cortex and enlargement of the bone. (Reproduced with permission from Zimmerman, D. C., Dahlin, D. C., and Stafne, E. C.: Fibrous Dysplasia of the Maxilla and Mandible. Oral Surg., Oral Med. & Oral Path. *11*:55–68 [Jan.] 1958.)

The roentgenographic appearance of the lesions in which the osseous tissue is predominant and which are almost completely calcified is one of uniform increased radiographic density.

Dental roentgenograms of monostotic lesions of the maxilla that exhibit a cystic, mottled, and uniformly dense roentgenographic appearance are shown in Figure 16–1. Monostotic lesions involving the mandible are illustrated in Figure 16–2.

Lesions that reach an appreciable size and cause deformity produce thinning and expansion of the cortex, but rarely do they perforate it and produce new periosteal bone. Those that have their onset early in life may destroy the tooth germ, or prevent the eruption of teeth that have already formed. Roentgenographic evidence of agenesis and noneruption of the teeth in the region of the lesion should therefore provide a clue as to the approximate time that the lesion began to develop. The lesion also may cause resorption of the roots of erupted teeth on which it encroaches, and this is not an infrequent roentgenographic observation.

Serial roentgenograms have shown that the lesion becomes more calcified with increase in age of the patient; however, exceptions to this are not uncommon. Generally speaking, the osseous or more highly calcified lesions of fibrous dysplasia are found in older patients and in those in whom the lesion is of longer duration.

Most of the lesions are fairly well circumscribed, particularly smaller ones that have a cystic or mottled appearance. Those of uniform abnormal radiographic density and of more extensive size are prone to exhibit indefinite margins and borders. Certain roentgenograms, particularly of the maxilla, are deceiving concerning the limits and borders of the tumor. Roentgenograms of the maxillary sinus taken in Water's position often give the impression that the mass is diffuse and without definite borders, while the lateral view may reveal that it is well circumscribed.

Occlusal films of the maxilla and mandible of a patient with polyostotic fibrous dysplasia are shown in Figure 16–3. They were made for a man 32 years of age, in whom asymmetry of the face had first been noted at 8 years of age. The lesions involved the right side of the skull and the right maxilla and mandible. Surgical measures had been taken to reduce the deformity of the mandible at 13 years of age, and similar measures to reduce the deformity of the maxilla at 22 years of age. Several roentgenograms were available that dem-

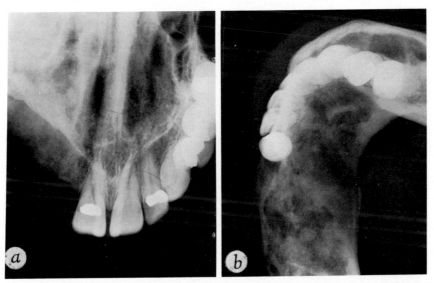

Figure 16–3 Polyostotic fibrous dysplasia. *a*, Occlusal view of the maxilla, showing lesion that is confined to one side only and is evidenced by increased radiographic density. *b*, Occlusal view of mandible, showing a thinned cortex, evidence of new bone formation within the lesion, and enlargement of the bone.

onstrate the extent of involvement of the bone. The occlusal films, while they do not reveal the limits of the lesion, are shown because they better visualize its architecture and internal structure, particularly in the view of the mandible. The occlusal view of the maxilla (Fig. 16–3a) demonstrates that the lesion does not extend across the median line, in which respect it differs from Paget's disease of the maxilla. In the mandible, fibrous dysplasia appears to have no respect for the midline, and often extends across it to involve the opposite side. The occlusal view of the mandible (Fig. 16–3b) reveals enlargement of the bone, which still has a relatively smooth surface and within which there are alternating areas of radiolucence and sclerosis. As a point of differential diagnosis, an ameloblastoma that would involve a mandible to this extent and reach such propor-

tions would at some point invariably perforate the thin cortex and extend at some distance into soft tissue, producing a lobulated and irregular surface.

The treatment of choice in fibrous dysplasia is almost always surgical. When the lesion is small and completely encapsulated, and removal can be accomplished without creating too large a surgical defect or loss of continuity of bone, this should be done. If the lesion is extensive and the limits of the involved bone make it impossible to remove it in its entirety, the lesion is simply trimmed surgically until a good aesthetic result is achieved. Whenever possible, it may be advisable to postpone operation for aesthetic purposes until after puberty, when the lesion tends to become static. According to Zimmerman and coworkers (1958), approximately 20% of the lesions continue to grow after treatment,

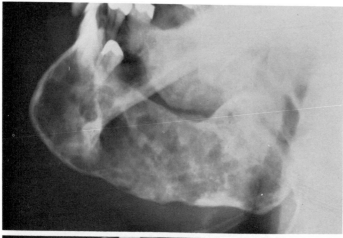

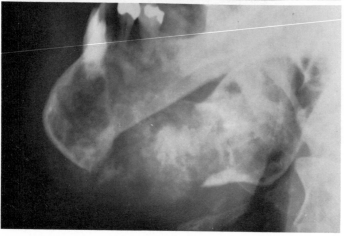

Figure 16–4 Fibrous dysplasia complicated by sarcoma. *Above,* Typical appearance of fibrous dysplasia, evidenced by continuous cortical plate. *Below,* Roentgenogram made more than 2 years later, showing destruction of cortex at lower border of mandible produced by superimposed osteogenic sarcoma. (Reproduced with permission from Tanner, H. C., Dahlin, D. C., and Childs, D. S.: Sarcoma Complicating Fibrous Dysplasia: Probable Role of Radiation Therapy. Oral Surg., Oral Med. & Oral Path. *14*:837–846 [July] 1961.)

except those treated by radical excision. Radiation therapy is ineffectual in fibrous dysplasia and may be a potential hazard. That irradiation can be an inciting factor in the development of sarcoma in these patients is highly suggestive. Tanner and co-workers (1961) reported four cases in which sarcoma complicated fibrous dysplasia. The lesions were confined to the facial bones in all four instances, and all of them had been irradiated.

Figure 16–4 shows roentgenograms from one of the cases reported by Tanner and colleagues (1961). The upper roentgenogram was made for a 32-year-old man who at 8 years of age received nine series of roentgen-ray treatments to the right side of the face for a fibro-osseous lesion. It revealed extensive involvement of the mandible, but a thin, continuous cortex was still present, which is consistent with fibrous dysplasia. The lower roentgenogram was made 2¼ years later, when the patient returned because of rapid enlargement of the right mandible. It revealed invasion and destruction of the cortex at the inferior border, caused by what proved to be a superimposed osteogenic sarcoma.

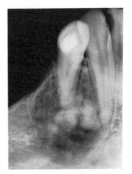

Figure 16–5 Ossifying fibroma (fibro-osteoma). Solitary, circumscribed fibrous lesion in which there is evidence of dense calcifications in the central portion.

OSSIFYING FIBROMA (FIBRO-OSTEOMA)

Fibro-osseous lesions that are considered neoplastic in origin by some authors (Pindborg, 1951; Sherman and Sternbergh, 1948; Thoma, 1956; Waldron, 1953) are referred to as ossifying fibroma or fibro-osteoma and, in some instances, as cementifying fibroma. They usually are described as well-circumscribed lesions that are most often solitary, but sometimes multiple, and

it is contended that they develop from cell rests in normal bone.

The following two illustrations are given because they are typical of cases that frequently have been illustrated and described as ossifying fibroma and fibro-osteoma. The roentgenogram shown in Figure 16–5 is that of a well-circumscribed solitary lesion in which there is evidence of dense calcification in the central portion. Figure 16–6 represents one that might be described as multiple in form, since the lesion that is situated posterior to the mandibular second molar appears to be separated by normal bone from the larger and more highly calcified one that is situated anterior to it. Microscopic examination of the lesion shown in Figure 16–5 might well lead to a diagnosis of cementifying fibroma, and similar examination of the one shown in Figure 16–6 to a diagnosis of ossifying fibroma; yet on the basis of such an examination, both of them justifiably could be placed in the category of fibrous dysplasia. That one can separate ossifying fibroma from fibrous dysplasia on the basis of the

Figure 16–6 Multiple form of ossifying fibroma as evidenced by the lesion in the third molar region, which is separated from the lesion that is situated anterior to it.

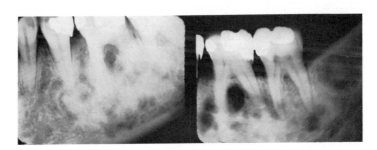

roentgenographic appearance is very doubtful.

CHERUBISM (FAMILIAL INTRAOSSEOUS SWELLINGS OF THE JAWS)

While the histologic appearance of familial fibrous enlargement of the jaws is somewhat similar to that of fibrous dysplasia, Caffey and Williams (1951) expressed the belief that the two entities should be considered separately because of the marked difference in their clinical pictures. Bruce and co-workers (1953) considered the former a separate entity and expressed the opinion that it does not meet entirely the rigid criteria for giant-cell tumor, for which it may be mistaken, nor does it fit snugly in the category of fibrous dysplasia.

Cherubism is characterized by benign, firm, painless swellings that occur bilaterally in the mandible, usually in the region of the angle. Other regions of the mandible also may be involved, and in some instances the tuberosity regions of the maxilla may be affected. The swellings may appear as early as 1 year of age, and the greatest expansion of the jaws occurs during the first and second years after onset. The tumors tend to cease growing shortly after puberty. With increase in age and size of the patient, the deformity produced becomes less noticeable, and by middle age the face may have returned to nearly normal appearance, even though the lesions, as such, may not have been reduced in actual size. There is a decided familial tendency for this condition to appear, and this has been reported by Jones and associates (1950), Caffey and Williams (1951), and Bruce and co-workers (1953).

During the stage of active growth and expansion of the lesions, the roentgenogram reveals multilocular, irregular cystic spaces in bone that are separated by fine septa, and there are thinning and expansion of the cortex. In some instances the cortex may be perforated and destroyed. The roentgenographic picture may be very similar to that seen in fibrous dysplasia and in some forms of central giant-cell tumor. Agenesis of the teeth in the involved region is almost a constant feature, and those teeth that are present may be prevented from erupting, or are forced to a location remote from their original position. On the basis of the roentgenogram, the multiple occurrence of the cystic lesions and the early age at which they are seen should lead one immediately to suspect cherubism, and particularly so if similar lesions have occurred in other members of the family.

The roentgenogram in Figure 16–7

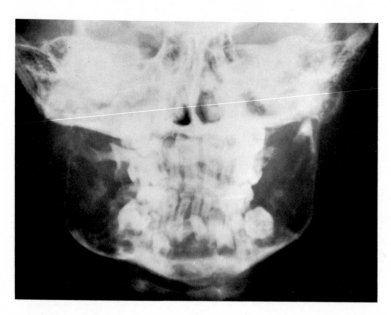

Figure 16–7 Cherubism (familial intraosseous swellings of the jaws) in a patient 5 years of age. Anteroposterior view, showing bilateral expansive cystic lesions of the posterior regions of the mandible. A similar lesion is also evident at the symphysis. (Reproduced with permission from Bruce, K. W., Bruwer, A., and Kennedy, R. L. J.: Familial Intraosseous Fibrous Swellings of the Jaws ("Cherubism"). Oral Surg., Oral Med. & Oral Path. 6:995–1014 [Aug.] 1953.)

was made for a white girl 5 years of age who had cherubism and whose father and grandfather had had a similar condition. This anteroposterior view reveals bilateral expansive lesions of the posterior regions of the mandible that extend upward into the rami, and another cystic lesion at the symphysis. The mandibular permanent second molars are absent. In addition to demonstrating the lesions present in the mandible, roentgenograms of the maxilla revealed that both tuberosities were involved.

With increase in age of the patient, the bony septa increase in width, and bony trabeculae form to the extent that the lesion may assume a greater degree of radiopacity than that of the surrounding normal bone.

Should the facial deformity persist, surgical treatment may be advisable and indicated, but for cosmetic reasons only. Unlike in true fibrous dysplasia, there appears to be no tendency for continued growth following surgical intervention, particularly after the lesion apparently has reached a quiescent state.

CEMENTOFIBROMA, CEMENTO-OSSIFYING FIBROMA, AND OSSIFYING FIBROMA

The cementoma, which was dealt with in Chapter 14 (Odontogenic Tumors), might justifiably be placed in the category of fibro-osseous lesions. In recent years, histologic studies have shown that a diagnosis based only on roentgenographic evidence is not reliable because many of these lesions are actually ossifying fibromas, including the periapical lesions. In a study of 43 cases in which clinical histories, roentgenograms, and microscopic sections were available, Waldron and Giansanti (1973) subdivided the lesions into three types, all considerably different from fibrous dysplasia: cementofibroma, cemento-ossifying fibroma, and ossifying fibroma. With the exception of three lesions, all were restricted to the tooth-bearing area. The authors concluded that the lesions

have their origin in cells of the periodontal membrane.

REFERENCES

Albright, F., Butler, A. M., Hampton, A. O., and Smith, P.: Syndrome Characterized by Osteitis Fibrosa Disseminata, Areas of Pigmentation and Endocrine Dysfunction, with Precocious Puberty in Females: Report of Five Cases. New England J. Med. 216:727–746 (Apr.) 1937.

Bernier, J. L.: The Management of Oral Disease: A Treatise on the Recognition, Identification, and Treatment of Diseases of the Oral Regions. 2nd ed. St. Louis, The C. V. Mosby Company, 1959.

Bruce, K. W., Bruwer, A., and Kennedy, R. L. J.: Familial Intraosseous Fibrous Swellings of the Jaws ("Cherubism"). Oral Surg., Oral Med. & Oral Path. 6:995–1014 (Aug.) 1953.

Caffey, J. and Williams, J. L.: Familial Fibrous Swelling of the Jaws. Radiology. 56:1–14 (Jan.) 1951.

Cahn, L. R.: Leontiasis Ossea. Oral Surg., Oral Med. & Oral Path. 6:201–212 (Jan.) 1953.

Gorlin, R. J. and Chaudhry, A. P.: Oral Melanotic Pigmentation in Polyostotic Fibrous Dysplasia, Albright's Syndrome. Oral Surg., Oral Med. & Oral Path. 10:857–862 (Aug.) 1957.

Jaffe, H. L.: Giant-Cell Reparative Granuloma, Traumatic Bone Cyst, and Fibrous (Fibro-osseous) Dysplasia of Jawbones. Oral Surg., Oral Med. & Oral Path. 6:159–175 (Jan.) 1953.

Jones, W. A., Gerrie, J., and Pritchard, J.: Cherubism—A Familial Fibrous Dysplasia of Jaws. J. Bone & Joint Surg. 32B:334–347 (Aug.) 1950.

Pindborg, J. J.: Fibrous Dysplasia or Fibro-osteoma: Report of Case. Acta radiol. 36:196–204 (Sept.) 1951.

Pugh, D. G.: Fibrous Dysplasia of Skull: Probable Explanation for Leontiasis Ossea. Radiology. 44:548–555 (June) 1945.

Schlumberger, H. G.: Fibrous Dysplasia (Ossifying Fibroma) of Maxilla and Mandible. Am. J. Orthodontics. 32:579–587 (Sept.) 1946.

Sherman, R. S. and Sternbergh, W. C. A.: Roentgen Appearance of Ossifying Fibroma of Bone. Radiology. 50:595–609 (May) 1948.

Tanner, H. C., Dahlin, D. C., and Childs, D. S.: Sarcoma Complicating Fibrous Dysplasia: Probable Role of Radiation Therapy. Oral Surg., Oral Med. & Oral Path. 14:837–846 (July) 1961.

Thoma, K. H.: Differential Diagnosis of Fibrous Dysplasia and Fibro-osseous Neoplastic Lesions of the Jaws and Their Treatment. J. Oral Surg. 14:185–194 (July) 1956.

Waldron, C. A.: Ossifying Fibroma of Mandible: Report of 2 Cases. Oral Surg., Oral Med. & Oral Path. 6:467–473 (Apr.) 1953.

Waldron, C. A. and Giansanti, J. S.: Benign Fibro-osseous Lesions of the Jaws: A Clinical-Radiologic-Histologic Review of Sixty-five Cases. II. Benign Fibro-osseous Lesions of Periodontal Ligament Origin. Oral Surg., Oral Med. & Oral Path. 35:340–350 (Mar.) 1973.

Zimmerman, D. C., Dahlin, D. C., and Stafne, E. C.: Fibrous Dysplasia of the Maxilla and Mandible. Oral Surg., Oral Med. & Oral Path. 11:55–68 (Jan.) 1958.

17

EFFECTS OF IRRADIATION UPON THE TEETH AND THEIR SUPPORTING STRUCTURES

ROGER E. CUPPS, M.D.

The effects of irradiation upon the teeth and jaws may be grouped under four headings: (1) direct effects, (2) indirect effects, (3) interference with normal development of bone, and (4) osteoradionecrosis.

The effects of irradiation may depend on its wavelength, the age of the patient at the time of exposure, and the susceptibility of the patient to irradiation. Other contributing factors are the volume of the tissue irradiated and the quantity of energy transferred to that volume.* The dosage per treatment, the number of fractions (doses) administered, and the overall duration of therapy also contribute to the effects produced.

DIRECT EFFECTS OF IRRADIATION ON TEETH

INTERFERENCE WITH NORMAL DEVELOPMENT OF TEETH (HUMAN)

Among those who have reported on the effects of irradiation on the developing

---

*The unit used to define absorbed energy is the rad; 1 rad represents absorption of 100 ergs per gram of absorber.

230

dentition in man are Rushton (1947), Stafne and Bowing (1947), Brown (1949), and Bruce and Stafne (1950). From the evidence revealed by their cases, one may assume that irradiation can injure a tooth germ to the extent that a tooth will not form and that there will be dwarfing of the permanent teeth, dwarfing of the roots of permanent teeth whose crowns have formed prior to the time of irradiation, premature completion of calcification of a tooth, and, in some instances, early eruption of the affected tooth. Usually, a combination of these defects occurs. Examples are illustrated in Figures 17–1, 17–2, and 17–3. Gorlin and Meskin (1963) also noted enamel hypoplasia in a patient who had received radiation therapy at 9 months of age.

Irradiation administered during the period of development can produce recognizable changes or even arrest of growth at any stage (Kimeldorf et al., 1963). Kimeldorf and co-workers emphasized that, because humans have deciduous and permanent dentitions, the stage of development when irradiation occurs is important in relation to the defect later seen. Leist (1926) found retardation of deciduous tooth eruption, as well as disturbance in the

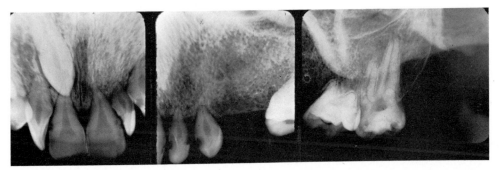

Figure 17–1   Roentgenograms made for a girl 15 years of age in whom teeth failed to develop as a result of radiation therapy. Beginning at 8 weeks of age, she had received radium treatments intermittently over a 4-year period for a hemangioma of the right side of the face and scalp. The right maxillary premolars were absent (both develop in a region that was irradiated prior to the normal time of onset of calcification of the premolars). The incisors, canine, and first molar had developed but were dwarfed. Interference with dental development was limited largely to the right maxillary teeth, because the radium packs were in more intimate association with them owing to the location of the lesion. (Reproduced with permission from Bruce, K. W. and Stafne, E. C.: The Effect of Irradiation on Dental System as Demonstrated by Roentgenogram. J. Am. Dent. A. *41*:684–689 [Dec.] 1950.)

usual sequence of eruption of the teeth, in three of six children whose mothers had received abdominal ionizing radiation during the second and third months of pregnancy. By destroying odontogenic cells, irradiation may destroy the tooth bud or it may change differentiation or stop further growth. This depends on the dosage administered.

INTERFERENCE WITH DEVELOPMENT OF TEETH (NONHUMAN)

Animal experiments show the tooth to be most radiosensitive in the period of early development. The odontogenic cells originate in both ectodermal and mesodermal layers of the developing embryo. Ameloblasts, which form enamel, are epithelial cells of ectodermal origin; odontoblasts are of mesodermal origin and form dentin. Kimeldorf and colleagues (1963) noted that mature odontoblasts were relatively resistant to irradiation except at very high dosage, but immature odontoblasts that still were differentiating would undergo destruction or complete necrosis, depending on dose. A less-than-lethal dose caused temporary cessation of normal dentin formation, and later a defect or niche could be seen in the dentin layer. The Kimeldorf

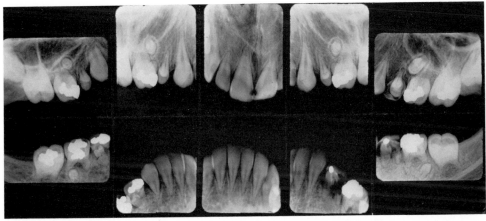

Figure 17–2   Roentgenograms illustrating dwarfing of teeth as a consequence of radiation therapy. These were made for a girl 11 years of age who at 2 years of age had received roentgen therapy for an extensive lymphangioma of the tongue. The anterior two-thirds of the tongue had been treated by insertion of radium seeds at 4 years of age. The roentgenogram reveals marked dwarfing of all the premolars and underdevelopment of the roots of the other permanent teeth present.

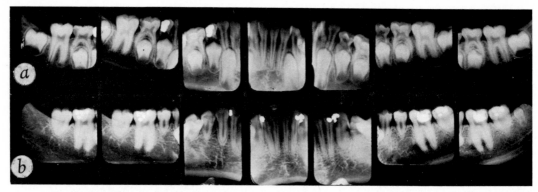

Figure 17–3   Arrested development of the roots of teeth caused by radiation therapy. Roentgenograms made for a girl 8 years of age *(a),* prior to irradiation for an adenocarcinoma of the thyroid, show the permanent teeth at a stage of development and calcification consistent with the chronologic age, the incisors and first molars being the only teeth that have undergone complete calcification. Roentgenograms made 9 years later *(b)* reveal that only the mandibular teeth were affected. The roots of the canines, premolars, and second molars are appreciably shorter than normal, and the overall length of the roots of these teeth is only slightly greater than the length reached 9 years previously. The process of calcification was not arrested completely, however, because the wide apical foramina has been closed and the root apices have a tapered form. The small size of the unerupted third molar in this instance might be attributed to irradiation. (Reproduced with permission from Stafne, E. C. and Bowing, H. H.: The Teeth and Their Supporting Structures in Patients Treated by Irradiation. Am. J. Orthodontics [Oral Surg. Sect.]. *33*:567–581 [Aug.] 1947.)

group noted that, as a result of irradiation, immature odontoblasts might alter their secretory function to form "osteodentin, an amorphous substance, rather than organized dentin." Ameloblasts are less affected by irradiation but, with higher dosages to the differentiating ameloblasts, they may fail to produce enamel thereafter.

Kimeldorf and co-workers (1963) described the radiobiologic mechanism of direct radiation injury to teeth as primarily an interference with the mitosis of proliferative tissue and an impairment of metabolic processes in differentiating secretory cells. The secretory functions in mature cells appear to be relatively insensitive to radiation injury. Nonetheless, examples of altered secretory function in differentiating cells have been reported. The formation of osteodentin by odontoblasts in several species and of keratin by ameloblasts in hamsters are examples of altered secretory function in incompletely differentiated cells (Kimeldorf et al., 1963). Burstone (1950) suggested that in mice irradiation may change some pulp connective tissue cells into osteoid-forming cells. English and associates (1955) described an unusual enamel formation produced by partially functional ameloblasts in irradiated swine. The occurrence of these abnormal secre-

tory products suggests a radiation-induced alteration in the metabolism of at least some of the cells that remained viable after exposure. If the damage after irradiation is reparable, there is a temporary retardation in growth, with repair being initiated by "persistent and viable remnants of odontogenic epithelium of enamel tissue" (Kimeldorf et al., 1963).

Kimeldorf and colleagues (1963) cautioned that "The importance to tooth damage of extraodontal radiation effects has not been established; exposure of the teeth without simultaneous irradiation of some potentially relevant tissue, such as supportive or vascular tissues, has not been made successfully."

INDIRECT EFFECTS OF IRRADIATION ON TEETH

DENTAL CARIES AS A RESULT OF IRRADIATION

When the major salivary glands lie within a radiation treatment field, all teeth risk the development of rampant caries. In the preantibiotic era, del Regato (1939) suggested that changes in the saliva led to the development of caries with characteristic changes peculiar to irradiation. Frank and co-workers (1965) showed that, when the salivary glands were irradiated, teeth outside the field of treatment were at risk for dental caries, as were those within the field, and that the dental defects acquired after irradiation had the histologic characteristics of dental caries whether the teeth were inside or outside the field of irradiation. With irradiation to the teeth and jaws, but not to the salivary glands, such dental defects did not develop.

Temporary or permanent xerostomia may result from irradiation of the parotid, submaxillary, or submandibular glands. Occasionally, symptomatic radiation parotitis occurs during the first day or two of radiation therapy. The condition appears to be dose-dependent. Less than a week after initiation of radiation therapy, there is a decrease in parenchyma and size of the salivary gland (English et al., 1955). Suggested causes are salivary duct obstruction and interstitial edema (Moss and Brand, 1969).

With salivary gland irradiation, there is a decrease in the amount of saliva and a change in the viscosity of the saliva; the remaining saliva becomes more acidic. More than 50 years ago, a lower pH of saliva from salivary glands that had been irradiated was reported. Current studies show a decrease in pH of saliva of patients undergoing radiation therapy when the salivary glands are within the treatment field. With a decrease in amount of saliva, there is loss of the continuous washing action of saliva over the teeth and, therefore, a loss of the washing away of both microorganisms and food particles. There is also less dilution and buffering of the acids produced by fermentation of trapped food particles. Some observers (e.g., Frank et al., 1965) have reported a change in color of the saliva to yellow or brown along with the change in viscosity. With this change in the character of the saliva, this material coats the teeth and provides a medium for bacterial culture. Frank and associates (1965) suggested that the origin of this viscid saliva is mucus secreted by the minor salivary glands that are disseminated in the oral mucous membrane.

Guerra (1973) is investigating the change in endogenous bacterial flora in the saliva and its role in producing dental caries. The biochemical changes in saliva after irradiation are also being evaluated in his ongoing studies.

Del Regato (1939) reported that patients whose salivary glands have been irradiated have a sensation of elongation of the teeth, as well as hypersensitivity of the teeth to cold, hot, or sweet foods. Masella and co-workers (1972) have stated that in teeth within the treatment field the pulp undergoes the same inflammatory reaction in response to radiation that other soft tissues do, and hyperemic pulp may become hypersensitive to thermal stimuli. With gingival recession, cementum can become exposed and this may explain the sensitivity to sweets; inflammation of the periodontal ligament could be the reason for the sensation of elongation.

The severity and permanence of the xerostomia depend on the total number of salivary glands irradiated and the relative contribution of the irradiated glands to resting and stimulated salivary flow. The dosage and the individual susceptibility to irradiation are also important.

The carious process attacks primarily the cervical part of the tooth, and cases have been seen in which entire crowns have been broken off or destroyed within a year after irradiation. The roentgenograms in Figure 17–4 show the cervical type of caries that may be characteristic of such cases.

PREVENTION AND TREATMENT OF RAMPANT CARIES

Rampant caries can no longer be justified as an unavoidable side-effect of head and neck irradiation. Dental consultation before beginning a program of radiation therapy that will include the salivary glands is mandatory for good patient care.

Dental prophylaxis is frequently required before irradiation. For patients

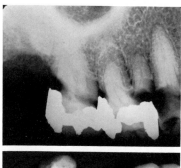

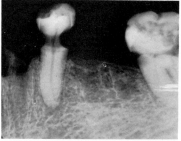

Figure 17–4 Cervical caries of teeth resulting from radiation therapy. These dental roentgenograms were made for a patient less than 1 year after first exposure to roentgen rays. They were selected from the left maxillary and right mandibular regions; the right mandibular premolar particularly shows the cervical type of caries that may be characteristic in such patients.

with adequate dentition, fluoride gel carriers are fabricated and the patient is instructed in their use. Fletcher and associates (1969) reported that use of a fluoride treatment program decreased the incidence of dental caries. The fluoride gel may be compounded by a pharmacist or is available from commercial suppliers (Masella et al., 1972). Topical applications of fluoride produce a dramatic response; almost 95% of the patients studied by Daly (1971) had complete relief of sensitivity to hot, cold, or sweet foods, as well as relief from sensitivity when brushing the teeth. The remaining patients experienced partial relief.

INTERFERENCE WITH NORMAL DEVELOPMENT OF BONE

Underdevelopment of the irradiated mandible, producing asymmetry of the face, has been reported by Dechaume and colleagues (1951), and Donohue and colleagues (1965) reported a case in which there was diminution in the size of the jaw.

Epiphyseal growth disturbances depend on both dosage and age of the child (Neuhauser et al., 1952). In this study, children 2 years old or younger showed the most severe changes. Between 2 and 6 years of age, fractionated orthovoltage treatment of 1000 to 2000 R produced only minor growth disturbances in the vertebrae, but larger doses were likely to produce growth disturbances. It appeared that less than 1000 R could be administered with little chance of producing a vertebral abnormality, regardless of age. Clinical experience reveals the same potential for radiation damage to the bones of the face and jaws in children.

From animal experiments, Gowgiel (1961) suggested that growth of alveolar bone or of the follicular sac was necessary for eruption of the tooth. Adkins (1966) experimentally produced growth retardation in the mandibles of rats with a single exposure to 1000 R of ionizing radiation.

OSTEORADIONECROSIS

Osteoradionecrosis is the devitalization of bone subjected to ionizing radiation either within a portal of radiation therapy or in the site of deposition of a radionuclide. Specific histologic criteria for bone necrosis have been available for over a decade (International Atomic Energy Agency, 1960) and are: (1) empty lacunae, (2) vessel injury, (3) development of irregular abnormal new bone, and (4) appearance of varying degrees of fibrosis.

Rubin and Casarett (1968) stated that irradiation is a predisposing influence that makes mature bone and cartilage more susceptible to damage by other noxious stimuli. Even after exposure to heavy irradiation, microscopic integrity of bone tends to be maintained, but with superimposed trauma or infection there may be gross disintegration. Factors known to affect osteoradionecrosis are: (1) excessive dosage, (2) infection, (3) trauma, and (4) the site irradiated.

EXCESSIVE DOSAGE

Therapeutic doses of ionizing radiation administered to vital structures are planned to be at levels that will be tolerated by the normal tissues within the field of treatment. The radiation tolerance of the most sensitive essential structure within the treatment area determines the dose level; should this amount be exceeded, both early and late complications may ensue. If this dosage level eradicates the malignancy within the area in a significant percentage of patients, such radiation therapy is said to be curative in intent; if not, the treatment is described as palliative.

For some anatomic regions the normal tissue tolerance levels have been documented (Roswit et al., 1972). For many organ systems these levels can only be approximated. It is believed that such factors as fractionation, volume irradiated, and overall time of treatment may be as important as the type of ionizing radiation

used and the overall (rad) dosage administered.

The normal tissue tolerances to radiation allow for biologic variation within the human species; tolerance has been described as that level which, with the technique in question, will produce irreversible damage in 5% of the patients within 5 years of treatment. In patients with cancer of the head and neck, Fletcher and co-workers (1969) found the rate of osteoradionecrosis to be 22% with tumor doses of 6000 rads or less and 78% with doses greater than 6000 rads. However, some of these patients had residual tumor or had surgery or other traumatic events within the irradiated area where necrosis eventually occurred. Also, they noted that initial treatment of the tumor with multiple therapeutic modalities, such as radium implants in addition to external radiation, increased the incidence of necrosis.

Ericson (1965) reported that, of 703 patients with head and neck malignancy ir-

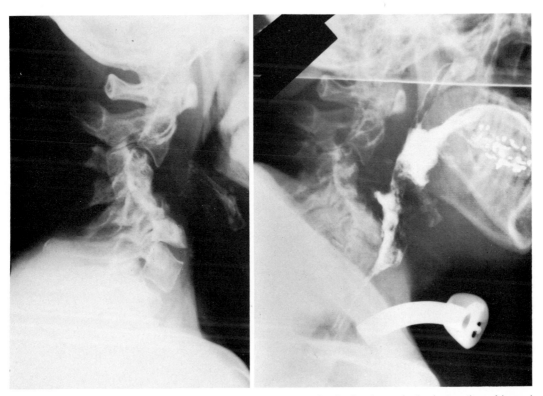

Figure 17–5 *Left,* Osteoradionecrosis involving the cervical spinal column. Lytic destruction of bone became apparent approximately 8 years after completion of orthovoltage radiation therapy. *Right,* Barium swallow reveals radionecrosis involving soft tissues in the neck. The abnormal mucosal pattern of the pharynx is demonstrated by the barium column. Note tracheostomy tube in place to maintain functional airway.

radiated between 1950 and 1962, 38 developed osteoradionecrosis. Of these 38 patients, only 5 received cobalt teletherapy, and the average dose calculated at a depth of 3 cm was 6450 R. Twelve patients treated with orthovoltage radiation therapy received an average dosage at 3 cm of 5250 R. Five patients had radium needle or radon seed treatment, and 16 had combined forms of treatment (dosage data not available). No radionecrosis was found with orthovoltage or supervoltage irradiation levels of less than 4000 R.

Excessive dosage to bone (Fig. 17–5) may result from the different wavelength characteristics of the form of ionizing radiation.

With a treatment beam of lower energy (kilovoltage), the energy absorption of the skin, muscles, and connective tissues may be one-third that of bone. Conversely, bone under a tumor and included within the orthovoltage treatment field often receives three times the dosage that the immediately adjacent tumor receives (Fig. 17–6).

With the higher energy (megavoltage) therapy equipment in common use since 1954 (cobalt) and the early 1960's (linear accelerators), the energy absorbed by the bone, soft tissues, and tumor is about the same. Details of radiation physics are presented in Part III of the Appendix.

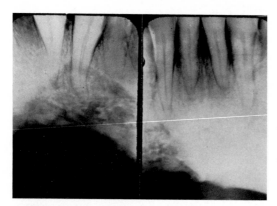

Figure 17–6 Osteoradionecrosis after radiation therapy for cancer of the skin. Osteoradionecrosis became evident 5 years after orthovoltage radiation therapy for what was said to be a cancer of the skin overlying the chin. Note destruction with sequestration of the bone of the inferior border of the mandible. Swelling and drainage were present, but the teeth gave a normal response to tests for vitality, and it is doubtful that they were in any way responsible for the condition. Histologic examination of bone revealed no evidence of malignancy.

Theoretically, one could set the dosage low enough to eliminate completely the risk of osteoradionecrosis, but there would be a corresponding risk of increasing the failure rate of tumor control. With current knowledge of fractionation techniques and equipment, a balance between benefit and damage must be achieved for each patient.

EXCESSIVE DOSAGE DUE TO RADIONUCLIDES

When taken by mouth, some radioactive substances may remain permanently in bone and emit radiations which, among other effects, produce osteoradionecrosis (Fig. 17–7). In the earliest recognized cases of necrosis of bone from this cause, the condition was due to the radioactive substance used for the painting of luminous watch dials; in this instance, the worker touched the brush containing the material to the tongue. The first case of radium osteoradionecrosis to be recognized was reported by Blum (1924) in a patient who came to him for treatment of osteomyelitis of the jaws. According to Hoffman (1925), Evans (1933), Heaney (1971), and Hempelmann (1971), resistance to infection in the bone is lowered, and osteomyelitis of the jaws, one of the first and outstanding features of the condition, occurs as a result of bacterial infection from the periodontal and periapical disease that is so commonly present.

In contrast to the bone-sparing effect of cobalt-60 external beam treatment, when radium or radon seeds are implanted in tumor adjacent to bone, increased radiation injury to bone may result (Dodson, 1962; MacComb, 1962).

The gamma radiations from radium (Ra) and radon (Rn) are used in the treatment of local tumor by implanting needles (Ra) or seeds (Rn) in a specific pattern. The pattern chosen depends on the size of the tumor, the margin of normal tissue to be included in the treatment plan, and the maximal and minimal dosage levels to be achieved. The ionization is closely confined to the area of the interstitial implant; however, if the radioactive sources are placed adjacent to bone, such as the mandible, intense and destructive ionization in the periosteum can occur.

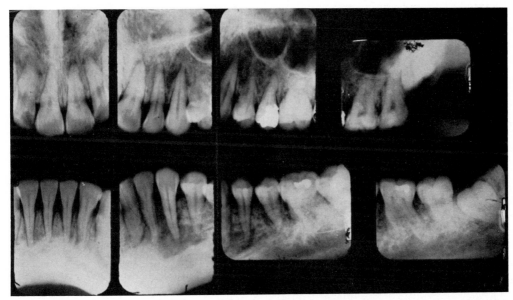

Figure 17-7 Osteoradionecrosis involving both jaws as a result of ingesting radioactive material. The opposite side was similarly involved. Evidence of osteoradionecrosis may be present in the dental roentgenograms in the absence of clinical symptoms. These roentgenograms were made for a patient 26 years of age who at that time had no other oral manifestations to suggest the presence of the condition. Irregular areas of bone destruction were evident throughout both jaws. Bordering some of the areas of destruction is bony sclerosis. The condition revealed by the dental roentgenogram led to a roentgenologic survey of the skeleton, which disclosed similar destructive lesions in the pelvic and other bones. Later, active osteomyelitis of the left mandible developed. (Reproduced with permission from Stafne, E. C.: Dental Roentgenologic Manifestations of Systemic Disease: Granulomatous Disease, Paget's Disease, Acrosclerosis and Others. Radiology. *58*:820–828 [June] 1952.)

Newer radioactive materials, such as iridium-192 and cesium-137, are currently being evaluated for interstitial therapy of malignant tumors.

INFECTION

Frequently, infection is the initiating factor in osteoradionecrosis of previously irradiated bone. Poor oral hygiene must be corrected prior to the time definitive radiation therapy is administered. Uncorrected severe periodontal disease markedly increases the risk of radionecrosis. Any persistent periodontal abscesses or scale provides ready sites for bacterial growth and subsequent infection (Fig. 17–8).

During the period of mucositis due to radiation therapy, the gingival area surrounding the teeth is at risk; after the acute reaction has subsided, any break in the mucosa provides a portal of entry for bacteria and places the irradiated bone in jeopardy.

Because the primary effect of ionizing radiation is to produce subendothelial hyperplasia in medium-sized vessels, the normal vascular reaction to infection is retarded or, depending on the dosage and the individual's response to his irradiation, missing. An infection that would induce capillary proliferation in unirradiated bone is less likely to be controlled by this means when the bone has received high-dosage radiation therapy. Especially vulnerable are bones such as the mandible in which the paucity of original vascularity does not allow development of an efficient collateral circulation after irradiation (Fig. 17–9). According to Ericson (1965):

Ewing postulated that osteoradionecrosis was due primarily to an interference of the nutritional supply of bone resulting from obliteration of the periosteal, nutrient, and capsular vessels. Watson and Scarborough emphasize the significance of the structural histology of bone to radiotherapy. The delicate canaliculi of bone, the Haversian canals and the nutrient vessels are all enclosed in a rigid framework thereby markedly increasing their susceptibility to irradiation. They point out that apparent hyalinization of lamellar bone with occluding of the canaliculi, obliterative sclerosis of the nutrient canals, and obstruction of the arterioles renders the bone devoid of circulation following irradiation. Wildermuth and Cantril state that Regaud

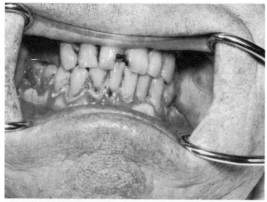

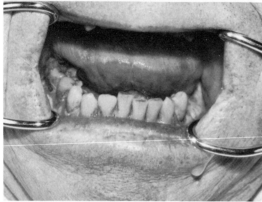

Figure 17–8 Teeth and poor oral hygiene seen at time of radiation therapy consultation for carcinoma of the base of the tongue. Note severe periodontal disease and scale. Extraction of nonrestorable teeth and correction of periodontal disease were recommended prior to instituting radiation therapy, to decrease risk of osteoradionecrosis.

found complete endarteritis in some of his cases of osteoradionecrosis. MacLennan and Meyer have also noted that endarteritis and periarteritis with fibrous thickening of the periosteal vessels' walls, disruption of the elastic fibers, and predisposition to thrombus formation are constant findings in radionecrotic bone.

Rubin and Casarett (1968) compared postradiation changes in the vessels of mature bone to those produced by aging. They found that, with increasing age, the active turnover or elaboration of osteoid and cartilage matrix decreased, resorption processes were relatively increased, and the fine vasculature and microcirculation were progressively decreased.

Because all tumors contain necrotic cells, the same infection hazard exists when tumor has invaded bone by direct extension. The incidence of osteoradionecrosis increases rapidly in this circum-stance. Rubin and Casarett suggested that when infection and tumor are known to be present in bone at the time of radiation therapy, the subsequent osteoradionecrosis should be termed "complicated osteoradionecrosis" in contrast to "simple osteoradionecrosis" if the bone in question was not involved but only heavily irradiated.

TRAUMA

A frequent initiating event in producing osteoradionecrosis is trauma. Initially the bone is damaged by the absorption of energy (ionization). Pathologic fractures may ensue with normal use of the irradiated bone when it has become osteoporotic or demineralized.

Before radiation therapy is started, nonrestorable teeth should be removed as atraumatically as possible. When necessary, alveoloplasty is performed to remove sharp spicules of bone that will delay healing. Adequate healing should precede the start of radiation therapy, or the risk of infection and subsequent osteoradionecrosis will be increased. Because the source of subsequent bone formation is the clot in the socket, Fletcher and colleagues (1969) warned that adequate time must be allowed for clot formation. In uncomplicated healing, 2 weeks is an adequate period. However, the clinical status of the patient and any contributing factors, such as diabetes, alcoholism, or negative nitrogen balance, must be considered.

Three additional factors noted by Fletcher and colleagues (1969) that increase the frequency of osteoradionecrosis in patients with dental extractions performed prior to radiation therapy were extraction of impacted teeth, multiple difficult extractions, and bone contouring to obtain primary closure.

Prostheses should be removed during each treatment and should not be worn by the patient from the time of onset to healing of the radiation mucositis. After radiation therapy, appropriate adjustment or new dentures is frequently necessary. The mucosa within the portal of treatment will be atrophic, thin, and less vascular. The

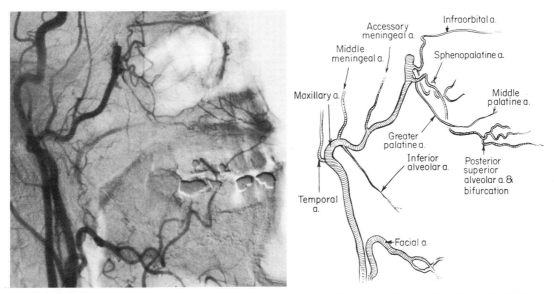

Figure 17-9 Arteriogram, made by the subtraction technique, illustrating the paucity of arterial blood supply to the mandible compared with the maxilla. The mandibular artery supply is through the inferior alveolar artery. (Arteriogram courtesy of Dr. O. W. Houser, Department of Diagnostic Radiology, Mayo Clinic, Rochester, Minnesota. Illustration after Edward Pernkopf.)

decision regarding the use of soft or hard denture bases for prostheses must be made on an individual basis by a qualified dentist. He must individualize the fitting of the prosthesis and be certain that the patient understands the necessity of regular follow-up examinations.

The period immediately after the patient starts wearing his prosthesis is the time of greatest hazard. Poorly fitting dentures in the irradiated patient may interrupt the mucosal integrity. If a mucosal abrasion due to a poorly fitting prosthesis appears and is treated by removal of the prosthesis and by appropriate antibiotics, infection should seldom proceed to osteoradionecrosis.

Ericson (1965) found no evidence that prostheses contributed significantly to his 38 cases of osteoradionecrosis. However, after development of the osteoradionecrosis, less than one-half of the patients could tolerate prostheses in the irradiated area. Fletcher and colleagues (1969) reported on the postradiation experiences of 81 patients with prostheses (64 complete, 17 partial); 5 patients developed bone necrosis, and 4 of these healed with conservative treatment. In one, necrosis was still evident at the time of publication.

After radiation therapy for head and neck cancer, surgical trauma, in the form of dental extractions, can initiate radionecrosis. Carl et al. (1973) found osteoradionecrosis after extractions to be a greater problem if a surgical procedure, such as a radical neck dissection, had been performed before the radiation therapy than if irradiation alone was used in the treatment of the malignancy. They related this to the decreased vascular supply to the mucosa and periosteum after radical neck dissection. If only two or three teeth were extracted at a time, with prophylactic antibiotic treatment and care to leave no sharp bony edges after extraction, most patients had uneventful, although occasionally delayed, healing. An exception to the normal healing process occurred when a small sequestrum of bone was present.

In Ericson's (1965) series, 11 of 38 patients developed osteoradionecrosis after dental extraction, even though some were receiving antibiotics prophylactically. Contrary to popular belief, radionecrosis does occur in the edentulous jaw; 14 patients developed osteoradionecrosis without evident precipitating causes (9 of these patients were edentulous).

For most patients with cancer of the

head and neck, the current recommendations are: remove nonrestorable teeth before radiation therapy, allow healing before beginning radiation therapy, and use judicious oral surgery in the postradiation period when needed.

SITE IRRADIATED

The close proximity of the tumor site to bone increases the likelihood of bone necrosis after radiation therapy (Fletcher et al., 1969). With irradiation of head and neck cancer, the mandible is the most frequent site of radionecrosis. In Ericson's (1965) series, 34 of the 38 cases of radionecrosis occurred in the mandible; in 17, fracture of the mandible ensued. The mandible has a poor blood supply, compared with the blood supply of the maxilla, and, after radiation therapy, it has less opportunity to establish a collateral circulation. Other bones within the irradiated region may be affected.

SYMPTOMS AND ROENTGENOGRAPHIC APPEARANCE

In establishing the diagnosis of osteoradionecrosis, it is helpful to consider both the patient's symptoms and the roentgenographic appearance of the lesion. The most frequent presenting symptom is severe pain. Because the patient with persistent or metastatic head and neck cancer has the same complaint, it is important to differentiate between the two entities. The onset of symptoms due to radionecrosis may be within 6 months to several years after the completion of radiation therapy. The shorter interval usually is found in patients with poor oral hygiene uncorrected before radiation therapy and, therefore, when infection is considered to be a significant contributing factor.

Postirradiation osteoporosis is the most common roentgenographic finding. This represents a loss, at the cellular level, of the normal balance between osteoblastic and osteoclastic activities. Osteolysis is favored by the relative radioresistance of the osteoclasts. Their numbers are increased compared with the more sensitive osteoblasts of the inner periosteum, which are decreased or absent. Because osteoblasts form osteoid, there is a corresponding decrease in active bone formation (Ewing, 1926; Stein et al., 1957; Meyer, 1958).

When teeth are present and the onset of osteonecrosis is at the alveolar crest, the first roentgenographic evidence may be destruction of the alveolar tooth sockets. In general, it would be difficult, if not impossible, to differentiate this from osteomyelitis of pyogenic origin. It also may be confused with recurrence of a malignant lesion associated with secondary involvement of bone.

Comparison of pretreatment and subsequent roentgenograms of the area frequently aids in arriving at the correct diagnosis. Disruption of the normal bony trabeculae is always present. Diffuse osteoporosis with areas of bony sclerosis is the common finding. In excluding metastatic disease, it is helpful if a roentgenographic bone survey or isotopic bone scan shows no other areas of involvement. Likewise, a lack of progression of the size of the lesion on serial roentgenograms argues against the diagnosis of metastasis.

Simple traumatic fracture is difficult to exclude on a roentgenographic basis; however, the sclerotic, rounded ends of the abutting fracture favor radionecrosis. The edges of the fracture site are initially sharp but gradually become rounded with increasing time and mechanical wear and tear on the bone. Remodeling and healing of irradiated bone are slow and often incomplete. Clinically, the absence of initiating pain argues against traumatic fracture. Additionally, the clinician is frequently able to discern other secondary changes due to radiation therapy, such as subcutaneous fibrosis or telangiectasia, in the area of fracture which help to support the diagnosis of osteoradionecrosis. The latter are less frequently seen with cobalt-60 therapy, due to the "skin-sparing effects" of the higher-energy gamma rays compared with lower-energy orthovoltage photons.

Sequestration is much slower in osteoradionecrosis than in osteonecrosis pro-

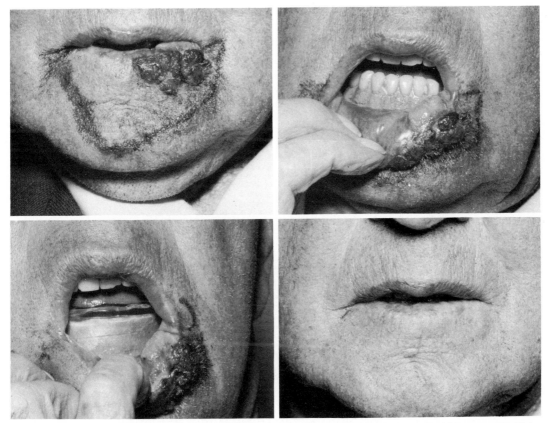

Figure 17–10 *Upper left,* Squamous-cell carcinoma involving lower lip in 81-year-old farmer with lifelong working exposure to sunlight. Area at risk is outlined in ink. *Upper right,* Lip everted to show extent of lesion. *Lower left,* Lead shielding placed during treatment to decrease to 5% the dosage to underlying structures. *Lower right,* Appearance 2 years after completion of treatment.

duced by infection or trauma only, and the process may extend over a period of many years.

The differentiation between osteoradionecrosis and metastasis may be difficult if discrete lytic areas are present within the injured bone. However, in such cases, when all else fails, one may resort to biopsy to establish the diagnosis. The hazard of re-irradiating an area of osteoradionecrosis is unacceptable.

PREVENTION AND TREATMENT OF OSTEORADIONECROSIS

With orthovoltage treatment, lead shields of appropriate thickness often can be placed to decrease to 5% or less the absorbed dose in bone and other supporting structures. Coating the shield with paraffin increases the distance, allowing for absorp-

tion of the characteristic radiation produced within the lead shield (Fig. 17–10).

With megavoltage beams, little intraoral shielding can be used because of both the thickness of the lead required to decrease absorption of energy beneath it and the distance required beneath the shield to allow absorption of scattered electrons. The best prevention with megavol-

Table 17–1. Mean Time of Onset of Radionecrosis After Treatment

MODALITY	PATIENTS (No.)	INTERVAL (Mo.)
Cobalt	5	18
Orthovoltage	12	47
Interstitial treatment (radium, radon seeds)	5	68
Combined surgery and irradiation	16	48

tage beams is careful and precise shaping of the portal to encompass only the necessary volume of tissue to be irradiated.

When metal restorations are present in the gingival region, the adjacent mucosa frequently have a brisk, painful, and temporary mucositis due to the low-energy secondary radiation produced by the interaction of photons with the metal of the restoration. However, the mucosa can be protected from this reaction by placing cotton rolls along the gumline during the treatment. If extensive restorations are planned, it may be wise to place acrylic restorations initially and then complete the final metal restorations at a later date (Masella et al., 1972).

The form of therapy chosen for osteora-

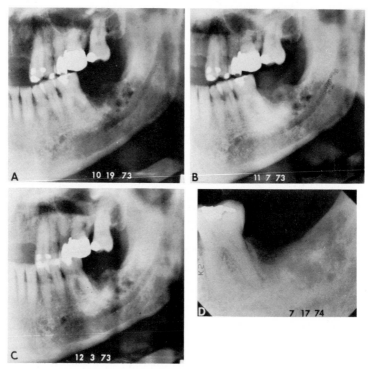

Figure 17–11   Roentgenograms illustrating successful treatment of osteoradionecrosis secondary to trauma. A 63-year-old man was first evaluated at the Mayo Clinic in May 1969 for treatment of a right posterior cervical lymph node metastasis. Review of the biopsy specimen revealed malignant lymphoma, histiocytic type with some nodular pattern. A course of radiation therapy, 2500 rads midplane tumor dose, was administered in 14 treatment days, utilizing a cobalt-60 teletherapy unit with a source-skin distance of 80 cm. Treatments were directed through parallel opposed neck fields, 13.5 by 20.5 cm. After 1 month's recuperation, an additional 2500 rads were administered over 14 treatment days for a total tumor dose, measured at the midline, of 5000 rads administered over 28 treatment days.

A, About 4 years after the end of radiation therapy, the patient returned for evaluation of tenderness in the left mandible following extraction of a lower left molar 6 weeks previously. The patient had not received antibiotics at the time of the extraction. Physical examination revealed edema of the left jaw and in the buccal space. Roentgenograms were compatible with the diagnosis of osteoradionecrosis. The prescribed treatment was application of moist, hot compresses four times daily and clindamycin hydrochloride hydrate, 150 mg three times daily, on a long-term basis. Within a few days, the buccal space swelling resolved completely. There was reportedly some firm periosteal elevation overlying the left mandibular body that was considered to be a smoldering osteomyelitis. The clindamycin therapy was continued.

B, Roentgenogram about 3 weeks later, at which time the oral surgeon noted complete granulation over the wound with the exception of a small area of exposed bone considered to be a sequestrum occurring at the most distal portion. The buccal infectious process was resolved and the patient was asymptomatic at that time. The clindamycin therapy was continued, and it was suggested that the patient return in 3 weeks. The moist compresses for jaw discomfort were continued, and the patient was given a syringe for irrigating the granulating socket.

C, At 1 month after *B,* the patient stated that he had no symptoms other than mild discomfort with wide opening of the jaw. Clinical examination was negative, and the roentgenogram revealed further resolution of the osteoradionecrosis. The clindamycin therapy was discontinued because of associated diarrhea.

D, At 7 months after *C,* roentgenogram demonstrates further remodeling of bone with decrease in the lytic component in the left mandible. At that time the patient was completely asymptomatic.

dionecrosis depends on its severity and the time of onset. Fletcher and colleagues (1969) found that bone necrosis appeared in 65% of patients within 1 year of initiating radiation therapy and in 87% within 2 years. Osteoradionecrosis seldom was seen to develop after 2 years. They also noted that 78% of the patients healed within 12 months after beginning treatment. In Ericson's (1965) series, onset of osteoradionecrosis was later (Table 17–1). Small areas showing early signs of necrosis often progress to complete healing with conservative therapy; attempts at surgical treatment may lead ultimately to jaw resection.

Conservative measures should always be tried first. An attempt should be made to bring infection under control. Grossly infected areas do not respond, and more aggressive procedures may be required. The same holds true for large areas of bone necrosis. Often, sequestra of bone will be extruded as foreign bodies. Zinc peroxide packs, topical application of 1% neomycin solutions, and systemic administration of antibiotics are recommended (Fletcher et al., 1969), as is gentle removal of loose spicules of bone appearing above the gingival crest. Good oral hygiene also is important (Fig. 17–11).

With failure of conservative techniques—as evidenced by the presence of continuing trismus, recurrent severe infection, or intractable pain—surgical removal of the osteoradionecrotic foci is advisable. Total or partial mandibular resection should be considered, but usually resection of bone should be carried back to unirradiated, healthy bone. At the time of operation, this area is readily identified because healthy bone will bleed vigorously when it is surgically divided. Resection through the irradiated area, leaving in situ a portion of irradiated mandible, frequently fails to alleviate the problem of radionecrosis.

PROGNOSIS

The patient's ultimate prognosis depends most often on the outcome of his malignancy. If the cancer is cured, the osteoradionecrosis can, in time, be controlled. Only one of MacComb's (1962) patients with osteonecrosis died as a result of osteonecrosis when the primary tumor was controlled.

REFERENCES

Adkins, K. F.: The Effect of Single Doses of X Radiation on Mandibular Growth. Brit. J. Radiol. 39:602–606 (Aug.) 1966.

Blum, T.: Osteomyelitis of the Mandible and Maxilla. J. Am. Dent. A. 11:802–805 (Sept.) 1924.

Brown, W. E., Jr.: Oral Manifestations Produced by Early Irradiation: Report of a Case. J. Am. Dent. A. 38:754–757 (June) 1949.

Bruce, K. W. and Stafne, E. C.: The Effect of Irradiation on the Dental System as Demonstrated by the Roentgenogram. J. Am. Dent. A. 41:684–689 (Dec.) 1950.

Burstone, M. S.: The Effect of Radioactive Phosphorus Upon the Development of the Teeth and Mandibular Joint of the Mouse. J. Am. Dent. A. 41:1–18 (July) 1950.

Carl, W., Schaff, N. G., and Sako, K.: Oral Surgery and the Patient Who Has Had Radiation Therapy for Head and Neck Cancer. Oral Surg., Oral Med. & Oral Path. 36:651–657 (Nov.) 1973.

Daly, T. E.: Dental Care of Head and Neck Cancer Patients Receiving Radiation Therapy. In Chalian, V. A., Drane, J. B., and Standish, S. M.: Maxillofacial Prosthetics: Multidisciplinary Practice. Baltimore, The Williams & Wilkins Company, 1971, pp. 196–207.

Dechaume, M., Canhepe, J., and Goudaert, M.: Action de la radiothérapie sur le développement des maxillaires, des germes dentaires et des glands salivaires. (Abstr.) Oral Surg., Oral Med. & Oral Path. 4:922, 1951.

Dodson, W. S.: Irradiation Osteomyelitis of the Jaws. J. Oral Surg. 20:467–474 (Nov.) 1962.

Donohue, W. B., Durand, C. A., and Baril, C.: Effects of Radiation Therapy in Childhood Upon Growth of the Jaws. Canad. Dent. A. J. 31:1–6 (Jan.) 1965.

English, J. A., Wheatcroft, M. G., Lyon, H. W., and Miller, C.: Long-Term Observations of Radiation Changes in Salivary Glands and the General Effects of 1,000 R. to 1,750 R. of X-ray Radiation Locally Administered to the Heads of Dogs. Oral Surg. 8:87–99 (Jan.) 1955.

Ericson, B. K.: Osteoradionecrosis of the Jaws. Thesis, Mayo Graduate School of Medicine (University of Minnesota), Rochester, 1965.

Evans, R. D.: Radium Poisoning: A Review of Present Knowledge. Am. J. Pub. Health. 23:1017–1023 (Oct.) 1933.

Ewing, J.: Radiation Osteitis. Acta Radiol. 6:399–412, 1926.

Fletcher, G. H., Daly, T. E., Castro, J. R., and Boone, M. L.: Management of Dental Problems in Irradiated Patients. Read at the Meeting of the Radiological Society of North America. Chicago, December, 1969.

Frank, R. M., Herdly, J., and Philippe, E.: Acquired Dental Defects and Salivary Gland Lesions After Irradiation for Carcinoma. J. Am. Dent. A. 70:868–883 (Apr.) 1965.

Gorlin, R. J. and Meskin, L. H.: Severe Irradiation During Odontogenesis. Oral Surg., Oral Med. & Oral Path. *16*:35–38 (Jan.) 1963.

Gowgiel, J. M.: Eruption of Irradiation-Produced Rootless Teeth in Monkeys. J. Dent. Res. *40*:538–547 (May-June) 1961.

Guerra, O. N.: Preliminary Report of an On-Going Research Study Presented at the 21st Annual Meeting of the American Academy of Maxillofacial Prosthetics. Hilton Palacio Del Rio Hotel, San Antonio, Texas, Oct. 23, 1973.

Heaney, R. P.: Radionuclide Bone Toxicity. In Beeson, P. B. and McDermott, W. (Eds.): A Textbook of Medicine. Ed. 13. Philadelphia, W. B. Saunders Company, 1971, pp. 1873–1874.

Hempelmann, L. H.: Radiation Injury. In Beeson, P. B. and McDermott, W. (Eds.): A Textbook of Medicine. Ed. 13. Philadelphia, W. B. Saunders Company, 1971, pp. 47–51.

Hoffman, F. L.: Radium (Mesothorium) Necrosis. J.A.M.A. *85*:961–965 (Sept. 26) 1925.

International Atomic Energy Agency: Radiation Damage in Bone, STI/PUB/27, p. 10. Karntner Ring, Vienna 1, 1960.

Kimeldorf, D. J., Jones, D. C., and Castanera, T. J.: The Radiobiology of Teeth. Radiat. Res. *20*:518–540 (Nov.) 1963.

Leist, M.: Odontologic Findings in 6 Children of Mothers Irradiated During Pregnancy with Roentgen Rays or Radium. Oesterr. Ztschr. Stomatol. *24*:448–452, 1926.

MacComb, W. S.: Necrosis in Treatment of Intraoral Cancer by Radiation Therapy. Am. J. Roentgenol. *87*:431–440 (Mar.) 1962.

Masella, R. P., Cupps, R. E., and Laney, W. R.: Dental Management of the Irradiated Patient. Northwest Dentistry. *51*:269–275 (Sept.–Oct.) 1972.

Meyer, I.: Osteoradionecrosis of the Jaws. Chicago, Year Book Medical Publishers, Inc., 1958, p. 51.

Moss, W. T. and Brand, W. N.: Therapeutic Radiology: Rationale, Technique, Results. Ed. 3. St. Louis, The C. V. Mosby Company, 1969, 564 pp.

Neuhauser, E. B. D., Wittenborg, M. H., Berman, C. Z., and Cohen, J.: Irradiation Effects of Roentgen Therapy on the Growing Spine. Radiology. *59*:637–650 (Nov.) 1952.

del Regato, J. A.: Dental Lesions Observed After Roentgen Therapy in Cancer of the Buccal Cavity, Pharynx and Larynx. Am. J. Roentgenol. *42*:404–410 (Sept.) 1939.

Roswit, B., Malsky, S. J., and Reid, C. B.: Severe Radiation Injuries of the Stomach, Small Intestine, Colon and Rectum. Am. J. Roentgenol. *114*:460–475 (Mar.) 1972.

Rubin, P. and Casarett, G. W.: Clinical Radiation Pathology. Vol. II. Philadelphia, W. B. Saunders Company, 1968, pp. 557–608.

Rushton, M. A.: Effects of Radium on Dentition. Am. J. Orthodontics (Oral Surg. Sect.). *33*:828–830 (Dec.) 1947.

Stafne, E. C. and Bowing, H. H.: The Teeth and Their Supporting Structures in Patients Treated by Irradiation. Am. J. Orthodontics (Oral Surg. Sect.). *33*:567–581 (Aug.) 1947.

Stein, M., Brady, L. W., and Raventos, A.: The Effects of Radiation on Extraction-Wound Healing in the Rat. Cancer. *10*:1167–1181 (Nov.–Dec.) 1957.

ORAL ROENTGENOGRAPHIC MANIFESTATIONS OF SYSTEMIC DISEASE

18

EUGENE E. KELLER, D.D.S.
EDWARD C. STAFNE, D.D.S.

The dental roentgenogram often provides information that is valuable in the recognition and diagnosis of systemic disease. Cahn (1950) has stated that roentgenographic patterns of the jaws are as frequently diagnostic of systemic disease as are the oral soft tissues. Shira (1953) has made an excellent contribution to the literature on manifestations of systemic disorders in the facial bones.

The effects of a disease may be manifested by accelerated or retarded formation, calcification, or eruption of the teeth. In addition, structural dental defects, changes in cancellous or cortical osseous pattern, and formation of lesions of the supporting bone may reflect systemic disease. These manifestations most often occur in diseases in which skeletal involvement is generalized, namely metabolic disturbances, granulomatous diseases, skeletal developmental disturbances of unknown cause, reticuloendotheliosis, Paget's disease of bone, and others. In general, abnormalities of formation, calcification, and eruption of the teeth occur in association with systemic disturbances that have their onset in infancy, childhood, or early adolescence; alterations in cancellous or cortical bone pattern,

in contrast, may occur at any time during life. In some instances, the dental roentgenographic findings may provide the first clue that leads to an early diagnosis of the disease. However, oral roentgenographic manifestations are not always present in a given patient, and the degree of expression is highly variable and may reflect the severity and duration of the systemic disease.

To determine abnormalities in development and eruption of teeth one must be familiar with the normal. The chronologic age for the beginning of calcification and the completion of enamel and dentin formation, as well as the age for eruption of individual teeth, has been well established by Schour and Massler (1941) and others. A chart prepared by Schour and Massler, showing development of the human dentition, is reproduced in Figure 18–1. This chart is reasonably accurate and can be quickly and readily referred to. However, basing their work on roentgenographic observations, Moorrees and colleagues (1963) studied the age variation of calcification stages of 10 permanent teeth. Their findings have provided a reproducible and reliable index. They documented that dental

245

DEVELOPMENT OF THE HUMAN DENTITION

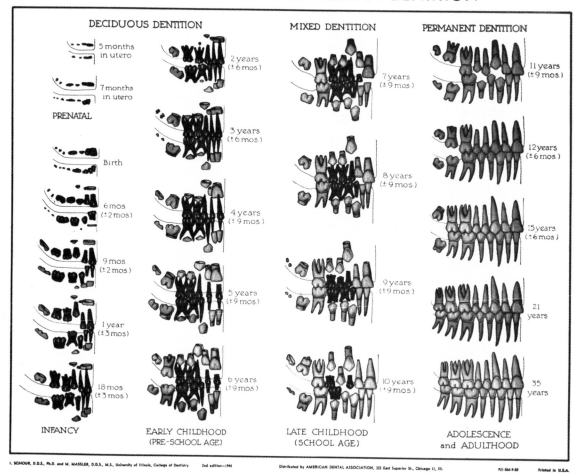

Figure 18–1 Normal development of human dentition. (This chart is reproduced by permission of the authors and publisher. It is the second edition of one that originally appeared in Schour, I. and Massler, M.: The Development of Human Dentition. J. Am. Dent. A. 28:1153–1160 [July] 1941.)

maturation occurs earlier in the female than in the male. Except for some rare and unusual anomalous conditions that are peculiar to the teeth and jaws, dental development generally conforms to chronologic skeletal development. The degree or stage of dental development can therefore be used as an index of the approximate skeletal age, much as the number of calcification centers in the wrist is utilized as an index of the degree of skeletal development. The stage of development of the carpal bones has long been used as an index for comparing skeletal maturation age with chronologic age, and charts depicting the stages of normal development have been prepared by Greulich and Pyle (1959) and others. A roentgenogram of the wrist of a patient 9½ years of age who had hypopituitarism is shown in Figure 18–2. It reveals that the carpal bones have reached a stage of development that is normally reached at 3 years of age. In abnormal skeletal development, the degree of dental development and the degree of carpal development, however, are not always consistent. More often, dental development is retarded or accelerated to a lesser degree than carpal development. In some instances, nevertheless, the variation between dental age and chronologic age has been as great as that between carpal age and chronologic age.

In determining the dental age, the stage of calcification of the teeth as re-

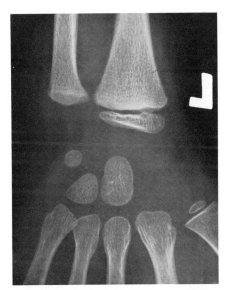

Figure 18–2 Roentgenogram of wrist used to determine skeletal age. Carpal age is about 3 years; chronologic age, 9½ years.

vealed by the roentgenogram is of more significance than the time of their eruption, since eruption may be altered by lack of growth or by quality of bone of the alveolar process. Furthermore, when the dental age is estimated, the third molars should be disregarded, because their time of development is too variable. The roentgenographic changes may vary appreciably, depending on the duration and severity of the systemic disease, or the characteristic roentgenographic picture of a disease may be altered by therapeutic measures. Many disturbances are amenable to treatment in varied degrees, so these alterations are not an uncommon finding.

Abnormalities of the teeth caused by systemic disease include alteration in number, structural defects of enamel, dentin, and cementum, and, in rare instances, variations in size.

ENDOCRINE DISTURBANCES

The teeth and jaws reflect endocrine dysfunction just as do other parts of the skeleton, and the dental defects produced may remain as a permanent record of the disorder. Any quantitative change in the hormones secreted by these glands, be it overproduction or underproduction, may lead to disturbances in growth and maturation of bones and teeth. According to Wilkins (1965), endocrine disorders that have an influence upon growth generally are produced by lack of or increased production of the pituitary growth hormone or hormones of the "target glands," namely the thyroid, gonads, or adrenal cortex, and also of other glands, such as the parathyroids, pancreas, and adrenal medulla, which are not directly regulated by the pituitary.

Any influence that endocrine dysfunction may have upon the teeth themselves is limited almost entirely to the period of their development, and this may be manifested by retarded or accelerated maturation, and in some instances by structural defects. Defects that occurred in the incisor teeth of rats deprived of their parathyroid glands first led Erdheim (1911) to the realization that secretion from these glands influences calcium metabolism.

Schour and Massler (1943) have stated that, because the teeth are highly specialized structures, they are valuable for analysis of endocrine dysfunction and often reflect effects with kymographic accuracy. In general, the size of the teeth is not altered in endocrine disturbances. Dwarfs do not have dwarfed teeth, nor are the teeth of a giant necessarily larger than those that might well be seen in persons of normal size.

The effects of endocrine disturbances upon the bone of the jaws are similar to those on other bones of the skeleton. Endocrine dysfunction during the period of growth and maturation may be manifested by retardation or acceleration of facial development. If overdevelopment of the skeleton occurs in an adult, the mandible, because of the normal persistence of growth cartilage of the condyle, may continue to develop, as in acromegaly.

If the quality or structure of the bone is altered, the intraoral dental roentgenogram is of value, for it often reveals mild demineralization and minimal alteration of trabecular pattern that may not be demonstrable in other roentgenograms. Keating (1947) has said, "The technical superiority of roentgenograms of the bone surrounding the teeth plus the special advantage provided by the uninvolved teeth as a gauge of density makes dental roentgenograms particularly useful in the recognition of mild degrees of skeletal involvement." Once the teeth are fully calcified, endogenous hypercalcification or demineralization does not occur (an exception is secondary dentin formation or localized idiopathic resorption secondary to local pathologic conditions); therefore there is no change in radiographic density. Thus, the teeth serve as a penetrometer, or a gauge of density, to aid in the recognition of cases in which osseous changes are present.

Alterations in the trabecular pattern are usually associated with decreased or increased radiographic density. Diseases in which fibrosis is a dominant feature, that is, hyperparathyroidism and Paget's disease of bone, are generally characterized by a fine lacelike pattern, while osteoporosis and rickets are evidenced by a decrease in the number of trabeculations and by reduced radiographic density. Changes that may take place are alteration in the thickness of the mandibular inferior cortex, obliteration of the narrow radiopaque lines that represent the borders of the maxillary sinuses and nasal fossae, and disappearance of the lamina dura that delineates the normal tooth sockets.

DISORDERS OF PITUITARY GLAND

The pituitary gland is situated within the sella turcica in the posterior cranial base and has an anterior and a posterior lobe. It controls the production, storage, or release of several hormones, some of which influence the secretion of hormones of other endocrine glands. The anterior lobe (adenohypophysis) produces somatotropin (STH), thyrotropin (TSH), adrenocorticotropin (ACTH), gonadotropin (luteinizing hormone [LH] and follicle-stimulating hormone [FSH]), and melanocyte-stimulating hormone (MSH). The posterior lobe (neurohypophysis) stores and controls the release of vasopressin and oxytocin, which are produced by cells of the supraoptic and paraventricular nuclei of the hypothalamus.

Hypopituitarism. In anterior pituitary insufficiency, the amount of effective growth hormone is decreased and there is a lack of growth of all tissues, somatic and skeletal. When the deficiency occurs early in life, pituitary dwarfism results. Pronounced retardation of facial growth is well documented in patients with anterior pituitary insufficiency (Keller, 1968; Spiegel et al., 1971). In general, the jaws are symmetrically and proportionally retarded in relation to each other and to the remainder of the skeleton. That an immature (skeletal open-bite) facial growth pattern is maintained was documented by Spiegel and associates (1971), who studied 25 patients by cephalometric analysis and found greater growth retardation in posterior facial height than in anterior facial height. Retarded growth and increased flexion of the cranial base also were documented. The size of the teeth is not affected; however, their formation, calcification, and subsequent eruption are significantly retarded. Although dental development is markedly delayed, it is consistently less so than skeletal (carpal) maturation (Keller, 1968), illustrating the difference in effects of hormone deficiency on dental and skeletal growth.

Loss of the anterior pituitary gland may be partial or complete. The clinical manifestations depend on the amount and type of functional tissue affected, and various degrees of somatotropin, gonadotropin, and thyrotropin deficiencies may exist. Considerable variation in the degree of dental and facial growth retardation is evident in large groups of patients.

Figure 18–3 shows roentgenograms of a 9¼-year-old boy with idiopathic anterior pituitary insufficiency. Pronounced growth retardation occurred at an early age, and skeletal (carpal) maturation age was 3½ years. Cephalometric analysis documented symmetric jaw growth retardation. All deciduous teeth except mandibular central incisors were retained in a class I occlusion. Dental development as evaluated roent-

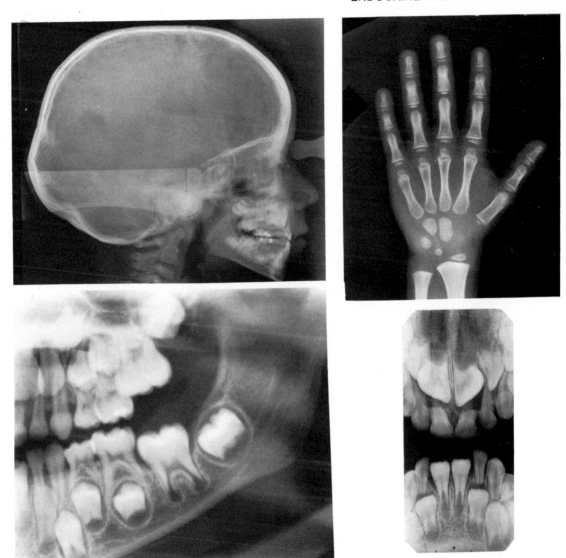

Figure 18–3 Anterior pituitary insufficiency (idiopathic) in 9¼-year-old boy; skeletal (carpal) maturation age, 3½ years; dental (calcification) age, 5 to 6 years. Cephalometric analysis documented symmetric jaw growth retardation maintaining a skeletal class I jaw relationship.

genographically by calcification stages was retarded (5 to 6 years), but not to the extent that skeletal (carpal) maturation was retarded.

In Figure 18–4 are roentgenograms of a 10-year-old boy with anterior and posterior pituitary insufficiency of known organic etiology (craniopharyngioma). Growth retardation in this patient had a slow, insidious onset during childhood. Skeletal (carpal) maturation age (5 years) and dental (calcification) age (6 to 7 years) were retarded but not to the same degree

as in the preceding patient; however, the relationship of skeletal and dental ages to chronologic age was approximately the same.

Figure 18–5 presents the dental roentgenograms of a 12½-year-old girl with idiopathic anterior pituitary insufficiency. All deciduous teeth were present except the mandibular central incisors, the eruption pattern of a 5- to 6-year-old girl. On the other hand, the dental age as determined by calcification stages was 8 years. This case illustrates how eruption of teeth and

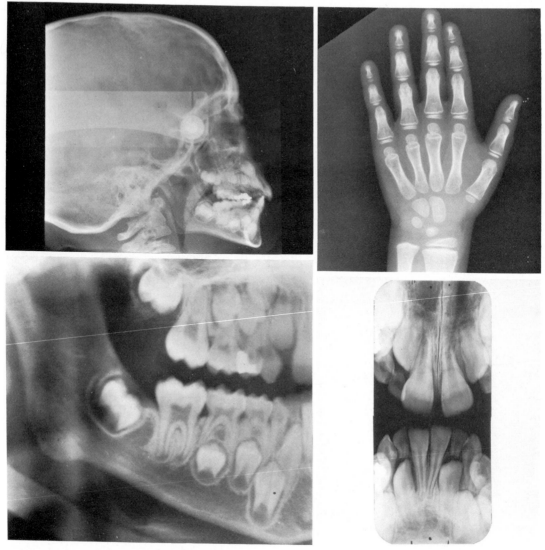

Figure 18–4 Anterior and posterior pituitary insufficiency of known etiology (craniopharyngioma) in 10-year-old boy; skeletal (carpal) maturation age, 5 years; dental (calcification) age, 6 to 7 years. Note enlarged sella turcica on lateral cephalogram secondary to enlarging craniopharyngioma. Growth retardation had a slow, insidious onset during early childhood in this patient.

their formation and calcification may be affected differently by endocrine factors.

Hyperpituitarism. In hyperpituitarism there is increased production of growth hormone, resulting in increased growth of those tissues that are capable of growth at the time of the hypersecretion. Growth hormone overproduction may be constitutional (idiopathic) or may result from a functioning pituitary neoplasm (acidophilic adenoma).

1. GIANTISM. If hyperfunction has its

onset during childhood or adolescence, when most tissues are growing actively, there is a relatively uniform overgrowth of all somatic and skeletal tissues, producing a fairly well-proportioned but abnormally large individual. Dental roentgenograms for a giant, made with standard-size films, are shown in Figure 18–6. The crowns of the teeth are of normal size. The roots of the posterior teeth are large in proportion to the crowns, largely owing to hypercementosis. This may be a reflection of func-

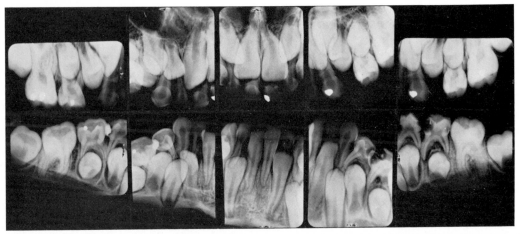

Figure 18–5 Anterior pituitary insufficiency in 12½-year-old girl; dental (calcification) age, 8 years; dental eruption pattern compatible with that of 6-year-old girl. (Reproduced with permission from Stafne, E. C.: Dental Roentgenologic Manifestations of Systemic Disease. I. Endocrine Disturbances. Radiology. *58*:9–22 [Jan.] 1952.)

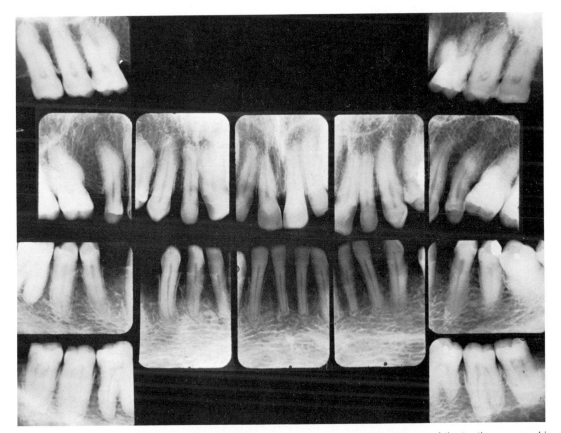

Figure 18–6 Hyperpituitarism (giantism). Abnormal spacing of teeth. The crowns of the teeth are normal in size, but the roots of the posterior teeth are abnormally large in proportion to the crowns, owing to secondary cementum deposition. (Reproduced with permission from Stafne, E. C.: Dental Roentgenologic Manifestations of Systemic Disease. I. Endocrine Disturbances. Radiology. *58*:9–22 [Jan.] 1952.)

tional and structural demands rather than a primary response to the hormone. There is abnormally wide spacing of the teeth, indicating an absolute increase in dental arch size. The trabecular pattern is normal; however, an overall increase in radiographic density is evident and most likely reflects osseous adjustments to increased myofunctional stimulus. The lateral view of the skull of the same patient (Fig. 18–7) shows an enlarged cranium, an enlarged sella turcica, a prominent frontal sinus, and a prognathic mandible. The mandible demonstrates an accentuation of the normal growth pattern that also can be seen in patients with acromegaly or hyperthyroidism.

2. ACROMEGALY. In acromegaly (hyperpituitarism of adult onset), growth occurs in those tissues in which growth potential persists in the adult: toes, fingers, cranium (external cortex), and mandibular condyle. According to Weinmann and Sicher (1947), the main feature of acromegalic change in the skull is enlargement of the mandible. This represents an extension of the normal growth pattern; an increase in "endochrondral-like" condylar growth results in increased ramus height with anterior and inferior positioning of the mandibular body and symphysis. This is followed by eruption of the teeth (secondary cementum deposition), to maintain occlusal contact, and deposition of alveolar bone with an increase of mandibular body height. The position of the maxillary complex in relation to the cranium remains unchanged, except for the vertical positioning of the teeth and alveolus, and a class III skeletal malocclusion is manifested. Lateral roentgenograms made by Mortimer and co-workers (1937) of a series of museum acromegalic crania all reveal prognathism. An increase in dental arch length does not occur (as in giantism); however, spacing may occur (predominantly in the anterior arch) secondary to flaring of teeth produced by the functional effects of macroglossia. According to Korkhaus (1933),

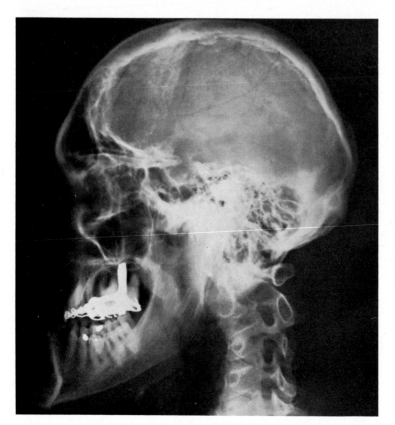

Figure 18–7 Hyperpituitarism (giantism). Lateral view of head of patient represented in Figure 18–6, showing disproportionate overgrowth of mandible as compared to other bones of the head. (Reproduced with permission from Stafne, E. C.: Dental Roentgenologic Manifestations of Systemic Disease. I. Endocrine Disturbances. Radiology. *58*:9–22 [Jan.] 1952.)

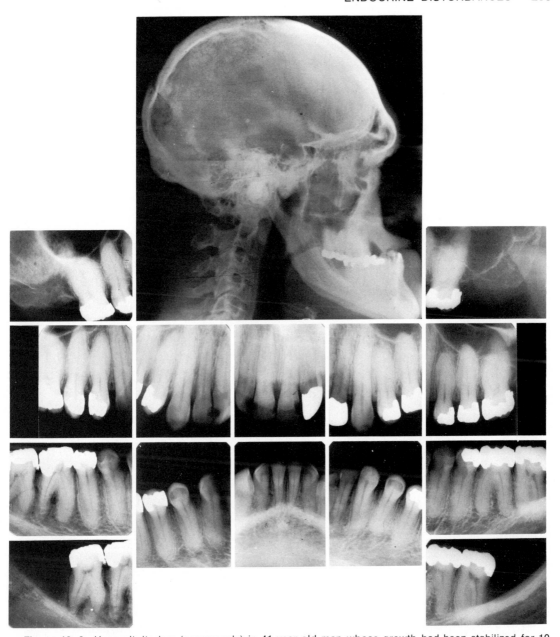

Figure 18–8 Hyperpituitarism (acromegaly) in 41-year-old man whose growth had been stabilized for 10 years after pituitary irradiation. Cephalometric roentgenogram illustrates an enlarged sella turcica, prognathic mandible, prominent frontal sinus (outer cortex), and thickened occipital protuberance. Intraoral roentgenograms illustrate hypercementosis on all posterior teeth and spacing of all anterior and maxillary bicuspid teeth.

this is one important feature of acromegaly and may serve to differentiate acromegalic prognathism from prognathism of genetic or hereditary etiology.

The dental and cephalometric roentgenograms of an acromegalic are presented in Figure 18–8. The cephalogram demonstrates enlarged sella turcica, mandible, frontal sinus, and occipital prominence. Intraoral roentgenograms reveal hypercementosis of all posterior teeth, spacing of all anterior and maxillary bicuspid teeth, and a normal trabecular pattern with some increase in overall radiographic density.

DISORDERS OF THYROID GLAND

The thyroid gland produces thyroxine and calcitonin. Its function is regulated, through a feedback mechanism, by thyrotropin produced by the pituitary gland. In addition to its energy-regulating function, thyroxine is essential for normal growth and maturation. Calcitonin, the hypocalcemic factor, is important in calcium homeostasis.

Hypothyroidism. In hypothyroidism, the decreased production of effective thyroxine results in various degrees of growth retardation, depending on the time of onset and the degree of deficiency. Three types of hypothyroidism are recognized according to time of onset: cretinism, present at birth; juvenile myxedema, onset during infancy or childhood; and adult myxedema, onset after puberty, in which case no skeletal growth retardation is apparent.

In a preadolescent patient, untreated hypothyroidism produces various degrees of facial and dental growth retardation. Cephalometric studies on 12 juvenile myxedema patients by Spiegel and associates

(1971) documented decreased facial height, immature facial growth pattern, decreased posterior cranial base length, and increased flexion of the cranial base. Development and eruption of the dentition are delayed. This delay in dental development was found in 15 other hypothyroid patients and was comparable in degree to the dental retardation in 29 patients with anterior pituitary insufficiency (Keller et al., 1970). Tooth size and dental calcification are normal.

The roentgenograms shown in Figure 18–9 were made for a 13½-year-old girl with juvenile myxedema. A majority of the deciduous teeth are present, and the eruption pattern is compatible with that of a 6- or 7-year-old girl. Dental development (calcification stage) was 8 years and skeletal (carpal) maturation was markedly retarded (age 6 years).

The roentgenograms shown in Figure 18–10, *left*, were made for an 8-year-old girl with infancy onset hypothyroidism. The cephalogram shows an immature facial growth pattern with symmetric retardation of jaw growth (maintaining class I dental occlusion). Skeletal (carpal) maturation delay was pronounced (age 1 year). All deciduous teeth were present and dental (calcification) age was 5 years. After 2 years of thyroid replacement therapy, roentgeno-

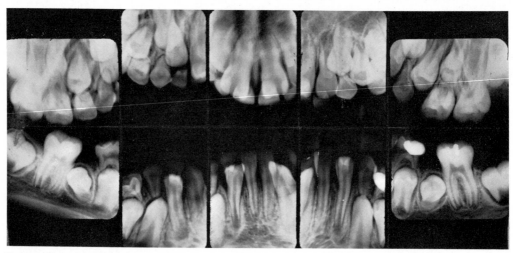

Figure 18–9 Hypothyroidism (infancy onset). A girl 13½ years of age in whom development of teeth corresponds to that of a child 6 or 7 years of age. (Reproduced with permission from Stafne, E. C.: Dental Roentgenologic Aspects of Systemic Disease. J. Am. Dent. A. *40*:265–283 [Mar.] 1950.)

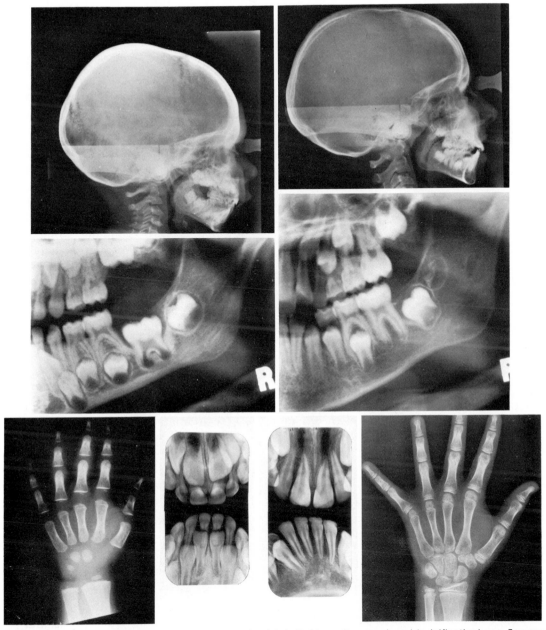

Figure 18–10 Hypothyroidism, infancy onset, in girl. *Left,* At age 8 years; dental (calcification) age, 5 years; skeletal (carpal) maturation age, 1 year. Cephalogram illustrates retarded facial growth with symmetric retardation of jaw growth and class I dental occlusion. All deciduous teeth are retained. Compare with $7\frac{1}{2}$-year-old patient with hyperthyroidism in Figure 18–12. *Right,* Same patient after 2 years of thyroid replacement therapy (age 10 years); dental (calcification) age, 9 years; skeletal (carpal) maturation age, 8 years. Note marked advancement of dental and facial development. Change in ratio of cortical to cancellous bone is shown by narrower inferior mandibular cortex and increased mandibular body height with development of alveolus and eruption of dentition.

grams showed a marked advance in dental and facial development (Fig. 18–10, *right*). Dental development advanced from 5 to 9 years and skeletal maturation advanced from $1\frac{1}{2}$ to 8 years. The panoramic roentgenogram revealed a change in the thickness of the mandibular inferior border cortex. A change in the ratio of cortical to cancellous bone was noted as the cortex narrowed, and the mandibular body height increased with the development of the alveolus and eruption of the dentition.

The delay in dental development in hypothyroidism seldom approaches the delay in skeletal (carpal) maturation, and the skeletal system generally responds more rapidly to thyroid replacement therapy than does the dental system (Keller et al., 1970). In one study (Keller et al., 1970), early adequate thyroid replacement therapy resulted in normal dental and facial development of 14 cretins diagnosed at birth, illustrating the importance of thyroxine in normal dentofacial growth.

Hyperthyroidism. In this condition there is increased secretion of biologically active thyroid hormones. When present in children, hyperfunction in some instances may accelerate osseous development. This can be detected only when the hyperthyroid state has existed for a significant length of time. Cephalometric studies (Keller, 1968; Spiegel et al., 1971) have demonstrated advanced facial growth in six hyperthyroid adolescent girls. Anterior facial height showed the greatest increase in growth and resulted in an open-bite skeletal growth pattern. Mild prognathism was noted in four of the six patients. Increased cranial base length (endochondral growth) and flexion were documented by Spiegel and associates (1971) in this group of patients.

Significant acceleration of the formation, calcification, and eruption of the dentition is a rare occurrence and, in hyperthyroidism, depends on the time of onset, severity, and duration of hyperfunction. In a study of 253 hyperthyroid children less than 15 years of age, Hayles and colleagues (1959) found that only 4.2% were less than 5 years old and that 81% were 10 to 14 years old. Thus, there is a marked increase in the incidence of hyperthyroidism just before or during adolescence. If hyperthyroid patients were exposed to hormone imbalance for longer periods at an earlier age (as occurs in hypothyroid patients), documentation of significant dental advancement might be more common in the literature. In a study of 15 hyperthyroid adolescents, Keller and associates (1970) found only 1 patient with significant dental advancement, 3 with significant dental delay, and the remainder with normal dental development (as indicated by the calcification stages established by Moorrees and associates [1963]).

The roentgenograms presented in Figure 18–11 were made for an 11-year-old girl with untreated hyperthyroidism. The dental development was advanced approximately 1½ years (the apices of the second bicuspids and second molars had begun to close). Skeletal (carpal) maturation was advanced 1 year. The cephalogram illustrates a mild prognathic tendency with advanced vertical and horizontal positioning of the mandible in relation to the cranial base (compare the hypothyroid patient in Figure 18–10, *left*). Uniform demineralization of bone with thinning of the inferior cortex of the mandibular body and the absence of the mandibular canal cortex was conspicuous in this patient and is compatible with altered calcium homeostasis in a longstanding hyperthyroid state.

The dental roentgenograms shown in Figure 18–12 were made for a 7½-year-old girl with untreated hyperthyroidism. Dental development was within normal limits for the age and sex, and skeletal (carpal) maturation was moderately advanced (age 10 years). The cephalometric analysis documented a skeletal open-bite growth pattern. Uniform demineralization of bone was evident (compare with Figure 18–10, *left*).

The illustrated cases document normal to mildly advanced dental development, demineralization of bone, and advanced facial growth with an open-bite skeletal growth pattern in adolescent patients with hyperthyroidism. These findings would not be evident in cases with onset after puberty, except for the generalized demineralization of bone that may be noted in adult cases of long standing.

DISORDERS OF PARATHYROID GLANDS

The principal function of the parathyroid hormone (PTH) is maintenance of normal concentrations of calcium and phosphate ions in the extracellular fluids. In-

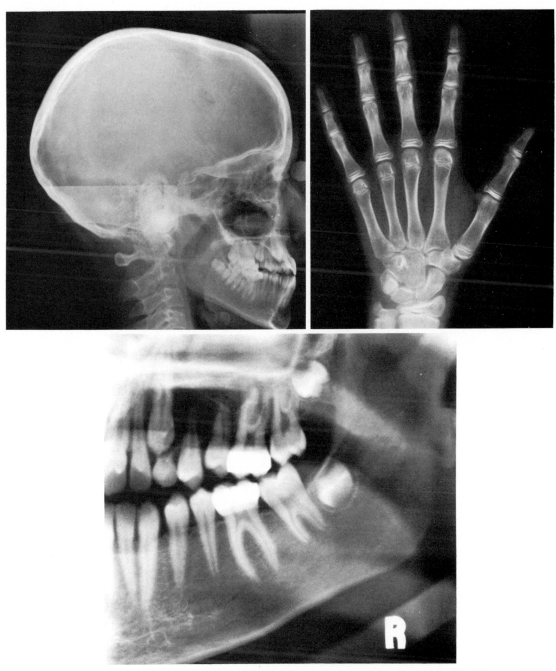

Figure 18–11 Untreated hyperthyroidism in 11-year-old girl; dental (calcification) age, 12 to 13 years; skeletal (carpal) maturation age, 12 years. Cephalogram illustrates skeletal class III jaw relationship. Note uniform demineralization of bone, thinning of inferior mandibular cortex, and absence of mandibular canal cortex.

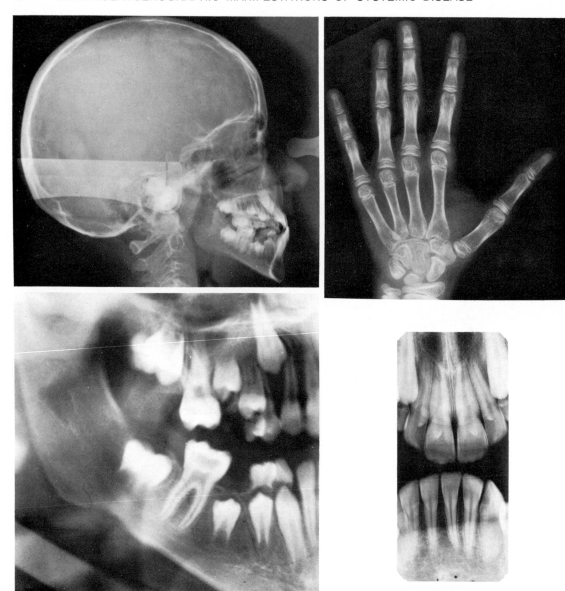

Figure 18–12   Untreated hyperthyroidism in 7½-year-old girl; dental (calcification) age, 8 years; skeletal (carpal) maturation age, 10 years. Cephalometric analysis revealed a skeletal class III jaw relationship with a skeletal open-bite growth pattern. Uniform demineralization of bone and thinning of inferior mandibular cortex are present as in Figure 18–11. Compare with 8-year-old patient with hypothyroidism in Figure 18–10, *left.*

fusion of PTH causes mobilization of calcium and phosphate from bone by osteoclastic activity; it also causes increased renal tubular reabsorption of calcium and decreased renal tubular reabsorption of phosphate (Peacock and Nordin, 1973).

Hypoparathyroidism.   Decreased renal tubular reabsorption of calcium in hypo-

parathyroidism produces hypocalcemia, which leads to increased neuromuscular excitability. Latent tetany is manifested by positive Chvostek and Trousseau signs. Increased renal tubular reabsorption of phosphate is also present and results in hyperphosphatemia. Various types of convulsive disorders are common, and paresthesias, mental retardation, photophobia, cataracts, and steatorrhea frequently accompany this endocrine disturbance (Bronsky et al., 1958). The etiology of hypoparathyroidism may be related to accidental removal of or damage to the glands in the course of thyroidectomy, or the condition may be idiopathic. In the latter instance, an autoimmune basis is suggested by the concomitant presence of chronic mucocutaneous candidiasis secondary to impaired cellular immunity.

Abnormalities of calcification observed in idiopathic hypoparathyroidism include the following: increase or decrease in bone density and microradiographic evidence of diminished bone resorption and formation (Jowsey, 1966); ectopic soft tissue mineralization (subcutaneous, basal ganglia); and enamel hypoplasia. Albright and Strock (1933) observed that hypoplasia of dentin may occur as evidenced by short underdeveloped roots and enlargement of the pulp canal. The dental and roentgenographic examinations may help to establish the approximate time of onset, because calcification defects are present in specific teeth at various levels corresponding to the onset of parathyroid dysfunction.

The dental roentgenograms shown in Figure 18–13 were made for a 17-year-old girl with idiopathic hypoparathyroidism. Enamel hypoplasia was noted on all premolars and second and third molars, with shortened roots and delayed formation and eruption of the second and third molars. The remaining teeth, which had undergone formation and calcification earlier, were unaffected. The onset of dental disturbance

in this patient could be established at 2 to 3 years of age, which corresponded with initial signs of increased neuromuscular excitability. Calcification of the basal ganglia was also present.

Pseudohypoparathyroidism. In this syndrome the clinical and laboratory findings are similar or identical to those of hypoparathyroidism, but administration of PTH fails to correct the hypocalcemia or the hyperphosphatemia. Histologically, the parathyroid glands are normal or hyperplastic. It is thought that PTH secretion is normal but that end-organ (renal tubules and osteoclasts) response is lacking. The condition is familial and of unknown etiology (Vaughan and McKay, 1975). Affected patients may have short stature; other skeletal abnormalities include bowing, exostosis, and a shortening of one or more of the metatarsal and metacarpal bones.

The dental roentgenographic findings are similar or identical to those in hypoparathyroidism: enamel hypoplasia, short underdeveloped roots, and delayed eruption or noneruption of affected teeth. The premolars and second molars are the teeth most frequently involved. Noneruption of several teeth is not uncommon (Ritchie, 1965). Croft and colleagues (1965) reported on the microscopic appearance of the hypoplastic enamel and dentin in this disturbance.

Hyperparathyroidism. Hyperparathyroidism may be "primary" or "secondary." The primary form results from secretion of more PTH than is needed to meet physiologic requirements. This surplus se-

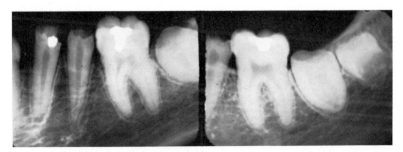

Figure 18–13 Hypoparathyroidism, with hypoplasia of enamel. All the premolars and the second and third molars were involved. Other teeth were unaffected. The defects of enamel suggest that the glandular disturbance had its onset at 2 to 3 years of age. (Reproduced with permission from Stafne, E. C.: Dental Roentgenologic Aspects of Systemic Disease. J. Am. Dent. A. *40*:265–283 [Mar.] 1950.)

cretion is caused either by parenchymal hyperplasia or by functional benign (adenoma) or malignant (carcinoma) neoplasms of the parathyroid glands. Secondary hyperparathyroidism results from excessive secretion of PTH to compensate for another metabolic disturbance. In general, the metabolic disturbances that produce retention of phosphate or depletion of calcium will cause hyperplasia and increased metabolic activity of the parathyroid glands. The following discussion deals only with primary hyperparathyroidism.

Identifiable bone disease is not always present because increased dietary intake of calcium may offset increased renal loss; however, when skeletal features of hyperparathyroidism are evident, the jaws are invariably involved. Pugh (1952) found that one-third of the patients show sufficient osseous changes to make possible a roentgenographic diagnosis. The evidence is decreased radiographic density and transformation of the normal trabecular pattern into fine, lacelike trabeculae. Areas of fibrosis, where the trabeculae are mostly destroyed, appear cystlike; where the areas of radiolucency are more circumscribed, reparative giant-cell lesion formation may be present.

There is a definite predilection for the formation of giant-cell lesions (brown tumor) in the jaws, particularly in disease of long duration. The condition now is recognized more often in the earlier stages and the incidence of tumor formation has decreased. Rosenberg and Guralnick (1962) reported giant-cell lesions of the jaws as a presenting finding in 4.5% of a series of 220 cases.

Changes in cortical bone include disappearance of the narrow radiopaque lines that delineate the borders of the nasal fossae, maxillary sinus, and inferior alveolar canal and thinning or absence of the wider radiopaque lines that normally represent the cortical bone of the alveolar crest and the inferior border of the mandible.

The lamina dura may be completely or partially absent, depending on the severity of skeletal involvement. There is no alteration in radiographic density in the teeth, and they stand out in marked contrast to the radiolucent demineralized bone. The lamina dura was absent in 40% of the cases studied by Rosenberg and Guralnick (1962). With disappearance of the lamina dura, the roots of the teeth appear to be spindle-shaped and present a roentgenographic picture similar to that of extracted teeth. The cementum that covers the roots of the teeth is not as radiopaque as dentin, so that it becomes less distinct when the lamina dura disappears and there is decreased radiographic density of the surrounding bone. Hence, the spindle-shaped appearance of the roots observed in hyperparathyroidism usually can be explained on the basis of an optical illusion rather than on the basis of demineralization of the cementum. In successfully treated cases, the lamina dura is restored and the roentgenographic image of the root again returns to its normal configuration and contour.

The dental roentgenograms in Figure 18–14A were made for a patient 20 years of age who had primary hyperparathyroidism produced by a functioning adenoma of the parathyroid gland. They show a marked decrease in radiographic density of bone, absence of the radiopaque lines that delineate the maxillary sinuses, absence of the lamina dura, and spindle-shaped roots of the teeth. Figure 18–14B shows roentgenograms made for the same patient 6 months after surgical treatment; radiographic landmarks have returned to normal.

Roentgenograms illustrating more precisely the absence and reappearance of the

Figure 18–14 Hyperparathyroidism. *A*, Marked reduction in radiographic density of bone in both jaws and absence of lamina dura. The teeth are of normal radiographic density. *B*, Six months after successful surgical treatment, when the lamina dura has reappeared and the bone has returned to normal density. (Reproduced with permission from Stafne, E. C.: Dental Roentgenologic Aspects of Systemic Disease. J. Am. Dent. A. *40*:265–283 [Mar.] 1950.)

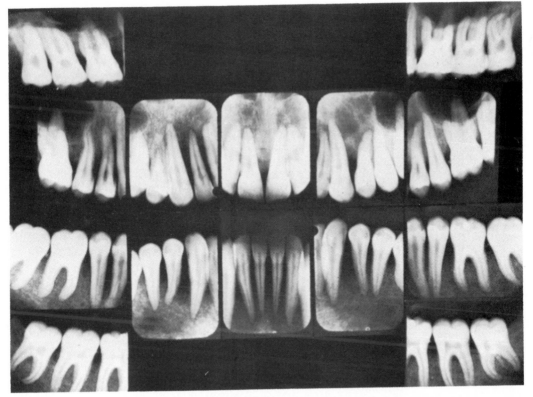

A

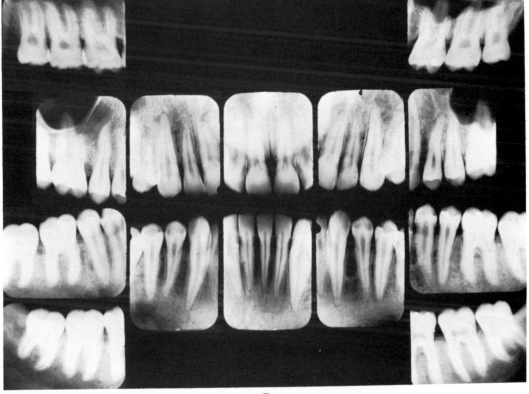

B

Figure 18–14 See opposite page for legend.

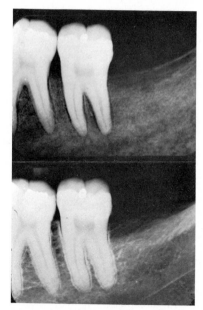

Figure 18–15 Hyperparathyroidism. *Above,* Absence of lamina dura. *Below,* Return to normal following removal of adenoma of parathyroid gland.

lamina dura in hyperparathyroidism are shown in Figure 18–15. The lower roentgenogram was made 3 years after surgical treatment.

The dental roentgenograms presented in Figure 18–16 illustrate primary hyperparathyroidism with accompanying central giant-cell lesions (brown tumor) in the mandible. The upper illustration reveals multiple cystic spaces in the mandible, which represent tumors that recurred after surgical treatment based on the assumption that the tumors were of local origin. The lower roentgenograms, made 5½ months after removal of an adenoma of the parathyroid gland, demonstrate remineralization of the cystic lesions by dense bone without local surgical intervention. Not all central giant-cell lesions of the jaws are associated with hyperparathyroidism, but their occurrence should raise the possibility of metabolic bone disease, even though the cortical and cancellous bone surrounding the cystic lesions may have a normal roentgenographic appearance (Chaudhry et al., 1958). The roentgenographic appearance of affected bones may change decidedly after successful treatment of the primary metabolic disease (Bramley and Dwyer, 1970; Kennett and Pollick, 1971); bone in which fibrosis has not been too extensive may return to normal, leaving no evidence of previous changes. Regions in which the trabeculae have been extensively or completely destroyed may be replaced by sclerotic bone (Fig. 18–16). The roentgenographic changes after treatment may help to confirm successful treatment of the metabolic disorder.

DISORDERS OF ADRENAL GLANDS

The adrenal glands are situated over the superior pole of each kidney. Each

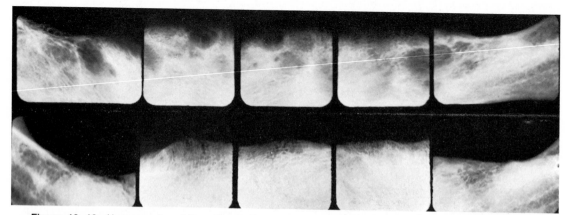

Figure 18–16 Hyperparathyroidism. *Above,* Cystic spaces in the mandible which were occupied by giant-cell tumors. *Below,* Five and a half months after removal of a parathyroid adenoma, the cystic cavities have been replaced by dense bone of increased radiographic density. (Reproduced with permission from Stafne, E. C.: Dental Roentgenologic Manifestations of Systemic Disease. I. Endocrine Disturbances. Radiology. *58*:9–22 [Jan.] 1952.)

gland has two functional components, the cortex and the medulla. The adrenal medulla produces catecholamines (epinephrine and norepinephrine) which, among other functions, serve as the postganglionic neurohormone mediators of the sympathetic nervous system. The adrenal cortex produces numerous steroid compounds that have multiple functions, including regulatory roles in maintaining fluid and electrolyte balance (mineralocorticoids) and carbohydrate, protein, and fat metabolism (glucocorticoids). The adrenal cortex also produces androgens that influence secondary sexual development, advance skeletal and somatic growth and maturation processes, and accelerate epiphyseal calcification during puberty.

Disease entities caused by alterations in the hormone secretions of the adrenal gland and producing roentgenographically detectable dental changes are Cushing's disease and the adrenogenital syndrome. Exogenous hypercortisonism secondary to administration of corticosteroids above physiologic requirements also produces such changes.

Adrenogenital Syndrome (Incomplete Sexual Precocity). In the adrenogenital syndrome there is increased production of adrenal androgens, either because of adrenocortical hyperplasia (secondary to a defect in the biosynthesis of cortisol) or because of the presence of a functioning benign or malignant neoplasm of the adrenal cortex. In the adult, onset of hypersecretion results in feminization in the male and virilism in the female. In the congenital form, precocious growth and maturation occur and pseudohermaphroditism may be present. A child who receives late or no treatment will exhibit marked sexual, somatic, and skeletal development at an early age, but will ultimately be of

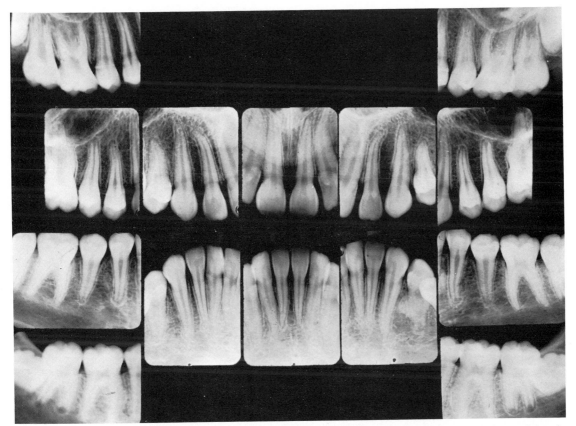

Figure 18–17 Adrenogenital syndrome. Girl 9 years of age whose dental age is about 13 years and thus is advanced 4 years over the chronologic age. The carpal age was consistent with a chronologic age of 16 years.

short stature because of premature closure of epiphyseal (endochondral) growth sites. Numerous authors have reported advanced dental development in this group of patients (Garn et al., 1965; Gorlin et al., 1960; Wagner et al., 1963); however, recent studies by Sklar (1966) and by Keller and colleagues (1970) of 24 patients with the adrenogenital syndrome have documented normal dental development. They concluded that the dental system is not no-ticeably affected by factors that greatly accelerate osseous and sexual maturation; however, four of their late-treated patients exhibited advancement of approximately 2 years, suggesting a potential for accelerated dental development.

The dental roentgenograms shown in Figure 18–17 illustrate moderate advancement of dental development in a 9-year-old girl with adrenocortical hyperplasia and pseudohermaphroditism.   17-Ketosteroid

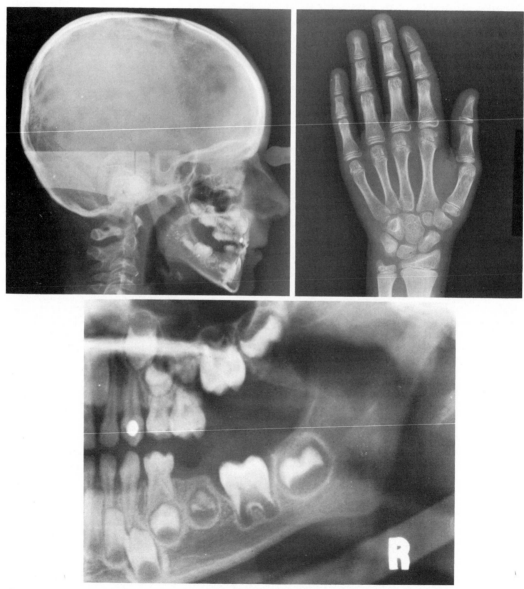

Figure 18–18 Adrenogenital syndrome (adrenocortical hyperplasia) in a 5¹/₂-year-old boy; dental (calcification) age, 5 years; skeletal (carpal) maturation age, 12¹/₂ years. Note that facial and dental development is compatible with chronologic age in the presence of a 7-year advancement of skeletal (carpal) maturation.

excretion was 56.4 mg per 24 hr, and skeletal (carpal) maturation was markedly advanced (16-year-old girl). The apices of the second bicuspids and second molars had begun to close, indicating a dental calcification age of 12 to 13 years, an increase of 3 to 4 years over the chronologic age.

Figure 18–18 illustrates normal dental and facial development in a 5½-year-old nontreated boy with adrenocortical hyperplasia and macrogenitosomia praecox. Skeletal (carpal) maturation was markedly advanced (age 12½ years), but dental calcification age was consistent with the chronologic age.

There is controversy about the effects of excess adrenal androgens on facial growth. Cohen (1959) and Seckel (1950) reported advanced facial growth in patients exposed to excess androgens; however, a recent cephalometric study (Keller, 1968) of eight cases of adrenogenital syndrome documented normal facial growth with one exception: the anterior positioning of the mandible in relation to the cranial base was consistently and significantly advanced. Spiegel and associates (1971) evaluated the same group of patients and documented advanced growth and increased flexion of the cranial base, as well as anterior placement of the mandible in relation to the maxilla. This may indicate a selective effect of androgens on endochondral ossification (cranial base and mandibular condyle) in contrast to intramembranous ossification of the middle portion of the face.

The roentgenograms shown in Figure 18–19 were made for an 11½-year-old girl with adrenocortical hyperplasia who had received late and inadequate treatment. Skeletal (carpal) maturation was markedly advanced (age 17½ years) and essentially complete, but dental development (age 12½ years) was consistent with the chronologic age. Cephalometric evaluation documented mandibular prominence in relation to the maxilla.

Cushing's Syndrome. Cushing's syndrome is characterized by increased production of glucocorticoids, owing to hyperplasia or to functional tumors of the adrenal cortex. The cortical hyperplasia may be secondary to increased production of adrenocorticotropic hormone as a result of a functioning basophilic pituitary adenoma or to increased production of corticotropin-releasing factor by the hypothalamus. Evidence of abnormal carbohydrate metabolism (obesity), retarded skeletal and somatic growth, and decreased musculature may exist in varying degrees. Decreased osteoid formation and bone mineralization may also be seen, depending on the degree and duration of hypersecretion. According to Levine and Weisberg (1950), Cushing's syndrome is accompanied by generalized demineralization of bone in 64% of females and in 75% of males. Decrease in bone mass occurs most commonly in the pelvis, ribs, and vertebrae.

The jaws have not been adequately studied, and therefore the relative incidence of change at this site is not known. Increased radiolucency of the jaws has been seen, however; roentgenograms from such an instance are shown in Figure 18–20. They were made for a 47-year-old woman who also had generalized demineralization and multiple compression fractures of the vertebral bodies. Uniform demineralization was evident in both jaws, with thinning of the cortices and partial obliteration of the radiopaque lines that define the borders of the maxillary sinus. The lamina dura also was affected.

Hypercortisonism. The term "hypercortisonism" connotes the effects of administration of cortisone, or related synthetic adrenocortical hormones, in amounts greater than physiologic requirements for a significant period (Slocumb et al., 1957). One of the undesirable side-effects of such excessive administration of cortisone or one of the newer synthetic analogs is a decrease in bone formation manifested roentgenographically by varying degrees of uniform radiolucency. Clinically, the vertebral column and pelvis are most commonly involved (Soffer, 1956), and bone structure may be weakened to such a degree that pathologic fracture occurs (Curtiss et al., 1954). Cortisone affects metabolism of bone at three sites: (1) the bone itself, (2) the renal tubules, and (3) the gastrointestinal

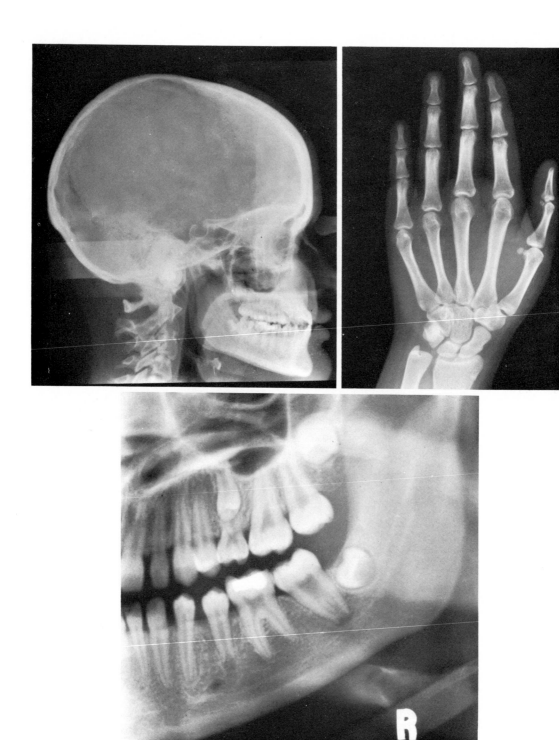

Figure 18–19 Adrenogenital syndrome (adrenocortical hyperplasia) in 11½-year-old girl; dental (calcification) age, 12 to 13 years; skeletal (carpal) maturation age, 17½ years. Note marked advancement of carpal maturation (which was essentially complete). Dental development was within normal limits. The cephalogram illustrates mandibular prominence in relation to the maxilla.

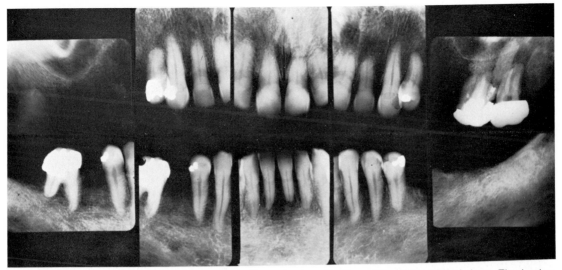

Figure 18–20 Cushing's syndrome, with uniform demineralization of the bone of both jaws. The lamina dura is only faintly discernible. (Reproduced with permission from Stafne, E. C.: Dental Roentgenologic Manifestations of Systemic Disease. I. Endocrine Disturbances. Radiology. *58*:9–22 [Jan.] 1952.)

tract. The changes that occur in bone are attributed to decreased formation of osteoid, the protein matrix in which hydroxyapatite crystals are deposited. Administration of cortisone also may increase renal tubular excretion of phosphate. In addition, absorption of calcium from the gastrointestinal tract may be restricted, as evidenced by increased fecal excretion of calcium. Histologically, bony trabeculae are reduced in thickness and number.

In the jaws, the effects of hypercortisonism are manifested roentgenographically by fine, indistinct trabeculae and thinning or obliteration of thin cortical outlines such as the lamina dura (Stafne and Lovestedt, 1960). These features are illustrated in dental roentgenograms of a 45-year-old man who had received corticosteroids above physiologic requirements without interruption for 8 years (Fig. 18–21). Roentgenographic changes seen in exogenous hypercortisonism are similar or identical to those in endogenous hypercortisonism (Cushing's syndrome); a uniform increase of radiolucency and a thinning of cortical outlines are observed.

DISORDER OF PANCREATIC HORMONE SECRETION

The pancreas has both endocrine and exocrine functions. The endocrine function is related to insulin production by the islets of Langerhans.

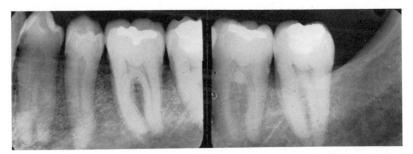

Figure 18–21 Osteoporosis of the mandible associated with hypercortisonism as evidenced by the absence of the lamina dura and by fine, indistinct trabeculae. (Reproduced with permission from Stafne, E. C. and Lovestedt, S. A.: Osteoporosis of the Jaws Associated with Hypercortisonism. Oral Surg., Oral Med. & Oral Path. *13*:1445–1446 [Dec.] 1960.)

Diabetes Mellitus. Absence or decreased production of biologically effective insulin causes diabetes mellitus, a disorder of carbohydrate metabolism. Hyperglycemia, glycosuria, polyuria, and polydipsia, associated with abnormal metabolism of carbohydrates, protein, and fat and with generalized vascular disease (diabetic microangiopathy), characterize the condition. Not all cases of diabetes mellitus are due to defects in the islets of Langerhans, because endocrine glands other than the pancreas may have an influence on the metabolism of carbohydrates (Drash, 1975).

Diabetes mellitus in itself does not cause periodontal disease; however, diabetics or patients with an increased blood glucose concentration (>200 mg per dl) tend to have an increased incidence and severity of periodontal disease (United States National Center for Health Statistics,

1969). In addition, the diabetic microangiopathy (thickened and disrupted capillary basement membrane) of the periodontium (Frantzis, 1970) may alter the effectiveness of treatment of periodontitis in this group of patients. Frantzis (1970) postulated that the vascular alterations in diabetics may enhance the susceptibility of the periodontium to periodontitis and ". . . serve as etiologic factors in pathologic bone resorption and increased severity of soft-tissue damage in the periodontal disease process of diabetics."

Periodontitis was not detected roentgenographically in 12 juvenile diabetics (Keller, 1968); however, one would not expect clinically detectable periodontitis until the metabolic defect and subsequent vascular changes have been established for a significant length of time. The dental roentgenograms shown in Figure 18–22

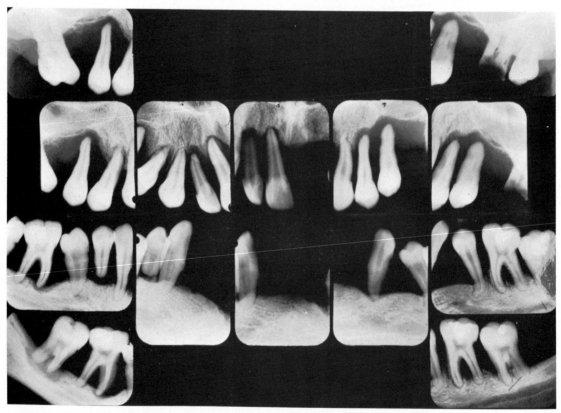

Figure 18–22 Hypoinsulinism (diabetes mellitus). There is marked destruction of alveolar bone. Many remaining teeth are attached to soft tissue only. Note also increased density of remaining basal bone. (Reproduced with permission from Stafne, E. C.: Dental Roentgenologic Aspects of Systemic Disease. J. Am. Dent. A. *40*:265–283 [Mar.] 1950.)

were made for an 18-year-old man in whom the diagnosis of diabetes mellitus had been established for 12 years. Extensive loss of alveolar bone is present in all quadrants. In this patient, significant radiopacity of the remaining alveolar and basal bone may reflect reduced vascularity; due primarily to the vascular changes of diabetes mellitus (Frantzis, 1970) or secondarily to longstanding sepsis (condensing osteitis).

DISORDERS OF GONADAL HORMONE SECRETION

Primary sexual development, including spermatogenesis in the male and ovulation in the female, is controlled by pituitary gonadotropins (follicle-stimulating hormone). Secondary sexual development in the male is controlled in part by androgens produced by the testicular Leydig cells under the influence of pituitary luteinizing hormone. Secondary sexual development in the female is controlled in part by estrogens from the graafian follicles produced under the influence of pituitary follicle-stimulating hormone. Adrenal androgens also affect secondary sexual development in both sexes.

A majority of the primary gonadal disorders are due to defective embryonic development of the gonads, which results in aplasia, hypoplasia, or dysplasia of the gonads. Secondary gonadal dysfunction may result from absence of pituitary gonadotropins in pituitary-hypothalamic disorders. Gonadal insufficiency does not noticeably affect skeletal development unless it appears before puberty. The term "eunuchoidism" is used to describe the condition of adults who have not undergone sexual maturation. They are tall in stature as a result of prolonged epiphyseal growth. Schour and Massler (1943) described the face of a eunuchoid giant as childlike in its proportions, but oversized. Primary gonadal disorders, such as gonadal dysgenesis (Turner's syndrome), may be associated with a variety of somatic anomalies, of which short stature is the most common. Skeletal anomalies of various types also may be present, including fusion of the cer-

vical vertebrae, cubitus valgus, deformity of the wrists, and short fingers and toes. The most common cranial defects are micrognathia and bradycephalia.

What influence the gonadal hormones may have on development of the dentition is uncertain. Muracciole (1956) found normal tooth eruption in castrated mice. Sklar (1966) studied seven patients with Turner's syndrome (variant of gonadal aplasia) and noted normal to slightly delayed dental development. A cephalometric analysis of the same group of patients by Spiegel and associates (1971) documented minimally retarded facial and cranial base growth; however, the anteroposterior index indicated prominence of the mandible in relation to the maxilla (both were retruded in relation to the cranial base). Seipel and associates (1954) reported malocclusion and disturbances of facial development (pseudoprognathic profile) in monkeys receiving large doses of testosterone. They noted that hypertrophy of the masticatory and tongue musculature in these animals complicated the evaluation and may have affected the final mandibular position. In contrast, they failed to note facial growth alterations (except for a less-prominent zygomatic arch) in castrated monkeys.

Precocious Puberty. This term is applied only to those patients in whom sexual development begins before 9 years of age in girls or 11 years of age in boys. In the majority of instances the condition is the so-called idiopathic ("complete" or "constitutional") type which, for unknown reasons, appears to be initiated by a normal hypothalamic-pituitary-gonadal-adrenal mechanism that has been activated at an unusually early age. Primary and secondary sexual development progresses along normal patterns. Spermatogenesis occurs in males, and ovulation and menstrual cycles may be established in females, introducing the possibility of pregnancy. Neurogenic precocious puberty resembles idiopathic precocious puberty, except that in the former a demonstrable lesion of the central nervous system initiates the onset of sexual maturation.

The causes of "incomplete" or "non-

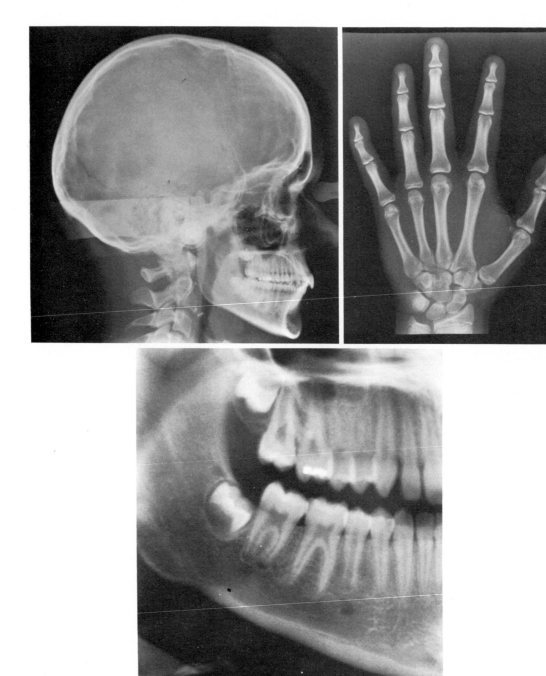

Figure 18–23   Precocious puberty (constitutional) in a 9-year-old girl; complete sexual maturation occurred at 2 years of age; dental (calcification) age, 12 to 13 years; skeletal (calcification) maturation age, 15 years. Serial injections of medroxyprogesterone had been given from 2½ to 9 years of age. Note advanced skeletal (facial and carpal) development in relation to chronologic age; dental development also is mildly advanced. Compare with 9-year-old boy with skeletal growth retardation of pituitary origin (Fig. 18–3).

constitutional" precocious puberty are most often tumors of the ovaries and testes, or hyperplasia or tumors of the adrenal gland (see Adrenogenital Syndrome, p. 263). In these patients androgens of gonadal and adrenal origin inhibit the secretion of pituitary gonadotropins, and spermatogenesis and ovulation do not occur.

In patients with constitutional precocious puberty, skeletal maturation is markedly accelerated, but dental development is normal (Keller et al., 1970). However, some patients with the same diagnosis who have received serial injections of medroxyprogesterone acetate from an early age have demonstrated a consistent though moderate advancement of dental development. One such case is illustrated in Figure 18–23. This 9-year-old girl had reached complete sexual maturation at 2 years of age and had started receiving medroxyprogesterone at 2½ years. At the time of our evaluation her chronologic age was 9 years, skeletal (carpal) maturation age was 15 years, and dental development was compatible with that of a 12- to 13-year-old girl (the second molars and second bicuspids had begun root closure). Facial development was also significantly advanced for her chronologic age.

Spiegel and associates (1971) and Keller (1968) documented advanced facial growth in relation to chronologic age in 13 females with constitutional precocious puberty. When facial growth measurements were compared with skeletal age (maturation) measurements, which were greatly advanced, there was considerable retardation. This discrepancy is to be expected, because these patients attain their pubertal growth early but the duration of growth is short. Skeletal height is similarly reduced in adults who undergo early maturation. A tendency for anterior placement of the mandible in relation to the maxilla also was noted by both groups. An adult skull containing deciduous teeth was a typical finding, again emphasizing the relative immunity of the dentition to hormones that accelerate osseous development and maturation.

The roentgenograms shown in Figure 18–24 were made for a boy 5¼ years of age who had experienced rapid growth and sexual maturation. The eruption pattern and the formation of incisors were advanced by 2 years; however, in the cuspids through the second molars, formation and calcification age were compatible with his chronologic age, illustrating the different effects of hormonal factors on individual teeth.

Delayed Puberty. Delayed sexual maturation may occur in boys or girls in

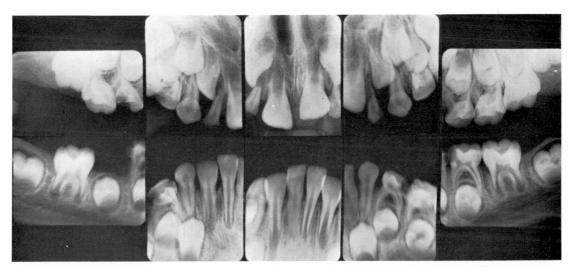

Figure 18–24 Idiopathic precocious puberty. Boy 5¼ years of age with premature eruption of the teeth. The formation and eruption of the incisors was advanced 2 years (7 years); however, calcification age of cuspids through second molars was compatible with chronologic age, illustrating differential effects on the individual teeth. (Reproduced with permission from Stafne, E. C.: Roentgenologic Manifestations of Systemic Disease in Dentistry. Oral Surg., Oral Med. & Oral Path. *6*:483–493 [Apr.] 1953.)

variable degrees but is much more common in boys. The fact that adequate maturation ultimately is attained suggests that the primary problem among these patients is in the timing rather than in hormone production. Often there is a familial pattern of delayed puberty.

Many of the patients are children who have consistently been of smaller than average stature and have demonstrated delays of 2 to 4 years in skeletal development. With the onset of puberty, somatic growth may progress rapidly, or there may be gradual sexual maturation with slow growth continuing for a long time. Many patients eventually attain full adult height; others remain small in stature.

There is a significant delay in dental development; this delay was equal to or greater than the delay in skeletal maturation in patients studied by Keller et al. (1970). The mean dental delay in this group was 2.3 years, in contrast to mean delays of 3.3 and 3.8 years in patients with juvenile myxedema and idiopathic anterior pituitary insufficiency, respectively. Cephalometric analysis of patients with delayed puberty has documented a general retardation of facial growth in relation to chronologic age, with the posterior facial height being affected to a greater extent than the anterior facial height and an immature skeletal growth pattern being retained (Spiegel et al., 1971).

The roentgenograms in Figure 18–25 were made for a 13½-year-old boy with delayed puberty and short stature. The skeletal (carpal) maturation age was 8½ years and dental (calcification) age was 10 years. Facial growth was retarded in relation to chronologic age. This patient reached normal puberty at a later date and attained normal sexual and skeletal development (compare with 9-year-old girl with precocious puberty, Figure 18–23).

RICKETS

In rickets, generalized radiolucent lesions of bone are present and result from failure of osteoid to mineralize completely. This lack of mineralization (rickets) is a manifestation of several metabolically unrelated disturbances. Among these are vitamin D deficiency (dietary), renal tubular dysfunction (vitamin D-resistant rickets; hypophosphatemia), chronic renal insufficiency (renal rickets), depressed alkaline phosphatase activity (hypophosphatasia), and malabsorption syndromes (Fraser and Salter, 1958). Regardless of etiology, clinical rickets is manifested in varying degrees on dental roentgenograms as uniform thinning or absence of cortical bone (lamina dura, alveolar crest, nasal fossa cortex, maxillary antrum cortex, inferior mandible cortex, mandibular canal cortex) and uniform alteration (thinning or absence) of the trabeculae of cancellous bone.

VITAMIN D-DEFICIENCY RICKETS

Rickets resulting from a deficiency of dietary vitamin D is uncommon when the socioeconomic status is good. A vitamin D-deficient diet combined with a lack of exposure to ultraviolet light from the sun produces clinical rickets. Many patients with mild vitamin D-deficiency rickets undergo spontaneous healing on exposure to sunlight.

In addition to rachitic osseous changes, dental disturbances may be present, including hypoplasia of enamel, dentin dysplasia, and deficient cementum formation. Follis and co-workers (1943) found the greatest incidence of vitamin D-deficiency rickets to be between 3 months and 3 years of age. In this age group enamel hypoplasia is relatively common and may be demonstrated by roentgenograms prior to eruption of the involved teeth (Fig. 18–26). Enamel hypoplasia may be associated with other local and systemic disturbances.

VITAMIN D-RESISTANT RICKETS (HYPOPHOSPHATEMIA)

Hypophosphatemia is a form of rickets that is resistant to therapeutic doses of vitamin D. Serum calcium concentrations are almost always within normal limits, but serum phosphate levels are persistently

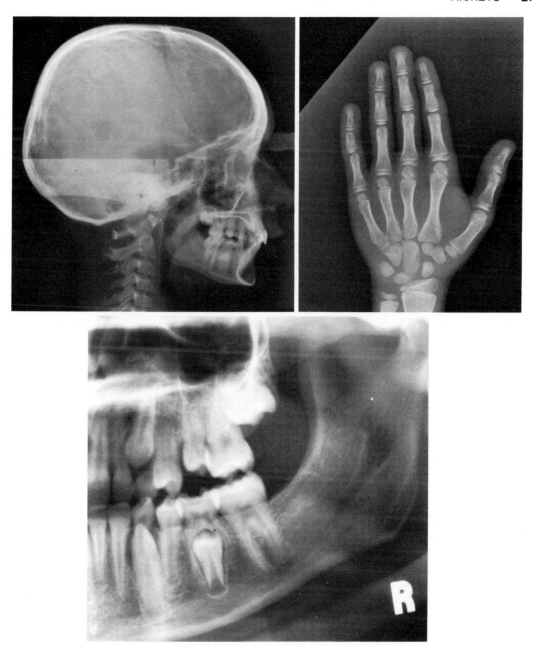

Figure 18–25 Delayed puberty in 13½-year-old boy; dental (calcification) age, 10 years; skeletal (carpal) maturation age, 8½ years. This patient eventually attained normal sexual development and average skeletal height.

low. The latter is secondary to impairment of renal tubular reabsorption of inorganic phosphate. Generalized deficient mineralization of osteoid results in severe growth retardation, bone deformities, and typical rachitic roentgenographic changes. These changes may not be observed clinically until 1 or 2 years of age or even later.

The condition is almost always familial. In most instances it is inherited as a dominant characteristic; however, in some families it is transmitted as an X-linked dominant and there are also some sporadic cases (Winters et al., 1958).

Dental findings include a high incidence of spontaneous dental abscesses,

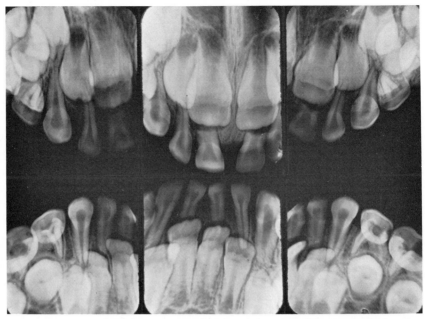

Figure 18–26 Enamel hypoplasia of permanent incisors and canines demonstrated prior to eruption of the teeth involved.

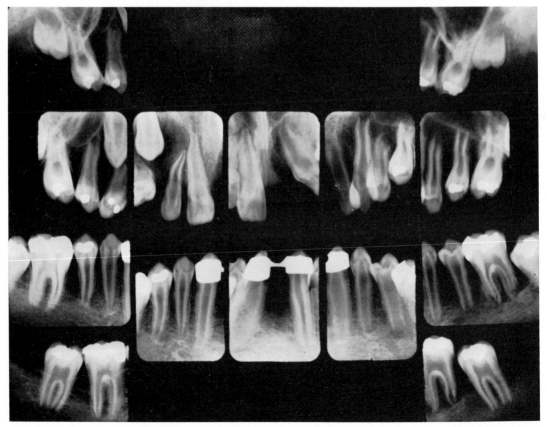

Figure 18–27 Vitamin D-resistant rickets (hypophosphatemia) in a boy 15 years of age, showing retarded apical closure, osseous lesions, and abnormally large pulp chambers.

quantitative and qualitative ("interglobular dentin") defects of dentin formation (Tracy et al., 1968, 1971), enamel hypoplasia (Gigliotti et al., 1971), enlarged pulp chambers, and delay of apical calcification and closure.

The pathogenesis of spontaneous dental abscesses is uncertain and may result from pulp involvement secondary to microscopic enamel and dentin defects (Harris and Sullivan, 1960) or may be periodontal in origin from defective cementum formation. Roentgenographically the

osseous lesions may be quite extensive and may be present as diffuse, poorly defined rarefactions, at times involving the entire root surface and suggesting a periodontal rather than a pulpal pathogenesis.

The pulp chambers usually remain excessively large. After intensive vitamin D therapy, the walls may become abnormally radiopaque from hypercalcification of newly formed secondary dentin.

Figure 18–27 presents dental roentgenograms made for a 15-year-old boy with hypophosphatemia. Apical calcification

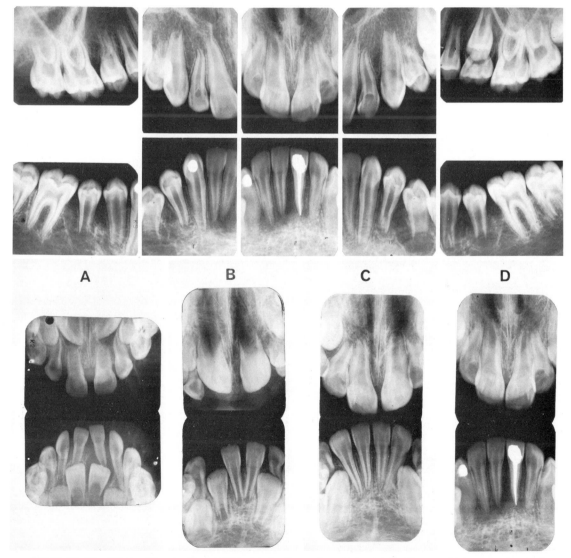

A   B   C   D

Figure 18–28 *Upper,* Vitamin D-resistant rickets (hypophosphatemia) in 13-year-old boy, demonstrating enlarged pulp chambers, indistinct lamina dura, indistinct nasal fossa and alveolar crest cortex, and mandibular incisor periapical radiolucency. *Lower,* Anterior periapical roentgenograms of same patient illustrated at ages 4 (A), 7 (B), 10 (C), and 13 (D). Note periapical abnormality present at ages 4 and 13.

and subsequent closure were delayed on all teeth. Pulp chambers were uniformly enlarged, and several diffuse alveolar osseous radiolucencies were evident. In addition, typical cortical and cancellous rachitic bone changes were noted.

Dental roentgenograms made for a 13-year-old boy with hypophosphatemia are shown in Figure 18–28. Vitamin D therapy had been continuous since 2 years of age. There was a history of spontaneous dental abscesses, and a series of anterior roentgenograms demonstrated periapical radiolucency of both deciduous and permanent incisors. There was no history of trauma. Enlarged pulp chambers, indistinct lamina dura, absence of the outline of the nasal fossa, alveolar crest, and mandibular canal cortex, and altered trabecular pattern are apparent in this patient. Complete api-

cal closure was absent, except for the mandibular incisors and first molars.

OSTEOMALACIA

Osteomalacia is simply rickets that occurs after the linear growth of the skeleton has stopped. Almost all cases of osteomalacia are due to defective absorption of vitamin D and calcium from the intestinal tract. Steatorrhea secondary to adult celiac disease, cystic fibrosis of the pancreas, or bile duct malfunction results in malabsorption of fat-soluble vitamins; large losses of vitamin D and calcium occur in the feces. Deficient absorption over a long period leads to osteomalacia (Follis, 1966). Pugh (1951) described the roentgenographic picture as uniform generalized demineralization, often with an absence of trabecular bone structure.

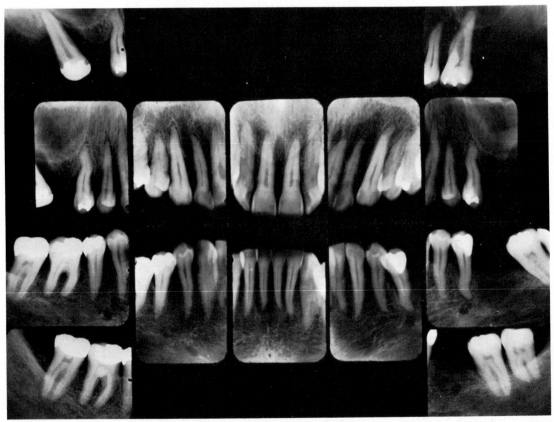

Figure 18–29 Osteomalacia due to sprue. Uniform demineralization of both jaws, with almost complete disappearance of the radiopaque lines that depict the lamina dura, alveolar crest, maxillary antrum, and mandibular canal cortex. (Reproduced with permission from Stafne, E. C.: Dental Roentgenologic Manifestations of Systemic Disease. III. Granulomatous Disease, Paget's Disease, Acrosclerosis and Others. Radiology. *58*:820–829 [June] 1952.)

Because the disease begins after dental development is complete, the teeth are not affected, but their supporting bone may undergo rachitic changes similar to those that occur in other bones. A dental roentgenogram made for a patient 56 years of age who was suffering from sprue is shown in Figure 18–29. It illustrates rachitic changes in the jaws as evidenced by uniform radiolucency. The narrow radiopaque lines that depict the walls of the maxillary sinus and nasal fossa are almost completely obliterated, and the lamina dura is only faintly distinguishable.

RENAL RICKETS AND RENAL OSTEODYSTROPHY

Chronic renal glomerular and tubular dysfunction may lead to clinical rickets in children and to evidence of osteomalacia in adults. The renal disorder produces a marked hyperphosphatemia with a secondary decrease in intracellular calcium concentration. Hypocalcemia develops, which initiates increased PTH secretion and secondary hyperparathyroidism. The skeletal manifestations resemble the osseous lesions of rickets and hyperparathyroidism. Histologically, however, the bone lesions may be more characteristic of hyperparathyroidism and may not show the lack of mineralization of osteoid seen in rickets (Harrison, 1961). The compensatory hyperparathyroidism may be manifested by typical roentgenographic changes (Walsh and Karmiol, 1969).

When renal rickets occurs in childhood, characteristic features may include short stature, rachitic skeletal deformity, and retarded development and calcification of the dentition. The dental roentgenograms made for a 14-year-old boy with renal failure and skeletal rickets are shown in Figure 18–30. Retarded calcification of the mandibular second molars is apparent. Cortical bone delineating the nasal fossa, maxillary sinus, and tooth socket (lamina dura) is indistinct or absent. The trabecular pattern of both jaws is very fine, uniformly radiolucent, and consistent with that seen in hyperparathyroidism.

The dental roentgenograms shown in Figure 18–31 were made for an adult with long-standing renal insufficiency and secondary hyperparathyroidism (parathyroid hyperplasia). Decalcification of the jaws was so extensive that a roentgenogram made with the customary exposure failed to identify mineralization in some areas; the

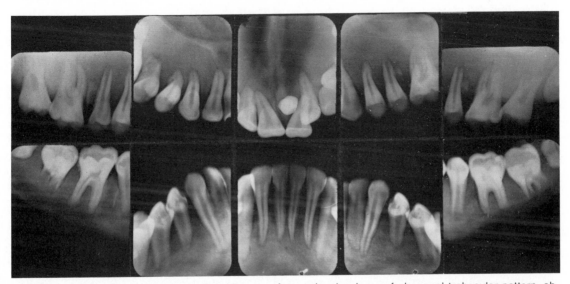

Figure 18–30 Renal rickets in a boy 14 years of age, showing bone of abnormal trabecular pattern, absence of lamina dura, and retarded calcification of mandibular second molars. (Reproduced with permission from Stafne, E. C.: Dental Roentgenologic Aspects of Systemic Disease. J. Am. Dent. A. *40*:265–283 [Mar.] 1950.)

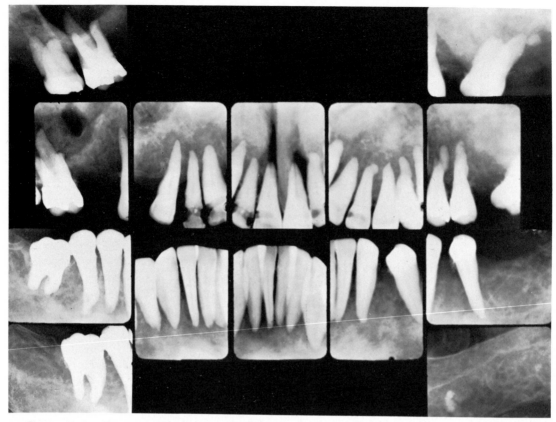

Figure 18–31 Renal osteodystrophy, characterized by alteration of trabecular pattern, absence of lamina dura, and spindle-shaped appearance of dental roots similar to that seen in primary hyperparathyroidism. (Reproduced with permission from Stafne, E. C.: Roentgenologic Manifestations of Systemic Disease in Dentistry. Oral Surg., Oral Med. & Oral Path. 6:483–493 [Apr.] 1953.)

illustrated roentgenograms were taken at a greatly reduced exposure to demonstrate the minimally mineralized bone, and at this exposure the teeth appear abnormally radiopaque. This patient exhibits complete absence of cortical outlines (including the lamina dura) and the alteration of trabecular pattern typical of that seen in hyperparathyroidism.

HYPOPHOSPHATASIA (LOW PHOSPHATASE RICKETS)

Hypophosphatasia is a hereditary disorder belonging to the general category of inborn errors of metabolism. It is characterized by impaired mineralization of bone, decreased alkaline phosphatase activity, premature loss of deciduous teeth, and increased secretion of phosphatidylethanolamine in the urine. The serum phosphate level is normal, but the serum calcium level may be increased in severely affected patients. Roentgenologically and histologically the changes in bone are similar in many respects to those of rickets. The disorder appears to be inherited as a simple recessive trait (Baysal, 1965).

The clinical manifestations may vary greatly in severity. They may be present at birth, appear in infancy, or remain undetected until a later age. The prognosis is fairly good for patients who survive early childhood. In older children the first sign may be growth failure, orthopedic deformity, or premature loss of deciduous teeth. Premature exfoliation of teeth was the chief complaint in five of seven cases of childhood hypophosphatasia reviewed by Beumer and associates (1973) and is considered a salient feature of the disease (Bruckner et al., 1962).

Microscopically, exfoliated teeth have enlarged pulp chambers and impaired cementogenesis (absent or poorly calcified) and dentinogenesis (excessive width of predentin and increased amounts of interglobular dentin). The cementum defect undoubtedly contributes to the premature exfoliation.

Two groups (Beumer et al., 1973; Kjellman et al., 1973) have reported horizontal alveolar bone loss without evidence of inflammatory periodontal disease in their patients. The significance of this is unknown but may be related to lack of periodontal fiber attachment and of functional osseous stimulus secondary to impaired cementogenesis.

The dental findings in two patients have been reported by Baer and associates (1964). Dental roentgenograms (Fig. 18–32) made for one of these patients show enlarged pulp chambers, horizontal bone loss, and exfoliating incisors, which are characteristic dental manifestations of hypophosphatasia.

CYSTINOSIS

Cystinosis is a rare congenital disturbance of protein metabolism characterized by deposition of cystine crystals throughout the reticuloendothelial system and other tissues, notably the kidneys and cornea. Cystine deposits in the renal tubular cells result in defective reabsorption of phosphate. Aminoaciduria, phosphaturia, and proteinuria secondary to progressive renal insufficiency produce severe growth retar-

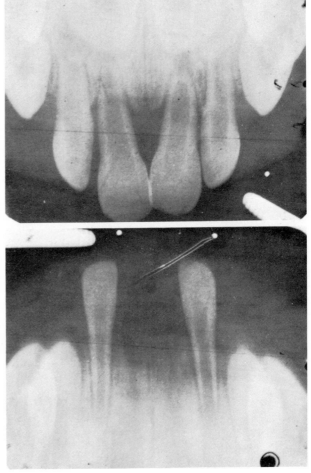

Figure 18–32 Hypophosphatasia. Roentgenograms made for a boy 2½ years of age, showing maxillary primary incisors with abnormally large pulp chambers and horizontal alveolar bone loss. The mandibular central incisors had been lost previously. (Reproduced with permission from Baer, P. N., Brown, N. C., and Hamner, J. E., III.: Hypophosphatasia: Report of Two Cases with Dental Findings. Periodontics. 2:209–215 [Sept.–Oct.] 1964.)

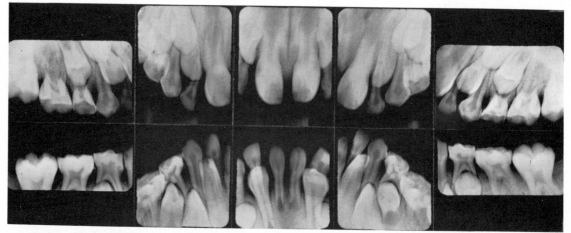

Figure 18–33 Cystinosis in a patient 10 years of age in whom eruption of teeth was retarded about 3 years. Retarded dental (calcification) age, alveolar bone loss, indistinct lamina dura, bell-shaped incisor roots, and altered trabecular pattern are apparent.

dation and renal rickets. When they occur, roentgenographic osseous alterations are nonspecific and indistinguishable from those of other forms of active rickets. Retarded development and eruption of the teeth is conspicuous. Nazif and Osman (1973) reviewed three cases of cystinosis and noted the following roentgenographic changes in all cases: retarded dental calcification age, absence of lamina dura, enlarged pulp chambers, and periapical and interradicular rarefactions. Interdental bone loss and bell-shaped incisor roots were noted in two cases. In addition, hypermineralization of alveolar bone after calciferol therapy was documented.

The roentgenograms in Figure 18–33 were made for a 10-year-old boy with cystinosis and severe growth retardation. The deciduous incisors did not begin to erupt until age 4, and the permanent central incisors and first molars had just begun to erupt at age 10. The roentgenograms reveal retarded dental calcification age, interdental horizontal bone loss, indistinct lamina dura, altered trabecular pattern, and bell-shaped incisor roots.

IDIOPATHIC, SENILE, AND POSTMENOPAUSAL OSTEOPOROSIS

"Osteoporosis" denotes a deficiency of bone tissue per unit volume of bone as an organ. The bone that remains is considered to be normal by histologic criteria. There is no clear evidence of osteoclastic or osteoblastic dysfunction. The external dimension of the bone does not change. The decrease in bone mass expresses itself as reduction in thickness and increase in porosity in normally compact bone, and as loss of trabeculae in cancellous bone.

Age changes in bone follow a fairly definite pattern. After complete skeletal maturity is attained, bone enters a phase of quiescence. Turnover in structure is low, and cortical bone is thick, dense, and fully mineralized. However, after 35 years of age the bone mass begins to decrease, and this decrease continues steadily until death. Available estimates indicate that bone mass decreases by 5 to 10% per decade (Heaney, 1975).

The condition referred to as "senile osteoporosis" is characterized by greater loss of bone mass than occurs in normal age changes in bone. This loss may be extreme and may be associated with other complications, of which fracture is the most common. In the two decades from age 50 to age 70, the disease occurs predominantly in women. The prevalence in elderly men (at about age 80) is similar, but in them the disease usually is less severe. In the dental roentgenogram, senile osteoporosis is evidenced by decreased radiopacity of bone (as a result of thinning of the cortex and lamina dura) and by sparsity of trabeculae. Roentgenograms, made of a patient 66 years of age, that demonstrate these features are shown in Figure 18–34. A skeletal survey revealed that the vertebrae and other bones of the skeleton also were osteoporotic. That the alteration in bone might be associated with some other condition should be considered; in this case, clinical investigation for hyperparathyroidism and other possible systemic causes gave negative results.

It has been suggested (Jowsey, 1974) that approximately one-fourth of all white females in the United States develop clinically significant osteoporosis and that the disease is related to the menopause.

PROGERIA (HUTCHINSON-GILFORD SYNDROME)

Progeria is a rare condition characterized by dwarfism and signs of premature senility. Usually it becomes manifest before 1 year of age. Senile changes include loss of hair and subcutaneous fat, and precocious development of arteriosclerosis. Among other characteristics are receded chin, beaked nose, malocclusion, and retarded eruption of the teeth (Album and Hope, 1958). The bones are small and delicate, but there appears to be no significant arrest in bone maturation.

The cause of progeria is obscure; however, Talbot and associates (1945) have

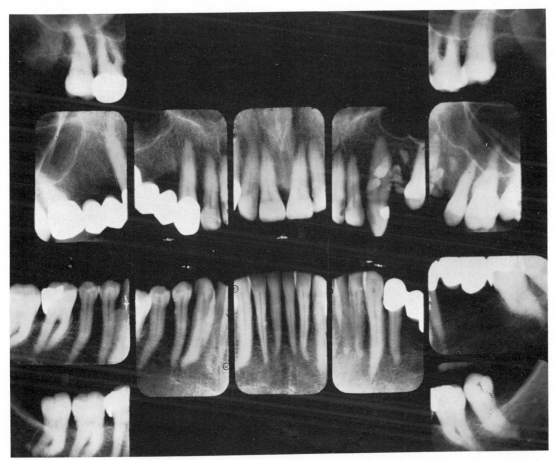

Figure 18–34 Senile osteoporosis in a patient 66 years of age, showing bone of reduced radiographic density, sparse trabeculae, and thinning of lamina dura.

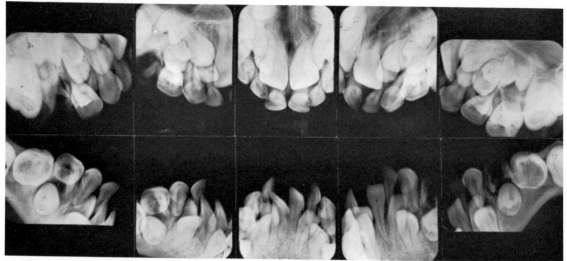

Figure 18–35 Progeria. Roentgenogram made at 10 years of age, showing prolonged retention of the primary teeth and retarded eruption of the permanent teeth.

suggested that the condition is a metabolic disturbance in which, even with adequate amounts of food, all calories appear to be used for energy metabolism with nothing left for growth and subcutaneous fat. Most often, the patient dies of coronary artery disease before adolescence.

The dental roentgenogram shown in Figure 18–35 was made for a girl 10 years of age who had progeria. She had weighed 8½ pounds at birth, and growth and gain in weight had been normal until 13 months of age. The primary teeth had not begun to erupt until 15 months of age. Clinical examination showed that she still had all her primary teeth except the mandibular central incisors. The roentgenogram revealed that the roots of most of the primary teeth were not undergoing normal resorption. The teeth of the permanent dentition were of normal size, and all except the mandibular central incisors were unerupted. Because the jaws were small, the teeth were crowded, and many were diverted from their usual position for normal eruption. Development of the teeth was within normal limits for the chronologic age. The mandibular second premolars were congenitally absent.

Eruption of the teeth is retarded approximately 3 to 4 years; this may be owing in large measure to their crowded condition and to failure of the roots of the primary teeth to undergo resorption. On microscopic examination of two teeth obtained at autopsy of a 10½-year-old boy, Gardner and Majka (1969) found the most significant observation to be accelerated formation of secondary dentin, apparently a manifestation of the premature aging associated with the disorder.

CONGENITAL, DEVELOPMENTAL, AND HEREDITARY ABNORMALITIES

In several entities there is a disturbance of skeletal development for which the cause is unknown. In many of these, inheritance factors are important. In some instances, symptoms may be present at birth; in others they may develop during childhood or adolescence. Associated dental disturbances may be manifested largely by faulty structure of the teeth, interference with normal development and eruption of the teeth, and malocclusion. In general, the dental disturbance is more severe in the conditions that are congenital.

There are many syndromes with which dental abnormalities are associated, and only a limited number of them are included in this chapter. For further information on this subject, the publications by Gorlin and Pindborg (1964) and by Gorlin and Goldman (1970) are recommended.

CLEIDOCRANIAL DYSOSTOSIS

Cleidocranial dysostosis is characterized by complete or incomplete aplasia of the clavicles, delayed ossification of the fontanels, malformation of the craniofacial bones, and abnormalities of the jaws and teeth. On occasion other bones may be either overdeveloped or stunted. There is a decided tendency to hereditary transmission.

Abnormality of the jaws and teeth is almost a constant feature. It is characterized by delayed resorption of the roots of the primary teeth, failure of eruption of many of the permanent teeth, formation of supernumerary dental structures, and underdevelopment of the maxilla. Another abnormality is failure of cellular cementum to form. Rushton (1956) found that cellular cementum was absent in eight of nine teeth from five patients who had the disease. He did not attribute failure of eruption of teeth to absence of cellular cementum, for cementum also was absent in fully

erupted teeth. Rushton's observation can be confirmed in a measure by the roentgenogram, for evidence of hypercementosis is conspicuously lacking in cleidocranial dysostosis.

The roentgenograms shown in Figure 18–36 were made for a patient who had clavicular and craniofacial defects and also involvement of the terminal phalanges of the thumbs and toes. The roentgenogram shown in the upper part of Figure 18–36 was made at the age of 10 years. Most of the primary teeth were still present. All the permanent teeth, including the first and second molars, for which there were no predecessors, still remained unerupted. There were four supernumerary premolars, one being situated in each quadrant. Orthodontic measures had been instituted in an effort to expand the underdeveloped maxillary arch. While the primary teeth invariably are lost by the time the patient reaches adult life, most of the permanent teeth fail to erupt. This tendency is evident in the roentgenogram (Fig. 18–36) made when the

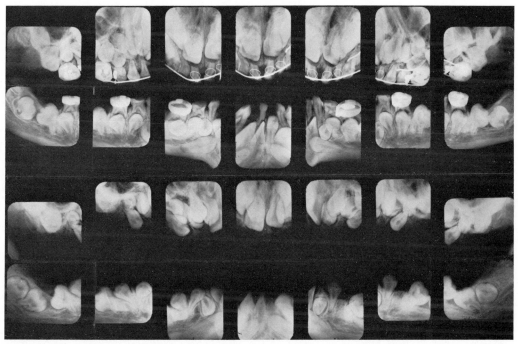

Figure 18–36 Cleidocranial dysostosis. *Above,* Appearance at 10 years of age, showing four supernumerary premolars, prolonged retention of primary teeth, and noneruption of permanent teeth. *Below,* Appearance at 15 years of age, showing noneruption of teeth. (Reproduced with permission from Millhon, J. A. and Austin, L. T.: Dental Findings in Four Cases of Cleidocranial Dysostosis. Am. J. Orthodontics [Oral Surg. Sect.]. *30*:30–40 [Jan.] 1944.)

patient had reached 15 years of age, when there was partial and full eruption of a few teeth only.

A dental roentgenogram made for a boy 15 years of age (Fig. 18–37) illustrates the marked tendency to formation of supernumerary teeth. Thirteen such teeth were present, and the occlusal views (Fig. 18–38) show their position in relation to the normal teeth.

HYPERTELORISM

Greig (1924) described hypertelorism as a definite variety of craniofacial dysostosis. It is a congenital malformation of the skull that is characterized by abnormally great separation of the eyes, and by broadening and deformity of the nose. According to Washington (1957), other malformations that have been observed are absence of the anterior part of the nasal septum, incomplete development of the alveolar process of the maxilla, and underde-

velopment of the mandibular ramus. The deformity may occur in mild form and has no associated disturbances. Some examples of ocular hypertelorism also are found in cleidocranial dysostosis and Crouzon's craniofacial dysostosis (Caffey, 1972).

Very little information is available concerning the effect of hypertelorism upon the teeth. From a review of the literature and observations by one of the authors (Stafne) in two cases, it appears that there is a tendency toward congenital absence of teeth. If this is so, it is in contradistinction to dental anomalies associated with craniofacial abnormalities of cleidocranial dysostosis, in which not only the normal number of teeth but also supernumerary dental structures are present.

A dental roentgenogram made for a patient 9 years of age (Fig. 18–39) who had hypertelorism revealed an absence of two lateral incisors, three premolars, and one second molar from the maxilla, and of one canine, two premolars, and two second

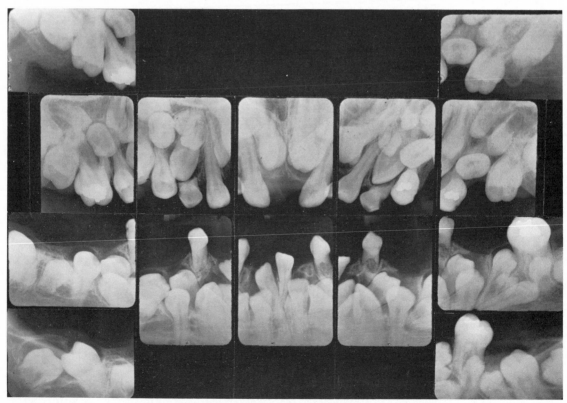

Figure 18–37 Cleidocranial dysostosis in a boy 15 years of age who has 13 supernumerary teeth. Most of them are premolars and are smaller, on the average, than normal teeth.

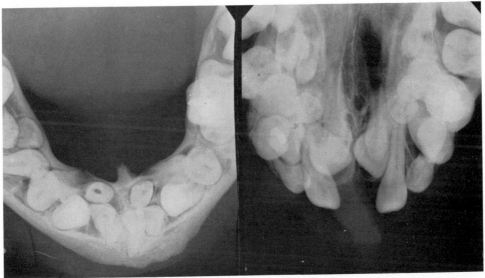

Figure 18–38 Cleidocranial dysostosis. Occlusal views of case represented in Figure 18–37, which reveal that the supernumerary teeth are palatal and lingual to the normal teeth. Those in the maxilla appear as though they are forming a second arch.

molars from the mandible. The maxillary arch was abnormally broad and short, causing marked malocclusion.

CONGENITAL HEMIHYPERTROPHY OF THE FACE (FACIAL GIANTISM)

Congenital hemihypertrophy originates in some developmental abnormality early in the growth of the ovum, and the overgrowth is detectable at birth. One-half of the entire body may be involved; however, the hypertrophy may be limited to only one portion (such as the trunk, an extremity, or the head), in which event it is called "segmental hypertrophy" (Ward and Lerner, 1947). When the overgrowth includes several systems—muscular, skeletal, vascular, and nervous—it is classified as total hypertrophy.

The incidence of mental deficiency in hemihypertrophy is said to be from 15 to

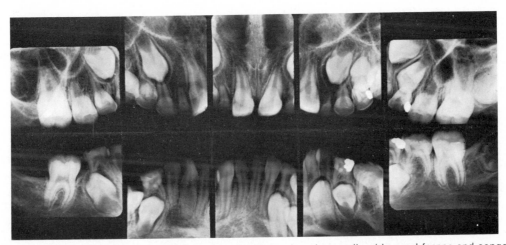

Figure 18–39 Hypertelorism. Patient 9 years of age showing abnormally wide nasal fossae and congenital absence of teeth in both jaws. (Reproduced with permission from Stafne, E. C.: Dental Roentgenologic Manifestations of Systemic Disease. II. Developmental Disturbances. Radiology. *58*:507–516 [Apr.] 1952.)

20%. Reports of a familial tendency are exceedingly rare.

In hemihypertrophy of the face, both skeletal and soft tissues are most often involved. According to Pagenstecher (1906), the histologic structures of the enlarged parts are larger and coarser than normal. The muscles have coarse fibers and the venous bed is richly developed. The sebaceous and sweat glands may be larger and the hair thicker than normal. Not all structures necessarily participate, nor do the affected ones enlarge or hypertrophy to the same degree.

Enlargement of the cheek with resulting asymmetry of the face first calls attention to the condition. Other parts that usually are enlarged on the involved side are the lips, nostril, ear, and tongue. The surface of the tongue is irregular and the papillae enlarged over the hypertrophied portion. When skeletal structures are involved, overgrowth of the jaws is a prominent feature.

The characteristic dental abnormalities are premature development and eruption, macrodontia, and congenital absence of teeth (Burke, 1951; Stafne and Lovestedt, 1962). The second premolars are the teeth most frequently absent. Teeth that may be larger than the corresponding teeth on the opposite side are, in order of frequency, the canines, the first premolars, the second premolars, and the first molars. Unlike bone and soft tissues, the teeth are unique in that their form and size are determined early and thereafter are not modified. A consideration of the teeth on the affected side therefore is essential, for it establishes the condition as a congenital one. The presence of the dental abnormalities is a significant finding and is very important in the differential diagnosis of congenital hemihypertrophy of the face from other conditions that produce enlargements of the face, particularly tumors.

The dental roentgenogram shown in Figure 18–40 was made for a boy 5½ years of age who had hypertrophy of the right side of the face. The enlargement had been noted shortly after birth. The primary teeth on the left side are still in place, and the stage of development of the permanent teeth is consistent with the chronologic age. Except for the maxillary central and lateral incisors, the teeth on the involved side have developed prematurely and are several years in advance of the chronologic age. The canines, first premolars, and maxillary first molar are appreciably larger than the corresponding teeth on the uninvolved side. The right mandibular lateral incisor and both second premolars are absent.

Since it is necessary to diagnose facial

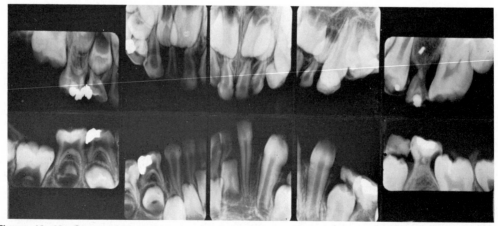

Figure 18–40 Congenital hemihypertrophy of the face (facial giantism) of the right side in a boy 5½ years of age. There are premature development and eruption of the teeth on the involved side, and several teeth are larger than corresponding teeth on the left. (Reproduced with permission from Stafne, E. C.: Dental Roentgenologic Manifestations of Systemic Disease. II. Developmental Disturbances. Radiology. *58*:507–516 [Apr.] 1952.)

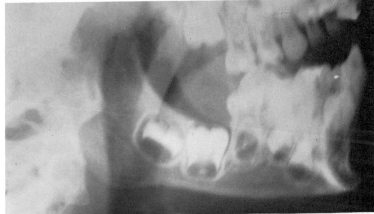

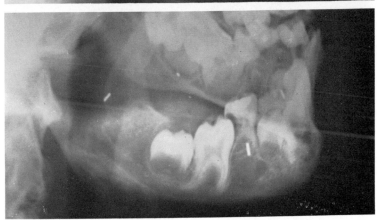

Figure 18–41 Congenital hemihypertrophy of the face. Lateral-view roentgenograms of the jaw from the case illustrated in Figure 18–40. *Above,* Left side of mandible, which is normal. *Below,* Right or affected side, showing enlarged mandible and premature development and eruption of teeth. (Reproduced with permission from Stafne, E. C.: Dental Roentgenologic Manifestations of Systemic Disease. II. Developmental Disturbances. Radiology. *58*:507–516 [Apr.] 1952.)

giantism early in infancy, at a time when it is difficult or impossible to obtain satisfactory intraoral roentgenograms, the extraoral lateral-view roentgenogram of the jaw is of invaluable aid. It may demonstrate enlargement of the mandible and premature development and calcification of the primary molars and the permanent first molar, and

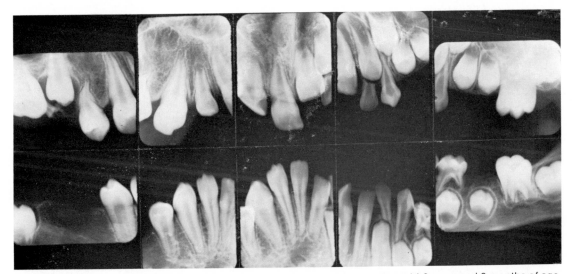

Figure 18–42 Congenital hemihypertrophy of the left side of the face in a girl 6 years and 2 months of age. The roentgenogram shows premature development and eruption of teeth and abnormally large canines and maxillary premolars on the affected side.

thereby permit an early diagnosis to be made. Figure 18–41 shows lateral-view roentgenograms of the left and right sides of the mandible of the patient represented in Figure 18–40. The molars on the right (Fig. 18–41) have reached a stage of development that is well in advance of those on the left and, in addition, the mandible is appreciably larger on the right than on the left.

The roentgenogram shown in Figure 18–42 was made for a girl 6 years of age who had hypertrophy of the left side of the face. She had marked enlargement of the cheek, lips, nose, tongue, and jaws on the involved side. Her left ear was slightly

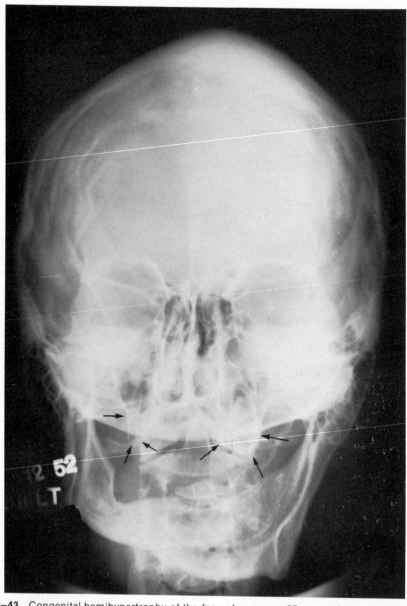

Figure 18–43 Congenital hemihypertrophy of the face of a woman 35 years of age. Roentgenogram of the head showing, on the involved side, hyperostosis of the frontal and parietal bones and pronounced overgrowth of the mandible. The alveolar process of the maxilla (arrows) is also appreciably larger on the right than on the left. (Reproduced with permission from Stafne, E. C. and Lovestedt, S. A.: Congenital Hemihypertrophy of the Face (Facial Giantism). Oral Surg., Oral Med. & Oral Path. *15*:184–189 [Feb.] 1962.)

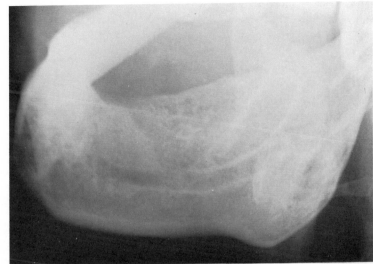

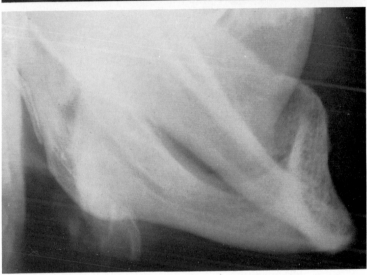

Figure 18–44 Lateral views of the mandible illustrating the disproportion in size between the left and the right side in the case represented in Figure 18–43. The involved side *(above)* is about twice the size of the normal side. (Reproduced with permission from Stafne, E. C. and Lovestedt, S. A.: Congenital Hemihypertrophy of the Face (Facial Giantism). Oral Surg., Oral Med. & Oral Path. *15*:184–189 [Feb.] 1962.)

larger than her right one, but it had a normal form and pattern. She had a speech difficulty because of the enlarged tongue and malocclusion, and she also was mentally retarded. Asymmetry of the face was noticed at birth, and the physician observed erupting cusps of the teeth on the enlarged side at the time of delivery.

The roentgenogram revealed that the stage of development and eruption of the teeth on the right was consistent with the chronologic age of the patient. On the involved side the incisors, canines, and first premolars were completely erupted, except for the maxillary lateral incisor. The crowns of both canines and of the maxillary first and second premolars were appreciably larger than those of the corresponding teeth on the right.

The roentgenogram of the head shown in Figure 18–43 reveals the extent of deformity and hypertrophy of bones that may characterize hemihypertrophy of the face. It was made for an edentulous woman 35 years of age who had an enlargement of the right side of the face that had been noted at birth. At the midline the anomalous bone of the involved side of the skull is sharply demarcated from that of the normal side. There is osteomatous thickening of the right frontal and parietal bones. The alveolar process of the maxilla is three times as wide as that on the opposite side, and the mandible is appreciably larger.

Figure 18–44 shows the disproportion in size of the two sides of the mandible. On the involved side *(above)* the vertical dimension of the body of the mandible is more than twice that of the normal side *(below)*. The diameter of the mandibular canal is significantly greater, and the enlargement appears to be in direct proportion to the abnormal increase in size of the mandible. The presence of the abnormally large canal should serve to differentiate this congenital overgrowth of the jaw from enlargements caused by fibrous dysplasia, Paget's disease, and some tumors.

Obviously, facial hemihypertrophy presents difficult dental problems. When the teeth are present, malocclusion is a major complication. If the patient becomes edentulous, there may be inadequate space for the insertion of artificial dentures, or it may not be possible to construct them to the desired occlusal plane. In such instances, surgical reduction of the enlarged alveolar processes should be the most satisfactory solution.

FACIAL HEMIATROPHY (HEMIHYPOPLASIA)

Facial hemiatrophy may be congenital or acquired. The exact cause is obscure. In the congenital form there may be underdevelopment and varied degrees of aplasia of the zygomatic arch, mastoid process, temporal bone, maxilla, and mandible, causing marked asymmetry of the face. The auditory canal may be absent, and the external ear may be rudimentary or completely lacking. A not uncommon feature is agenesis of the condyle, and in some instances the ramus and a portion of the body of the mandible may fail to form as well (Fig. 18–45). In contrast to facial hemihypertrophy, the development and eruption of the teeth often are retarded (Fig. 18–46). In some patients, the teeth on the involved side may be smaller than normal (Burke, 1957; Rushton, 1951).

Facial hemiatrophy that has its onset several years after birth may not influence dental development; however, the atrophy of the skin and subcutaneous tissues affects the underlying muscles and bone, with the result that the jaws may be atrophied and cause malocclusion and noneruption of the teeth.

OSTEOPETROSIS (MARBLE BONES, ALBERS-SCHÖNBERG DISEASE)

Osteopetrosis is characterized by increased density of the cortical and spongy portions of the entire osseous system. The marrow cavity may be encroached upon to the point of obliteration. In general, the structural contours of the bones are preserved (McCune and Bradley, 1934). The

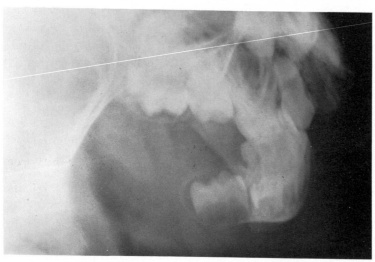

Figure 18–45 Facial hemiatrophy (congenital) in a child 4½ years old, showing agenesis of condyle, ramus, and a portion of the body of the mandible. There was also partial agenesis of the malar bone, and the external ear was rudimentary.

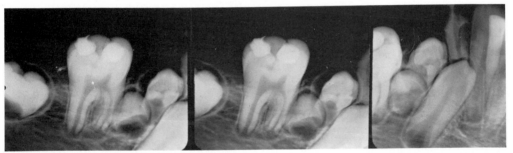

Figure 18–46 Facial hemiatrophy in a patient 10 years of age. The mandibular premolars and second molar have reached a stage of calcification that normally is attained at the chronologic age of 6 years.

disturbance is of mesenchymal origin; the most widely accepted concept is that the fundamental defect is a faulty differentiation of hematogenic and osteogenic tissue. The abnormal density of bone is in large measure due to reduced osteoclastic activity. Among complications that may arise are anemia and enlargement of the spleen, liver, and lymph nodes.

Because of the disproportion of mineral and organic substances, and a purposeless arrangement of the bone trabeculae, the bones are fragile and subject to fracture. Resistance to infection is decreased, and owing to the common occurrence of superimposed periodontal and periapical infection, the jaws, particularly the mandible, are vulnerable to osteomyelitis. Among those who have reported cases of osteomyelitis associated with osteopetrosis are Bloom (1943) and Linsey (1944). In the latter case, the infection led to complete loss of the mandible.

Clinically osteopetrosis is usually classified according to two types: (1) infantile, or malignant, and (2) adult, or benign. In the infantile type the disturbance is apt to be severe and the mortality rate high. The adult type follows a relatively slow course, and may be carried into adult life without clinical evidence of its presence (Piatt et al., 1956). It is compatible with reasonably normal living, and may cause few if any symptoms. Often the disease is first detected incidentally on roentgenologic examination, and this might well be on dental examination.

The hereditary character of osteopetrosis appears to be well established. It is transmitted as a simple recessive mendelian character; therefore several cases of the disease may appear in successive generations of the same family.

The roentgenographic appearance of the bones is one of homogeneity and increased radiopacity. There is prominent thickening of the base of the skull, and the paranasal sinuses are narrowed, or partially effaced. Roentgenograms of the jaws may show partial or complete obliteration of the marrow cavities. The condition has been called "marble bones" because of its white, uniform roentgenographic appearance, and not because of the degree of hardness of the bones.

The roentgenogram shown in Figure 18–47 was made for a man 40 years of age who knew he had the disease and was aware of the complications that might arise incidental to the extraction of teeth. It revealed a uniform and homogeneous opacity of both jaws with almost complete obliteration of the marrow spaces. The bone of the mandible was extremely radiopaque, so that the roots of some of the teeth were barely visible. The patient's mother, a brother, and two of four children also were known to have the disease. All were asymptomatic, and the condition had first been detected by dental roentgenograms made for the brother some years previously.

Any effect that osteopetrosis may have upon the teeth occurs in the congenital form of the disease. Deformed and stunted roots on which the cementum is sparse and of irregular thickness are the most common dental defects. Also, Bergman and co-workers (1956) observed hypoplasia of the enamel which varied from that of hypoplastic pits to that of gross malformation of the crowns.

A roentgenogram that illustrates a disturbance of development of the roots is shown in Figure 18–48. It was made for a man 28 years of age who had osteopetrosis. The roots of all the teeth present were underdeveloped and dwarfed. The bone of the jaws was abnormally dense, particularly in the mandible, where the marrow spaces appeard to be completely obliterated in the anterior and premolar regions. A brother who also had osteopetrosis had a similar dental anomaly, and as a result had lost his teeth at an early age.

OSTEOGENESIS IMPERFECTA (FRAGILITAS OSSIUM)

Osteogenesis imperfecta is a disturbance of mesenchymal development char-

acterized primarily by brittle bones and possibly associated with blue scleras and deafness. It has a definite familial tendency.

Two varieties of the disease usually are described: (1) a fetal, or infantile, form and (2) an adolescent, or tardy, form. The fetal form is apt to be severe, and those afflicted seldom survive into adult life. The tardy form is milder, and a wide spectrum of severity exists. Most often the tendency to fracture regresses with puberty and skeletal maturity, although fractures tend to recur in later life. Stool and Sullivan (1959) reported the case of a woman who sustained a fracture at 95 years of age. Five members in three generations of the patient's family had the disease, and a daughter had had a fracture at 59 years of age.

Dental development may be disturbed in the fetal or infantile form, and the incidence is relatively high. Heys and coworkers (1960) found that 8 of 13 families

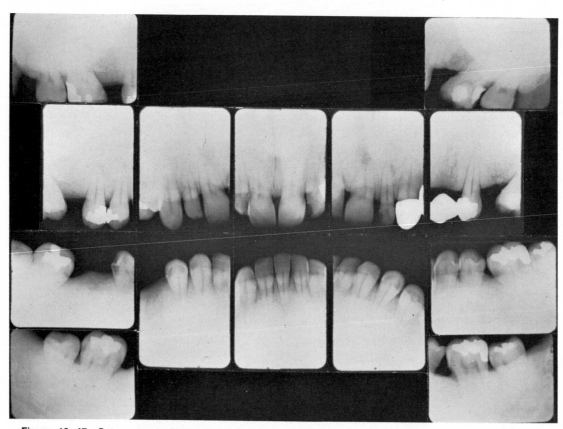

Figure 18–47 Osteopetrosis. Dental roentgenogram showing extreme radiopacity of the bone of both jaws.

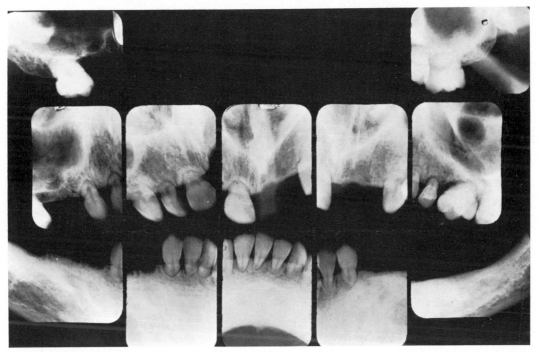

Figure 18–48 Osteopetrosis in a man 28 years of age, showing bone of abnormal density and dwarfed roots of the teeth. (Reproduced with permission from Stafne, E. C.: Dental Roentgenologic Aspects of Systemic Disease. J. Am. Dent. A. *40*:265–283 [Mar.] 1950.)

with osteogenesis imperfecta also had an associated dentinogenesis imperfecta. The dental abnormality is in most respects similar to that of hereditary dentinogenesis imperfecta (opalescent dentin), a dental anomaly that is not necessarily associated with systemic disease and has been dealt with in a previous chapter. As in hereditary opalescent dentin, abnormal color of the teeth and dentinal dysplasia may be noted; however, the dentinal dysplasia exhibits a wider and more varied pattern. Teeth that are of abnormal color may have pulp cavities that are not abnormally reduced in size. In some patients, obliteration of the pulp chamber may be confined to a few teeth, and these are most often the incisors and first molars. The size of the pulp chamber usually is reduced later in the stage of tooth development than it is in hereditary opalescent dentin, in which obliteration occurs almost simultaneously with calcification of the tooth. The roots of the teeth also are more prone to approach normal size. The primary teeth are affected more often than the permanent teeth; in

this respect the condition differs from hereditary opalescent dentin, in which the dentitions are affected consecutively in nearly all patients.

The color of the teeth is varied. It has been described as opalescent, translucent, white, diffuse gray, pink, yellow, and brown. The teeth that have been erupted for some time, and especially those that have been worn away by attrition, take on darker hues. Dissimilar colors may be evident in the same person, the variation most often existing between the anterior and the posterior teeth.

Excellent descriptions of the histologic aspects of the involved teeth have been provided by Becks (1931) and Pindborg (1947). Among those who have reported on the clinical features are Mittelman (1950) and Stafne (1952).

Roentgenograms from three cases are presented to illustrate varied degrees of obliteration of the pulp cavities. One in which the pulp cavities are seen to be almost completely obliterated in all the teeth is shown in Figure 18–49. It was made for a

may be assoc c microdontia p 22

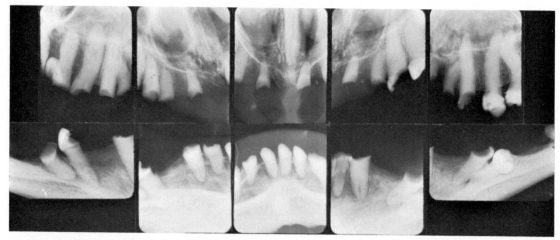

Figure 18–49 Dentinogenesis imperfecta associated with osteogenesis imperfecta. Roentgenogram made for a boy 17 years of age, showing obliterated pulp cavities of all the teeth and rapid destruction of the crowns of the teeth by attrition.

boy 17 years of age who had blue scleras and had sustained the first of numerous fractures at 2 years of age. The enamel of such teeth may be soft, and in this patient the crowns of some of the teeth that have been in occlusion are completely worn away by attrition.

The roentgenogram shown in Figure 18–50 illustrates a case in which the pulp chamber had been eradicated in a limited number of teeth. It was made for a boy 14 years of age who had blue scleras and who

had experienced approximately 40 fractures, the first occurring at 1 year of age. The pulp cavities of the mandibular incisors had been obliterated, but in the other teeth present there was partial obliteration in some and no reduction in size of others. The roots of the teeth were of normal size and form. The maxillary lateral incisors and the mandibular first premolars were congenitally absent, but this is not a feature of the disease.

A roentgenogram that illustrates a wide

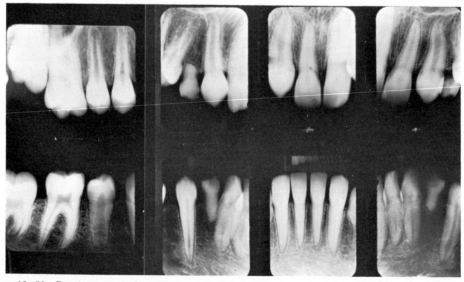

Figure 18–50 Dentinogenesis imperfecta associated with osteogenesis imperfecta, showing varied degrees of obliteration of the pulp cavities.

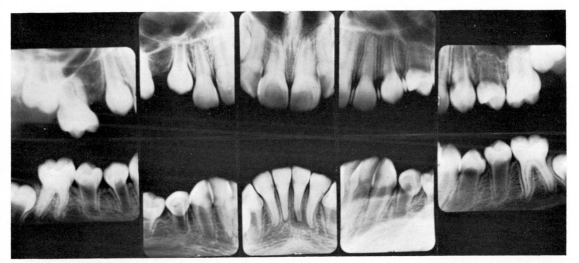

Figure 18–51 Dentinogenesis imperfecta associated with osteogenesis imperfecta. The roentgenogram reveals obliteration of the pulp cavities of the incisors and first molars, and abnormally large pulp cavities (shell teeth) in the premolars. (Reproduced with permission from Stafne, E. C.: Dental Roentgenologic Manifestations of Systemic Disease. II. Developmental Disturbances. Radiology. 58:507–516 [Apr.] 1952.)

variation in the size of the pulp cavities is shown in Figure 18–51. It was made for a girl 8 years of age who had blue scleras and had sustained more than 20 fractures, the first at 11 days of age. All the teeth had translucent, amber color. The pulp cavities of the incisors and first molars have been obliterated; however, those of the premolars are still extremely large and have the roentgenographic appearance of the so-called shell teeth reported by Rushton (1954). He found that these teeth had a thin peripheral layer of dentin in which the tubules became dilated and abruptly disappeared. There was absence of odontoblasts, and the enormous pulp cavities contained coarse collagen fibers. He suggested that the teeth might represent an extreme variant of dentinogenesis imperfecta. The roentgenogram shown here is perhaps rare in that it exhibits in the same individual both extreme variants of dentinal dysplasia.

In osteogenesis imperfecta the severity of the disease and the degree of dental disturbance do not seem to be definitely correlated.

ACHONDROPLASIA

A disturbance in the development and formation of cartilage is the primary feature in achondroplasia. Because of the lack of growth at the epiphyses of the long bones, the extremities are short in comparison with the torso, so that, in extreme cases, a very familiar form of dwarfism is produced. Other characteristics are a prominent forehead, a saddle nose, and a retruded maxilla. Malocclusion is not uncommon, and interference with dental development is most often manifested by retarded eruption and noneruption of the teeth.

A dental roentgenogram made for an achondroplastic dwarf 30 years of age is shown in Figure 18–52. It revealed 20 embedded permanent teeth and five embedded primary molars that had undergone almost complete resorption. The presence of so many unerupted teeth is also typical of cleidocranial dysostosis.

ECTODERMAL DYSPLASIA

Ectodermal dysplasia is a developmental disturbance that is characterized by partial or total absence of hair, faulty fingernails, scantiness or absence of sweat glands, and partial or complete absence of the teeth. The degree of dental aplasia no doubt depends on the time of onset of the disturbance. If the disease occurs early in fetal life, there may be total aplasia. If it

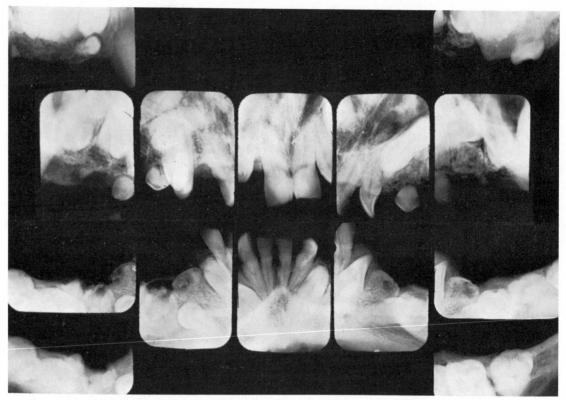

Figure 18–52 Achondroplasia in a man 30 years of age, showing 20 embedded permanent teeth and five embedded primary teeth. (Reproduced with permission from Stafne, E. C.: Dental Roentgenologic Aspects of Systemic Disease. J. Am. Dent. A. *40*:265–283 [Mar.] 1950.)

occurs later in fetal life, the primary teeth may remain unaffected, but a few or all of the permanent teeth may fail to form. Of the permanent teeth, the anlagen of the incisors, canines, and first molars are the first to be laid down. Therefore they are the teeth that are most apt to remain unaffected. Cook (1939) reported a case in which only the permanent maxillary canines and first molars were present. Guil-

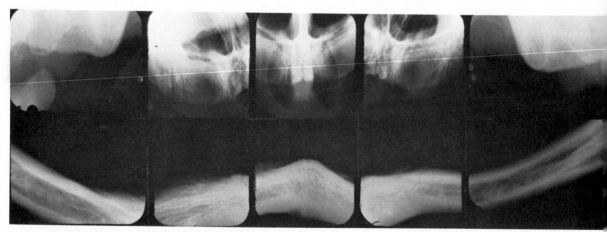

Figure 18–53 Ectodermal dysplasia in a man 22 years of age, associated with total dental aplasia. (Reproduced with permission from Lovestedt, S. A.: Examples of Dental Dysplasia. Am. J. Orthodontics [Oral Surg. Sect.]. *33*:625–629 [Aug.] 1947.)

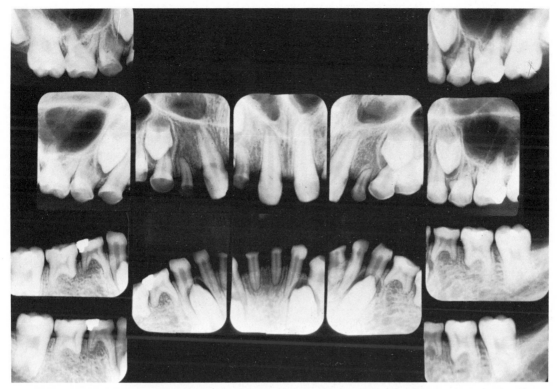

Figure 18–54 Ectodermal dysplasia in a boy 10 years of age, associated with partial anodontia. (Reproduced with permission from Stafne, E. C.: Dental Roentgenologic Aspects of Systemic Disease. J. Am. Dent. A. *40*:265–283 [Mar.] 1950.)

ford (1883), Lovestedt (1947), Thoma and Allen (1940), and Sarnat and co-workers (1953) reported cases in which there was total anodontia.

A dental roentgenogram made for a man 22 years of age who had ectodermal dysplasia and total dental aplasia is shown in Figure 18–53. Both jaws were underdeveloped in the vertical dimension, and the roentgenographic appearance was very similar to that of edentulous jaws in which the alveolar ridge has undergone complete resorption following extraction of the teeth. The size of the arches closely approached that of the normal jaw, and artificial dentures had been worn satisfactorily for 14 years.

A dental roentgenogram made for a boy 10 years of age who had ectodermal dysplasia and partial anodontia is shown in Figure 18–54. All the primary teeth except the maxillary lateral incisors were still present. The roentgenogram revealed that

the only teeth of the permanent dentition that had developed were the maxillary central incisors, canines, and first molars, and the mandibular canines and first molars.

MISCELLANEOUS DISEASES

SYPHILIS

One of the first general conditions with which definite association of dental abnormalities was established is syphilis. The most prominent of these abnormalities are those of size and form of the teeth: the screwdriver-shaped crown and notched incisal edge of permanent maxillary central incisors described by Hutchinson, and the "mulberry molars," both of which may occur in congenital syphilis. Since these teeth do not erupt before the patient is 6 to 7 years of age, it is well to know that an appreciable portion of the crowns has

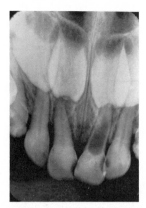

Figure 18–55 Congenital syphilis. Roentgenogram made at 4 years of age, demonstrating unerupted Hutchinson's central incisors. (Reproduced with permission from Stafne, E. C.: Roentgenologic Interpretation. In Grossman, L. I.: Lippincott's Handbook of Dental Practice. Ed. 2. Philadelphia, J. B. Lippincott Company, 1952, p. 70.)

formed at 1 year of age. The presence of the anomalous crowns can therefore be demonstrated at an early age with the roentgenogram, thereby providing information that may be of value in differential diagnosis several years prior to eruption of the teeth. A roentgenogram made for a patient 4 years of age, illustrating screwdriver-shaped maxillary central incisors as described by Hutchinson, is shown in Figure 18–55. A roentgenogram demonstrating fully erupted Hutchinson's central incisors and the typical constricted crowns and cusps of the first molars (mulberry molars) is shown in Figure 18–56.

While constriction of the crowns or the cusps of the teeth may be peculiar to con-genital syphilis, the dental stigmas show wider variations than is generally known. Such defects result from direct injuries to the ameloblasts and odontoblasts owing to spirochetal infection. Boyle (1932), Burket (1937), and Bradlaw (1953) have demonstrated the presence of *Treponema pallidum* in the developing tooth germs of persons suffering from congenital syphilis. Sarnat and Shaw (1943), in a study of 73 patients who had congenital syphilis, found that 22 of them, or 30%, had dental defects in the form of either enamel dysplasia or morphodifferentiation. In some instances, enamel dysplasia of the primary dentition was present. Brauer and Blackstone (1941), in a study of 38 children, found that 2 of them had hypoplasia of the enamel of the primary molars.

It is generally conceded that a high incidence of dental abnormalities is associated with congenital syphilis and that these are not necessarily limited to the typical Hutchinson incisor and mulberry molar. A case in point is that of a boy 17 years of age who had congenital syphilis and also had amelogenesis imperfecta for which no history of familial tendency to this anomaly could be elicited. The dental roentgenogram, shown in Figure 18–57, reveals that the unerupted as well as the erupted teeth are all almost completely devoid of enamel. Whether the enamel dysplasia in this instance could be attributed to congenital syphilis is problematic.

Bone infections occur both in congenital and in tertiary syphilis and may take the form of localized osteitis caused by a

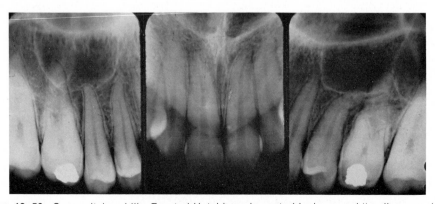

Figure 18–56   Congenital syphilis. Erupted Hutchinson's central incisors and "mulberry molars."

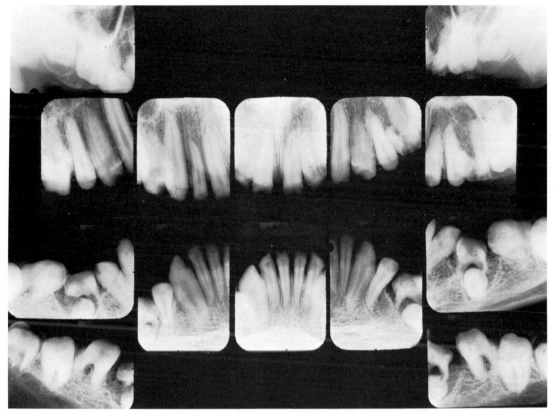

Figure 18–57   Congenital syphilis associated with amelogenesis imperfecta.

gumma, or the form of osteomyelitis. In the jaws the gumma most frequently occurs in the anterior part of the hard palate, where it may cause destruction of bone and perforation into the nasal cavity.

HISTIOCYTOSIS X (RETICULOENDOTHELIOSIS)

Lichtenstein (1953) advanced the concept that conditions previously designated as Letterer-Siwe disease, Hand-Schüller-Christian disease, and eosinophilic granuloma are interrelated manifestations of a single malady, and suggested the term "histiocytosis X." The three conditions are similar histologically, and according to Dahlin (1957) there is so much overlapping in clinical and pathologic manifestations that attempts at strict classification of individual cases are futile. The disease is characterized by the formation of granulomatous lesions in which there are large

accumulations of histiocytes and usually a variable number of eosinophilic leukocytes.

Certain features have been responsible for the tendency to divide the disease into three separate entities. These are (1) the acute, sometimes rapidly fatal expression of the condition as seen in Letterer-Siwe disease; (2) the disseminated nature of the condition and its possible association with exophthalmos and diabetes insipidus as seen in Hand-Schüller-Christian disease; and (3) the tendency of the condition to manifest itself as solitary or multiple lesions of bone as seen in eosinophilic granuloma.

The hard and soft tissues of the oral cavity are often involved. Blevins and coworkers (1959) found that oral and dental manifestations were presenting symptoms or developed later in 34 of 66 cases of histiocytosis X. The diagnosis was confirmed histologically (not necessarily in the jaws) in 27 of the 34 cases, and in 12 of these, oral involvement was the most significant clinical feature and the chief reason for seeking dental and medical service. Sleeper (1951) found that 62% of 39 patients with Hand-Schüller-Christian disease included oral symptoms among their complaints.

The chief oral manifestations of the disease are inflammation and swelling of the gingiva, loosening and sloughing of the teeth, destruction of alveolar bone, retardation of healing or failure of wounds to heal after extraction, and formation of osteolytic lesions in the jawbones. These signs simulate in large measures those of other lesions that may involve the jaws, including benign and malignant tumors. Biopsy, therefore, is extremely important as an aid in differential diagnosis (Kruger et al., 1949).

Minimal roentgen therapy is effective in destroying the lesion (Dealy and Sosman, 1956). A single treatment is directed to a given region, and is repeated as judged necessary. The low dosage used (usually not exceeding 300 R) is not likely to harm the developing dentition. Curettement alone may suffice to eliminate the lesion,

and this may be indicated for readily accessible solitary lesions.

Hand-Schüller-Christian Disease. This disease usually occurs in early life. The bones most often affected are the pelvis, ribs, scapulas, calvaria, and jaws; it is not unusual for the lesions to appear first in the jaws. Lesions of the jaws have a predilection for the periapical region or dentin papilla of developing teeth. With expansion of the lesions, the dental crypt or alveolar socket, as the case may be, is destroyed, and the partially developed teeth eventually are exfoliated. During the process of exfoliation, the roentgenographic appearance is that of teeth floating in space, which is distinctive and diagnostic of the disease.

The dental roentgenogram shown in Figure 18–58 was made for a boy 8 years of age who had Hand-Schüller-Christian disease. The first lesion had appeared in the calvaria 4 years previously. There was a history of successive sloughing of several of the primary and permanent teeth. The roentgenogram revealed destructive lesions of the maxilla on the right and in both posterior regions of the mandible. Three mandibular primary molars and their per-

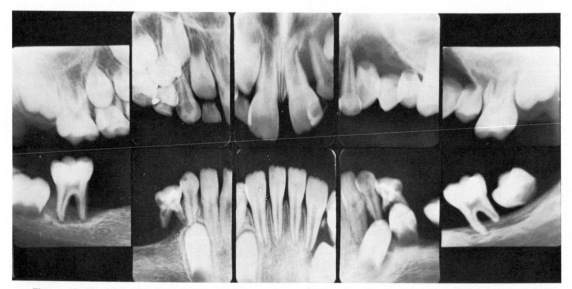

Figure 18–58 Hand-Schüller-Christian disease in a boy 8 years of age, showing destruction of the alveolar process in the right maxilla and posterior regions of the mandible. The teeth in the involved regions are being exfoliated, including some that are only partially developed. (Reproduced with permission from Stafne, E. C.: Dental Roentgenologic Aspects of Systemic Disease. J. Am. Dent. A. *40*:265–283 [Mar.] 1950.)

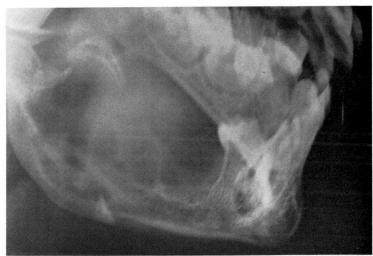

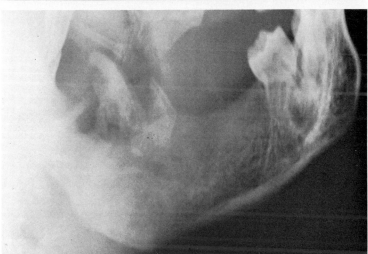

Figure 18–59 Hand-Schüller-Christian disease. *Above,* Lesion involving ramus of mandible. *Below,* Nine months after roentgen therapy, lesion has undergone healing.

manent successors had been lost, and teeth undergoing sloughing were the right maxillary canine and premolars, the mandibular primary first molars, the permanent first molars, and the right first premolar and second molar.

Some of the mandibular lesions cause diffuse and extensive destruction of bone which roentgenographically may simulate that produced by malignant tumors (Fig. 18–59). However, unlike that of sarcoma and other malignant tumors of the jaw, the destruction appears to be limited to alveolar bone and does not extend downward to invade and destroy the inferior border of the mandible. Furthermore, it is doubtful that an initial lesion in the mandible ever arises

in bone that is inferior to the mandibular canal.

Eosinophilic Granuloma of Bone. So-called eosinophilic granuloma occurs most often in older children and adults, and may be solitary or multiple. The lesions tend to be confined to bone, but it is not certain whether, some time later, tissues other than bone may be involved as well. The initial lesions may appear in the jawbones, and in some instances they may be limited solely to that region.

Figure 18–60 *(upper part)* shows a roentgenogram made for a boy 3 years 8 months of age who for several months past had had inflamed swellings of the soft tissues adjacent to both of the primary max-

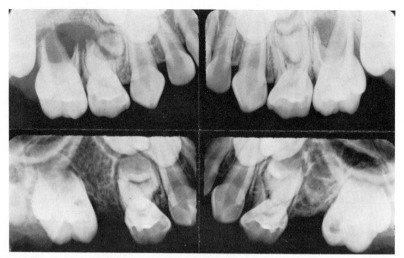

Figure 18–60 Eosinophilic granuloma. *Above,* Destructive lesions involving the primary second molars. *Below,* Roentgenogram made 1 year after roentgen therapy, showing onset of calcification of the permanent right second molar.

illary second molars that on biopsy proved to be eosinophilic granuloma. The dental roentgenogram revealed destruction of bone involving the trifurcation of both molars, the lesion on the left having destroyed most of the bone supporting the roots of the tooth. A roentgenologic survey did not disclose lesions elsewhere in the skeleton. The lesions responded favorably to roentgen therapy and rapidly disappeared. As a result, the roots of the involved teeth became denuded and they had to be extracted about 4 months after therapy. Eleven months after therapy the alveolar bone in the region where the lesions had been present appeared normal (Fig. 18–60, *lower*). The right permanent second premolar was developing, as evidenced by the presence of a tooth bud and onset of calcification of the crown. On the left there was as yet no evidence of a tooth bud, and it was likely that it had been destroyed by the lesion rather than by the low dose of radiation administered.

Early recognition and roentgen therapy of childhood eosinophilic granulomas of the jaws will save many teeth of both dentitions that would slough if no measures were taken to destroy the lesions.

When eosinophilic granuloma occurs in the jaws of an adult whose teeth are present, the clinical course is fairly charac-

teristic. The disease appears primarily as a periodontal lesion that causes extensive destruction of alveolar bone, loosening of the tooth, and failure of the wound to heal normally after extraction or sloughing of the tooth. Only one region may be involved, but more often the lesions in the jaws are multiple. Microscopic examination of the lesions is essential for correct diagnosis, particularly if a roentgenologic survey does not reveal lesions in the calvaria or elsewhere in the skeleton.

The roentgenograms in a case in which the disease has followed a typical course are shown in Figure 18–61. The patient was a man whose teeth first began to slough at 31 years of age. The left mandibular premolars had become very loose and had to be extracted. Over a period of 3½ years thereafter he had had successive loss of all the mandibular teeth except the incisors, loss of the right posterior maxillary teeth, and loss of the left maxillary third molar. The patient said he had received several courses of antibiotic therapy that helped little to arrest the progress of the disease. The roentgenogram (Fig. 18–61, *upper part*) revealed osteolytic lesions of both sides of the mandible and in the left maxillary molar region. Microscopic examination of the lesion of the left side of the mandible confirmed a diagnosis of eo-

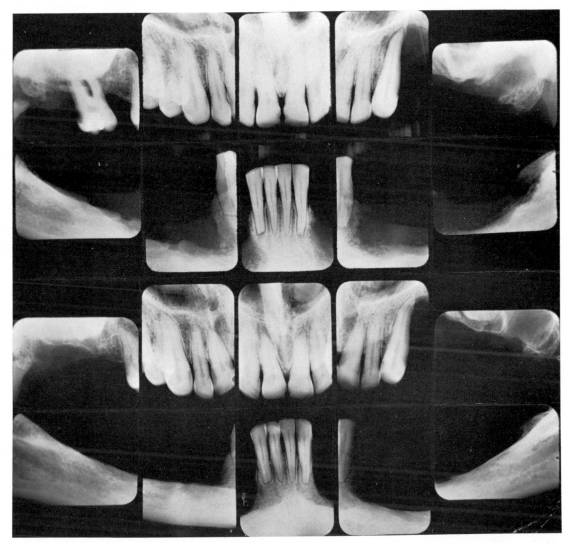

Figure 18–61 Eosinophilic granuloma of the jaws. *Above,* Appearance 3½ years after onset of successive sloughing of posterior teeth, showing nonhealing of alveolar bone. *Below,* Appearance 9 months after roentgen therapy, showing complete healing of lesions.

sinophilic granuloma. A roentgen survey did not reveal similar lesions elsewhere in the skeleton. A roentgenogram made 9 months after roentgen therapy disclosed that the bone lesions had healed completely, including those not treated surgically (Fig. 18–61, *lower part*).

A patient 22 years of age who had multiple eosinophilic granulomas involving the calvarium, jaws, and other bones gave a history suggesting that the first symptoms of the disease and osseous lesions appeared in the jaw. The right mandibular second and third molars became loose and

were extracted 3 years before a correct diagnosis was made. The wound at the site of the extraction had never healed completely, and a dental roentgenogram revealed the presence of an osteolytic lesion (Fig. 18–62, *upper part*). Several months after roentgen therapy, which included treatment of the lesion in the mandible, the cavity formerly occupied by the granuloma had completely filled with bone (Fig. 18–62, *lower part*). While curettement might have sufficed to eliminate the lesion, this case illustrates further the efficacy of roentgen therapy.

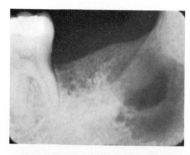

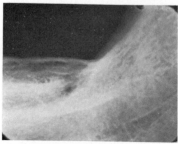

Figure 18–62 Eosinophilic granuloma. *Above,* Evidence of osteolytic lesion in third molar region of mandible. *Below,* Several months after roentgen therapy the cavity formerly occupied by the lesion has become completely filled with bone. (Reproduced with permission from Stafne, E. C.: Roentgenologic Manifestations of Systemic Disease in Dentistry. Oral Surg. Oral Med. & Oral Path. 6:483–494 [Apr.] 1953.)

PAGET'S DISEASE (OSTEITIS DEFORMANS)

Paget's disease, or osteitis deformans, is a disease of the skeleton that usually occurs after middle age, although it has occurred in persons less than 20 years of age. The cause of the disease is not known. It may be limited to a part or all of a single bone, but in the disseminated form it may involve almost all the bones. The progressive and advanced types may be accompanied by deformities and fractures. The incidence of involvement of the jaws is relatively high (Stafne and Austin, 1938); the maxilla alone is affected most often, and both the maxilla and the mandible rarely (Clark and Holte, 1950; Stafne, 1946). The involved jaw may become abnormally large, resulting in malocclusion and a grotesque appearance. The initial lesion is one of destruction by resorption; later an excessive amount of bone of inferior quality is deposited.

The roentgenographic appearance depends on the stage at which the condition is seen. In the early osteolytic or resorptive stage the radiographic density of the bone is decreased, and the trabecular pattern is altered into one that has a ground-glass appearance. These osteolytic lesions are more apt to occur and persist in the regions immediately surrounding the roots of the teeth. The lamina dura around the teeth in the involved regions is absent, and there may be evidence of resorption of the roots of the teeth in rare instances. Resorption of the roots of the teeth in the early stages of Paget's disease has been pointed out by Rushton (1938) and Cooke (1956). Such evidence of root resorption is shown in a dental roentgenogram made for a patient who had involvement of many bones, including the mandible (Fig. 18–63). There was also pronounced radiolucency of bone, along with absence of the lamina dura.

As the disease progresses, osteoblastic may exceed osteoclastic activity, so that apposition exceeds resorption of bone. In the progressive and advanced forms of the disease, therefore, the roentgenogram presents evidence of alternating regions of fibrosis and osteosclerosis, the latter being more prominent. In the maxilla, gradual encroachment upon and reduction in the

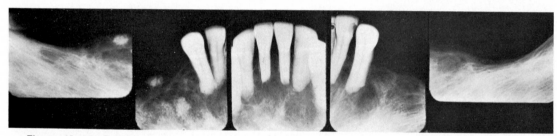

Figure 18–63 Paget's disease of the mandible. Early or resorptive stage, evidenced by radiolucence of bone and resorption of roots of teeth.

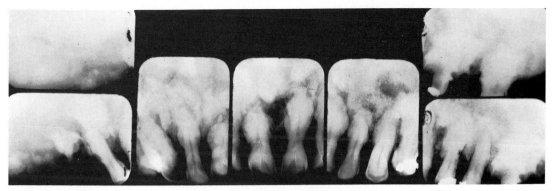

Figure 18–64 Paget's disease of the maxilla. Advanced stage, showing predominance of osteosclerosis, obliteration of maxillary sinuses, hypercementosis, and absence of lamina dura.

size of the maxillary sinuses may be associated with the increased osteoblastic activity; also, poorly differentiated cementum is deposited on the roots of the teeth. Another characteristic feature is the absence of the lamina dura which, once it has been obliterated, never returns in Paget's disease. A roentgenogram in a case of advanced Paget's disease of the maxilla is shown in Figure 18–64, and one of the mandible in Figure 18–65. In both instances, marked enlargement and deformity were present.

The formation of an excessive amount of poorly differentiated cementum on the roots of teeth in Paget's disease has been noted by Seldin (1933), Cahn (1937), and others. This excess of hyperplastic cementum apparently is peculiar to Paget's disease and, when present, is of value in suggesting a diagnosis, for it serves as a

point of differentiation from other osseous lesions that may involve the jaws.

The formation of new osseous tissue on the surface of bones, which is characteristic of Paget's disease, can be seen rarely in dental roentgenograms. However, in the mandible the layers of bone that have been formed may be in evidence on the edentulous alveolar crest, and can be demonstrated on the inferior border if the film is placed sufficiently far downward to include it. Laminated bone on the surface of the mandible in a case of Paget's disease is shown in Figure 18–66.

The most serious and important complication associated with Paget's disease of bone is the possible occurrence of osteogenic sarcoma, of which there is a higher incidence than that which is found in normal bone. In a series of 24 cases of

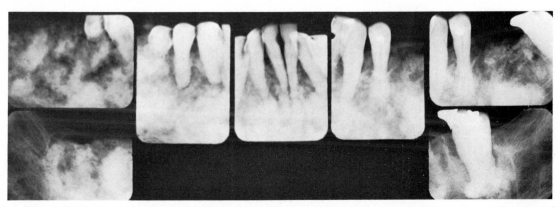

Figure 18–65 Paget's disease of the mandible. Advanced stage, showing alternating areas of fibrosis and osteosclerosis, and absence of lamina dura.

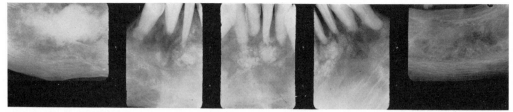

Figure 18–66 Paget's disease of the mandible, showing fine layers of bone on the crest of the alveolar ridge and on the inferior border of the mandible.

Paget's disease of the jaws studied by Tillman (1962), there were 2 well-documented cases of osteogenic sarcoma. In 9 of the 24 cases the diagnosis of Paget's disease had been made by the dentist who first noted the changes in the jaw.

SCLERODERMA (ACROSCLEROSIS)

Scleroderma is characterized by hardness and rigidity of the skin and subcutaneous tissues. It may occur in the diffuse (acrosclerotic) form, in which the entire surface of the skin may be involved and in which the disease is limited chiefly to the face, shoulder girdle, upper part of the thorax, and fingers (O'Leary and Waisman, 1943), or in the "coup de sabre" form, in which the lesions approximate at times the terminal distribution of a nerve. In some instances, scleroderma may be associated with resorption of bone, particularly of the distal phalanges, where such resorption may be attributed to continuous pressure of the involved skin.

A dental roentgenologic finding that appears to be peculiar to scleroderma, and particularly to acrosclerosis, and that occurs in approximately 10% of cases, is abnormal widening of the periodontal-membrane space (Stafne and Austin, 1944). This space is created by a thickening of the periodontal membrane as a result of an increase in the size and number of collagen fibers. The enlarged space is almost uniform in width,

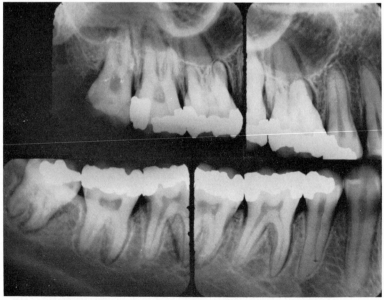

Figure 18–67 Acrosclerosis. Roentgenogram showing abnormal increase in width of periodontal-membrane space. The teeth on the opposite side were similarly involved. (Reproduced with permission from Stafne, E. C.: Dental Roentgenologic Aspects of Systemic Disease. J. Am. Dent. A. *40*:265–283 [Mar.] 1950.)

surrounds the entire root of the tooth, and makes the tooth appear as if it is being extruded rapidly from its socket. The increased size of the periodontal space, however, is created at the expense of the alveolar socket. There is roentgenographic evidence of resorption and destruction of the lamina dura, which are followed by sclerotic changes in the walls as evidenced by the wide, radiopaque line that eventually outlines the limits of the enlarged socket (Fig. 18–67). The change that takes place seems to have a predilection for the posterior teeth. Cases in which associated periodontal changes have been present have been reported by Krogh (1950), Mitchell and Chaudhry (1957), and Traiger (1961).

The localized variety of linear scleroderma that involves the face, forehead, and tongue may be associated with atrophy of the alveolar process and dental abnormalities in the direct line of involvement. Looby and Burket (1942) reported a case in which the maxillary alveolar process was depressed and the left central incisor failed to erupt on the involved side.

A girl 15 years of age who had linear scleroderma of the right side of the face also had atrophy of the gingivae that was confined to the right maxillary and mandibular lateral incisors, leaving the roots of these teeth partially denuded. A roentgenogram (Fig. 18–68) revealed a wide radiolucent space surrounding the roots, suggesting involvement of the periodontal membrane and also resorption of the crest of the alveolar bone supporting these teeth.

INFANTILE CORTICAL HYPEROSTOSIS (CAFFEY-SMITH SYNDROME)

Infantile cortical hyperostosis is a clinical entity of obscure cause that was first described by Caffey and Silverman (1945). It is characterized by sudden onset, tender soft-tissue swellings of the face, thorax, or extremities, and roentgenologic evidence of periosteal bone formation underlying the soft-tissue swellings. It also is often associated with fever. Its onset is most often at from 1 to 4 months of age, although there is evidence that it may occur prior to birth. Bennett and Nelson (1953) demonstrated roentgenographically that the condition was present in a stillborn fetus. Hyperostosis usually is no longer visible in the roentgenogram 12 months after onset. However, Caffey (1952) observed a chronic type of infantile cortical hyperostosis, with late crippling residuals in the skeleton, in which the thickened cortical walls were converted into thin walls, resulting in a dilated medullary cavity. Burbank and co-workers (1958) found varied degrees of residual deformity of the mandible in 8 of 11 patients. According to Van Buskirk and co-workers (1961), the condition has a familial tendency; they reported that it occurred in 11 members of a family in two generations.

Characteristically, the mandible is invariably involved. Therefore, roentgenographic examination of the mandible is most important in arriving at a correct diagnosis. The roentgenographic appearance is one of enlargement, increased radiopacity, and evidence of new bone formation on the surface. The apposition of new bone on the surface may occur in layers, and this is best visualized in the lateral views, as shown in Figure 18–69, *above.* This roentgenogram was made for a boy 5 months of age who had bilateral involvement of the mandible and involvement of the right humerus. The mandible was enlarged, and the laminated character of the hyperostosis can be seen at the inferior border. The anteroposterior

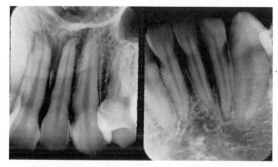

Figure 18–68 Linear scleroderma. Roentgenogram of the right maxillary and mandibular incisors, showing resorption of the alveolar crest and a wide radiolucent space surrounding the roots of these teeth.

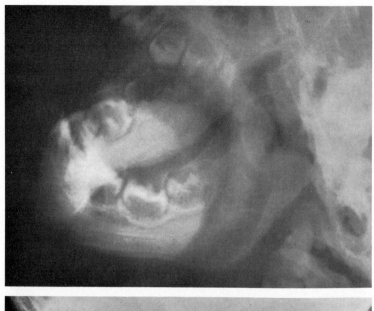

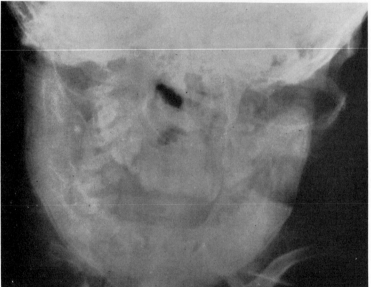

Figure 18–69   Infantile cortical hyperostosis. *Above,* Lateral view of the mandible of a patient 5 months of age, showing enlargement and laminated character of new bone formation. *Below,* Anteroposterior view, illustrating abnormal enlargement of entire mandible.

view (Fig. 18–69, *below*) demonstrates the marked uniform enlargement of the entire mandible, although the laminated character of the bone is not as clearly visualized.

Conditions with which infantile cortical hyperostosis might be confused are cellulitis, osteomyelitis, and acute parotitis.

GARDNER'S SYNDROME

The salient features of a familial condition known as Gardner's syndrome (see also p. 194) are multiple polyposis of the colon, multiple epidermoid cysts, the presence of desmoid tumors, and the presence of osteomas (Gardner and Richards, 1953; Weiner and Cooper, 1955). Not all of the last three features are necessarily evident, but there is a significant association of one or more of them with multiple polyposis of the colon.

The most common site for occurrence of osteomas is the mandible, where they take the form of irregular masses attached to the surface of the rami, angles, or body. They may be attached by a broad base or they may be pedunculated. The central portion of the jaws may exhibit multiple areas of increased opacity. In the skull the osteomas form on the surface of the external table, and they also may project into the sinuses. In the long bones they develop on the surface of the cortex, or as irregular thickenings of the cortex.

A woman 29 years of age whose roentgenograms are shown in Figures 18–70 and 18–71 was one of three members of a family with features of Gardner's syndrome. The other two members were the patient's mother and a brother. Also, a younger brother and a 3-year-old daughter had osteomas of the mandible. The genetic aspects of this family have been reported by Smith (1958). A roentgenologic survey of the skeleton of the patient revealed osteomas of the jaws, the calvaria, and the cortex of long bones. The dental roentgenogram disclosed multiple areas of hypercalcification or enostosis in the central portion of both the maxilla and the mandible. Figure 18–70 shows a large osteoma attached to the angle of the left side of the mandible and multiple areas of hypercalcification within the jaw. Figure 18–71 reveals an additional osteoma attached to the lateral aspect of the right ramus and an osteoma in the left frontal sinus.

Apparently the osteomas of the jaws most frequently appear early in life, and often are detected because of some deformity of the jaws or face. These patients are then frequently seen by the dentist or physician long before any symptomatic difficulty with the colon is apparent. In view of the association of osteomas of the jaws with multiple polyposis of the colon, it seems reasonable to suggest that these patients undergo an examination of the large bowel.

MULTIPLE BASAL-CELL NEVI, JAW CYSTS, AND SKELETAL DEFECTS

A clinical syndrome characterized by cysts of the jaws, multiple basal-cell tumors of the skin, and a high incidence of skeletal anomalies has been well established by Gorlin and Goltz (1960). At least two of the manifestations, namely, basal-cell tumors and cysts of the jaws, must be present to establish a diagnosis. The defects of the skeleton and other deformities of ectodermal and mesodermal origin may not be obvious in all patients.

The skin lesions associated with the syndrome usually manifest themselves early in life, often in childhood, and have been diagnosed as basal-cell nevus and epithelioma adenoides cysticum. These tumors are multiple and frequently appear as hundreds of individual lesions, particularly over the trunk and face.

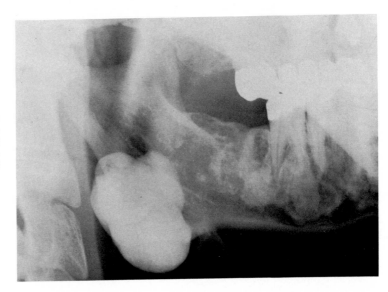

Figure 18–70 Gardner's syndrome. Lateral view of the mandible, showing an osteoma attached at the angle and areas of hypercalcification in the central portion of the body of the mandible.

The cysts of the jaws may be unilocular or multilocular, and most often the occurrence is multiple. In almost all of them the cyst lining is keratinized (keratocysts), a type of cyst in which there is a very high incidence of recurrence after removal (Browne, 1970). They may be of the dentigerous type, in which the crown of a tooth is situated within the lumen of the cyst, or of the primordial type, in which calcified dental structures are not present. According to Gorlin and Pindborg (1964), there may be numerous cysts scattered throughout the jaws, varying from microscopic size to several centimeters in diameter. The cysts are confined to the jaws and have not been found in other bones of the skeleton.

The most common of the associated developmental skeletal anomalies are those that involve the ribs and vertebrae.

The syndrome has a definite familial or hereditary tendency, but no sex predilection. Anderson and Cook (1966) examined the medical record of a 38-year-old woman who suffered from the syndrome. They found that of 19 relatives studied, 9 had the syndrome and 8 of these had a total of 32 odontogenic cysts, two-thirds of which occurred in the mandible.

Embryologic and histogenetic consid-

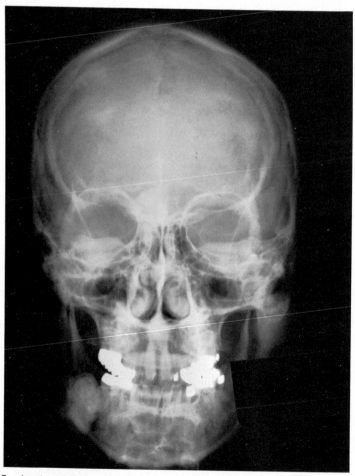

Figure 18–71 Gardner's syndrome. Posteroanterior view of the case represented in Figure 18–70, revealing an additional osteoma that is attached to the lateral surface of the ramus on the right side, and an osteoma in the left frontal sinus. (Reproduced with permission from Smith, W. G.: Multiple Polyposis, Gardner's Syndrome and Desmoid Tumors. Dis. Colon & Rectum. *1*:323–332[Sept.–Oct.] 1958.)

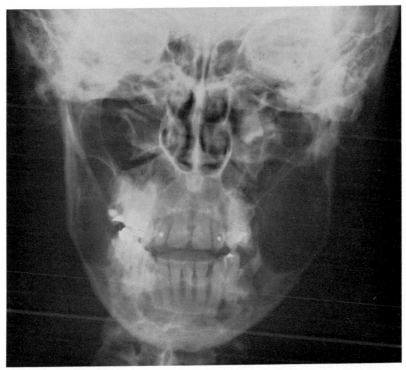

Figure 18–72 Multiple cysts of the jaws associated with basal-cell nevus syndrome. The roentgenogram reveals bilateral cysts of the mandible and one in the right maxilla. (Reproduced with permission from Maddox, W. D., Winkelmann, R. K., Harrison, E. G., Jr., Devine, K. D., and Gibilisco, J. A.: Multiple Nevoid Basal Cell Epitheliomas, Jaw Cysts and Skeletal Defects: A Clinical Syndrome. J.A.M.A. *188*:106–111 [Apr. 13] 1964.)

erations may explain the close relationship between basal-cell tumors of the skin and the cysts of the jaws. The formation of the cutaneous appendages (hair and glandular structures) and odontogenesis are closely related developmental processes. In both processes the epithelial cells possess the qualities of pluripotentiality. Maddox and colleagues (1964) therefore suggested that the formation of basal-cell tumors from pluripotential cells of the epithelial anlagen, and of odontogenic cysts from pluripotential cells of the dental lamina, may be related pathologic processes in patients predisposed to the syndrome. They reported 12 cases and in 1 of them encountered an ameloblastoma, which indicates that potentially aggressive lesions of odontogenic origin also may occur. A roentgenogram made for one of their patients (a 27-year-old woman) that exhibits multiple cysts of the jaws is shown in Figure 18–72. It revealed bilateral cysts of the mandible and another in the right maxilla. Six

months subsequent to removal of these cysts, other cysts appeared in the left maxilla.

Many of the patients first seek the services of the dentist because of symptoms referable to the cysts of the jaws. Therefore, he may have the first opportunity to bring the syndrome to light. The cysts may become quite expansive and destructive, and there is a marked tendency for recurrence, possibly from adjacent microcysts.

REFERENCES

Albright, F. and Strock, M. S.: The Association of Acalcification of Dentine and Hypoparathyroidism in Rats and the Cure of Same with Parathormone, with Some Correlated Observations in Man. (Abstr.) J. Clin. Invest. *12*:974 (Sept.) 1933.

Album, M. M. and Hope, J. W.: Progeria: Report of a Case. Oral Surg., Oral Med. & Oral Path. *11*:985–998 (Sept.) 1958.

Anderson, D. E. and Cook, W. A.: Jaw Cysts and the Basal Cell Nevus Syndrome. J. Oral Surg. *24*:15–26 (Jan.) 1966.

Baer, P. N., Brown, N. C., and Hamner, J. E., III: Hypophosphatasia: Report of Two Cases with Dental Findings. Periodontics. 2:209–215 (Sept.-Oct.) 1964.

Baysal, M. C.: Premature Loss of Deciduous Teeth in Identical Twins with Congenital Hypophosphatasia. Dent. Digest. 71:536–539 (Dec.) 1965.

Becks, H.: Histologic Study of Tooth Structure in Osteogenesis Imperfecta. Dent. Cosmos. 73:437–454 (May) 1931.

Bennett, H. S. and Nelson, T. R.: Prenatal Cortical Hyperostosis. Brit. J. Radiol. 26:47–49 (Jan.) 1953.

Bergman, G., Borggren, M. B., and Engfeldt, B.: Studies on Mineralized Dental Tissues. VII. Dental Changes Occurring in Osteopetrosis: Continued Studies. Acta odont. scandinav. 14:81–101 (Sept.) 1956.

Beumer, J., III, Trowbridge, H. O., Silverman, S., Jr., and Eisenberg, E.: Childhood Hypophosphatasia and the Premature Loss of Teeth: A Clinical and Laboratory Study of Seven Cases. Oral Surg., Oral Med. & Oral Path. 35:631–640 (May) 1973.

Blevins, C., Dahlin, D. C., Lovestedt, S. A., and Kennedy, R. L. J.: Oral and Dental Manifestations of Histiocytosis X. Oral Surg., Oral Med. & Oral Path. 12:473–483 (Apr.) 1959.

Bloom, H. J.: Osteopetrosis: Report of Case. J. Oral Surg. 1:340–346 (Oct.) 1943.

Boyle, P. E.: The Histopathology of the Human Tooth-Germ in Congenital Syphilis. (Abstr.) J. Dent. Res. 12:425–426 (June) 1932.

Bradlaw, R. V.: Dental Stigmata of Prenatal Syphilis (Herman L. Reiss Memorial Lecture). Oral Surg., Oral Med. & Oral Path. 6:147–158 (Jan.) 1953.

Bramley, P. and Dwyer, D.: Primary Hyperparathyroidism: Its Effect on a Mother and Her Children. Oral Surg., Oral Med. & Oral Path. 30:464–471 (Oct.) 1970.

Brauer, J. C. and Blackstone, C. H.: Dental Aspects of Congenital Syphilis. J. Am. Dent. A. 28:1633–1639 (Oct.) 1941.

Bronsky, D., Kushner, D. S., Dubin, A., and Snapper, I.: Idiopathic Hypoparathyroidism and Pseudohypoparathyroidism: Case Reports and Review of the Literature. Medicine (Baltimore). 37:317–352 (Dec.) 1958.

Browne, R. M.: The Odontogenic Keratocyst: Clinical Aspects. Brit. Dent. J. 128:225–231 (Mar.) 1970.

Bruckner, R. J., Rickles, N. H., and Porter, D. R.: Hypophosphatasia with Premature Shedding of Teeth and Aplasia of Cementum. Oral Surg., Oral Med. & Oral Path. 15:1351–1369 (Nov.) 1962.

Burbank, P. M., Lovestedt, S. A., and Kennedy, R. L. J.: The Dental Aspects of Infantile Cortical Hyperostosis. Oral Surg., Oral Med. & Oral Path. 11:1126–1137 (Oct.) 1958.

Burke, P. H.: True Hemihypertrophy of the Face. Brit. Dent. J. 91:213–215 (Oct. 16) 1951.

Burke, P. H.: Unilateral Facial Hypoplasia Affecting Tooth Size. Brit. Dent. J. 103:41–44 (July 16) 1957.

Burket, L. W.: Histopathologic Study in Congenital Syphilis. Internat. J. Orthodontia. 23:1016–1031 (Oct.) 1937.

Caffey, J.: On Some Late Skeletal Changes in Chronic Infantile Cortical Hyperostosis. Radiology. 59:651–657 (Nov.) 1952.

Caffey, J.: Pediatric X-ray Diagnosis. Vol. 1. Ed. 6. Chicago, Year Book Medical Publishers, 1972, p. 52.

Caffey, J. and Silverman, W. A.: Infantile Cortical Hyperostoses: Preliminary Report on New Syndrome. Am. J. Roentgenol. 54:1–16 (July) 1945.

Cahn, L. R.: Paget's Disease of Bone. Arch. Clin. Oral Path. 1:141–144, 1937.

Cahn, L. R.: Metabolic Diseases of the Jaw Bones. New York State Dent. J. 16:485–490 (Nov.) 1950.

Chaudhry, A. P., Hayes, P. A., and Gorlin, R. J.: Hyperparathyroidism Involving the Mandible: Report of a Case J. Oral Surg. 16:247–251 (May) 1958.

Clark, H. B., Jr. and Holte, N. O.: Paget's Disease Simulating Osteomyelitis of the Mandible: Case Report. Northwest Dentistry. 29:247–249 (Oct.) 1950.

Cohen, I. C.: Evaluation of Dentofacial Growth and Maturation of Children with Precocious Male Sexual Development. Unpublished study, May 8, 1959.

Cook, T. J.: Hereditary Ectodermal Dysplasia of Anhidrotic Type. Am. J. Orthodontics. 25:1008–1010 (Oct.) 1939.

Cooke, B. E. D.: Paget's Disease of the Jaws: Fifteen Cases. Ann. Roy. Coll. Surgeons England. 19:223–240 (Oct.) 1956.

Croft, L. K., Witkop, C. J., Jr., and Glas, J.-E.: Pseudohypoparathyroidism. Oral Surg., Oral Med. & Oral Path. 20:758–770 (Dec.) 1965.

Curtiss, P. H., Jr., Clark, W. S., and Herndon, C. H.: Vertebral Fractures Resulting From Prolonged Cortisone and Corticotropin Therapy. J.A.M.A. 156:467–469 (Oct. 2) 1954.

Dahlin, D. C.: Bone Tumors: General Aspects and an Analysis of 2276 Cases. Springfield, Illinois, Charles C Thomas, Publisher, 1957, 224 pp.

Dealy, J. B., Jr. and Sosman, M. C.: Irradiation Therapy in Hand-Schüller-Christian's Disease. Oral Surg., Oral Med. & Oral Path. 9:1295–1296 (Dec.) 1956.

Drash, A.: Diabetes Mellitus. In Vaughan, V. C., III and McKay, R. J.: Nelson Textbook of Pediatrics. Ed. 10. Philadelphia, W. B. Saunders Company, 1975, pp. 1259–1271.

Erdheim, J.: Zur Kenntnis der parathyreopriven Dentin-Veränderung. Frankfurt. Ztschr. Path. 7:238–248, 1911.

Follis, R. H., Jr.: Rickets and Osteomalacia. In Harrison, T. R.: Principles of Internal Medicine. Ed. 5. New York, McGraw-Hill Book Company, Inc., 1966, vol. 1, pp. 383–389.

Follis, R. H., Jr., Jackson, D., Eliot, M. M., and Park, E. A.: Prevalence of Rickets in Children Between 2 and 14 Years of Age. Am. J. Dis. Child. 66:1–11 (July) 1943.

Frantzis, T. G.: The Ultrastructure of Capillary Basement Membranes in the Attached Gingiva of Diabetic and Nondiabetic Patients with Periodontal Disease. Thesis, Mayo Graduate School of Medicine (University of Minnesota), Rochester, 1970.

Fraser, D. and Salter, R. B.: The Diagnosis and Management of the Various Types of Rickets. Pediat. Clin. North America. May, pp. 417–441, 1958.

Gardner, D. G. and Majka, M.: The Early Formation of Irregular Secondary Dentine in Progeria. Oral Surg., Oral Med. & Oral Path. 28:877–884 (Dec.) 1969.

Gardner, E. J. and Richards, R. C.: Multiple Cutaneous and Subcutaneous Lesions Occurring Simultaneously with Hereditary Polyposis and Osteomatosis. Am. J. Human Genet. 5:139–147 (June) 1953.

Garn, S. M., Lewis, A. B., and Blizzard, R. M.: Endocrine Factors in Dental Development. J. Dent. Res. *44* (Suppl. 1):243–258 (Jan.-Feb.) 1965.

Gigliotti, R., Harrison, H., Reveley, R. A., and Drabkowski, A. J.: Familial Vitamin D-Refractory Rickets. J. Am. Dent. A. *82*:383–387 (Feb.) 1971.

Gorlin, R. J. and Goldman, H. M.: Thoma's Oral Pathology. Ed. 6. St. Louis, The C. V. Mosby Company, 1970.

Gorlin, R. J. and Goltz, R. W.: Multiple Nevoid Basal-Cell Epithelioma, Jaw Cysts and Bifid Rib: A Syndrome. New England J. Med. *262*:908–912 (May) 1960.

Gorlin, R. J. and Pindborg, J. J.: Syndromes of the Head and Neck. New York, McGraw-Hill Book Company, Inc., 1964, p. 406.

Gorlin, R. J., Chaudhry, A. P., and Kelln, E. E.: Oral Manifestations of the Fitzgerald-Gardner, Pringle-Bourneville, Robin, Adrenogenital, and Hurler-Pfaundler Syndromes. Oral Surg., Oral Med. & Oral Path. *13*:1233–1244 (Oct.) 1960.

Greig, D. M.: Hypertelorism. Edinburgh M. J. *31*:560–593 (Oct.) 1924.

Greulich, W. W. and Pyle, S. I.: Radiographic Atlas of Skeletal Development of the Hand and Wrist. Ed. 2. Stanford, California, Stanford University Press, 1959, 256 pp.

Guilford, S. H.: A Dental Anomaly. Dent. Cosmos. *25*:113–118 (Mar.) 1883.

Harris, R. and Sullivan, H. R.: Dental Sequelae in Deciduous Dentition in Vitamin D Resistant Rickets: Case Report. Aust. Dent. J. *5*:200 (Aug.) 1960.

Harrison, H. E.: Rickets. In McQuarrie, I.: Brennemann's Practice of Pediatrics. Hagerstown, Maryland, W. F. Prior Company, Inc., 1961, vol. 1, chap. 36, pp. 1–63.

Hayles, A. B., Kennedy, R. L. J., Beahrs, O. H., and Woolner, L. B.: Exophthalmic Goiter in Children. J. Clin. Endocrinol. *19*:138–151 (Jan.) 1959.

Heaney, R. P.: Osteoporoses. In Beeson, P. B. and McDermott, W.: Cecil-Loeb Textbook of Medicine. Ed. 14. Philadelphia, W. B. Saunders Company, 1975, pp. 1826–1830.

Heys, F. M., Blattner, R. J., and Robinson, H. B. G.: Osteogenesis Imperfecta and Odontogenesis Imperfecta: Clinical and Genetic Aspects in Eighteen Families. J. Pediat. *56*:234–245 (Feb.) 1960.

Jowsey, J.: Quantitative Microradiography: A New Approach in the Evaluation of Metabolic Bone Disease (Editorial). Am. J. Med. *40*:485–491 (Apr.) 1966.

Jowsey, J.: Personal communication, 1974.

Keating, F. R., Jr.: Hyperparathyroidism. Am. J. Orthodontics (Oral Surg. Sect.). *33*:116–128 (Feb.) 1947.

Keller, E. E.: A Radiographic Analysis of Dental, Skeletal, and Facial Development in Patients with Various Endocrine and Metabolic Diseases. Thesis, Mayo Graduate School of Medicine (University of Minnesota), Rochester, 1968.

Keller, E. E., Sather, A. H., and Hayles, A. B.: Dental and Skeletal Development in Various Endocrine and Metabolic Diseases. J. Am. Dent. A. *81*:415–419 (Aug.) 1970.

Kennett, S. and Pollick, H.: Jaw Lesions in Familial Hyperparathyroidism. Oral Surg., Oral Med. & Oral Path. *31*:502–510 (Apr.) 1971.

Kjellman, M., Oldfelt, V., Nordenram, A., and Olow-Nordenram, M.: Five Cases of Hypophosphatasia with Dental Findings. Internat. J. Oral Surg. *2*:152–158, 1973.

Korkhaus, G.: Changes in Form of Jaws and in Position of Teeth Produced by Acromegaly. Internat. J. Orthodontia. *19*:160–174 (Feb.) 1933.

Krogh, H. W.: Dental Manifestation of Scleroderma: Report of Case. J. Oral Surg. *8*:242–244 (July) 1950.

Kruger, G. O., Jr., Prickman, L. E., and Pugh, D. G.: So-called Eosinophilic Granuloma of Ribs and Jaws Associated with Visceral (Pulmonary) Involvement Characteristic of Xanthomatosis. Oral Surg., Oral Med. & Oral Path. *2*:770–779 (June) 1949.

Levine, R. and Weisberg, H. F.: Cushing's Syndrome. In Soskin, S.: Progress in Clinical Endocrinology. New York, Grune & Stratton, 1950, pp. 160–167.

Lichtenstein, L.: Histiocytosis X. Integration of Eosinophilic Granuloma of Bone, "Letterer-Siwe Disease," and "Schüller-Christian Disease" as Related Manifestations of a Single Nosologic Entity. A.M.A. Arch. Path. *56*:84–102 (July) 1953.

Linsey, E. V.: Osteopetrosis with Suppuration and Eventual Resection of Mandible: Report of Case. J. Oral Surg. *2*:369–374 (Oct.) 1944.

Looby, J. P. and Burket, L. W.: Scleroderma of Face with Involvement of Alveolar Process. Am. J. Orthodontics (Oral Surg. Sect.). *28*:493–498 (Sept.) 1942.

Lovestedt, S. A.: Examples of Dental Dysplasia. Am. J. Orthodontics (Oral Surg. Sect.). *33*:625–629 (Aug.) 1947.

Maddox, W. D., Winkelmann, R. K., Harrison, E. G., Jr., Devine, K. D., and Gibilisco, J. A.: Multiple Nevoid Basal Cell Epitheliomas, Jaw Cysts and Skeletal Defects: A Clinical Syndrome. J.A.M.A. *188*:106–111 (Apr. 13) 1964.

McCune, D. J. and Bradley, C.: Osteopetrosis (Marble Bones) in an Infant: Review of Literature and Report of a Case. Am. J. Dis. Child. *48*:949–1000 (Nov.) 1934.

Mitchell, D. F. and Chaudhry, A. P.: Roentgenographic Manifestations of Scleroderma: Report of a Case. Oral Surg., Oral Med. & Oral Path. *10*:307–309 (Mar.) 1957.

Mittelman, J. S.: Osteogenesis Imperfecta (Odontogenesis Imperfecta): Report of a Case. Oral Surg., Oral Med. & Oral Path. *3*:1562–1564 (Dec.) 1950.

Moorrees, C. F. A., Fanning, E. A., and Hunt, E. E., Jr.: Age Variation of Formation Stages for Ten Permanent Teeth. J. Dent. Res. *42*:1490–1502 (Dec.) 1963.

Mortimer, H., Levene, G., and Rowe, A. W.: Cranial Dysplasias of Pituitary Origin. Radiology. *29*:135–157 (Aug.); 279–295 (Sept.) 1937.

Muracciole, J. C.: Influence of Gonads on Tooth Development. Rev. Asoc. Odont. Argent. *44*:111–117 (Mar.) 1956.

Nazif, M. and Osman, M.: Oral Manifestations of Cystinosis. Oral Surg., Oral Med. & Oral Path. *35*:330–338 (Mar.) 1973.

O'Leary, P. A. and Waisman, M.: Acrosclerosis. Arch. Dermat. u. Syph. *47*:382–397 (Mar.) 1943.

Pagenstecher, E.: Einseitige angeborne Gesichtshypertrophie. Deutsche Ztschr. f. Chir. *82*:519–529, 1906.

Peacock, M. and Nordin, B. E. C.: Plasma Calcium Homeostasis. Ciba Found. Symp. *11*:409–428, 1973.

Piatt, A. D., Erhard, G. A., and Araj, J. S.: Benign Osteopetrosis: Report of 9 Cases. Am. J. Roentgenol. *76*:1119–1131 (Dec.) 1956.

Pindborg, J. J.: Dental Aspects of Osteogenesis Imperfecta. Acta path. et microbiol. scandinav. 24:47–58, 1947.

Pugh, D. G.: Roentgenologic Diagnosis of Diseases of Bone. New York, Thomas Nelson & Sons, 1951, pp. 41–43.

Pugh, D. G.: The Roentgenological Diagnosis of Hyperparathyroidism. Surg. Clin. North America. Aug., pp. 1017–1030, 1952.

Ritchie, G. M.: Dental Manifestations of Pseudohypoparathyroidism. Arch. Dis. Child. 40:565–572 (Oct.) 1965.

Rosenberg, E. H. and Guralnick, W. C.: Hyperparathyroidism: A Review of 220 Proved Cases, with Special Emphasis on Findings in the Jaws. Oral Surg., Oral Med. & Oral Path. 15 (Suppl. 2): 84–94, 1962.

Rushton, M. A.: The Dental Tissues in Osteitis Deformans. Guy's Hosp. Rep. 88:163–171 (Apr.) 1938.

Rushton, M. A.: Early Case of Facial Hemiatrophy. Oral Surg., Oral Med. & Oral Path. 4:1457–1460 (Nov.) 1951.

Rushton, M. A.: A New Form of Dentinal Dysplasia: Shell Teeth. Oral Surg., Oral Med. & Oral Path. 7:543–549 (May) 1954.

Rushton, M. A.: An Anomaly of Cementum in Cleidocranial Dysostosis, Brit. Dent. J. 100:81–83 (Feb. 7) 1956.

Sarnat, B. G. and Shaw, N. G.: Dental Development in Congenital Syphilis. Am. J. Orthodontics (Oral Surg. Sect.). 29:270–284 (May) 1943.

Sarnat, B. G., Brodie, A. G., and Kubacki, W. H.: Fourteen-year Report of Facial Growth in Case of Complete Anodontia with Ectodermal Dysplasia. J. Dis. Child. 86:162–169 (Aug.) 1953.

Schour, I. and Massler, M.: The Development of the Human Dentition. J. Am. Dent. A. 28:1153–1160 (July) 1941.

Schour, I. and Massler, M.: Endocrines and Dentistry. J. Am. Dent. A. 30:595–603 (Apr. 1); 763–773 (May 1); 943–950 (June 1) 1943.

Seckel, H. P. G.: Six Examples of Precocious Sexual Development. II. Studies in Growth and Maturation. Am. J. Dis. Child. 79:278–309 (Feb.) 1950.

Seipel, C. M., Van Wagenen, G., and Anderson, B. G.: Developmental Disturbances and Malocclusion of the Teeth Produced by Androgen Treatment in the Monkey (Macaca mulata). Am. J. Orthodontics. 40:37–43 (Jan.) 1954.

Seldin, N. A.: Paget's Disease – A Clinical Case. Dent. Cosmos. 75:691–692 (July) 1933.

Shira, R. B.: Manifestations of Systemic Disorders in Facial Bones. J. Oral Surg. 11:286–307 (Oct.) 1953.

Sklar, E.: The Effects of Endocrine Dysfunction on Dental Development and Maturation. Thesis, Mayo Graduate School of Medicine (University of Minnesota), Rochester, 1966.

Sleeper, E. L.: Eosinophilic Granuloma of Bone: Its Relationship to Hand-Schüller-Christian and Letterer-Siwe's Diseases, with Emphasis upon Oral Symptoms and Findings. Oral Surg., Oral Med. & Oral Path. 4:896–918 (July) 1951.

Slocumb, C. H., Polley, H. F., Ward, L. E., and Hench, P. S.: Diagnosis, Treatment and Prevention of Chronic Hypercortisonism in Patients with Rheumatoid Arthritis. Ann. Int. Med. 46:86–101 (Jan.) 1957.

Smith, W. G.: Multiple Polyposis, Gardner's Syndrome and Desmoid Tumors. Dis. Colon & Rectum. 1:323–332 (Sept.-Oct.) 1958.

Soffer, L. J.: Diseases of the Endocrine Glands. Ed. 2. Philadelphia, Lea & Febiger, 1956, pp. 365–368.

Spiegel, R. N., Sather, A. H., and Hayles, A. B.: Cephalometric Study of Children with Various Endocrine Diseases. Am. J. Orthodontics. 59:362–375 (Apr.) 1971.

Stafne, E. C.: Paget's Disease Involving Maxilla and Mandible: Report of Case. J. Oral Surg. 4:114–115 (Apr.) 1946.

Stafne, E. C.: Dental Roentgenologic Manifestations of Systemic Disease. II. Developmental Disturbances. Radiology. 58:507–516 (Apr.) 1952.

Stafne, E. C. and Austin, L. T.: A Study of Dental Roentgenograms in Cases of Paget's Disease (Osteitis Deformans), Osteitis Fibrosa Cystica and Osteoma. J. Am. Dent. A. 25:1202–1214 (Aug.) 1938.

Stafne, E. C. and Austin, L. T.: Characteristic Dental Finding in Acrosclerosis and Diffuse Scleroderma. Am. J. Orthodontics (Oral Surg. Sect.). 30:25–29 (Jan.) 1944.

Stafne, E. C. and Lovestedt, S. A.: Osteoporosis of the Jaws Associated with Hypercortisonism. Oral Surg., Oral Med. & Oral Path. 13:1445–1446 (Dec.) 1960.

Stafne, E. C. and Lovestedt, S. A.: Congenital Hemihypertrophy of the Face (Facial Giantism). Oral Surg., Oral Med. & Oral Path. 15:184–189 (Feb.) 1962.

Stool, N. and Sullivan, C. R.: Osteogenesis Imperfecta in a 95-Year-Old Woman. Proc. Staff Meet., Mayo Clin. 34:523–529 (Oct. 28) 1959.

Talbot, N. B., Butler, A. M., Pratt, E. L., MachLachlan, E. A., and Tannheimer, J.: Progeria: Clinical, Metabolic and Pathologic Studies on a Patient. Am. J. Dis. Child. 69:267–279 (May) 1945.

Thoma, K. H. and Allen, F. W.: Anodontia in Ectodermal Dysplasia. Am. J. Orthodontics. 26:503–507 (May) 1940.

Tillman, H. H.: Paget's Disease of Bone: A Clinical, Radiographic, and Histopathologic Study of Twenty-four Cases Involving the Jaws. Oral Surg., Oral Med. & Oral Path. 15:1225–1234 (Oct.) 1962.

Tracy, W. E. and Campbell, R. A.: Dentofacial Development in Children with Vitamin D-Resistant Rickets. J. Am. Dent. A. 76:1026–1031 (May) 1968.

Tracy, W. E., Steen, J. C., Steiner, J. E., and Buist, M. B.: Analysis of Dentine Pathogenesis in Vitamin D-Resistant Rickets. J. Oral Surg. 32:38–44 (July) 1971.

Traiger, J.: Scleroderma: Its Oral Manifestations. Oral Surg., Oral Med. & Oral Path. 14:117–121 (Jan.) 1961.

United States National Center for Health Statistics: Selected Examination Findings Related to Periodontal Disease Among Adults: United States, 1960–1962. Ser. 11. No. 33. Washington D. C., Government Printing Office, 1969, p. 31.

Van Buskirk, F. W., Tampas, J. P., and Peterson, O. S., Jr.: Infantile Cortical Hyperostosis: An Inquiry into Its Familial Aspects. Am. J. Roentgenol. 85:613–632 (Apr.) 1961.

Vaughan, V. C. III and McKay, R. J.: Nelson Textbook of Pediatrics. Ed. 10. Philadelphia, W. B. Saunders Company, 1975, pp. 1323–1324.

Wagner, R., Cohen, M. M., and Hunt, E. E., Jr.: Dental Development in Idiopathic Sexual Precocity, Congenital Adrenocortical Hyperplasia, and Adrenogenic Virilism. J. Pediat. 63:566–576 (Oct.) 1963.

Walsh, R. F. and Karmiol, M.: Oral Roentgenographic Findings in Osteitis Fibrosa Generalisata Associated with Chronic Renal Disease. Oral Surg., Oral Med. & Oral Path. 28:273–281 (Aug.) 1969.

Ward, J. and Lerner, H. H.: A Review of the Subject of Congenital Hemihypertrophy and a Complete Case Report, J. Pediat. 31:403–414 (Oct.) 1947.

Washington, J. A.: Hypertelorism. In McQuarrie, I.: Brennemann's Practice of Pediatrics. Hagerstown, Maryland, W. F. Prior Company, Inc., 1957, vol. 4, chap. 31, pp. 1–3.

Weiner, R. S. and Cooper, P.: Multiple Polyposis of the Colon, Osteomatosis and Soft-Tissue Tumors: Report of a Familial Syndrome. New England J. Med. 253:795–799 (Nov. 10) 1955.

Weinmann, J. P. and Sicher, H.: Bone and Bones: Fundamentals of Bone Biology. St. Louis, The C. V. Mosby Company, 1947, pp. 188–206.

Wilkins, L.: The Diagnosis and Treatment of Endocrine Disorders in Childhood and Adolescence. Ed. 3. Springfield, Illinois, Charles C Thomas, Publisher, 1965, p. 23.

Winters, R. W., Graham, J. B., Williams, T. F., McFalls, V. W., and Burnett, C. H.: A Genetic Study of Familial Hypophosphatemia and Vitamin D Resistant Rickets with a Review of the Literature. Medicine. 37:97–142 (May) 1958.

19

THE TEMPOROMANDIBULAR JOINT

JOSEPH A. GIBILISCO, D.D.S.

Preauricular or temporomandibular joint pain, clicking, swelling, popping, bony crepitation, chronic subluxation, trauma to the jaws or facial bones, facial asymmetry, possible arthritis or connective tissue disease, and trismus or limited motion are among the more common indications for roentgenographic examination of the temporomandibular joints. Because many roentgenographic techniques are complex and require sophisticated, expensive machines, the practitioner is reluctant to add roentgenographic examination of the

temporomandibular joints to his diagnostic process. However, many dentists are now practicing in medical-dental facilities, medical groups, or hospitals where the services of the Department of Diagnostic Radiology and the skill of the radiologist are available. This has enabled many dentists to further their interest in bone and joint pathology.

Recent technical advances in equipment have resulted in improved visualization of calcified structures. Similarly, improvements in technique have decreased

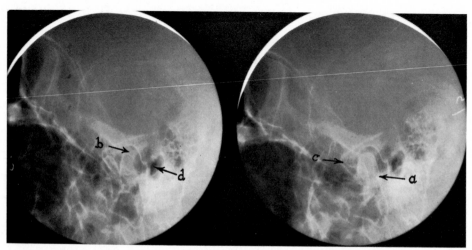

Figure 19-1 Standard lateral views of a normal left temporomandibular joint. Note regularity of articulating surfaces and free, adequate motion. *Left,* Mouth open. *Right,* Mouth closed. *a,* Condyle. *b,* Glenoid fossa. *c,* Articular tubercle. *d,* External auditory meatus.

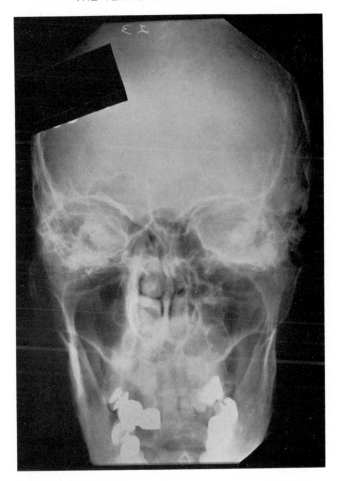

Figure 19–2 Anteroposterior view of the skull used in conjunction with lateral views of the temporomandibular joints to determine bilateral symmetry and to permit better examination of the pterygoid fossa and the medial aspects of the preauricular region. This view is also important in the examination of an injured patient or one with a calcification of neoplasm.

superimposition so that it now is possible to observe the bony parts clearly and accurately, thus increasing the possibility of identifying previously undetected pathologic changes.

For most patients who suffer a fracture of the joint or mandible, lateral oblique views usually suffice; however, there is a strong possibility of overlooking other bony fractures. The minimal number of films for an adequate survey of the mandible and jaws must include the oblique lateral transcranial projection as well as the anteroposterior view of the skull (Shore, 1960) (Figs. 19–1 and 19–2). One lateral view of the joint should be taken with the patient's teeth in occlusion and one should be taken with his mouth open as wide as possible. A calibrated Tolman block (Tolman and Eppard, 1968) is placed between the teeth to ensure that the patient has not closed or

decreased the degree of opening. (See Appendix, Part I.) The view taken with the teeth in contact demonstrates the relationship of the condyle in the glenoid fossa, the degree of joint space, and whether or not there are any morphologic variations between right and left condyles. Usually the condyle is found centered within the glenoid fossa. It is also advisable to compare the joint space of the right and left condyles in this roentgenogram. The view taken with the patient's mouth open wide shows the degree of motion of the condyle, its relationship to the articular eminence, and whether or not there are bony degenerative changes on the condyle or the articular eminence.

There are so many limitations to the lateral projections that the anteroposterior view is essential. This more comprehensive projection of the head is usually taken

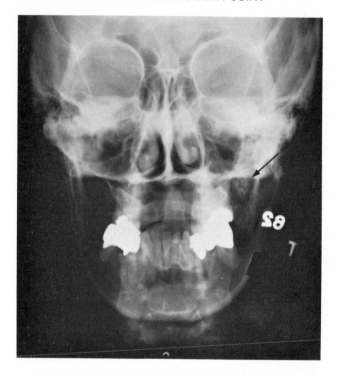

Figure 19–3 Partially calcified mass in the region of the left pterygoid fossa. This mass is situated posteriorly in the nasopharynx just bordering the pterygoid fossa on the left.

with the patient's mouth in occlusion. It demonstrates best the position of the condyle in the medial lateral view. This roentgenogram also permits additional study of symmetry, aids in the possible detection of a neoplasm or other lesion, and more accurately defines the outline of a condylar fracture. The value of such an anteroposterior view can be vividly illustrated by observing the presence of a large mass situated in the left pterygopalatine fossa (Fig. 19–3). This patient had a long-standing history of pain in the left temporomandibular joint and previously had had several lateral-view roentgenograms made. The tumor was not seen until the anteroposterior view was utilized. The specimen removed from the patient and a portion of the condyle are seen in Figure 19–4.

Despite the apparent thoroughness of the combined lateral and anteroposterior views, these still do not represent complete roentgenography of the temporomandibular joints. Lateral and anteroposterior views are considered routine films, or what radiologists may refer to as "scout" films. They are often sufficient, but on occasion merely indicate that further specialized views are required.

Many patients, probably the majority, complaining of distress in the temporomandibular joint do not demonstrate any destructive bony changes roentgenographically. The pain the patient is experiencing is often associated with factors that are producing discomfort in the muscles of

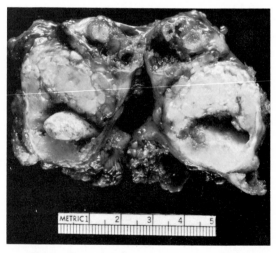

Figure 19–4 Gross specimen removed from the region of the pterygoid fossa. Pathologic report is of a chondrosarcoma with zones of calcification arising from the neck of the mandible.

mastication. These cases are often uncomplicated. Nonetheless, roentgenographic examination is indicated. There are other patients who do demonstrate varying degrees of bony destruction or alteration, and the roentgenographic findings are often diagnostic for a particular disease entity.

The roentgenograms and clinical records of 630 Mayo Clinic patients with abnormal temporomandibular joint roentgenograms seen over a period of 9 years were reviewed (Clark et al., 1972), and the study was summarized as follows:

... Abnormal temporomandibular joint roentgenograms were three times more frequent in women than in men. The highest incidence of temporomandibular joint abnormalities in both men and women was between the ages of 40 and 70 years. The complaint of pain did not necessarily correlate with roentgenographic evidence of bone changes. The condylar articular surface was the first bony surface of the temporomandibular joint to show roentgenographic evidence of destructive disease. Of the 222 patients who had bony crepitus, 164 had roentgenographic evidence of bone change. A decreased range of condylar motion was the most frequently reported abnormality in patients whose temporomandibular joint roentgenograms showed no evidence of bone alteration. ...

While there are a number of systemic complications that may produce degenerative disease of the temporomandibular joints, one disease, rheumatoid arthritis, is seen with such frequency that it serves to demonstrate many of the pathologic alterations that can occur in this joint. Usually, the patient with generalized rheumatoid arthritis who manifests inflammatory changes in the temporomandibular joints complains of pain and limitation of motion in either one or both of these joints. According to Russell and Bayles (1941), rheumatoid arthritis involves the temporomandibular joint in about 50% of patients and quite commonly limits opening of the mouth. Hatch (1967) reported a study of 100 cases in Mayo Clinic patients with a diagnosis of rheumatoid arthritis. He found that 58 of these patients had temporomandibular joint symptoms. The patients frequently described dull, deep-seated, localized pain over the involved joint as well as limitation

of motion. Severe limitation and pain were most noticeable to the patient on awakening in the morning. No swelling was palpable in any of the 58 patients. Slight to moderate stiffness was noted in 23, tenderness of the external pterygoid muscle in 35, and crepitus palpable as a grating or grinding sensation in 18 patients who also had minimal or no temporomandibular joint dysfunction. Roentgenograms of the temporomandibular joints were studied in 40 of the 58 patients. Of the 40 patients, 22 showed definite roentgenographic evidence of severe to moderate irregularity of the condylar surfaces and 18 showed no roentgenographic abnormality.

A clear, unobstructed view of the condyle is necessary in patients with rheumatoid arthritis or in those whose history suggests destructive changes of the condyle (Updegrave, 1957). Often the lack of clarity is due to superimposition of the intervening structures; therefore, tomography is of special value. This technique results in a roentgenogram that demonstrates a plane section of a part of any given point with the surrounding shadows blurred. This method of projecting plane sections of solid objects is a most useful aid in precise localization of pathologic changes on the surface of the condyle or the articular eminence. Tomography permits examination of the joint at various levels of penetration and with more accuracy. It is defined as a roentgenographic technique for viewing a selected plane with the elimination of outlines of the structures situated in planes above or below it. Modifications in tomography are numerous. It is similar to or often synonymous with planigraphy or planography, laminography, sectional roentgenography, and stratigraphy. A tomogram of a patient demonstrating destructive changes in the left condyle but a normal right condyle is shown in Figure 19–5.

Destructive bony changes, limited condylar motion, and loss of temporomandibular joint space are the three most useful characteristics in roentgenographic diagnosis of disease of this joint. The patient with rheumatoid arthritis involving the temporomandibular joint frequently dem-

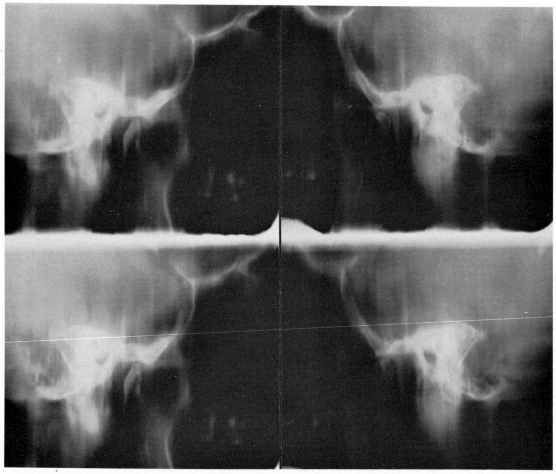

Figure 19–5 Tomograms of the temporomandibular joints. The articular surface of the condyle of the mandible on the left is irregular and deformed. This is a degenerative change. The condyle on the right is normal.

onstrates all three of these features (Fig. 19–6).

The clinical significance of loss of joint space is not completely understood. It is occasionally related to malocclusion of long duration, which may produce a flattening or a wearing of the articular disk. Loss of joint space is commonly associated with systemic arthritis. Interpretation of limited motion or of changes in joint space or position of the condyle within the glenoid fossa is highly empirical.

Limitation of motion may have a number of sources. It may be due to a disease process such as rheumatoid arthritis in which jaw excursions become painful, to dislocation of the jaw, to a lengthy and difficult dental procedure, to jaw surgery, or to injury sustained during an athletic contest. There are reported cases in which limitation of motion has been found to have a psychogenic origin (Fig. 19–7). Ankylosis, which produces complete limitation of motion of the temporomandibular joint, is not common. However, when ankylosis occurs, it is usually not difficult to determine its cause.

Bony crepitus of the temporomandibular joint is a frequent complaint. Yet roentgenograms seldom reveal any bone changes. Many patients with crepitation deny having any discomfort from it and are generally not disturbed by the "noise." There are some patients, however, who express considerable fear that the "cracking noise" they hear and feel represents a

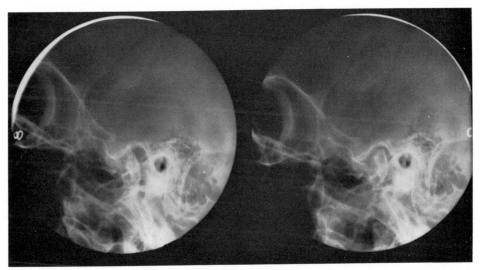

Figure 19–6   Temporomandibular joint demonstrating loss of joint space, limitation of motion, and destructive condylar changes.

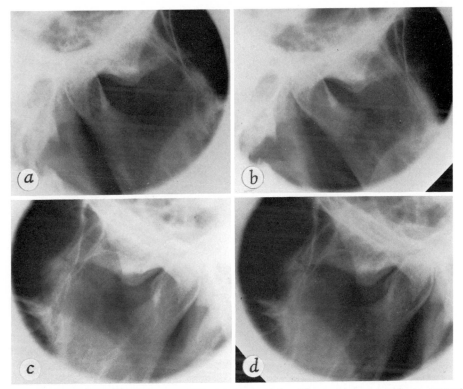

Figure 19–7   Limited motion of the temporomandibular joint. The patient was able to separate incisal edges less than 1 cm. There was no history of other joint disease, nor was there any clinical evidence of a dental origin. Note absence of pathologic changes in the temporomandibular joints. A psychogenic basis was established. The patient's general health was good. *a* and *b*, Right temporomandibular joint. *a*, Mouth open. *b*, Mouth closed. *c* and *d*, Left temporomandibular joint. *c*, Mouth open. *d*, Mouth closed.

sinister disease. In any event, the "noisy temporomandibular joint" should be examined roentgenographically.

"Clicking" is another source of disturbance to many patients. If clicking is the only presenting complaint and if the clinical history fails to reveal any other significant contribution, then roentgenograms are of little value; but again, they are essential to the complete diagnosis. A roentgenogram of a patient complaining of clicking of the joint is illustrated in Figure 19–8. This event probably occurs when the condyle passes over the anterior edge of the articular disk. One could speculate that, in the younger patient with such symptoms, condylar hypoplasia may later develop, but there is no evidence to substantiate this. Clicking usually occurs at the end of opening of the mouth to its normal extent and again during the closing cycle.

Difficulties encountered in roentgenographic technique make it extremely hazardous to attempt to correlate the clinical and roentgenographic findings of either popping or clicking joints. Malocclusion is considered a frequent offender, and correction of this discrepancy often eliminates the problem. Painful clicking may be noted in severe cases of recurrent or chronic subluxation. These patients find it difficult to return the condyle to the glenoid fossa after excessive opening of the mouth. If a dislocation occurs, the condyle passes beyond the articular tubercle, often becomes impacted in the infratemporal fossa in front of the tubercle, and cannot reenter the glenoid cavity until the dislocation has been reduced. If the dislocation is unilateral, the jaw deviates to the unaffected side (Copland, 1960).

Treatment should be considered for those patients who present with both pain and clicking. We have found that these symptoms can be relieved by correction of a pre-existing malocclusion. In most cases, an increase in the vertical dimension ("opening the bite") is required. Until recently, roentgenography was of little assistance in the development of the treatment plan. Cineradiography is most helpful when available. The moment and location of the clicking can be observed in the cine film. Video taping of the jaw excursions allows a frame-by-frame analysis of the film. The degree of occlusal correction is established, and its potential effectiveness can be demonstrated by further cineradiographic technique.

The most frequent eccentric mandibular movement found in joint dysfunction is deviation of the mandible on opening. This occurs when condylar movements are unequal. The jaw then deviates to the side on which movement is more limited. Deviation also occurs when there is unilateral condylar hyperplasia or when there is a tumor in the region of the temporomandibular joint fossa. Roentgenographic examination of these patients is most informative.

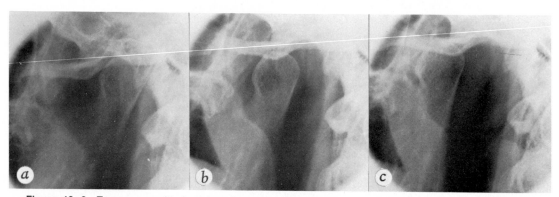

Figure 19–8 Temporomandibular joint of a patient with clicking. Roentgenograms were taken *(a)* with the mouth closed, *(b)* at the initial point of clicking on opening, and *(c)* at the end of the opening cycle. Note normal anatomic findings. Clicking occurs just at the point where the condyle of the mandible moves against the articular tubercle of the temporal bone.

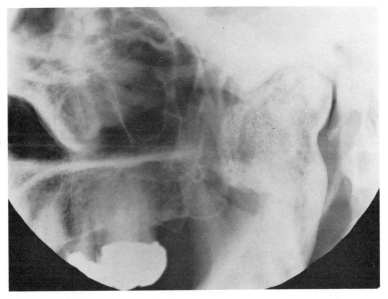

Figure 19–9 Osteoma of the condyle.

The roentgenogram seen in Figure 19–9 shows an osteoma of the right condyle in a woman 40 years of age who had first noticed swelling in the right side of her face 16 years previously. She had had gradual deviation in occlusion. A year preceding examination, trismus and pain had developed on the affected side. The roentgenogram shows a greatly enlarged condyle with evidence of trabecular bone in its center. At its outer border there is a wall of dense, laminated bone. Increased density and slight enlargement of the mandible on the same side suggested an osteoma, which

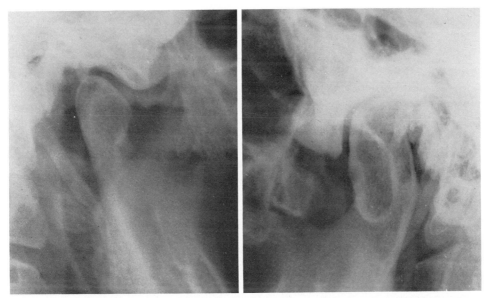

Figure 19–10 Temporomandibular joints in a patient with the findings of congenital hemihypertrophy. The right condyle is of normal size and form, as is the glenoid fossa. The left condyle is abnormally large, particularly in length. The condyloid tubercle is very prominent. There is marked hypertrophy and deformity of the articular tubercle. The abnormality limited movement of the condyle and did not permit a gliding motion in opening or closing of the mouth or in other movements of the mandible. (Reproduced with permission from Stafne, E. C. and Lovestedt, S. A.: Congenital Hemihypertrophy of the Face (Facial Giantism). Oral Surg., Oral Med. & Oral Path. *15*:184–189 [Feb.] 1962.)

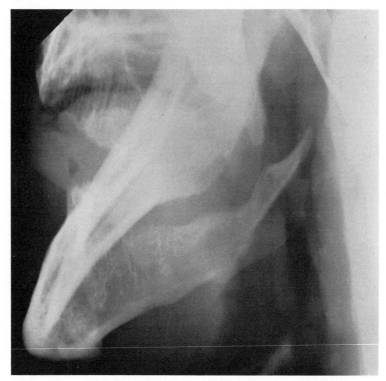

Figure 19–11 Lateral view of the mandible, showing condylar agenesis.

the lesion proved to be on microscopic examination.

Stafne and Lovestedt (1962) have described changes in congenital hemihypertrophy of the face. One of their patients illustrates the changes that can be seen in the temporomandibular joints. Figure 19-10 shows the hypertrophy of a condyle as described by these authors.

An interesting variation is seen in Figure 19–11, which is from a patient who presented with agenesis of the condyle and manifested other problems of underdevelopment as well. Marked asymmetry of the face and irregular mandibular excursions were prominent clinical signs.

Anomalies of the mandible and temporomandibular joint are fairly common.

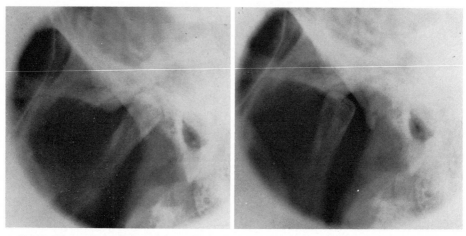

Figure 19–12 View of the left temporomandibular joint, showing small, narrow condyle. Patient was asymptomatic and jaw functioned normally.

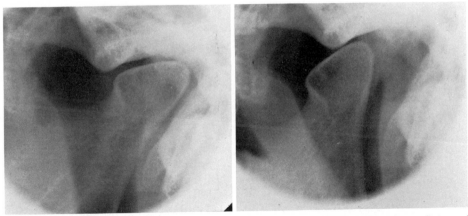

Figure 19–13 Lateral view of the left temporomandibular joint in a patient with a large, flat condylar surface and without symptoms.

Temporomandibular joints vary widely in shape and form. Fortunately, most variations seen in roentgenograms are not of major clinical significance. Figures 19–12 and 19–13 show two such variations in patients who were seen routinely during the course of general medical and dental examinations. They were not experiencing temporomandibular joint dysfunction or complaining of distress.

There are numerous other indications for utilizing roentgenograms of the head, skull, or jaws. Occasionally these roentgenograms reveal incidental but unrelated variations in the region of the temporoman-

dibular joint that are of interest. One such oddity is demonstrated in Figure 19–14, which shows a small bony fragment found incidental to other investigation. Another oddity was recorded and is demonstrated in Figure 19–15. This patient, however, did experience slight discomfort during the opening cycle.

One of the recent major developments in the field of dental roentgenology has been the use of orthopantomography, which employs a principle of laminography to the facial region. The word "panorama" is defined as an unobstructed view or prospect over a wide area, permitting a compre-

Figure 19–14 Lateral view of a jaw showing ramus of mandible and condyle, with small bony fragment. Small bony fragments may be found incidentally in the investigation of other problems. This small fragment was due to trauma. Definitive treatment is not indicated in the absence of symptoms.

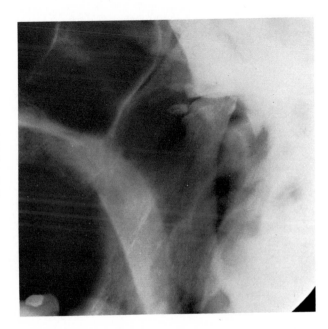

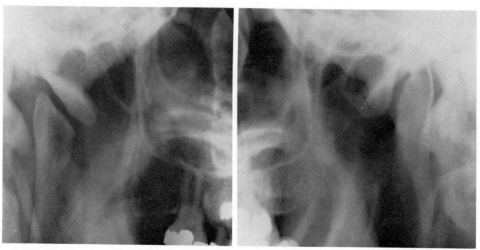

Figure 19–15 Views of right and left temporomandibular joints. The patient had discomfort, particularly during the opening cycle. Note prominent large articular tubercle. The anterior articulating surface of the condyle may demonstrate early pathologic change.

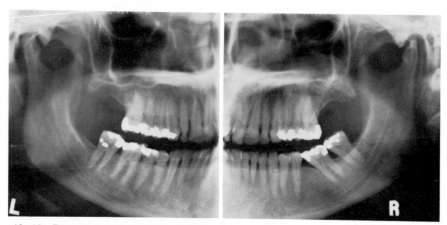

Figure 19–16 Panoramic roentgenogram which shows slight destructive changes in both condyles.

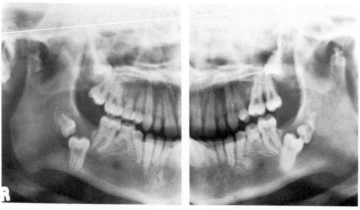

Figure 19–17 Panoramic roentgenograms of 17-year-old girl with lipochondrodystrophy.

hensive survey. There are several dental x-ray units that use variations of this principle of panoramic viewing. This type of roentgenogram has limited usefulness for precise diagnosis of temporomandibular joint disease, but it is a useful additional method for gross survey. It provides good roentgenographic coverage of injuries of the jaws, particularly fractures of the ramus and the condyle, but does not provide an accurate view of the relationship of the condyle to the fossa. This type of roentgenography is applicable in a number of dental investigations. However, it does distort or exaggerate the condyle. Many practitioners are adding this type of examination to their standard roentgenographic procedures and are occasionally noting variations in the temporomandibular joint. During such a survey in a patient who was being seen for other dental reasons, bilateral condylar alteration was noted (Fig. 19–16). Additional roentgenograms of the temporomandibular joints were taken and the patient's condylar disease was verified. Figure 19–17 shows the panoramic roentgenograms in another case. This patient, a 17-year-old girl, had lipochondrodystrophy, with marked degeneration of both condyles, congenital absence of several permanent teeth, and cystic development associated with unerupted mandibular molars. There also were changes in the hands and wrists, epiphyses of the hips and shoulders, and vertebrae. (See Roentgenographic Techniques in Appendix, Part I.)

REFERENCES

Clark, J. L., Mayne, J. G., and Gibilisco, J. A.: The Roentgenographically Abnormal Temporomandibular Joint. Oral Surg., Oral Med. & Oral Path. *33*:836–840 (May) 1972.

Copland, J.: Diagnosis of Mandibular Joint Dysfunction. Oral Surg., Oral Med. & Oral Path. *13*:1106–1129 (Sept.) 1960.

Hatch, G. S.: Clinical and Radiographic Findings of the Temporomandibular Joint in Patients with Rheumatoid Arthritis. Thesis, Mayo Graduate School of Medicine (University of Minnesota), Rochester, 1967.

Russell, L. A. and Bayles, T. B.: The Temporomandibular Joint in Rheumatoid Arthritis. J. Am. Dent. A. 28:533–539 (Apr.) 1941.

Shore, N. A.: The Interpretation of Temporomandibular Joint Roentgenograms. Oral Surg., Oral Med. & Oral Path. *13*:341–350 (Mar.) 1960.

Stafne, E. C. and Lovestedt, S. A.: Congenital Hemihypertrophy of the Face (Facial Giantism). Oral Surg., Oral Med. & Oral Path. *15*:184–189 (Feb.) 1962.

Tolman, D. E. and Eppard, D. G.: An Aid to the Roentgenographic Examination of the Temporomandibular Joint. Am. J. Roentgenol. *103*:674 (July) 1968.

Updegrave, W. J.: Roentgenographic Observations of Functioning Temporomandibular Joints. J. Am. Dent. A. *54*:488–505 (Apr.) 1957.

20 INJURIES TO TEETH, JAWS, AND ZYGOMAS

EASTWOOD G. TURLINGTON, D.D.S.

TRAUMATIZED TEETH

Injuries to the teeth are most common in younger persons, who are predisposed to minor trauma. Hallett (1953), in reporting a series of 1000 traumatized teeth, noted the greatest incidence in the age group eight to eleven years, with the peak at age nine. The maxillary incisors are the teeth most prone to injury. Individuals with class II malocclusion are five times more subject to injury of the anterior teeth, owing to the procumbency of the incisors (Hallett, 1953).

The specific type of injury sustained by a tooth varies from minor to major. It is desirable to have a knowledge of these variations, for the treatment more often than not is predicated on the nature of the injury and its possible sequelae. Bennett (1963) has provided a classification of injured teeth which, though simple, is fully encompassing and provides an index on which to base treatment. His classification is as follows:

Class   I. Traumatized tooth without coronal or root fracture
    A. Tooth firm in alveolus
    B. Tooth subluxed in alveolus
Class II. Coronal fracture
    A. Involving enamel
    B. Involving enamel and dentin
Class III. Coronal fracture with pulpal exposure

Class IV. Root fracture
    A. Without coronal fracture
    B. With coronal fracture
Class V. Avulsion of tooth (Figs. 20–1 through 20–3)

In any incident in which injury to the teeth is evident or suspected, roentgenograms should be made to determine whether injury in fact has occurred and, if so, to identify the site and the extent of the injury. Frequently it is equally important to note concomitant findings regarding the tooth or teeth in question, for these findings alone or combined with data concerning the injury can influence treatment. Particular attention should be paid to the proximity of the pulpal tissues to the frac-

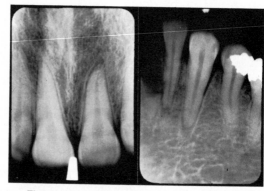

Figure 20–1 Class I injury. *Left,* Right central incisor firm in alveolus with increased width of periodontal ligament. *Right,* Cuspid displaced within alveolus.

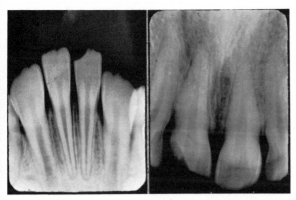

Figure 20–2 Class II injury. *Left,* Fracture of mesial angle of right central incisor involving enamel. *Right,* Fracture of coronal portion involving enamel and dentin.

ture line when a coronal fracture is present, the degree of apical involvement, the extent of root development (noting whether the pulp canal is open or closed), possible root fracture, evidence of subluxation of the tooth within the bony alveolus, and evidence of fracture of the alveolar process.

Not to be overlooked in dealing with injury to the teeth are concomitant lacerations of the lips and perioral tissues, and examination of the soft tissues should include roentgenograms of these areas. It is not uncommon to find portions of fractured teeth or other foreign bodies embedded within the lips that may subsequently cause adverse tissue responses and require surgical intervention. Occlusal projections of the lips and periapical projections with the films interposed between the soft and hard tissues will reveal the presence of radiopaque foreign bodies within the soft tissues (Fig. 20–4).

The scope of the roentgenographic examination is determined by the extent and the nature of the injuries. If, for instance, concomitant injuries to the jaws are suspected, the examination should be more encompassing than when it can reasonably be presumed that the injury is a local one and that intraoral roentgenograms of the teeth and adjacent bone will suffice. It is better to err in making the roentgenographic survey too extensive than too conservative.

In a class I injury, a tooth may be temporarily loosened and painful, but with no more serious trauma than this the pulpal tissues remain viable. In such a situation there is no roentgenographic evidence of damage except possibly an increase in width of the periodontal ligament space. The pulp may become necrotic immediately or after a variable period, and in the absence of any other abnormality, there will be no roentgenographic changes.

Evidence of tooth fracture depends on one or more of several roentgenographic appearances; however, absence of positive findings for fracture cannot absolutely rule out its existence. Roentgenologic examination is only one portion of the investigation, for equally important is the clinical assessment. The roentgenographic survey and clinical examination serve adjunctive

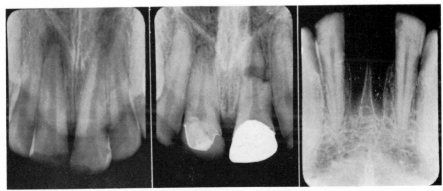

Figure 20–3 *Left,* Class III injury. Coronal fracture involving pulp, with resulting periapical infection. *Center,* Class IV injury. Oblique fracture of root of right central incisor. *Right,* Class V injury. Avulsion of central incisors secondary to trauma.

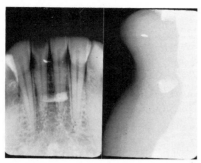

Figure 20–4 *Left,* Foreign bodies noted on periapical projection. *Right,* Localization of foreign bodies within lip revealed on lateral projection of soft tissues.

and collaborative purposes, one to the other. It would be erroneously presumptive to accept a negative roentgenologic finding as valid without conclusive support from the physical findings. This is applicable to all injuries, but particularly to a suspected injury of the teeth and jaws because of the physical limitations inherent in obtaining certain directions and projections of the central beam of x-rays when they are utilized in the jaw region. When the results of the initial roentgenographic examination are negative but the physical findings are positive, additional projections at different angles should be obtained in an effort to substantiate the presence of injury.

Though roentgenograms have limitations, fortunately most fractures of the teeth are demonstrable by this means. Not infrequently, the fracture of one tooth is associated with the fracture of another nearby; therefore, one should not relax after the identification of one fracture but should instead be alert to possible concomitant and approximating injury. It is thus desirable to

continue studying the roentgenograms after conclusively demonstrating one fracture.

Evidence of a radiolucent line between tooth segments, the fracture line, is positive for tooth fracture; however, it does not necessarily indicate a recent or unhealed fracture. The displacement of tooth fragments and the disruption of the continuity of the tooth surface are other notable signs of fracture. Frequently one may see, crossing the tooth, a gray shadow that represents the fracture line and is produced by either the direction of the x-ray beam or the oblique nature of the fracture with resulting superimposition of tooth structure (Fig. 20–5).

Displacement of adjacent tooth parts is a strong indication of fracture. Such displacement may take the form of a distraction of the parts so that the line of fracture is evident. Should the displacement be laterally or anteroposteriorly directed, then a steplike deformity on the surface of the tooth may be produced. Most root fractures of the anterior teeth occur at the midportion of the root. Rarely, deformity of the root follows fracture because of the limiting confines of the bony alveolus. More frequently, the coronal segment is displaced from its normal alignment. Comminuted tooth fractures are unlikely and, if present, are usually the result of an excessively heavy blow. Oblique fractures of the root can sometimes be mistaken for comminution, particularly when the fracture extends obliquely from the labial or buccal to the palatal or lingual surface, or vice versa, in such a way that two radiolucent lines are apparently traversing the root and thus are

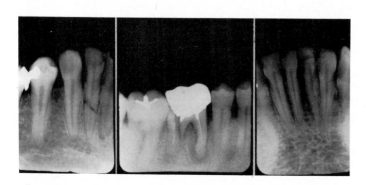

Figure 20–5 *Left,* Radiolucent line traversing root of lateral incisor denoting fracture. *Center,* Disruption in continuity of distal root of first molar due to fracture. *Right,* Coronal oblique fracture of right central incisor revealed by gray radiolucent line.

thought to represent two fractures (Fig. 20–6).

Occasionally coronal fractures may appear erroneously on roentgenograms to involve the pulp chamber. This appearance can be attributed to the oblique extension of the fracture line from the labial to the palatal or the lingual surfaces in such a manner that the shadow of the cleavage line appears to pass through the pulp chamber, when in fact it passes coronal to the chamber.

Serial roentgenograms made after tooth injury are of value in ascertaining post-traumatic bone changes. They are of additional value in trauma of incompletely formed teeth to assess the degree of further root development, the maturation of the apical tissues, and the eruption of the tooth (Fig. 20–7). Union between segments of a fractured tooth is usually not the rule, and resorption and subsequent rounding of the edges of adjacent segments at the fracture site are not uncommon (Fig. 20–8).

After initial trauma to a tooth, an area of radiolucency frequently appears at the apex and ultimately may disappear; if this occurs, the area was due to hyperemia. Should it persist or enlarge, then one can assume that the pulp is necrotic and that periapical infection is likely. Secondary to trauma, the continuity of the apical vessels may be interrupted, causing a necrotic or partially viable pulp. Some teeth so affected may appear roentgenographically normal, while others may later manifest ev-

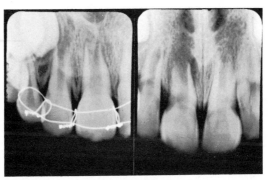

Figure 20–7 *Left,* Traumatized left lateral and central incisors with incomplete root development. *Right,* Six months following injury, denoting abnormal maturation of lateral incisor root and cessation of development of central incisor root with evidence of periapical inflammation.

idence of apical osteitis due to secondary infection.

Minimal injury to a developing tooth is usually of no consequence, and development continues normally. However, trauma sufficiently severe to alter the position of the tooth within the bony alveolus may cause multiple deformities. Such deformities can assume the form of dilaceration of the root, abortion of further growth, and other bizarre configurations in tooth morphology.

There are two normal findings in intraoral roentgenograms that may lead to the false-positive diagnosis of a tooth fracture. One of these is a demonstrated radiolucency that traverses the root and is due to the superimposition upon the root of the nutrient vascular canals within the alveolar bone. The other is noted primarily in the anterior region and is caused by the superimposition upon the root of the alveolar bone crest with a resulting change in roentgenographic density.

INJURIES OF THE JAWS

When one is confronted with a patient who has sustained facial injuries, the question of bony involvement arises. Though the trauma has been adjudged to be relatively minor, it is not uncommon to unearth roentgenographically fractures that were clinically unsuspected. Thus, roentgeno-

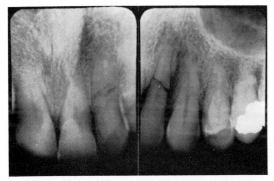

Figure 20–6 *Left,* Apparently comminuted fracture of root of lateral incisor. Simulation due to obliqueness of fracture. *Right,* Projection from different angle reveals presence of a single fracture.

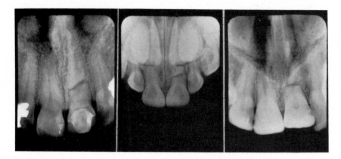

Figure 20–8 Root fractures without evidence of union and persistence of fracture line two years or more after injury.

graphic examination must be of sufficient scope that the findings combined with the knowledge acquired from clinical examination make it possible to rule out or to confirm with reasonable certainty the existence of a jaw fracture. Conversely, on occasion, a clinically suspected fracture may be undemonstrable roentgenographically. Suffice it to say that neither examination can stand alone, but, as previously pointed out, a correlation of the two in an adjunctive manner is mandatory.

Innumerable roentgenologic projections can be utilized in an examination of the mandible and the maxilla. Not to be omitted are the periapical views, which can enhance the study of the teeth and the alveolar bone. Additionally, the occlusal roentgenograms can be used advantageously to demonstrate many areas of the jaws, and they frequently yield results not procurable from other intraoral and ex-

traoral projections. The introduction of panoramic techniques has provided an excellent supplemental medium of roentgenographic examination that can be used almost universally in the investigation of jaw injuries. A word of caution, however, should be interjected regarding the panographic and lateral projections in an examination of the body and the symphysis regions of the mandible. Owing to the almost perpendicular projection of the central x-ray beam relative to the mandible, oblique fractures running in a lateral to a medial direction may go undetected unless there is superior or inferior displacement of the parts (Fig. 20–9). Similarly, fractures with overriding segments may prove difficult to demonstrate unless there is superoinferior displacement.

An examination of the mandible should include, as a basic minimum, bilateral oblique lateral views of the body and

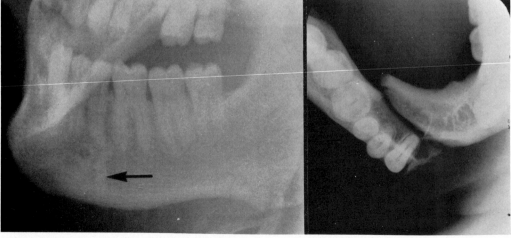

Figure 20–9 *Left,* Fracture of right mandible in cuspid-bicuspid region, with minimal evidence except for slightly increased density secondary to overlap in bicuspid region. *Right,* Occlusal projection of same fracture, revealing displacement and oblique direction of fracture.

ramus, with the views of the ramus to include the condyle, and the posteroanterior projection or the anteroposterior projection of the mandible. The Towne view is often of value in assessing the status of the condyles, condylar necks, and rami, because superimposition of the mastoid and zygoma over the condylar neck region in the straight posteroanterior projection often makes interpretation difficult. The Towne view eliminates this superimposition, thus giving good visualization of the condylar area and rami. The reverse Towne projection may be utilized, though the mandible becomes a little less distinct in the definition of the condyles. These projections should be supplemented, when indicated, by occlusal, oblique posteroanterior projections of the mandible and lateral and anteroposterior projections of the condyle and temporomandibular joint.

The maxilla should be examined roentgenographically in the same manner; however, in obtaining the proper views one must of necessity employ those that will alleviate superimposition of the dense parts of the petrous portion of the temporal bone and mastoid processes on the area to be examined. Projections by which this can be accomplished include the lateral projection of the skull, which presents the facial bones in a sagittal view. The posteroanterior oblique projection of the face (Water's view) is one of the most useful in an examination of the middle third of the face, giving a good view of the orbits, zygomas (though they are somewhat foreshortened), maxillary and frontal sinuses, pyriform fossae, and nasal septum. The angle of the central beam may be altered and directed caudally in the occipitomental projection so as to displace the petrous portion of the temporal bone further downward. The submental-vertical projection can be used to advantage to demonstrate the zygomatic arches and to give a good view of the hard palate, the palatine bones, and the lower border of the mandible. The occlusal films may be rewarding in demonstrating fractures of the alveolar process and the palate, as well as in revealing antral involvement. Examples of these various projections are illustrated and described in Part I of the Appendix.

INTERPRETATION OF EXTRAORAL ROENTGENOGRAMS

There are generally two prerequisites to the proper interpretation of roentgenograms. These are a thorough understanding of the normal roentgenographic anatomy and a basic understanding of the technique employed in obtaining the particular projection needed to reveal inherent distortion, superimposition, and the occurrence of phenomena that could lead to an erroneous diagnosis. It is equally important to develop a systematic pattern in the appraisal of a roentgenogram, rather than to use a haphazard approach by which one's attention may be directed toward an obvious fracture and thereby distracted from some of the more subtle and indistinct evidences of other concomitant fractures. Some of the projections could present inherent anatomic structures or spaces that can simulate fractures and are worthy of note. In viewing the lateral oblique view of the mandible, it must be remembered that the palatolingual and palatopharyngeal air spaces may be superimposed over the mandible in such a way as to form lines that closely resemble fractures. Additionally in this view, superimposition of the hyoid bone on the mandible may be confusing, as also may be an abnormally long styloid process, if the structure lies over or near the mandible (Fig. 20–10). The intervertebral spaces, as evidenced on the posteroanterior projections, may overlie the symphyseal region of the mandible and the maxillary region and may mimic an alveolar process, a symphysis fracture of the mandible, or a Le Fort type I fracture of the maxilla. Because of the projection angle in the Towne view, the condylar neck is brought to lie adjacent to the distorted and prominent zygomatic process of the frontal bone, and, because of this approximation, the appearance can simulate that of a fracture-dislocation of the condyle with medial displace-

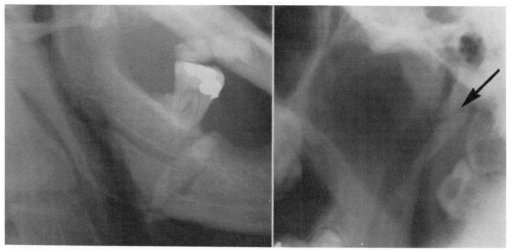

Figure 20–10 *Left,* Superimposition of pharyngeal air space upon ramus resembling a vertical fracture. (Note mandibular body fracture with superimposition of segments.) *Right,* Styloid process in proximity to posterior border of condylar neck and ramus could be misconstrued as a fracture of the mandible.

ment (Fig. 20–11). The upper orbital margin is projected downward over the midportion of the mandibular rami in this projection and thus may lead to misinterpretation.

The lateral and anteroposterior projections of the mandibular condyle deserve careful scrutiny, since it is frequently difficult in the injured patient to obtain roentgenograms with absolute clarity. It is helpful in tracing the continuity of the condylar neck on the lateral projection to follow the posterior border of the ramus upward so as to establish the direction before superimposition obscures the condylar region. Similarly, in viewing the posteroanterior projections, the lateral border of the ramus should be traced upward so as to afford orientation before it merges into an obscured area.

Because of the amount of information available from the Waters view and the extent of the anatomy confined within it, particular emphasis must be placed on surveying the bony margins systematically. This is best accomplished by dividing the inter-

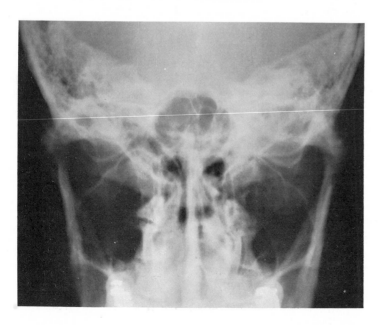

Figure 20–11 Towne projection, with distortion of zygomatic processes of frontal bones simulating fractures of mandibular condyles.

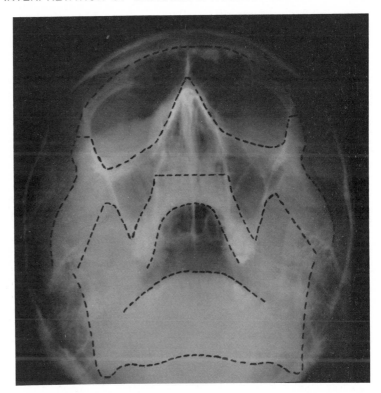

Figure 20–12 Waters' projection, with lines traced to serve as guides in surveying bony anatomy.

pretation into four phases by area and by following four curvilinear lines, as outlined by McGrigor and Campbell (1950). The first line follows from one zygomaticofrontal suture along the superior orbital margin, across the glabella to the superior orbital margin and the zygomaticofrontal suture of the opposite side. One should keep in mind that there is normally a shadow at the zygomaticofrontal suture. Fractures of the frontal sinus are usually demonstrable, though fractures of the cribriform plate of the ethmoid may be obscure. The second line courses from the superior aspect of the zygomatic arch and zygoma to the zygomaticofrontal suture along the inferior orbital margin, across the frontal process of the maxilla, the lateral wall of the nose through the septum, and then on to a like course on the opposite side. The third line passes from the mandibular condyle across the sigmoid notch and the tip of the coronoid process to the lateral and medial antral walls at the level of the nasal floor and on to a similar course on the opposite side. The fourth line traces the occlusal plane of the upper and lower teeth or, if the patient

is edentulous, the crest of the alveolar ridges, in order to detect any discrepancy. A fifth line may be noted—this is the lower border of the mandible and the posterior aspect of the rami (Fig. 20–12).

Comparable attention must be given to the interpretation of the lateral projection of the facial bones. Again one must follow the multiple bony margins as outlined in this view, and particular attention should be directed to those areas in which fractures are most likely to occur. The area of the glabella, through the orbital plate of the ethmoid and to the bone of the pterygoid laminae of the sphenoid, should be carefully evaluated. Attention should be given to the region passing from just above the anterior nasal spine posteriorly above the dense line of the nasal floor and the palate toward the tuberosity of the maxilla and the lower region of the pterygoid laminae, since this is an area predisposed to fracture (Fig. 20–13).

The submental-vertical projection can yield information regarding the zygomatic arches, hard palate, palatine bones, pterygoid laminae, sphenoid sinuses, and

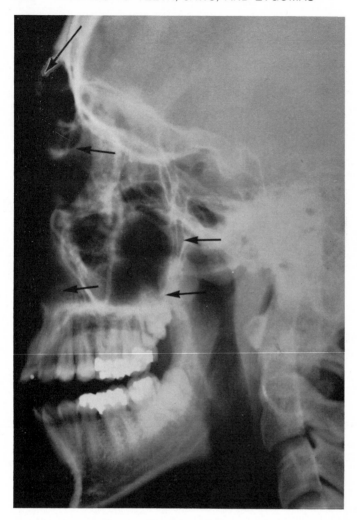

Figure 20–13 Lateral projection of facial bones, with arrows at sites prone to fracture.

cranial bone. Additionally, the continuity of the lower border of the mandible can be followed, and often good visualization of the mandibular condyles can be obtained.

ROENTGENOGRAPHIC EVIDENCE OF FRACTURES

There are three basic roentgenographic signs that solely or in combination are evidence of fracture: a demonstrable fracture line, a displacement of adjacent bony segments, and a deformation of normal bony shape and contour.

Roentgenographic evidence of a line of separation or a line of change is unequivocal proof of a fracture. Such a fracture line is produced by the passage of the central x-ray beam through the line of separation and is most clearly evident when the fracture is parallel to the axis of the central beam of the x-rays (Fig. 20–14). When the fracture is oblique or the x-ray projection is passed obliquely through the fracture, the line becomes less distinct. In certain instances, because of the obliqueness of the fracture and the inability of the x-rays to pass parallel to it, roentgenographic findings may be falsely negative (Fig. 20–9). Occasionally a fracture may be impacted sufficiently to cause superimposition of the trabeculae and thereby obscure the fracture line or cause an area of slightly increased radiopacity at the fracture site.

Displacement, the second basic roentgenographic sign of fracture, results

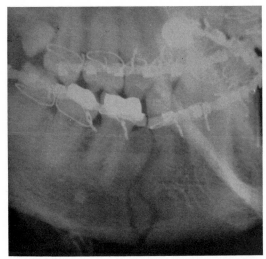

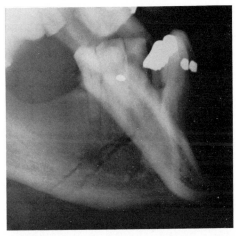

Figure 20–16 Two radiolucent lines produced by a single fracture running obliquely from lateral to medial cortices of mandible.

Figure 20–14 Sharply defined radiolucent line at fracture site produced by x-ray beam passing parallel to fracture site.

from a malalignment or an interruption in the normal continuity of the bony surface. If disruption is marked, this finding is obvious; if minimal, the evidence is subtle and, when present, usually assumes the form of a slight steplike deformity of the bony surface (Fig. 20–15).

Deformity, the third basic roentgenographic sign of fracture, is evidenced by any abnormal variation in bone morphology. Obviously an appreciation of normal roentgenographic anatomy is essential if a valid interpretation of an existing bony deformity is to be realized.

One situation that merits attention in the interpretation of roentgenograms is the image produced in oblique fractures of the mandible that pass from the lateral to the medial cortex or vice versa. On lateral projections this variety of fracture may produce two radiolucent lines, which may be erroneously assumed to be two fractures (Fig. 20–16).

Fractures of the mandible and the maxilla will be considered separately. Though the principles of interpretation apply equally to both, each poses problems peculiar to the bone involved.

Figure 20–15 Fracture of body of mandible, with minimal displacement as evidenced by steplike deformity in inferior border.

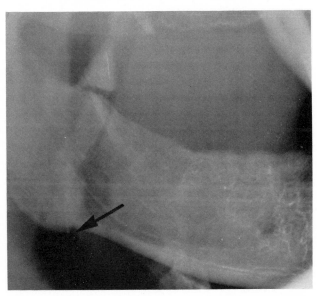

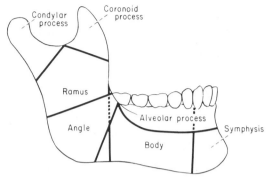

Figure 20–17 Anatomic division of mandible used in describing sites of fracture.

FRACTURES OF THE MANDIBLE

Though fractures of the lower jaw may occur in any region, they have a predilection for certain sites. The sites commonly involved are the condylar process, the coronoid process, and the angle, body, and symphysis regions of the mandible (Fig. 20–17). A single fracture of the lower jaw is found at times; however, it is more common to find two or more resulting from injury.

Fractures of the alveolar process are less frequent in the mandible than in the maxilla. They usually are confined to the anterior segment of the mandible and are rare in the bicuspid-molar region Roentgenographic demonstration of alveolar process fractures is best obtained by means of intraoral dental roentgenograms supplemented by occlusal projections (Fig.

20–18). Particular attention should be paid to the roots of the involved teeth to confirm or deny the presence of root fracture.

The classification of fractures into simple, compound, comminuted, and "greenstick" (complete or incomplete) is applicable to the mandible. Most can be detected roentgenologically, exclusive of the compound versus the closed variety. Too, it may be difficult to determine whether a fracture is complete or incomplete. "Greenstick" fractures are rare in the mandible because of the "hoop" configuration of the jaw, the presence of teeth within it, and the reaction of this anatomic entity to forces imposed on it. Such fractures are prone to occur in children rather than in adults. Comminution usually can be depicted roentgenographically, though, as previously explained, medial to lateral fractures can yield false-positive evidence of comminution (Fig. 20–19).

Displacement and deformation are best considered together, since they are normally closely associated in a cause-effect relationship. Several factors exerting an interrelated effect act to produce displacement and deformation. Stated briefly, these are the site and the direction of the fracture line and the action that muscles exert on the bony segments to which they are attached. To determine the presence and the extent of displacement it is necessary to obtain roentgenographic projections through the fracture site at right angles;

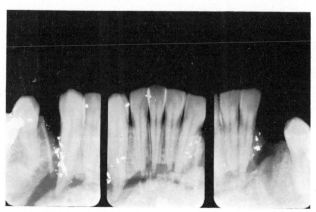
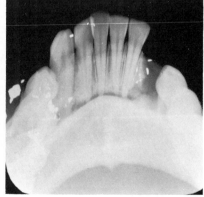

Figure 20–18 *Left,* Periapical projections of an alveolar process fracture of mandible complicating a fracture through symphysis. *Right,* Occlusal projection of the alveolar process fracture.

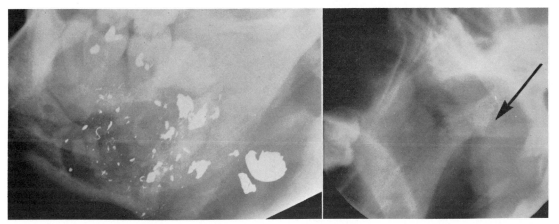

Figure 20-19   *Left,* Severely comminuted fracture of mandible secondary to gunshot wound. *Right,* Greenstick subcondylar fracture of mandible in an adolescent.

not uncommonly, particularly in the angle region, a lateral view fails to reveal the lateral displacement of the proximal segment (Fig. 20–20). The direction of the fracture line dictating the presence or the absence of displacement is clearly exemplified in the angle of the mandible. Here, when the fracture extends obliquely from the anterior to the posterior, the proximal segment (ramus) tends to be displaced in a superior and lateral direction secondary to the force of muscle pull. This situation is referred to as an "unfavorable" fracture (Fig. 20–21). Conversely, when the fracture runs obliquely in a superoposterior to an inferoanterior direction, the proximal segment becomes locked beneath the distal

segment and thereby resists the muscle pull and thwarts the displacement forces (Fig. 20–22).

Oblique fractures in the body of the mandible that pass in an anteroposterior direction may have the anterior end on the lateral or medial aspect, and the proximal end on the opposite side. Such a fracture can escape detection on lateral projection, for there is no clear fracture line and the fracture may be evidenced by only a step in the inferior border if some vertical displacement is present (Fig. 20–23, *left*). However, anteroposterior and occlusal projections usually reveal the presence of fracture, for normally one of the segments is displaced either medially or laterally (Fig.

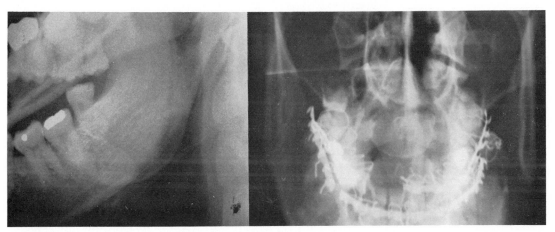

Figure 20-20   *Left,* Fracture through body in third molar region, with displacement of proximal segment superiorly and anteriorly. *Right,* Lateral displacement of proximal segment, which was inapparent on lateral projection.

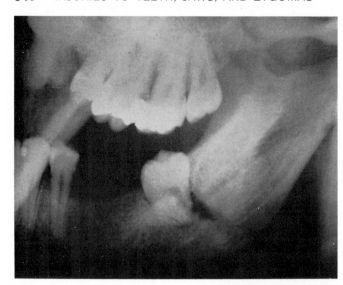

Figure 20–21 Unfavorable fracture of mandible with superior displacement of ramus.

Figure 20–22 Fracture through angle of mandible running obliquely from posterior to anterior, thereby preventing displacement of ramus superiorly.

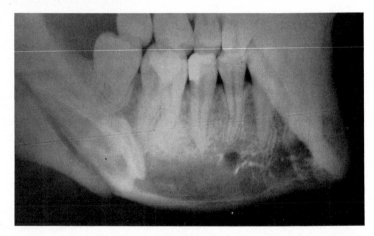

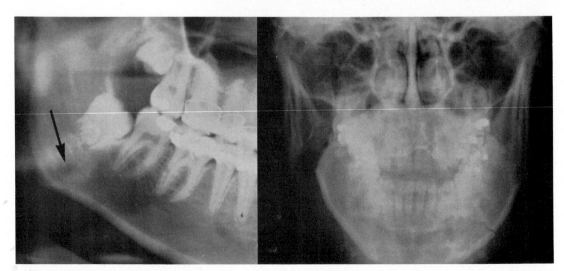

Figure 20–23 *Left,* Fracture passing obliquely through angle of mandible, with minimal displacement evident and with ill-defined fracture line. (Note increased radiopacity due to fragment overlap.) *Right,* Anteroposterior projection of fracture, disclosing lateral displacement.

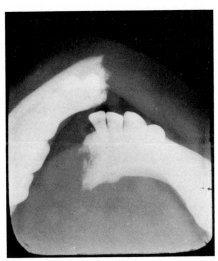

Figure 20–24 Symphysis fracture with collapse and overriding of segments.

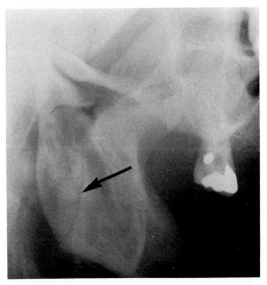

Figure 20–26 Vertical fracture of mandibular ramus in combination with a subcondylar fracture.

20–23, *right*). Similarly, fractures extending obliquely through the body of the mandible from the outer cortex medially and inferiorly without displacement may remain undetected on lateral views, since it is impossible for the central rays to pass parallel to the cleavage line. Fractures extending in a reverse direction present identical problems in roentgenographic interpretation.

Another instance in which direction influences displacement and deformation is that in which the route of fracture passes from the outer cortex anterior to the inner cortex and allows the proximal segment to deviate medially because of the action of the internal pterygoid and suprahyoid muscles. Bilateral fractures of the body of the mandible cause inferior displacement and deformation of the anterior segment secondary to the action of the suprahyoid muscle groups. The symphysis region, when involved in obliquely directed fractures, tends to displace, with the segments overriding in a telescoping fashion. This fracture-displacement is difficult to ascertain on lateral and anteroposterior projections and can best be demonstrated on occlusal views (Fig. 20–24). In injuries that preclude intraoral insertion of the occlusal film, an extraoral projection of the chin obtained with the occlusal film can be revealing.

Fractures of the coronoid process either alone or in combination with other fractures of the mandible are rare and of little consequence. Identification of such a fracture is usually a serendipitous event, since clinical findings are typically lacking (Fig. 20–25).

Fractures involving the ramus occur more commonly in the region of the angle, though no part of this segment of the mandible is immune to injury. Vertically and horizontally directed fractures are second and third, respectively, in order of frequency. Most fractures of the ramus are

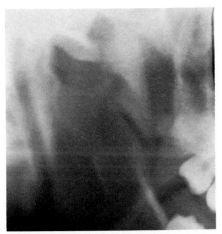

Figure 20–25 Fractured mandibular coronoid process.

simple, but comminuted ones occur if sufficient force is directed to the region. Vertical fractures normally run from the depth of the sigmoid notch at varying degrees of obliqueness to the posterior border (Fig. 20–26).

CONDYLAR FRACTURE

Fracture of the mandibular condyle occurs often enough from trauma to the lower jaw to alert one to suspect it in every instance of such trauma, and an investigation is indicated in all cases to rule out or confirm a fracture at this site. Bilateral condylar fractures are considerably less common than unilateral ones, and the latter are frequently found in conjunction with a contralateral fracture of the body of the mandible.

Condylar fractures are generally described as being intracapsular or extracapsular. The incidence of intracapsular fracture is negligible. Such fractures involve the articular surface; thus, the majority probably escape detection unless specific projections are made to study the temporomandibular joint. Intracapsular fractures are more likely to occur in infancy and childhood.

Extracapsular fractures may involve any portion from immediately beneath the condylar head to the junction of the condylar neck with the ramus at the level of the

depth of the sigmoid notch (Fig. 20–27). The commonest site of fracture is at the base of the condylar neck. Most fractured condyles are displaced from the glenoid fossa or occupy an altered position within it, and this displacement may assume any direction, with the majority being tipped medially. Posteroanterior views of the condyles are invaluable in demonstrating a fracture-dislocation, for in lateral views the true nature of the fracture escapes detection except for the low condylar neck fracture with inferior displacement; the fracture is missed in lateral views because of the overlapping of the condylar neck by the ramus and the superimposition of the cranial structures (Figs. 20–28 and 20–29). There are isolated reports of fractures in which the condyle is forced into the middle cranial fossa; obviously, this results from severe trauma. On occasion the fracture is transverse, but usually the cleavage line begins at the depth of the sigmoid notch and passes obliquely in a posteroinferior direction.

FRACTURES OF THE MAXILLA

Fractures of the maxilla may involve the alveolar process, the body of the maxilla, and the maxilla and approximating facial bones, or they may be present as a portion of a craniofacial dysjunction. These

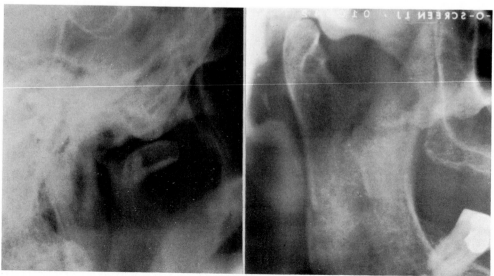

Figure 20–27 *Left,* High subcondylar fracture-dislocation. *Right,* Low subcondylar fracture-dislocation.

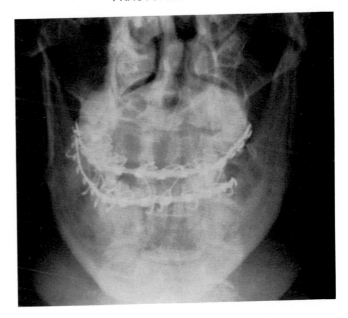

Figure 20–28 Anteroposterior view of bilateral fracture-dislocations of mandibular condyles with medial displacement.

may occur solely or in varying combinations one with another. Worthy of note is the so-called blow-out fracture of the floor of the orbit, which involves the superior maxillary antral wall alone with no other maxillary involvement.

Roentgenologic analysis of maxillary and middle face fractures is a good deal more difficult and less rewarding than is that of the mandible. This difficulty is attributable to the inherent limitations in revealing roentgenographically the bony structures and their deviation from normal in this region. Thus, it is again imperative to emphasize and correlate the clinical and roentgenographic examinations.

CLASSIFICATION OF MAXILLARY FRACTURES

The fact that certain areas of the maxilla show predisposition to fracture provides information by which a classification can be formulated. Knowledge of the classic fracture sites is of benefit in both diagnosis and treatment. Granted, there is no fixed rule to dictate the region in which the fractures will be contained; however, this appreciation serves as a useful guide if one realizes that the typical fractures may occur in varying combinations and in degrees of severity.

The sites and segments prone to frac-

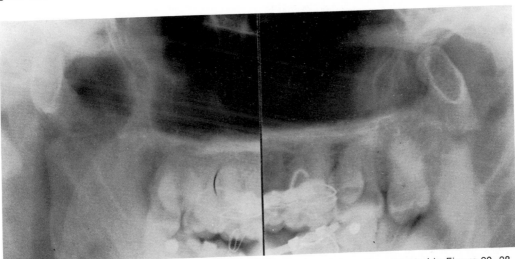

Figure 20–29 Lateral projections of subcondylar fracture-dislocations demonstrated in Figure 20–28.

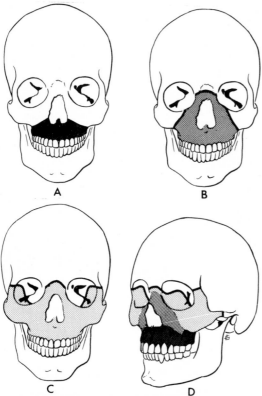

Figure 20–30 Schematic representation of maxillary fractures. *A*, Le Fort type I. *B*, Le Fort type II. *C*, Le Fort type III. *D*, Lateral oblique view of maxillary fractures.

ture permit formulation of classifications: (1) the alveolar process, (2) the horizontal maxillary fracture (Le Fort type I), (3) the pyramidal maxillary fracture (Le Fort type II), (4) the craniofacial dysjunction (Le Fort type III), and (5) the "blow-out" fracture of the orbit. As noted previously, these may occur in a myriad of combinations and involvement (Fig. 20–30).

Alveolar Process Fracture. Alveolar process fractures are more likely to occur in the maxilla than in the mandible, owing to the procumbency of the incisor and cuspid teeth. This region is the one most frequently involved, though any of the alveolar segments may be affected.

Generally, fractures of the alveolar process are well demonstrated on intraoral projections and are represented by a regular to an irregular radiolucent line. At times, the nutrient bony channels containing arterioles may be prominent and may simulate the radiolucencies of alveolar process fracture (Fig. 20–31). Other than this, there is little to complicate the roentgenographic evidence of this variety of fracture.

Injury to the teeth or the roots in the involved area is not an infrequent finding and may assume the form of root fracture, change in position relative to the bony alveolus, complete displacement of the tooth, or one of many injuries to the coronal portion. Fractures in the molar and bicuspid regions can implicate the walls of the maxillary antra; however, some difficulty may be met in demonstrating this with periapical projections, owing to the superimposition of the zygomatic processes of the maxilla. The panographic and Waters projections may help confirm the existence of a fracture. In the Waters view, particularly, it is possible to demonstrate the presence or the absence of opacification of the sinuses. Where antral injury is suspected, the presence of an opacity within the antrum gives strong, though presumptive, evidence of antral involvement. Such a finding is secondary to the fracture of the antral walls with subsequent hemorrhage into the antral cavity, which causes the opacity evidenced on the roentgenogram. The occlusal projections, too, provide an excellent means of assessing fractures of the maxillary alveolar process.

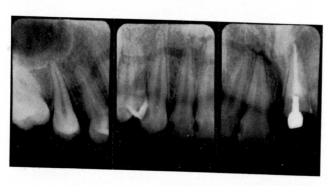

Figure 20–31 Maxillary alveolar process fracture as evidenced by radiolucent line.

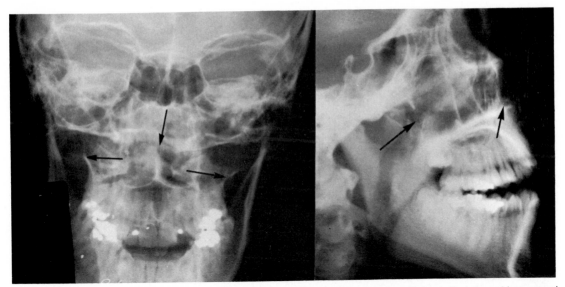

Figure 20-32 *Left,* Le Fort type I maxillary fracture involving lateral and medial antral walls and bony nasal septum. *Right,* Lateral projection of Le Fort type I fracture, evidencing inferior and posterior displacement of maxilla.

Le Fort Type I Fracture (Horizontal). When fracture of the maxilla is suspected, a systematic study of the roentgenograms is essential. The visual evaluation should proceed so as to follow the border of the involved bones in order to determine any displacement or discontinuity of the normal outline. Attention should be sharply focused at the sutural junctions of the facial bones. Additionally, an appreciation of the sites of predilection is worthwhile so that particular emphasis can be given to these regions.

The Le Fort type I fracture normally traverses the width of the maxilla, involving the lateral and nasal walls of the antra and the pterygoid plates at the junction of the lower one third with the upper two thirds (Fig. 20–32). This injury is frequently associated with depressed zygomatic fractures, as well as with fracture of the bony components of the nasal septum. The disjoined segment is commonly displaced posteriorly and inferiorly. With marked displacement, identification of the fracture lines is relatively easy in the lateral and posteroanterior projections. When displacement is minimal, positive roentgenographic evidence may depend on the demonstration of malalignment of the bony margins. Owing to the thinness of the bone, displacement is best demonstrated when the border approximates an air cavity, such as the sinuses, orbits, or nasal cavity. Another area to be noted roentgenographically is the maxillary antra. After trauma, opacity indicates hemorrhage into the antral cavity, which may be assumed to have resulted from the interruption of the integrity of the antral walls secondary to fracture.

On occasion, horizontal maxillary fractures may be unilateral, involving the lateral and nasal walls of the antrum, along with the pterygoid plates on one side and the midpalatal suture (Fig. 20–33). Occlusal projections are of value in demonstrating the palatal fracture line.

Le Fort Type II Fracture (Pyramidal). Classically, the Le Fort type II fracture involves the suture lines between the body of the maxilla and the frontal and lacrimal bones, perisuturally the zygomaticomaxillary interfaces, and also the infraorbital rim and floor of the orbit. The nasal bones, too, are often affected. The fracture lines usually follow points of weakness that exist in the nasal bones at the junction of the thick upper end with the thinner inferior portion forming the upper margin of the anterior nasal aperture. They then extend across both sides of the frontal process of the maxilla and cross the lacrimal bones, running obliquely superoinferiorly. The course then assumes an inferior, lateral,

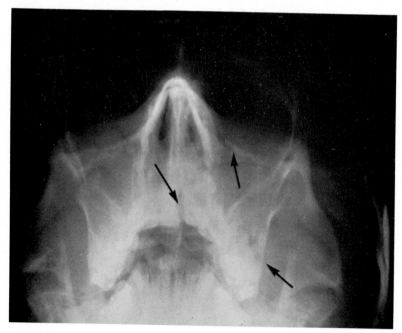

Figure 20–33 Unilateral right maxillary fracture with minimal displacement and involvement of infraorbital rim.

and anterior direction, crossing the inferior orbital floor in the region of the zygomaticomaxillary suture. The fracture line progresses downward through, or close to, the infraorbital foramen and traverses the lateral antral wall, approximating the zygomaticomaxillary suture. After passing the malar buttress, it courses posterosuperiorly to the pterygomaxillary fissure to run through the pterygoid plates at their midportion (Fig. 20–34).

A frequent associated finding is the fracture of one of the zygomas, with varying degrees of displacement and occurring in conjunction with the gross fracture of the zygomatic arch. In the roentgenographic determination of the Le Fort type II fracture, attention should be directed to the lateral antral walls in the region of the zygomaticomaxillary suture, to the infraorbital rim, and to the area of the nasal bones and frontal process of the maxilla on the posteroanterior projections. The nasal and frontal process regions and the posterior walls of the maxilla, which are usually clearly defined, should undergo careful scrutiny on the lateral projections.

Le Fort Type III Fracture (Craniofacial Dysjunction). The most severe fracture involving the maxilla is craniofacial dysjunction. It is usually considered to represent fracture through or near the fronto-maxillary and nasal bone sutures, the frontozygomatic suture, the zygomatic arch, the floor of the orbit, the ethmoids, and the lacrimal bones. The normal pathway of the fracture line extends above the zygoma and begins at the frontonasal region, with possible disruption of the cribriform plate and ethmoids, crosses the nasal bones and the frontal process of the maxilla at the respective suture lines, extends across the upper portion of the lacrimal bones, posteriorly traversing the orbital plates of the ethmoids with comminution, and then passes inferiorly and laterally to the posterior aspect of the inferior orbital fissure. The line courses across the posterior aspect of the maxilla and across the roots of the pterygoid plates. From the anterolateral portion of the inferior orbital fissure, the fracture passes across the lateral wall of the orbit to the junction of the zygoma, with the greater wing of the sphenoid separating the zygoma at the frontozygomatic suture. The fracture is completed as it extends through the zygomatic arch. The fracture line follows a similar course on the contralateral side (Fig. 20–35).

Usually this class of maxillary fracture is complicated by additional fractures, such as further fracture at the junction of the zygoma with the maxilla, displacement fracture of the zygomatic arch, superim-

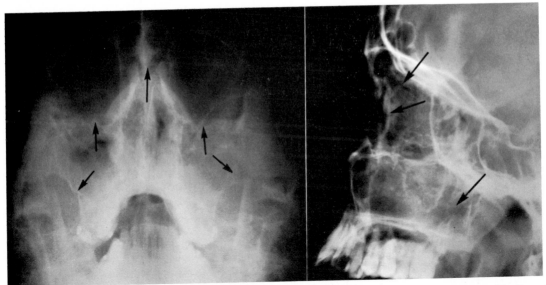

Figure 20–34   *Left,* Le Fort type II fracture of maxilla as noted on Water's projection. (Note opacification of antra.) *Right,* Lateral projection of skull, with fracture sites of Le Fort type II seen in sagittal view.

posed fracture of the Le Fort type I, and involvement of the nasal bones and septum, all of which may demonstrate mild to severe comminution and displacement. With increased complexity of this injury, it is often more difficult to make a specific roentgenographic identification of many of the fracture sites, and again a thorough knowledge of the areas of predilection to fracture is important.

Fracture of the Orbital Floor ("Blow-Out" Fracture).   When sufficient force is applied to the ocular region, the resultant energy is transmitted via the globe and orbital contents to the surrounding vault of bone. Since the inferior orbital floor is the weakest portion of the bony orbital cavity, the force causes a downward rupture of this eggshell-like bony plate into the maxillary antrum. Then some of the inferior orbital contents, such as fat and a portion of the inferior rectus muscle, may herniate through the resulting defect in the floor. Such an injury is best illustrated on Waters' projection and lateral views of the maxillary sinuses (Fig. 20–36). However, on occasion, hemor-

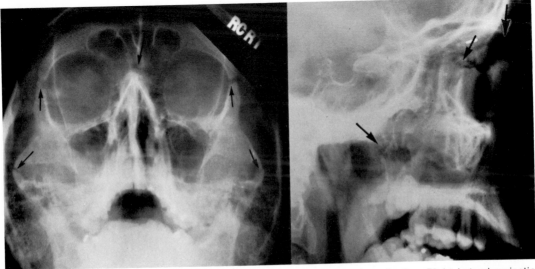

Figure 20–35   *Left,* Le Fort type III fracture of maxilla as seen in Water's projection. *Right,* Lateral projection of Le Fort type III fracture of maxilla.

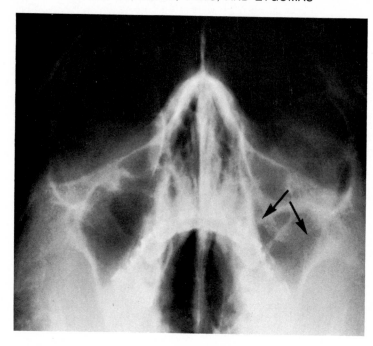

Figure 20–36 Fracture of right orbital floor with herniation of some of the inferior orbital contents into maxillary antrum.

rhage into the antrum, with resulting roentgenographic opacity, can lead erroneously to negative findings. In such an instance, tomograms of the antrum may be necessary to confirm the diagnosis.

FRACTURES OF THE ZYGOMA

Although the zygoma is not generally considered an integral portion of the jaws, the incidence of injury to the zygomas as a consequence of maxillofacial trauma, singularly or in combination with jaw injuries, is sufficiently significant to merit consideration of the roentgenologic findings associated with fractures of the zygoma. The zygomatic bone, commonly known as the malar bone, lends prominence to the cheek and forms a buttress of the facial skeleton, serving in the latter instance to distribute a portion of the masticatory force to the cranial base. This dense, strong structure has multiple articulations with other facial and cranial bones and, because of its anatomy and inherent strength, trauma to the zygoma is unlikely to fracture the bone but most probably will result in fracture beyond its periphery or at its sutural interfaces. An intimate knowledge of the osseous anatomy of the zygoma and its articulations as well as of the orbit and its contents is essential in order to interpret the presenting signs and symptoms secondary to trauma and to correlate these with the roentgenographic findings, so that a proper diagnosis may be established.

Because of the variety of fractures of the zygoma within its anatomic confines, consideration of fracture of the zygomaticomaxillary complex is more appropriate. Typically, although there may be many variations, a blow to the zygoma results in a fracture beyond the zygomaticomaxillary suture that will course upward across the anterolateral wall of the antrum, through the infraorbital foramen, over the rim of the orbit, and then posteriorly across the orbital floor until it meets the lateral extremity of the inferior orbital fissure. Here it will join with the fracture that passes behind the zygomatic buttress across the posterolateral antral wall, completing a circle. Fracture also can occur through the lateral wall of the orbit, passing through the zygomaticofrontal suture and extending inferiorly between the greater wing of the sphenoid and zygoma to the lateral extremity of the inferior orbital fissure, where it meets the zygomaticomaxillary fracture. Additionally, a fracture can occur through the zygomatic arch at about its midpoint (Fig. 20–37).

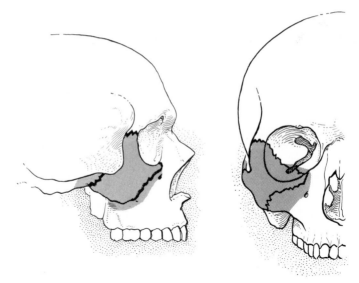

Figure 20–37 Schematic representation of the course of a typical zygomatic fracture.

CLASSIFICATION OF ZYGOMATIC FRACTURES

Efforts to classify zygomatic fractures have been directed toward correlation of the anatomic displacement and functional impairment. An anatomic classification devised by Knight and North (1961) is shown in Table 20–1.

ROENTGENOGRAPHIC FINDINGS

Several roentgenographic projections may be utilized for accurate assessment of

Table 20–1. Zygomatic Fractures: Classification of Knight and North

Group	Description	Incidence (%)
I	No significant displacement; fracture visible on roentgenogram	6
II	Arch fracture; medial buckling of arch	10
III	Unrotated body fracture; downward and inward displacement but no rotation	33
IV	Medially rotated body fracture; downward, inward, and backward displacement with medial rotation	11
V	Laterally rotated body fracture; downward, medial, and backward displacement with lateral rotation	22
VI	All cases in which additional fractures cross the main fragment	18

the extent of injury and degree of displacement after trauma to the zygomaticomaxillary complex. Evaluation of these roentgenograms should proceed in a systematic fashion. The regions of the zygomaticofrontal and zygomaticomaxillary sutures, the lateral wall of the antrum, and the zygomatic arch should receive special emphasis when the various roentgenograms are viewed. The most valuable single view is Waters' projection, which demonstrates the zygomas, the zygomatic arches, the orbital margins, and the antra. In addition to noting disruption in the continuity of the zygoma and its articulations, one should closely inspect the infraorbital rim for a "step deformity," and the right and left antra should be compared for relative opacification that signifies disruption in the antral walls (Fig. 20–38).

The submental-vertical projection is useful in visualizing the zygomatic arches; however, if sufficient exposure is used to demonstrate the cranial base, definition of the arches may be obscured (Fig. 20–39). These views are illustrated and an explanation of the anatomy is provided in Part I of the Appendix. The semiaxial, Titerington position is helpful in further visualizing the zygomatic arches, the lateral walls of the maxilla, and, particularly, the orbital margins (Fig. 20–40). Roentgenograms obtained for stereoscopic viewing are superior for interpretation, and tomograms are

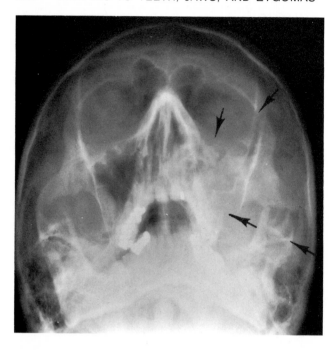

Figure 20–38 Fracture of right zygoma with lateral and inferior displacement, as noted in Waters' projection.

most useful in visualizing areas in which superimposition of other structures obviates clear definition (Figs. 20–41 and 20–42).

UNION OF FRACTURES

The use of roentgenograms to determine the presence of, or lack of, bony union in the postreduction and fixation period is not without fallacy. Normally, in long bones it is possible to demonstrate the callous formation roentgenographically, which serves as a guide to the efficacy and progress of treatment. Such is not the case when the mandible and facial bones are involved. Only rarely is it possible to identify the callous formation following reduction of mandibular fractures, and it is impossible when the facial bones are considered.

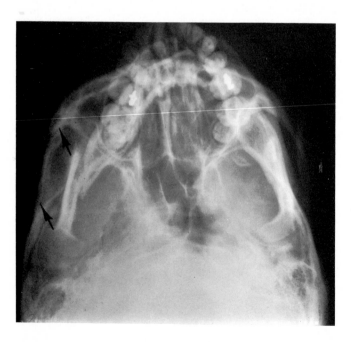

Figure 20–39 Fracture of right zygomatic arch with medial displacement in submental-vertical projection. A right mandibular fracture is also present.

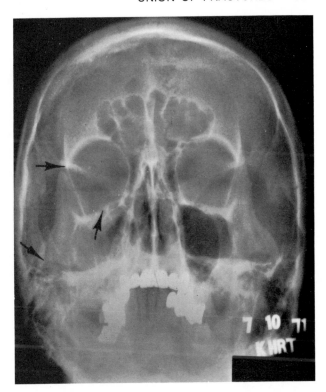

Figure 20–40 Semiaxial projection, demonstrating fracture sites at the left frontozygomatic suture, inferior orbital rim, and zygomatic arch.

Roentgenographic evidence of union is not present until long after clinical union is noted. Thus the determination of bony union depends on the clinical and not on the roentgenographic findings.

Evidence of fracture, particularly of the mandible, may persist on the roentgenograms for months to years after clinical and functional union (Fig. 20–43). Fractures in children and adolescents tend to heal more rapidly than those in adults; consequently, the roentgenograms may yield confirmatory evidence of union earlier.

At the outset, most fracture lines appear with slightly irregular margins; however, if the fracture is reexamined roentgenographically a few weeks later it will demonstrate a widened, more regular line. This is a normal finding, since the increased vascularity at the fracture site, a normal sequela of the healing process, promotes some demineralization near the edges of the fracture. As the course of healing

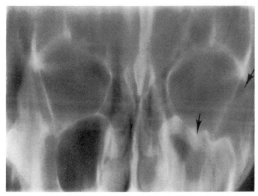

Figure 20–41 Posterior-anterior tomogram, demonstrating fractures through the right zygomaticofrontal suture and infraorbital floor. Opacification of right antrum is evident.

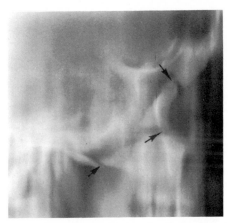

Figure 20–42 Tomogram, demonstrating fractures of the left lateral orbital rim and zygomatic arch with displacement.

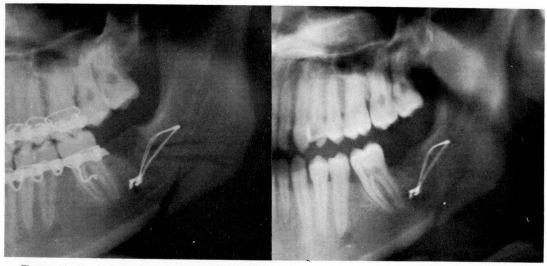

Figure 20–43 *Left,* Fracture line at time of treatment. *Right,* Fracture line five months after removal of fixation appliances.

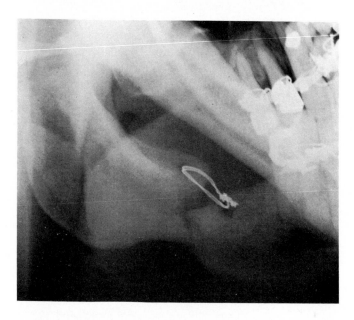

Figure 20–44 Nonunion of mandibular fracture with cortication, eburnation of ends of proximal and distal segments.

progresses and recalcification occurs, the width of the radiolucent line diminishes.

If nonunion occurs in the mandible, the margins of the fractured ends become rounded and smooth and lose their irregularity. Additionally, with the passage of time, increased density becomes evident at the margins, which ultimately become corticated (Fig. 20–44). This situation, in which increased mineralization of the margins follows nonunion, is commonly referred to as eburnation.

Roentgenograms of the facial bones shed even less light on the healing process in the postreduction phase of treatment than do those of the mandible, and serve only to reveal the position of the involved bones.

REFERENCES

Bennett, D. T.: Traumatised Anterior Teeth. Brit. Dent. J. *115*:309–311 (Oct. 15) 1963.
Hallett, G. E. M.: Cited by Bennett, D. T.
Knight, J. S. and North, J. F.: The Classification of Malar Fractures: An Analysis of Displacement as a Guide to Treatment. Brit. J. Plast. Surg. *13*:325–339, 1961.
McGrigor, D. B. and Campbell, W.: The Radiology of War Injuries. Part VI. Wounds of the Face and Jaw. Brit. J. Radiol. *23*:685–696 (Dec.) 1950.

POSTOPERATIVE ROENTGENOGRAPHIC EXAMINATION AND POSTSURGICAL DEFECTS

21

POSTOPERATIVE ROENTGENOGRAPHIC EXAMINATION

The necessity for postoperative roentgenographic examinations to observe the progress of repair and healing following surgical removal of cysts and tumors is taken for granted. In recent years routine examination following extraction of teeth has become a more common practice, and indications for doing so are obvious. Such an examination may reveal tooth fragments, foreign bodies, fracture of the alveolar process, injury to adjoining teeth, or other conditions that may prevent healing or cause retarded healing of the wound. The examination should be made as soon as convenient following the surgical procedure, since early detection and elimination of a retained root, foreign body, or detached bone fragment permits uneventful healing of the wound. Also, foreign bodies and retained roots are more easily removed early and prior to the time that they may become partially or completely embedded in bone.

The postoperative roentgenogram that shows no abnormality gives added assurance to the patient and also serves as a record should any question later arise as to whether the surgical procedure had been performed successfully.

The presence of fragments of silver alloy in the mandibular sockets is the most common finding in the postoperative roentgenograms. While most fragments do not cause unfavorable results, some do. Roots and other fragments of tooth structure that remain in the sockets should

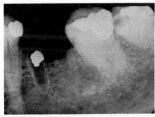 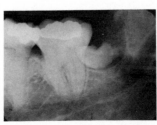 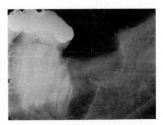

Figure 21-1 Postoperative roentgenograms revealing, *left,* silver alloy which has delayed healing of the mesial socket of a mandibular first molar; *center,* fragment of crown of mandibular third molar; and *right,* mesial root of a mandibular third molar.

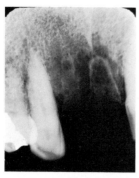
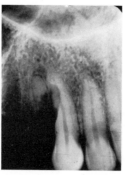
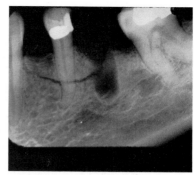

Figure 21-2 Postoperative complications causing pain. *Left,* Osteomyelitis as evidenced by destruction of bone beyond the limits of the alveolar socket. *Center,* Pulpitis of a canine caused by injury to its root by a surgical bur used in an attempt to recover the root of a first premolar. *Right,* Fracture of the alveolar process and loosening of the adjoining tooth.

always be removed, since they often become a source of residual infection or acute abscess (Fig. 21–1).

X-ray examination is indicated in all instances of severe postoperative pain. Such pain may accompany the onset of osteomyelitis, pulpitis that has resulted from injury to an adjoining tooth, fracture of the alveolar process (Fig. 21–2), and so-called dry socket. The roentgenographic appearance of a dry socket is usually normal.

The alveolar process is often fractured at the time of dental extraction, but if the fractured portion has not been much displaced and has not become detached from the mucoperiosteum, healing usually follows. Detached portions tend to slough, in which event they may delay healing for many weeks (Fig. 21–3). In some instances, healing takes place only after sequestrectomy is done. Sequestration that may follow electrocoagulation is shown in Figure 21–4.

POSTSURGICAL DEFECTS

Unlike other bones the jaws may be subjected to a large number of surgical procedures throughout life. The result of many of these surgical procedures may become a permanent record on the roentgenogram, which is evidenced by a radiographic density or trabecular pattern that varies from the pattern of the undisturbed surrounding bone. An alveolar socket may be replaced by bone that is not as dense as the adjacent bone, and the outline of the socket may still be visible many years after extraction of the tooth (Fig. 21–5, *left*). On the other hand, the bone that forms in the socket may be abnormally dense, resembling a dental root. The bone that forms in the space formerly occupied by a successfully treated cyst or tumor may vary both in density and in trabecular pattern. Most often the bone has a ground-glass appearance (Fig. 21–5, *right*).

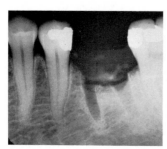
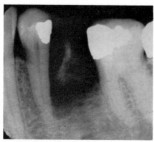
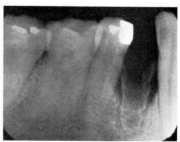

Figure 21-3 Sequestrations of bone which are a cause of retarded healing. The illustration on the right shows sloughing of the alveolar socket as a result of prolonged local treatment for relief of pain.

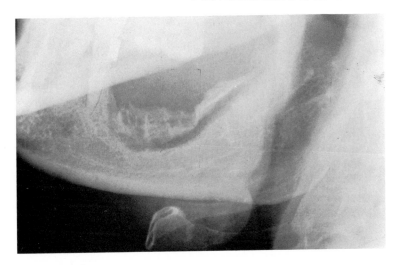

Figure 21–4 Sequestrum formed because of electrocoagulation for carcinoma. Biopsy at the time of sequestrectomy indicated that the carcinoma had not recurred.

In some defects that result from surgical procedures there is lack of the normal amount of bone — bone that may, of necessity, have been removed in the successful performance of the operation. The disclosure of such defects by the roentgenogram may, in some instances, cause confusion when a history of a previous surgical procedure is unavailable. One such defect is that which may follow removal of an embedded maxillary canine. In one instance, both the labial and palatal plate of bone had been removed at the time of odontectomy and, as a result, channels through the bone extending from one surface of the jaw to the other persisted. These channels were occupied by fibrous connective tissue, and were seen as areas of marked radiolucency (Fig. 21–6). A similar defect may be produced when apiectomy is performed on an anterior tooth, and the marked radiolucence near the apex of the root may suggest that the

root-canal therapy had been unsuccessful (Fig. 21–7, *left*). A rather unusual defect produced by a radical operation on the maxillary sinus is shown in Figure 21–7, *right*. A large opening that is devoid of bone extends transversely through the jaw, and the apex of the root of a second premolar presumably had been cut away at the time of operation.

Defects that are seen as indentations or concavities on the crest of the alveolar ridge may result when an appreciable portion of bone, including the alveolar socket, has been removed on the lingual as well as on the labial or buccal surface during extraction of a tooth (Fig. 21–8, *left*). No doubt some of these defects are produced when a forceps is applied in such a manner that it includes within its beaks an appreciable amount of alveolar process when the tooth is delivered.

If a maxillary sinus and a molar tooth

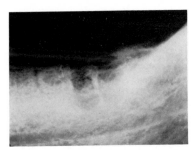 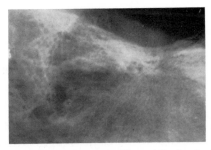

Figure 21–5 *Left,* Porotic bone in an alveolar socket 15 years after extraction of the tooth. *Right,* Bone of ground-glass appearance that has filled the space formerly occupied by a cyst.

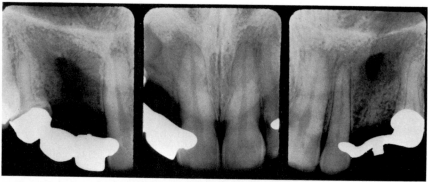

Figure 21–6 Radiolucent areas in the canine regions represent transverse channels through the jaw that were produced when the embedded canines were removed.

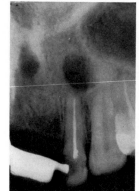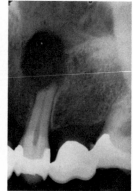

Figure 21–7 Postsurgical defects. *Left*, Transverse opening through the jaw produced at the time of apiectomy. *Right*, Defect produced by a surgical procedure on the maxillary sinus.

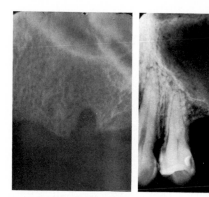

Figure 21–8 Postsurgical defects. *Left*, Defect produced by removal of buccal and lingual portions of the alveolar socket at the time of dental extraction. *Right*, Funnel-shaped opening into the maxillary sinus which is typical of antro-oral fistula of long standing.

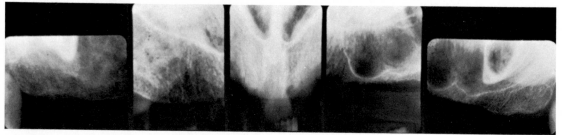

Figure 21–9 Alteration in appearance of maxillary sinus on the reader's left following a Caldwell-Luc operation. Note normal appearance of the undisturbed sinus on the right.

are in close contact with each other, it is not unusual for a portion of the floor of the sinus to remain attached to the root of the tooth and to come away with it when the tooth is extracted. Fortunately, such an incident rarely leads to an antro-oral fistula, and the extraction wound usually heals normally. Subsequent roentgenograms of the edentulous space will reveal an irregular defect in bone that interrupts the continuity of the floor of the maxillary sinus. If an antro-oral fistula results from antral exposure and is permitted to remain patent for any great length of time, a funnel-shaped opening leading from the sinus to the alveolar crest takes form; such an opening is characteristic of antro-oral fistula (Fig. 21–8, *right*). The shape of the opening is not altered following plastic closure of the fistula. It should be added that in some cases the defect produced by such a fistula

of long standing may not give a funnel-shaped appearance in the roentgenograms.

Alterations in bone that result from surgical procedures involving the maxillary sinus often are evident in dental roentgenograms of the maxilla, particularly those of the sinus that has been entered from an anterior or lateral approach. The most frequent change is that produced by a Caldwell-Luc operation, following which the wall of the sinus may become so thickened and sclerotic that the image of the sinus is almost completely obliterated (Fig. 21–9). This change is made more obvious when it is compared with the appearance of the undisturbed sinus on the opposite side. When this picture is encountered, a history of previous surgical treatment must be verified, however, for the picture may represent conditions other than postsurgical scarring.

22 FOREIGN BODIES IN AND ABOUT THE JAWS

Foreign bodies in the soft tissues as well as those within the jaws are frequently encountered incidental to routine dental roentgenographic examination, and most often when there are no symptoms referable to them. The soft tissues of the face probably contain more foreign bodies than do tissues elsewhere, for they are exposed, and are not covered by clothing that would be an obstruction to penetration of the skin.

The foreign bodies commonly found within the jaws are amalgam, gutta percha, cements, and dental instruments such as broaches, curets, and burs. Those in the soft tissues are more often hypodermic needles, pins, needles, shot, and a variety of metal fragments, many of them received in accidents. Some of them are placed in and about the jaws to serve a useful purpose.

The most common foreign body seen within the jaw is silver alloy or amalgam. Almost all foreign bodies of amalgam are found in the edentulous regions of the mandible. Since this alloy is fragile, the forceps or elevators that are used often fracture portions of the metal which by gravity than fall into the root socket or under the mucoperiosteum, where they invariably remain unnoticed, since in most instances these small fragments do not interfere with normal healing of the extraction wound. Those that lodge in the socket become completely surrounded by normal bone, and there is rarely evidence of infection or rarefaction of bone; therefore they are of no particular clinical significance. Permitting such fragments of alloy to remain in the

jaw following extraction is not to be encouraged, however. Postoperative roentgenograms will reveal their presence, and at a time when they can be removed with ease prior to healing of the socket. Those that do not enter the socket but lodge under the mucoperiosteum generally do not give trouble. If they are of appreciable size, the pressure of a denture on them may cause inflammation and discomfort, and indicate their removal. Often where small granular fragments of amalgam are situated under the mucoperiosteum or in the soft tissue, the overlying mucous membrane has a bluish purple color that may be a source of concern to the patient. It is

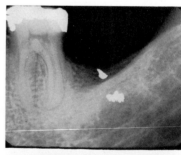

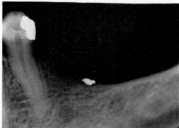

Figure 22–1 Silver alloy. *Above,* Two fragments within the bone. *Below,* A fragment in the mucoperiosteum.

often difficult to localize smaller particles of alloy, and surgical intervention rarely is indicated. Illustrations of foreign bodies of silver alloy are shown in Figure 22–1. In the upper illustration, two fragments of alloy are present and are completely embedded in and surrounded by normal bone; below, the fragment of alloy is situated in the soft tissue overlying the crest of the alveolar ridge, where it has produced an area of purplish discoloration of the mucous membrane of more than 1 cm in diameter, and also soreness and inflammation resulting from the pressure of an artifical denture that rested on it.

Examples of broken dental burs are shown in Figure 22–2, the upper one being in the maxillary region and the lower one in the mandibular molar region. Both of them no doubt were used during the extraction of teeth, for they are completely embedded in bone. The bone surrounding them appears to be normal.

Examples of broken curets are shown in Figure 22–3. The one shown above is near the crest of the alveolar ridge, with a fragment of amalgam anterior to it. They have prevented normal healing of the socket and are surrounded by inflammatory

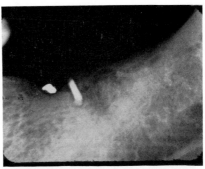
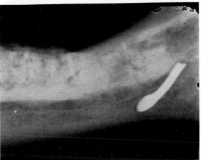

Figure 22–3 Broken dental curets situated within the bone of the mandible. The illustration above also reveals a fragment of silver alloy.

tissue, and their removal is indicated. The one shown below is completely embedded in bone and, in the absence of symptoms referable to it, there would be no indication for its removal. The presence of the beaks of broken forceps has been reported by Stanhope (1955) and others.

Dressings that contain radiopaque substances and are used in the postoperative treatment of extraction wounds are shown in Figure 22–4. The one on the left is an iodoform gauze dressing that was placed in the socket after removal of a mandibular third molar, and the roentgenogram was made 4 weeks postoperatively. The right one is a zinc oxide and eugenol dressing that was inserted for the relief of pain of a "dry socket." The roentgenogram was made 2 months after extraction of the tooth; it reveals that the dressing is being slowly forced toward the surface by the formation of new bone at the bottom of the socket. In both instances the patient had failed to return to have the dressing removed. With the present-day tendency to incorporate the medicament in

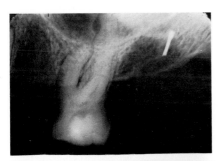
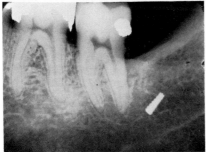

Figure 22–2 Dental burs situated within the bone of the jaws.

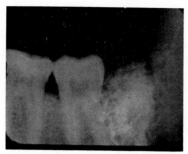
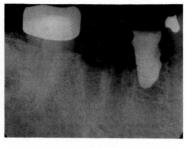

Figure 22–4   Postoperative dressings in dental sockets. *Left,* Iodoform gauze. *Right,* Zinc oxide and eugenol dressing.

a vehicle that is absorbable, such incidents are becoming much less frequent.

Lodgment of hypodermic needles in soft tissue as a result of breakage during the introduction of a local anesthetic agent occurred not uncommonly a few decades ago. As early as 1921 Blum reported 32 cases, of which 24 were associated with block of the inferior dental nerve, two with block of the infraorbital nerve, two with injections in the region of the tuberosity, and four with infiltrations. Fortunately, the breakage of needles now is relatively rare, for they are made of rustless alloys that are less fragile and bend readily so that the hazard of breakage is greatly reduced. Examples of broken hypodermic needles are shown in Figure 22–5. On the left is a needle that was broken during infiltration; in the center, one that was broken incidental to block of the inferior dental nerve; and on the right, one that remains after an injection in the region of the tuberosity. In all instances the needles had remained in the same location and without any untoward effects for periods of more than 20 years.

Sewing needles that are accidentally thrust under the skin and remain are not unusual; however, one rarely sees pins that are lodged in soft tissues, since the head prevents them from entering completely, and they are not as fragile as needles so that they are not easily broken. Roentgenograms that revealed two pins in the submaxillary duct are shown in Figure 22–6. They were made for a woman past middle age who had swelling and inflammation of the floor of the mouth. The occlusal view was made to rule out salivary calculi as a possible source of the swelling. The patient some years previously had done a great deal of sewing, and had had the habit of holding several pins in her mouth. The blunt head of the pins no doubt permitted them to enter the duct and move rapidly downward and posteriorly, for the patient was unaware of their presence. Whether the two pins had entered simultaneously or on different occasions is problematic. The lateral roentgenogram of the jaw was made at a right angle to the mandible to determine more accurately the location of the pins.

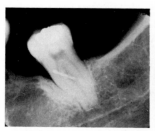
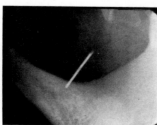
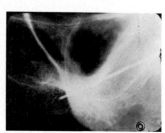

Figure 22–5   Broken hypodermic needles in various positions in relation to the jaws.

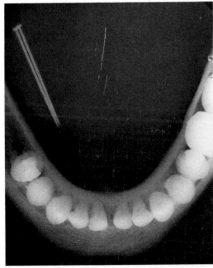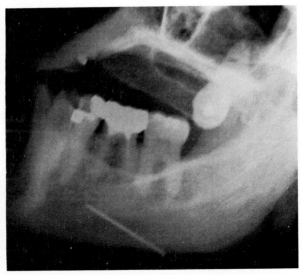

Figure 22–6   Two pins in the submaxillary duct. *Left,* Occlusal view. *Right,* Lateral view.

An occlusal view made for a man who had a firm swelling on the anterior part of the dorsal surface of the tongue revealed a radiopaque object at the site of the swelling (Fig. 22–7). On questioning, it was learned that following a blow to the face a filling from a maxillary anterior tooth had been dislodged and lost. The foreign object proved to be the missing gold inlay.

The roentgenogram in Figure 22–8 was made for a patient who had recently been injured by explosion of a box of dynamite caps. It reveals several shattered teeth and numerous small fragments of metal.

The presence of birdshot and bullets of small caliber is not an uncommon finding in the course of a routine dental roentgenographic examination. In the case of birdshot, the shape of the pellet often gives a clue as to its location. If the pellet is not altered, it is likely to be situated in the soft tissue of the face. With deeper penetration and impact with bone, the pellet is altered in shape and sometimes fragmented. Rifle bullets usually are altered in shape or shattered, since they invariably strike with sufficient velocity to impact with osseous structures. Three illustrations of birdshot pellets of varied size, unaltered shape, and situated in the soft tissues of the face are shown in Figure 22–9. A birdshot *(left)* and a rifle bullet *(right)* that have been altered in shape from impact with bone are shown in Figure 22–10.

Radiopaque foreign bodies may be introduced deliberately as a diagnostic or therapeutic measure, or for some other useful purpose. The radiopaque objects that are shown in Figure 22–11 are, *left,* iodized oil (Lipiodol) injected into the maxillary sinus as a diagnostic measure; *center,* bismuth paste injected into the soft tissue in the treatment of acute subperiosteal abscess; and *right,* radium seeds that have been implanted in the tissue lateral to the mandible as treatment for a carcinoma. Wires that were used incidental to surgical procedures are shown in Figure 22–12. In the illustration above are wires that were used in reducing a fracture of the mandible, and below are small-gauge wires that

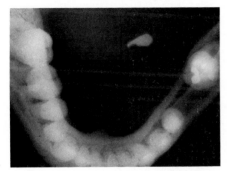

Figure 22–7   Gold inlay embedded in the tongue.

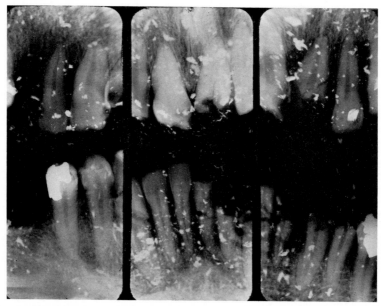

Figure 22–8 Metal fragments and shattered teeth from explosion of a box of dynamite caps.

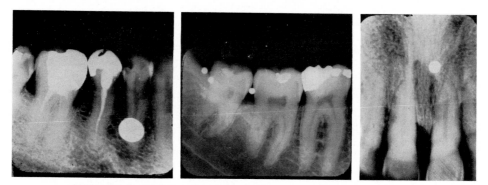

Figure 22–9 Birdshot of various sizes in the soft tissues of the face.

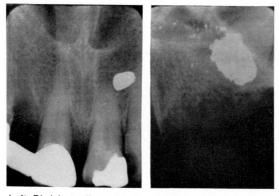

Figure 22–10 *Left,* Birdshot adjacent to bone. *Right,* Rifle bullet within the jawbone.

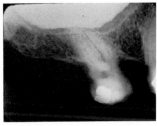
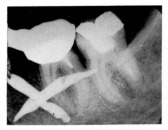
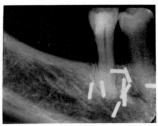

Figure 22–11   Radiopaque objects that have been introduced deliberately. *Left,* Iodized oil in the maxillary sinus. *Center,* Bismuth paste. *Right,* Radium seed implanted for treatment of malignant lesion.

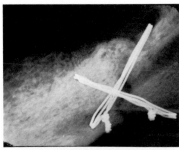

Figure 22–12   Wires used incidental to surgical procedures. *Above,* For reduction of a fracture. *Below,* For attachment of a surgical dressing to the face.

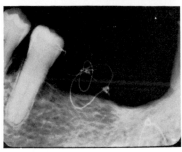

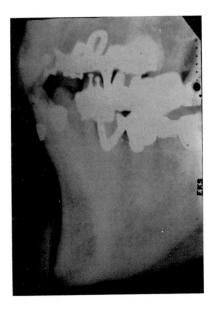

Figure 22–13   Cartilage implant over the anterior surface of the mandible.

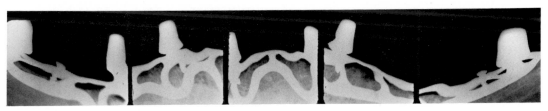

Figure 22–14   Metal framework of an implant denture.

were used to attach a postoperative surgical dressing firmly to the side of the face.

As with wires that are used in the reduction of fractures, there are other foreign bodies introduced that serve a useful purpose. Figure 22–13 shows cartilage that was implanted over the anterior surface of the mandible for cosmetic reasons. In Figure 22–14 are roentgenograms of a mandible showing the metal framework of an implant denture, beneath which the bone appears to be in good condition.

REFERENCES

Blum, T.: Foreign Bodies in and about the Jaws. Dent. Cosmos. 63:1227–1245 (Dec.) 1921.
Stanhope, E. D.: A Case of Retained Forceps Blade. Brit. Dent. J. 99:434 (Dec. 20) 1955.

ARTIFACTS

23

An artifact is a structure or appearance that is not normally present in the roentgenogram and is produced by artificial means. Artifacts may occur as a result of defects of the film and film packet, improper handling of the film packet, and accidents incidental to processing of the films.

Artifacts that result from imperfections in manufacture of the film and packet occur least frequently. Two of them are shown in Figure 23–1.

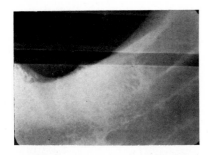

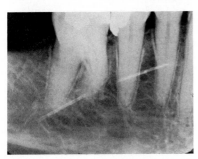

Figure 23–1 *Above,* Dark line of uniform width extending across the roentgenogram represents a double layer of emulsion. *Below,* Light line produced by a frayed margin of the lead-foil backing, which has become detached and is superimposed on the face of the film.

Improper handling of the film and packet accounts for most artifacts. The one that occurs most frequently is a double image that results from movement of the packet during the time of exposure (Fig. 23–2). Excessive bending of the film packet may produce cracking or defects in it that permit exposure to light. Such exposures cause dark markings on the developed film which may take the form of straight or crescent-shaped dark lines, or broader areas when the bending causes an opening at the margin of the packet (Fig. 23–3). As a result of excessive moistening by saliva, paper from the film packet may become attached to the film and produce white spots on it when it is developed (Fig. 23–4, *left*). Herringbone markings that appear in the roentgenogram (Fig. 23–4, *right*) represent the lead-foil backing which is embossed with this design. Such a picture is produced when the film packet has accidentally been placed in a reverse position.

Artifacts produced in the darkroom occur when water or other solutions used in processing are splattered on the film, or in

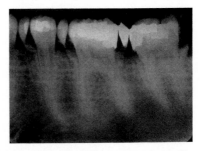

Figure 23–2 Double exposure resulting from movement of the film packet.

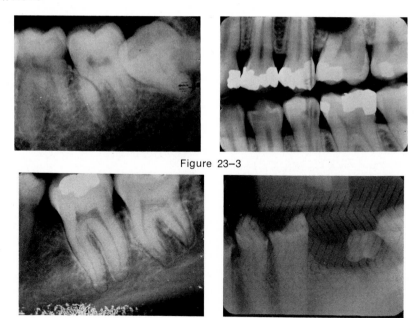

Figure 23–3

Figure 23–4

Figure 23–3 *Left,* Crescent-shaped dark line caused by bending of the film packet. *Right,* Dark vertical line across second premolars and dark area over root of maxillary first molar are caused by excessive bending of the film packet.

Figure 23–4 *Left,* White spots caused by paper from the film packet that has become attached to the film. *Right,* Herringbone markings that appear on the film when it is exposed with packet in reverse position.

some other way come in contact with it at the improper time. Some of them occur when the films come in contact with one another or with some other object. Water that is accidentally splattered on a film prior to its complete processing produces light spots in the roentgenogram that are usually round or oval, but are in some instances spindle-shaped. When superimposed on the teeth and bone they are rarely discernible; however, when superimposed on soft tissue only, they are visible. Those that appear on occlusal views made of the floor of the mouth may be mistaken for

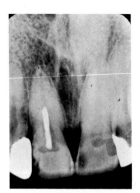

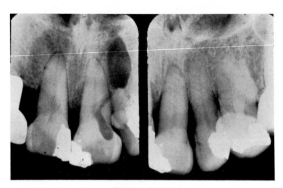

Figure 23–5

Figure 23–6

Figure 23–5 *Left,* Vertical white line on left central incisor caused by fixing solution that came in contact with the film. *Right,* Re-examination gave negative results.

Figure 23–6 *Left,* Dark markings over right incisors caused by developing solution that accidentally came in contact with the film. *Right,* Artifact does not appear in adjoining view.

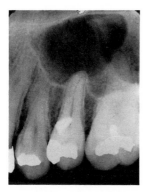

Figure 23–7 White marking on root of second premolar caused by a fragment of lead glass that was present in point of focusing tube.

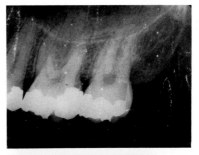

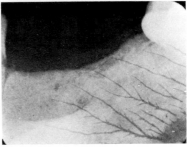

Figure 23–8 *Above,* Small white streaks caused by oil that was present in developing solution. *Below,* Tree-like dark markings produced by a small charge of static electricity.

salivary calculi. If fixing solution comes in contact with the film prior to its immersion into the developing solution, a light spot that is clearly visible appears on the developed film at the point of such contact (Fig. 23–5). When developing solution comes in contact with a portion of the film prior to its complete immersion, the area so exposed becomes overdeveloped and appears on the processed roentgenogram as an abnormally dark area (Fig. 23–6).

Foreign material may be present in a focusing cone which is sometimes used to aid in establishing correct angulation. It then appears in roentgenograms that are made when the tube is directed downward and the loose particles drop into the point of the cone (Fig. 23–7).

Foreign bodies and other foreign materials that are present in the developing solution may become attached to the film, thereby producing artifacts. The white streaks that appear in the roentgenogram shown in Figure 23–8, *above,* were caused by small particles of oil that adhered to the film as it was passed downward into a solution that accidentally had become contaminated with oil.

An artifact that is seen as a forked or tree-like marking and is produced by a small charge of electricity is shown in Figure 23–8, *below.* It is generated by friction which occurs at the time the film packet is being opened. According to Sweet and Porter (1935), it is more likely to occur during cold weather, when the atmosphere in the developing room is low in humidity owing to artificial heat.

Some artifacts may be a source of misinterpretation, since they closely resemble and may be mistaken for defects, fractures, and other pathologic conditions involving the teeth and bones. Those in which there is an associated defect in the emulsion usually can be identified by careful examination of the film under reflected light. If the identity of the artifact cannot be established, additional roentgenograms of the region should always be obtained.

REFERENCE

[Sweet, A. Porter S.]: Questions and Answers. Dental Radiography and Photography. 8:[no page numbers] March-April, 1935.

ROENTGENOGRAPHIC TECHNIQUES

DAN E. TOLMAN, D.D.S.

Two fundamental rules of roentgenography are that the central ray should pass through the region to be examined and that the film should be placed in a position so as to record the findings with the least amount of distortion. To obtain satisfactory roentgenograms of the teeth and jaws is one of the most involved and difficult technical problems in roentgenology.

The oral roentgenographic examinations to be dealt with in detail are those most frequently used in dentistry; namely the periapical, bite-wing, occlusal, and extraoral lateral jaw examinations. Other roentgenographic examinations to be discussed include panoramic, temporomandibular joint, cephalometric, sialographic, and cinefluorographic procedures. Also included are illustrations and diagrammatic representations of the lateral skull projection, Towne's projection, Water's projection, submental-vertical projection of zygomatic arches, and lateral projection of nasal bones. The technical procedures to be described are based on those employed for normal jaws. In the presence of certain traumatic, pathologic, and other abnormal conditions it is often necessary to deviate from the specified procedures.

PERIAPICAL EXAMINATION

The purpose of the intraoral periapical examination is to obtain a view of the apices of the roots of the teeth and their surrounding structures. Two basic techniques are employed at present for this examination: the paralleling technique and the bisecting-angle technique. Because of anatomic variations and limitations in some cases, certain modifications of one or the other of the two techniques may be necessary to obtain the desired view. Kilovoltage, milliamperage, and exposure time are variables that can influence the final product. These may be altered according to the type and thickness of the patient's tissues, the film selected, the equipment used, and the processing of the film (Updegrave, 1960). Because of these influencing factors and the manufacturers' specific recommendations for their products, values have not been included for these variables.

The choice of size of the film to use is largely applicable to both techniques, although greater use of a film that is narrower than the standard film may be necessary to attain true parallelism when an examination is made according to the paralleling technique. For children a film that is smaller than the standard-size film is available—one that is more easily accommodated in a small mouth.

PARALLELING TECHNIQUE

The paralleling technique also has been referred to as the "right-angle technique," the "long-cone technique," and the

"Fitzgerald technique." Dr. Gordon Fitzgerald (Fitzgerald, 1947, 1949) was largely responsible for developing the technique as a practical intraoral procedure.

The primary objective of the paralleling technique is to obtain a true roentgenographic orientation of the teeth with their supporting structures. This is accomplished by placing the film parallel to the long axis of the teeth. To attain parallelism, the film is moved away from the crowns of the teeth, while the edge of the film against the soft tissue is approximately in the same position in the palate or floor of the mouth as it is in the bisecting-angle technique. To avoid enlargement of the image as a result of moving the film away from the object, a long tube (16 to 20 inches) is employed. As a result, the rays that strike the object are the nearly parallel central rays, and the divergent rays that cause magnification and distortion of the image are largely eliminated. By employing the longer tubes and thereby increasing the target-film distance, the dose rate is decreased following the inverse square law. Therefore a greater exposure would be necessary in order that the dose to the film be adequate. The increased radiation hazard that would result from the use of a longer exposure is avoided by the use of a fast dental film.

To attain film-tooth parallelism, several methods and devices are used to aid in positioning the film packet and also to help hold it in place. A method that can be used is to place a cotton roll between the emulsion side of the film packet and the lingual surfaces of the crowns of the teeth and have the patient hold the packet in place with the thumb or index finger. Also, a long wood or plastic bite-block holder is useful in that the patient may close upon it and hold it in place after the film packet has been positioned at the desired distance from the lingual surfaces of the crowns of the teeth.

Special holders have been designed to fulfill the requirements for positioning of the film. One of them is the Rinn holder; one end of this device is used for positioning the film for the anterior region and the other is used for positioning the film for the posterior region. For the anterior region the holder is held in position by the patient; for the posterior region it can be held by the patient either with his finger or by his closing the upper and lower teeth on it.

Other film positioners include the XCP instruments, Precision x-ray instruments, Stabe bite block, and Emmenix film holder. Some of these instruments have been modified by the addition of an intraoral shield. There are situations in which these film holders are not applicable or cannot be used—for instance, in the severely traumatized patient who is unable to cooperate or the patient with systemic disease in whom intraoral roentgenographic examination is complicated. In these situations, the ability

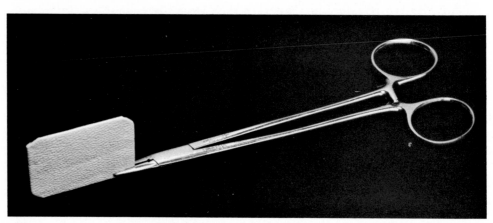

Figure I–1 Hemostat. Its small shank permits introduction and positioning of the film packet in the presence of trismus or inability to open the mouth normally. With rubber tubing slipped over its shank, it is often used for positioning and retention of the film in the paralleling technique.

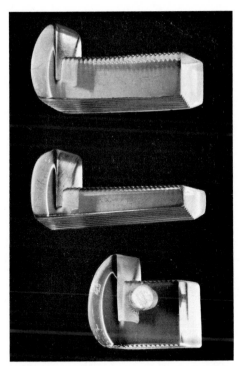

Figure I–2 Plastic bite-block film holders. *Top* and *center,* Long blocks used for retention of film for examination of the teeth of the maxilla and anterior region of the mandible. *Bottom,* Short block used for examination of the posterior teeth of the mandible. It can be used instead of the thumb and forefinger for retention of the film in all regions of the jaws with the bisecting-angle technique.

to use more than one technique may be important.

A hemostat serves as an excellent film holder, since the film packet can be held firmly between its beaks at varied positions so as to attain proper placement of the film. The hemostat may be held by the patient, or rubber tubing about 1 inch long may be slipped over the shank of the hemostat and positioned so that the patient may bite on the tubing and thereby hold the hemostat in place.

In addition to serving as an aid in attaining tooth-film parallelism, the hemostat is particularly useful for examination of patients who are unable to open the mouth sufficiently to permit the film packet to be introduced and positioned by means of the fingers or other methods. Because of the small size of the beak and shank of the hemostat, the film packet can be inserted

into the mouth and rotated into the proper position, even though the space between the upper and lower teeth is barely sufficient to accommodate the shank of the instrument. A film packet can be positioned by means of the hemostat for an examination of the anterior as well as the posterior teeth. Photographs of the hemostat, bite-block holders, and other positioners are shown in Figures I–1, I–2, I–3, and I–4.

The required vertical angulation of the x-ray tube is not excessive with the paralleling technique; therefore superimposition of the shadow of the malar bone and zygomatic process over the roots of the maxillary posterior teeth is frequently avoided. The technique permits accurate pointing of the central rays because they are directed at right angles to the surface of the film and not toward an imaginary line or plane.

Projection of the x-ray beam perpendicular to films that are placed parallel to the long axis of the teeth provides virtually correct orientation of all structures depicted. However, a central beam that is projected perpendicular to a film that must be placed a few degrees from absolute parallelism does not result in sufficient distortion of the images of the teeth and surrounding structures to affect the interpretive qualities of the roentgenogram (Waggener, 1951; Fixott and Neely, 1962). Because of variations in height and configuration of the palate, an adequate periapical view cannot always be obtained by adhering strictly to true parallelism. In this event, a projection at right angles to a film that is positioned away from the crown of the tooth but does not diverge from its long axis by more than 20° will provide a view of the periapical region, and with little longitudinal distortion (Barr and Grøn, 1959).

Some of the basic principles of the paralleling technique are illustrated in Figures I–5 to I–12. Although the standard-size film is shown in position for a projection of the maxillary anterior teeth in Figure I–5, it should be added that parallelism is more easily attained in this region by the use of the narrower films. This calls for one projection covering an area limited to the

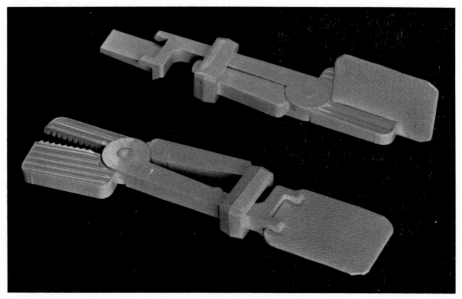

Figure I-3 Plastic film holder (Rinn). *Above,* Film positioned in holder for examination of the posterior teeth. *Below,* Film positioned in holder for examination of the anterior teeth.

central and lateral incisor and another limited to the canine region. A separate projection directed in a midsagittal plane at the central incisors will avoid superimposition of the image of the incisive canal and median suture of the palate over the apices of the roots of these teeth (Fig. I–13).

BISECTING-ANGLE TECHNIQUE

The bisecting-angle technique calls for variable angulations of the x-ray tube depending on the region of the jaws to be examined; therefore it is important that the patient's head be placed in the proper position. For an examination of the maxillary

Text continued on page 381.

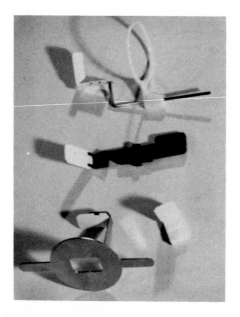

Figure I-4 Convenient film positioners for the paralleling technique include the XCP instruments. Precision x-ray instruments, Stable bite block, and Emmenix film holder. (Reproduced with permission from O'Grady, C. S. and Reynolds, R. L.: Paralleling Technic with a Short Cone: Shortcomings of This Procedure. Dent. Radiogr. Photogr. *46*:15–19, 1973.)

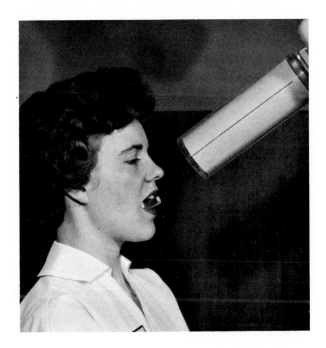

PARALLELING TECHNIQUE

Upper incisor region

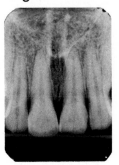

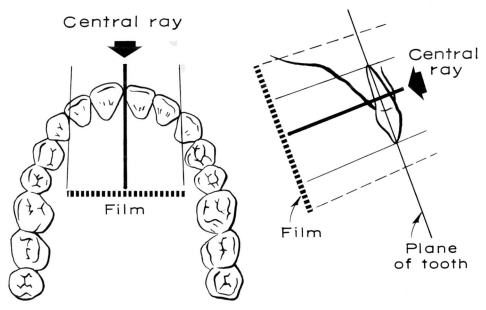

Central ray

Film

Central ray

Film

Plane of tooth

Figure I–5 To obtain a true roentgenographic orientation of the teeth with their supporting structures, the film is moved away from the crowns of the teeth, as shown in Figures I–5 through I–12. It is placed against the soft tissue and positioned as closely as possible to the long axis of the teeth. The central ray is directed at right angles, or perpendicular, to the surface of the film. A long tube (16 to 20 inches) and fast dental film are used.

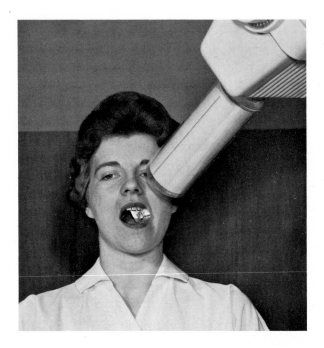

PARALLELING TECHNIQUE

Upper canine region

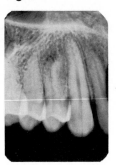

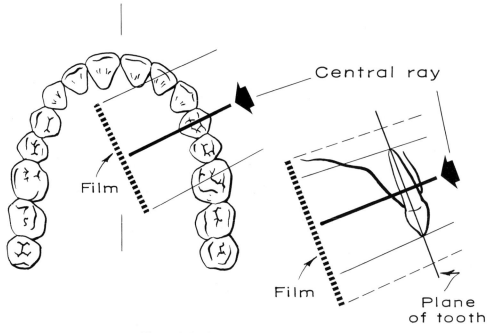

Central ray

Film

Film

Plane of tooth

Figure I–6 See legend for Figure I–5.

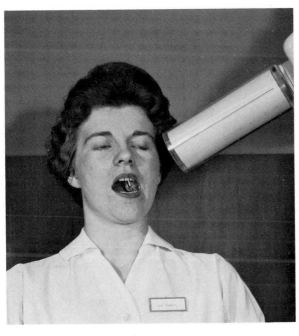

PARALLELING TECHNIQUE

Upper premolar-molar region

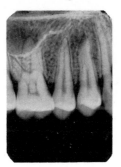

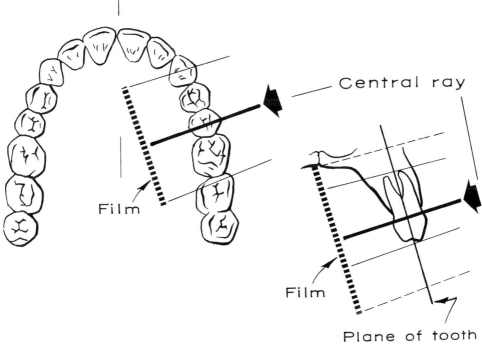

Central ray

Film

Film

Plane of tooth

Figure I–7 See legend for Figure I–5.

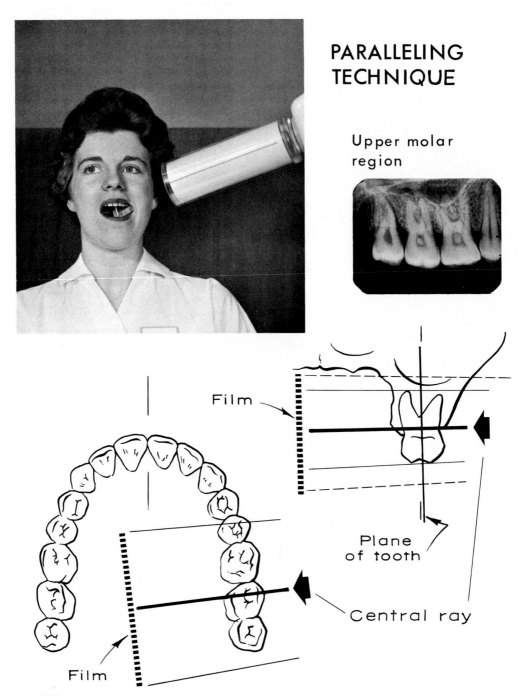

PARALLELING TECHNIQUE

Upper molar region

Film

Plane of tooth

Central ray

Film

Figure I–8 See legend for Figure I–5.

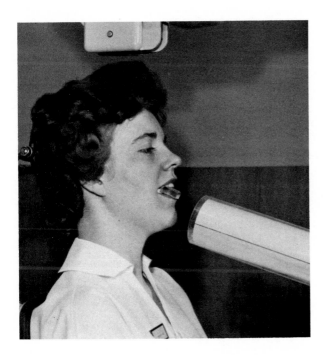

PARALLELING TECHNIQUE

Lower incisor region

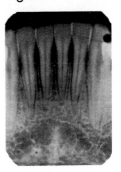

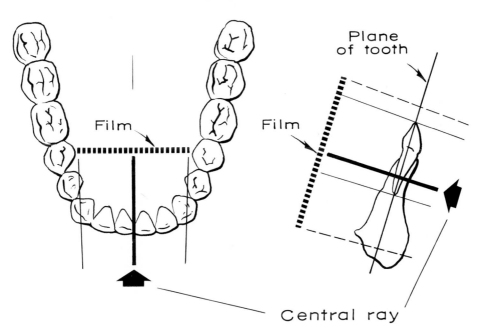

Figure I–9   See legend for Figure I–5.

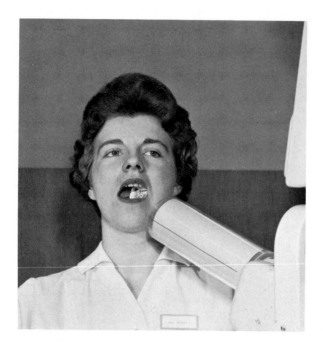

PARALLELING TECHNIQUE

Lower canine region

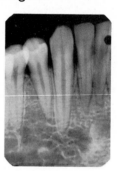

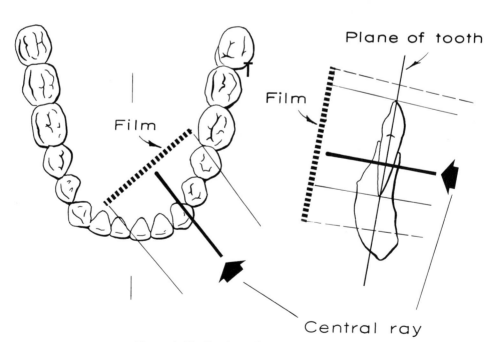

Figure I–10 See legend for Figure I–5.

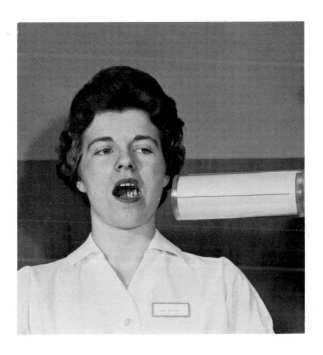

PARALLELING TECHNIQUE

Lower premolar-molar region

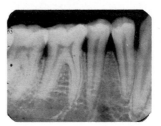

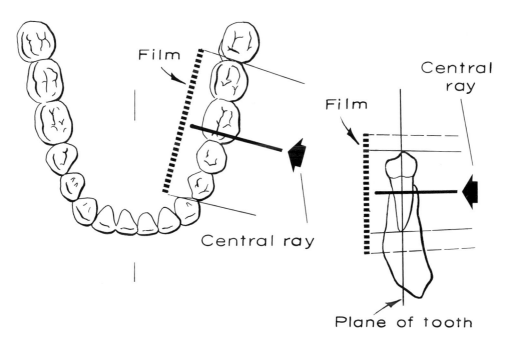

Figure I–11 See legend for Figure I–5.

PARALLELING TECHNIQUE

Lower molar region

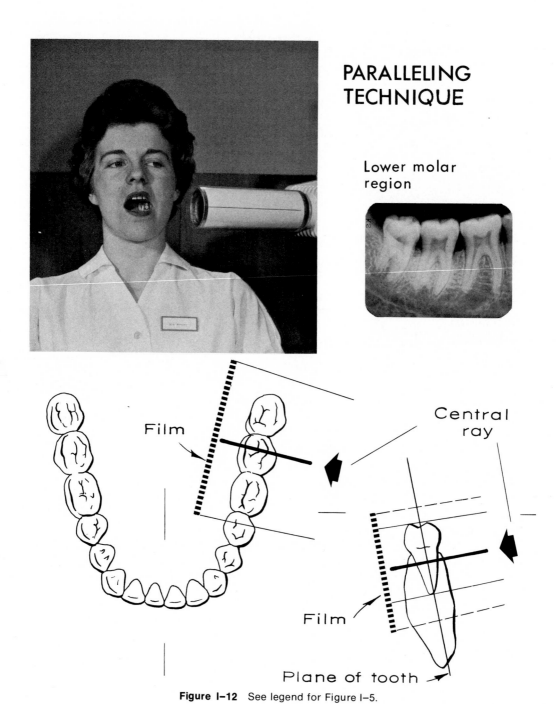

Figure I–12 See legend for Figure I–5.

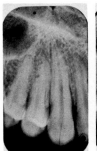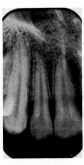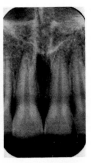

Figure I–13 Views of the maxillary anterior teeth obtained by the use of narrow film. *Left*, Canine projection. *Center*, Central-lateral incisor projection. *Right*, Central incisor projection.

regions the head should be positioned in the headrest so that the plane of occlusion is parallel to the plane of the floor of the room, and the sagittal plane is perpendicular to the plane of the floor. For the mandibular regions the head must be tilted directly backward to a position in which the plane of occlusion is parallel to the plane of the floor when the mouth is opened sufficiently to accommodate the forefinger of the patient or a bite-block film holder.

In the bisecting-angle technique the film is positioned in the mouth so as to contact the teeth and the soft tissues over their supporting structures. Although a film so positioned is close to the coronal portion of the tooth, it is at some distance from the apices of the roots because of the curvature of the palate and muscles attached to the lingual surface of the mandible. The film and the long axis of the tooth then form an angle, and an x-ray beam directed perpendicular to either the film or the long axis of the tooth will produce a markedly distorted image on the roentgenogram. To avoid distortions in the length of the image of the tooth, the bisecting-angle technique employs a geometric principle whereby the beam of radiation is directed at right angles to an imaginary line or plane that bisects the angle formed by the film and the long axis of the tooth. Since the ray passes through the tooth obliquely, distortion of the image is not completely eliminated.

The horizontal positioning of the x-ray tube in relation to the sagittal plane cannot be predetermined because of variations in the form and contour of the dental arch from one individual to another. A rule to follow is to direct the ray so that it will pass directly through the interproximal spaces of the teeth to be examined and thereby avoid overlapping or superimposition of the structures of the teeth on one another.

In positioning the x-ray tube at the proper vertical angle in relation to the horizontal plane, specific angles have been recommended for each region of the jaws, and these apply whether the thumb-and-forefinger method or the short bite-block film holder is used for film retention. Those who have described the technique are not all in complete accord as to the specific angles that should be used, and those recommended may vary a great deal, particularly in the anterior regions. Whichever recommendation is chosen, the student should adhere to the prescribed angle as a point from which to begin. It soon will become obvious that it is often necessary to deviate from the recommended angle in order to obtain a satisfactory roentgenogram. Most such deviations become necessary because of the wide anatomic variations of the palate from person to person. Where the vault of the palate is low the angle must be increased, and when the vault is higher than usual the angle must be decreased. The experienced person becomes very competent in noting and estimating the degree of divergence of the film from the long axis of the teeth and quickly arrives at the most favorable vertical angulation of the x-ray tube.

The position of the films and the angles that are recommended for each region of the jaws in a 14-film periapical examination are illustrated by photographs, roentgenograms, and drawings in Figures I–14 to I–21. The vertical angles suggested can be only approximate, but do serve as a point from which to begin the positioning of the x-ray tube. No less than 14 films should be used for a complete periapical examination, and a larger number may be not only desirable but also mandatory in some cases.

The long cone with the extended
Text continued on page 390.

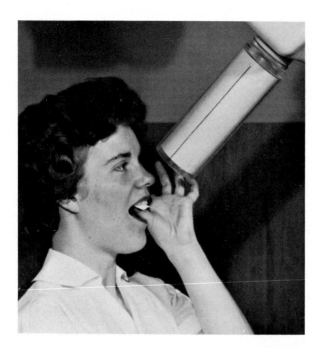

BISECTING–ANGLE TECHNIQUE

Upper incisor region

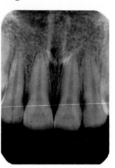

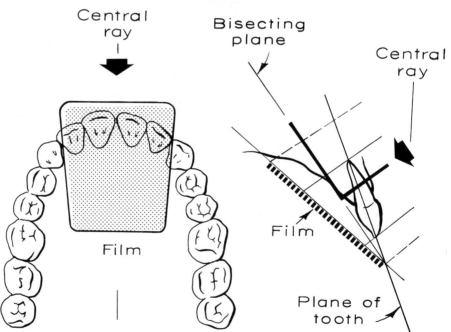

Figure I–14 For maxillary regions, the patient's head is positioned so that the plane of occlusion is parallel to the floor and the sagittal plane is perpendicular to the floor. The film is placed in contact with the crowns of the teeth and the soft tissues over their supporting structures. The central ray is directed at right angles to an imaginary line or plane which bisects the angle formed by the plane of the film and the long axis of the teeth, as shown in Figures I–14 through I–17.

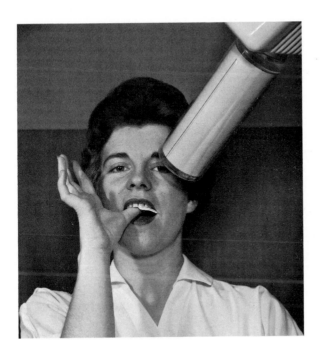

BISECTING-ANGLE TECHNIQUE

Upper canine region

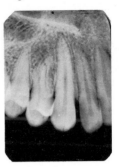

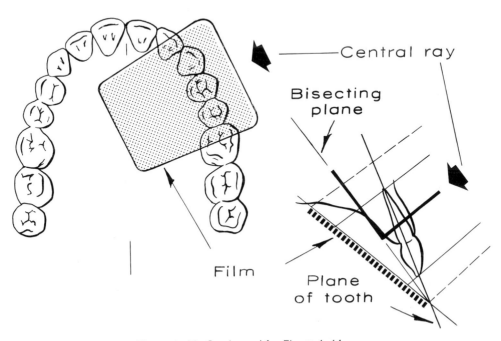

Central ray

Bisecting plane

Plane of tooth

Film

Figure 1–15 See legend for Figure 1–14.

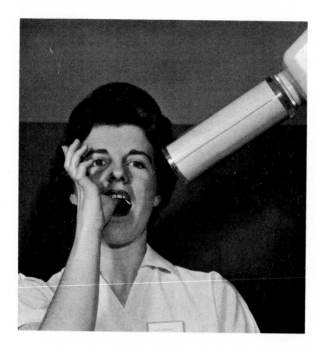

BISECTING–ANGLE TECHNIQUE

Upper premolar-molar region

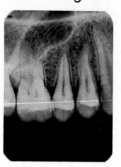

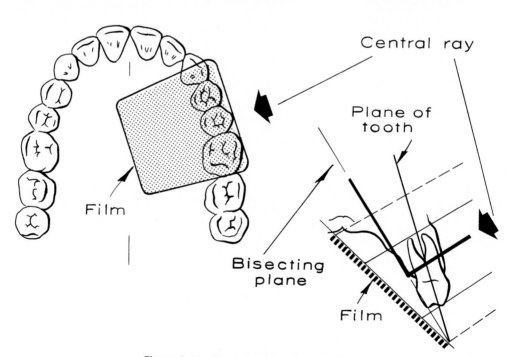

Figure I–16   See legend for Figure I–14.

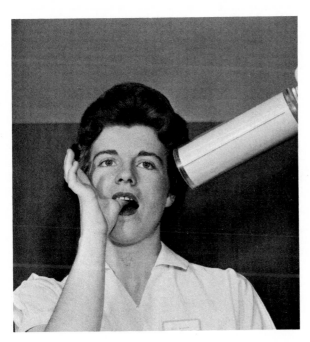

BISECTING–ANGLE TECHNIQUE

Upper molar region

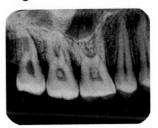

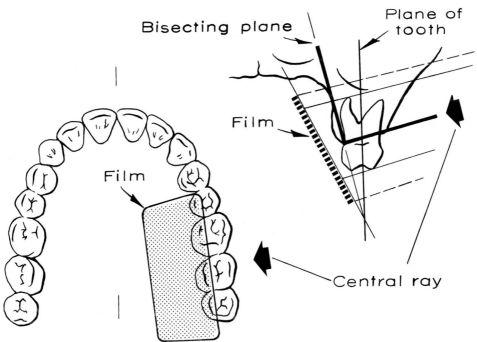

Figure I–17 See legend for Figure I–14.

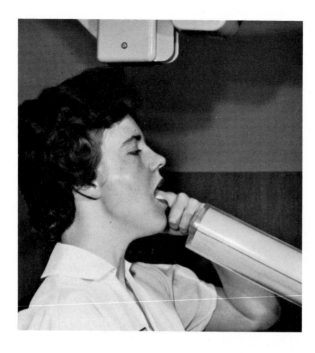

BISECTING–ANGLE TECHNIQUE

Lower incisor region

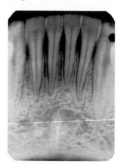

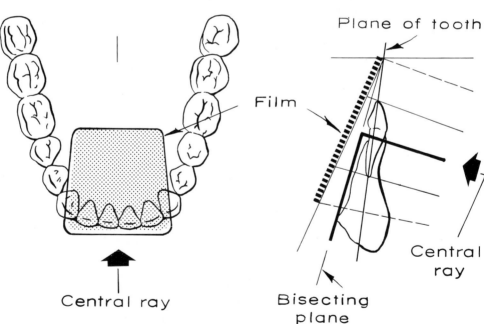

Figure I–18 For mandibular regions, the patient's head must be tilted backward until the plane of occlusion is parallel to the floor when the mouth is opened to accommodate digital retention of the film or bite-block film holder. The sagittal plane must be perpendicular to the floor. The film is placed in contact with the crowns of the teeth and the soft tissues. The central ray is directed at right angles to an imaginary line or plane which bisects the angle formed by the plane of the film and the long axis of the teeth, as shown in Figures I–18 through I–21.

BISECTING–ANGLE TECHNIQUE

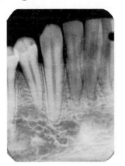

Lower canine region

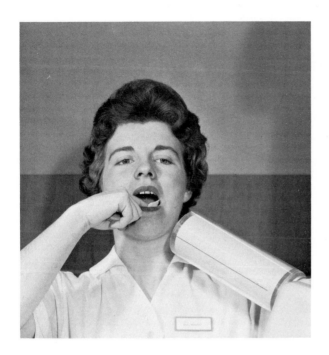

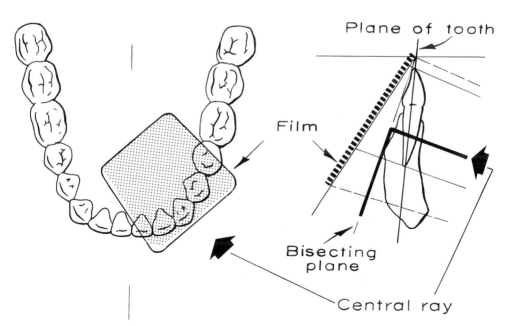

Plane of tooth

Film

Bisecting plane

Central ray

Figure 1–19 See legend for Figure 1–18.

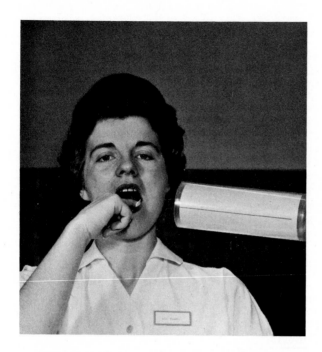

BISECTING– ANGLE TECHNIQUE

Lower premolar- molar region

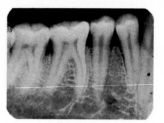

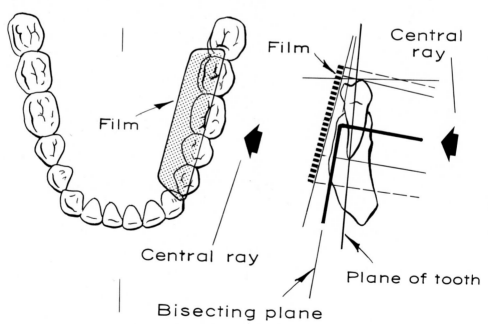

Figure I–20 See legend for Figure 1–18.

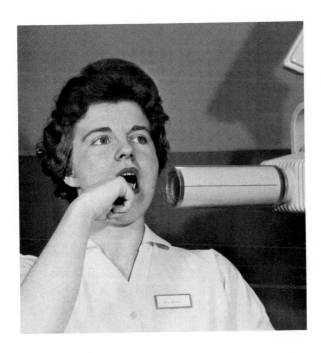

BISECTING–ANGLE TECHNIQUE

Lower molar region

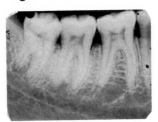

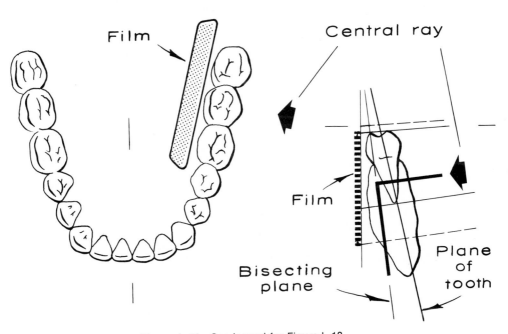

Film

Central ray

Film

Bisecting plane

Plane of tooth

Figure I–21   See legend for Figure I–18.

target-film distance also can be used for the bisecting-angle technique, and in that event the use of a fast film is required. An advantage of the long cone is that it permits more accurate pointing of the ray than does a short cone.

BITE-WING FILM EXAMINATION

The greatest value of the bite-wing film examination introduced by Raper (1925) is that it provides a view for detection of carious lesions of the proximal surfaces of the teeth, many of which cannot be detected by means of an explorer. It also reveals the size of the pulp chamber and the extent of penetration of proximal caries in relation to it. It provides a good view of the septal alveolar crest, and it is a means of determining the presence or absence of destructive changes that may involve the crest.

For the bite-wing film examination, the head of the patient is positioned in the headrest of the chair so that the plane of occlusion is parallel to the floor. The film, which has a tab attached to it from the emulsion side, is placed in the mouth with the tab extending outward between the upper and lower teeth. The patient is then instructed to close slowly while the film is being held parallel to the long axis of the teeth by means of the tab. For an examination of the posterior region the upper and lower teeth are closed firmly on the tab in centeric occlusion, and for the anterior region the tab is held between the incisal edges of the upper and lower teeth when they are in an end-to-end position. The central ray is directed at the point of contact of the upper and lower teeth, parallel to the proximal surfaces of the teeth, and at an angle of from 5 to 10° above the horizontal plane.

For the posterior teeth it is desirable to obtain two views on each side: one in which the film is placed posteriorly to include the interproximal space between the second and third molars, and the other in which it is placed far enough anteriorly to include the distal surfaces of the canines

(Fig. I–22). Such a bite-wing film examination of the posterior teeth should be included when a routine periapical examination is made, and space should be provided for the roentgenograms so that they can be inserted on the same film mount. For the anterior teeth, three views are necessary: one in which the film is positioned to the left of the midline to include the interproximal space between the cuspid and lateral incisor; one positioned in the midline; and the third positioned to the right of the midline to include the space between the cuspid and lateral incisor (Fig. I–23).

Often, routine periapical examination may not be indicated or needed for patients who have been under the surveillance of the dentist and have had such an examination at some time previously. In this event, a bite-wing film examination will suffice as a periodic check for the detection of new caries that may have developed. A total of seven exposures will provide a view of the proximal surfaces of all the teeth present. This examination is most efficient for detection of caries, is more economical than periapical examination, and reduces the amount of radiation to which the patient is subjected. Since it provides a good view of the alveolar crest, it may be useful also as a post-treatment examination in some cases of periodontal disease.

OCCLUSAL ROENTGENOGRAPHY

Of the films used to supplement the standard dental film, the occlusal film is perhaps the most helpful to the dentist. The occlusal film is about 3 by 2¼ inches in size and is packaged similarly to the standard intraoral dental film. It provides a more extensive view of the maxilla and mandible than does the standard film. Since it provides views that are at approximately right angles to those obtained by the standard intraoral dental and the extraoral lateral jaw films, it is an invaluable aid in determining the buccolingual extension of pathologic conditions, and provides additional information as to the extent and displacement of fractures involving the

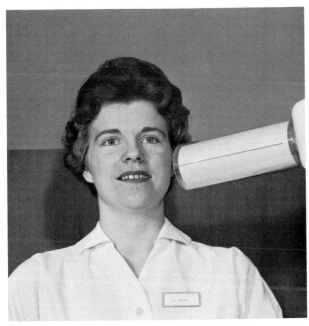

BITE-WING
FILM TECHNIQUE

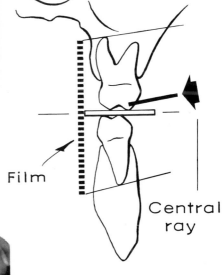

Film

Central
ray

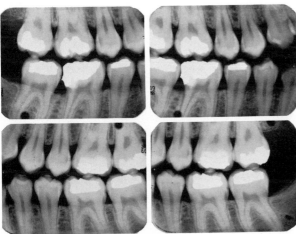

Figure I–22 The patient's head is positioned so that the plane of occlusion is parallel to the floor. The central ray is directed at the point of contact of the upper and lower teeth and parallel to their proximal surfaces, with the tube forming an angle of from 5 to 10° above the horizontal plane. For posterior teeth it is desirable to obtain two views on each side: one in which the film is placed posteriorly to include the interproximal space between the second and third molars, and the other far enough anteriorly to include the distal surfaces of the canines.

Figure I–23 Bite-wing film examination of the anterior teeth.

maxilla and mandible. It also is an aid in localizing foreign bodies, unerupted teeth, retained roots, and calculi in the submaxillary and sublingual salivary glands and ducts. Although a standard technique is recommended and should be adhered to in a routine examination, it often may be necessary to diverge from the normal placement of the film and the angulation of the central ray in order to obtain a desirable topographic view of a specific region or condition.

OCCLUSAL VIEWS OF THE MANDIBLE AND CONTIGUOUS STRUCTURES

For views of the mandible the film is placed in the mouth with the emulsion side of the film facing the floor of the mouth. It is moved backward until it comes in contact with the soft tissues of the retromolar region, and the patient is instructed to bite gently on the film to hold it in place. For the edentulous jaw, the film can be held in

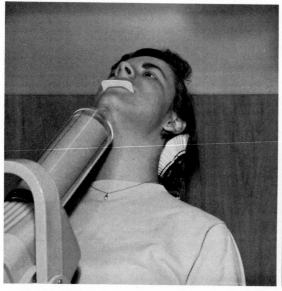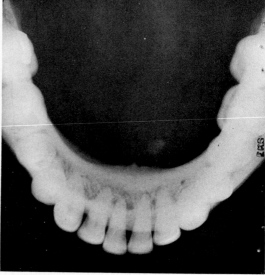

Figure I–24 *Left,* Position of head, film, and tube for examination of the anterior region of the mandible and the floor of the mouth. *Right,* Roentgenogram obtained according to this technique, which reveals a small stone in the salivary duct. Exposure factors: 80 kVp; 15 mA; target-film distance, 16 inches; and 5/10 second.

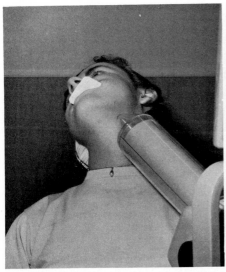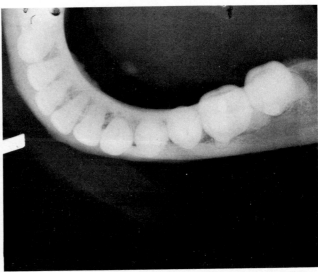

Figure I–25 *Left,* Position of head, film, and tube for examination of the posterior teeth and posterior portion of the mandible. *Right,* Roentgenogram made according to this technique. Exposure factors: 80 kVp; 15 mA; target-film distance, 16 inches; and 5/10 second.

place by the patient's forefingers for the lower jaws and thumbs for the upper jaws.

To obtain a view of the major portion of the floor of the mouth and the mandible, the head of the patient is tilted directly backward. The central ray is directed from a point in the midline beneath the chin parallel to the sagittal plane and perpendicular to the surface of the film (Fig. I–24, *left*). The roentgenogram obtained by this method provides a satisfactory view of the floor of the mouth and the anterior portion of the mandible. There is, however, an overlapping of the images of the posterior teeth (Fig. I–24, *right*).

To obtain a more satisfactory view of the posterior teeth and posterior portion of the mandible, the film is positioned laterally so that it is centered over the side of the mandible that is to be examined. The head is tilted away from the side to be examined, and the central ray is directed parallel to the long axis of the second premolar tooth (Fig. I–25, *left*). A roentgenogram obtained by this technique is shown in Figure I–25, *right*. Another way to obtain more of the posterior area is to position the occlusal film with the length across the posterior teeth.

The occlusal film is especially valuable for detecting and localizing calculi in the submaxillary and sublingual glands and ducts, since many of them are not revealed by the extraoral examination. Calculi situated in the anterior portion of the floor of the mouth are readily demonstrated by the methods described, but those situated near or in the submaxillary gland require special techniques for demonstration. For one of the methods, the film is placed laterally toward the side to be examined and held in place between the teeth. The head is tilted backward and toward the opposite side. The x-ray tube is positioned opposite the posterior border of the submaxillary gland, and the central ray is directed parallel to the lingual surface of the mandible upward and forward toward the nose (Fig. I–26, *left*). A roentgenogram that revealed a stone by this method is shown in Figure I–26, *right*.

Another method that has been very successful in demonstrating stones in the posterior region of the floor of the mouth is shown in Figure I–27, *left*. In this instance, the head of the patient is tilted forward and toward the opposite side, and the x-ray tube is positioned from over the shoulder of the patient. The central rays are then directed parallel to the lingual surface of the mandible from a point near the angle of

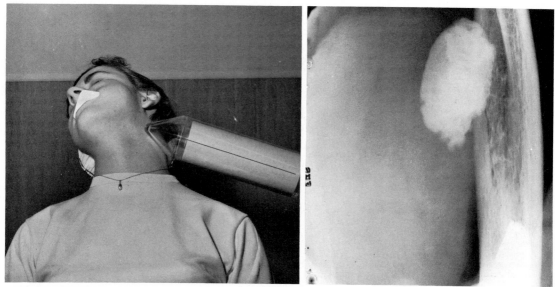

Figure I–26 *Left,* Position of head, film, and tube for examination to determine the presence or absence of calculi in the salivary glands and ducts. *Right,* Roentgenogram made according to this technique, which reveals calculus in the submaxillary gland. Exposure factors: 80 kVp; 15 mA; target-film distance, 20 inches; and 1 second. (Reproduced with permission from Levy, D. M., ReMine, W. H., and Devine, K. D.: Salivary Gland Calculi: Pain, Swelling Associated with Eating. J.A.M.A. *181*:1115–1119 [Sept. 29] 1962.)

the mandible and toward the nose. A roentgenogram made according to this technique is shown in Figure I–27, *center.*

OCCLUSAL VIEWS OF THE MAXILLA

In obtaining views of the maxilla, the head of the patient is placed in a vertical position and the film is held between the teeth with the emulsion side of the film toward the palate. The central ray is directed at the middle of the palate between the molar teeth with the point of the x-ray tube in the midline near the bridge of the nose (Fig. I–28, *left*). The roentgenogram made employing this technique gives a satisfactory view of the palate, but there

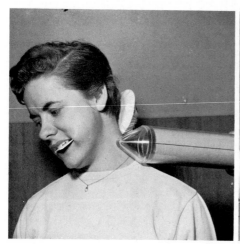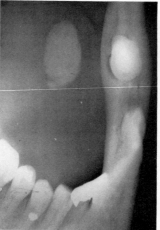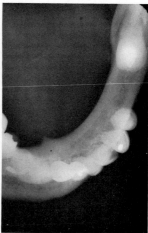

Figure I–27 *Left,* Technique for detecting calculi in the submaxillary gland and duct with the x-ray tube positioned over the shoulder of the patient. *Center,* Roentgenogram made according to this technique, which reveals a stone. *Right,* A projection that did not include a sufficient area of the floor of the mouth to disclose the stone. Exposure factors: 80 kVp; 15 mA; target-film distance, 20 inches; and 1 second.

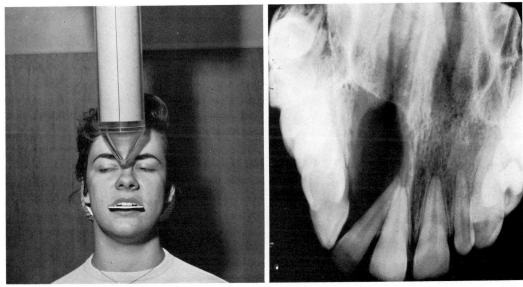

Figure I–28 *Left,* Position of head, film, and tube for examination of the palate and the anterior region of the maxilla. *Right,* Roentgenogram made according to this technique, which reveals a cyst in the anterior region of the jaw. Exposure factors: 80 kVp; 15 mA; target-film distance, 20 inches; and 8/10 second.

is marked overlapping of the posterior teeth (Fig. I–28, *right*). To obtain a true occlusal view, the tube is centered over the vertex so that the central ray is perpendicular to the surface of the film and directed to the midline of the palate between the molar teeth. Since the rays must pass through several opaque structures before reaching the teeth and palate, there may be considerable fogging of the film. To overcome this, the use of an occlusal cassette with intensifying screens will give a much better result.

An exposure that provides a view of

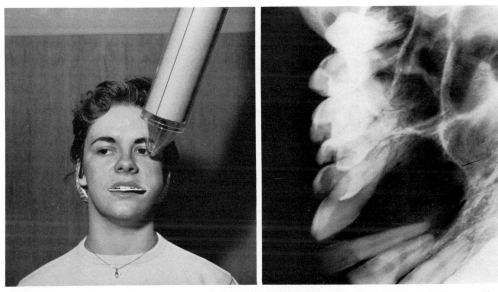

Figure I–29 *Left,* Position of film and tube for obtaining a unilateral view of the maxilla. *Right,* Roentgenogram made according to this technique. It provides a good view of the floor of the maxillary sinus and the molar teeth. Exposure factors: 80 kVp; 15 mA; target-film distance, 20 inches; and 8/10 second.

one side of the upper jaw from the incisor to the third molar region is made by moving the film laterally toward the side to be examined. The central ray is directed through the premolar region at a vertical angle of about 65° to the surface of the film (Fig. I–29, *left*). A roentgenogram made according to this technique is shown in Figure I–29, *right*.

Although the occlusal film is made primarily for use as an intraoral film, it may, because of its size, be conveniently used on occasion as an extraoral film (Silha, 1965). If the anterior portion of the mandible is to be examined, the film is held against the inferior border of the mandible beneath the chin. The central ray is directed in a sagittal plane at the midline of the chin and at an angle of about 75° to the occlusal plane (Fig. I–30, *above*). The roentgenogram obtained by this method

has been very useful in observing fractures of the anterior part of the mandible (Fig. I–30, *below*).

It also has been used as an extraoral film in the detection of calculi in the duct of the parotid gland. The film is positioned posterior to and at right angles to the surface of the cheek of the patient. The central beam is directed through the cheek perpendicular to the surface of the film, and the exposure is made when the patient is blowing the cheek outward (Fig. I–31, *left*). A roentgenogram made according to this method is shown in Figure I–31, *right*.

LATERAL JAW ROENTGENOGRAPHY

In examination of the mandible by means of the extraoral film, four views are used, each depending on the particular

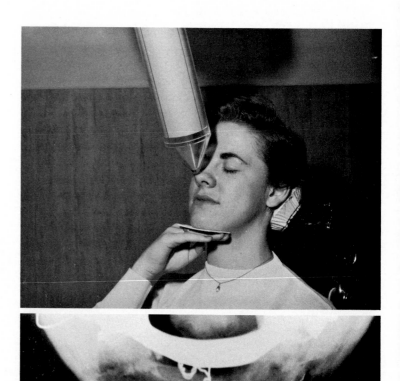

Figure I–30 *Above*, Position of film and tube when occlusal film is used extraorally for examination of the anterior region of the mandible. *Below*, Roentgenogram made according to this technique, which was used to observe progress of healing of a fracture in that region. Exposure factors: 80 kVp; 15 mA; target-film distance, 20 inches; and 1 second.

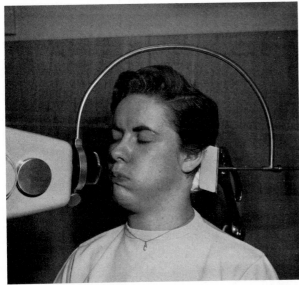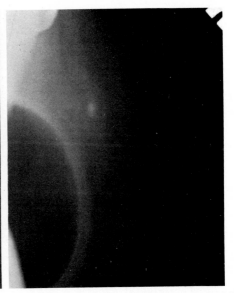

Figure I–31 *Left,* Position of film and tube when occlusal film is used extraorally for detection of calculi in the duct of the parotid gland. *Right,* Roentgenogram made according to this technique, which reveals a small calcareous deposit in the duct. Exposure factors: 70 kVp; 15 mA; target-film distance, 16 inches; and 1 second. (Reproduced with permission from Levy, D. M., ReMine, W. H., and Devine, K. D.: Salivary Gland Calculi: Pain, Swelling Associated with Eating. J.A.M.A. *181*:1115–1119 [Sept. 29] 1962.)

region of the jaw to be examined. These are (1) a view of the anterior region, (2) a view of the premolar-molar region, (3) a view of the mandibular ramus, and (4) a profile view, which is of aid in localizing broken needles, foreign bodies, and calculi in the salivary ducts. For these exposures the film is positioned with its border parallel to the inferior border of the mandible and at least 1 inch below it, and the film is centered over the region to be examined.

For a view of the anterior portion of

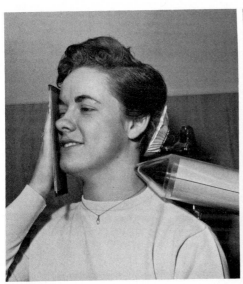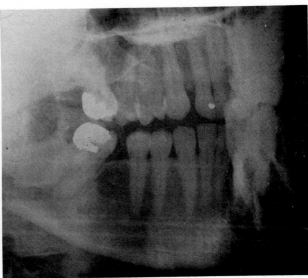

Figure I–32 *Left,* Position of film and x-ray tube for examination of the anterior region of one side of the mandible. *Right,* Roentgenogram made according to this technique. Exposure factors: 80 kVp; 15 mA; target-film distance, 23 inches; and 1/10 second, with intensifying screen.

the mandible, the head is flexed toward the side to be examined. The film is centered on the canine region and positioned on the face so that its anterior portion comes in contact with the nose and chin. The central ray is directed from a point below the angle of the mandible on the opposite side to the canine region of the side being examined, and perpendicular to the sagittal plane of the film (Fig. I–32, *left*). A roentgenogram made from this position will provide a satisfactory view of the incisor, canine, and premolar regions of the side examined (Fig. I–32, *right*).

For an examination of the premolar-molar region of the mandible, the film is centered on the first molar and parallel to the alignment of the posterior teeth, or parallel to the crest of the alveolar ridge if the jaw is edentulous. The central ray is directed from a point below the inferior border of the mandible on the opposite side to the first molar region of the side to be examined. The direction of the tube should be at right angles to the sagittal plane of the film (Fig. I–33, *left*). A roentgenogram made according to this technique is shown in Figure I–33, *right*.

To obtain views of the mandibular ramus, the film is positioned far enough posteriorly to include the condyle. To avoid superimposition of the cervical spine, the mandible is protruded and moved away from the side to be examined. The central ray is directed upward and posteriorly toward the center of the ramus from a point below the inferior border of the mandible of the opposite side and directly below the molar region (Fig. I–34, *left*). A roentgenogram made according to this technique is shown in Figure I–34, *right*.

The profile view is used chiefly as an aid in localizing foreign bodies, stones, and other radiopaque bodies in relation to the normal structures. With the head of the patient held erect, the film is placed against the face and is held perpendicular to the floor and parallel to the sagittal plane. The object is to superimpose one side of the jaw upon the other. Therefore, the central ray is directed so that it is perpendicular to the surface of the film. Figure I–35, *left*, shows the position of the tube for localization of an object in relation to the level of the mandible. A roentgenogram made by this technique and revealing a stone in the submaxillary gland is shown in Figure I–35,

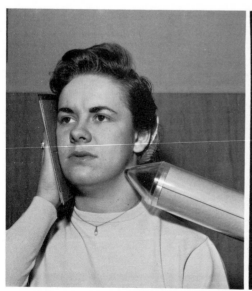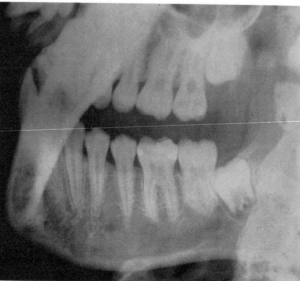

Figure I–33 *Left,* Position of film and x-ray tube for examination of the premolar-molar region of the mandible. *Right,* Roentgenogram made according to this technique. Exposure factors: 80 kVp; 15 mA; target-film distance, 23 inches; and 1/10 second, with intensifying screen.

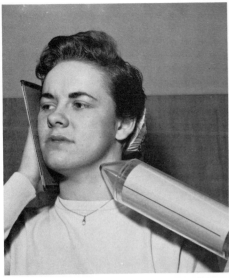
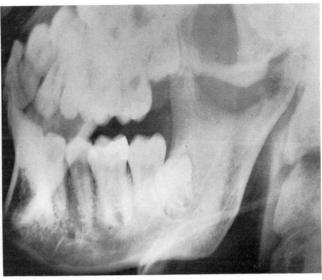

Figure I–34 *Left,* Position of film and tube for examination of the mandibular ramus. *Right,* Roentgenogram made according to this technique. Exposure factors: 80 kVp; 15 mA; target-film distance, 23 inches; and 1/10 second, with intensifying screen.

right. A similar true lateral view of the maxilla is often of value in locating highly misplaced teeth and other opaque bodies. In this instance, the central ray is directed transversely through the maxillary first molars and perpendicular to the surface of the film.

PANORAMIC ROENTGENOGRAPHY

Panoramic roentgenography produces a survey of the entire maxillary and mandibular dentoalveolar region on a single film. The indications and application for the use of this technique include screening

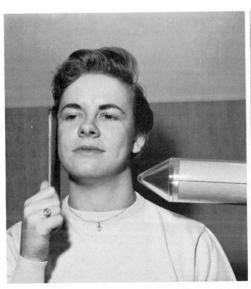
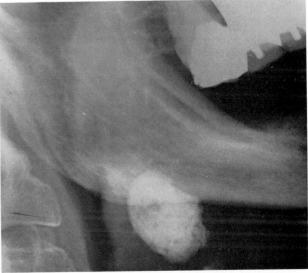

Figure I–35 *Left,* Position of film and tube as one of the projections that aid in localizing foreign bodies and broken needles in relation to the mandible. *Right,* Roentgenogram made by this method, which demonstrates a stone in the submaxillary gland. Exposure factors: 80 kVp; 15 mA; target-film distance, 23 inches; and 1/15 second, with intensifying screen.

of a large population, diagnosis of pathoses, treatment planning, evaluation of anomalies, and as one part of the follow-up evaluation in surgical or trauma cases.

Two different methods have been used to produce this survey. In one method an intraoral source of radiation is used to project the images onto a film positioned on the patient's face. In the other method both the source of radiation and the film are positioned extraorally. These methods have been described in detail by Blackman (1960), Blackman (1961), Kumpula (1961), Paatero (1961), Updegrave (1963), and Manson-Hing (1973). The second method, which utilizes the principles of curved-surface laminagraphy, has had three variations. In the most widely used variation the patient's head is stationary while the film and source of radiation (tube head) rotate around it. The patient is seated in the chair of the unit with his chin supported by the adjustable chin rest. It is important that the occlusal plane be parallel to the floor, that the lower border of the mandible be centered on the chin rest, and that the midsagittal plane be in alignment with the vertical center line of the chin support (Updegrave, 1966). A cotton roll usually is placed between the patient's incisors to prevent overlapping but may be omitted if a film with the teeth in occlusion is desired. The horizontal arm, supporting the film and the tube head, is then lowered into place (Fig. I–36).

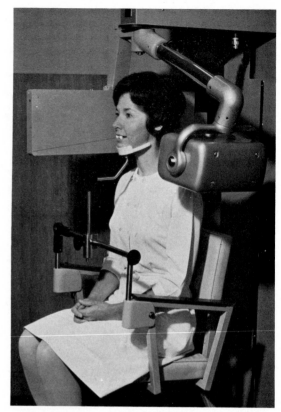

Figure I–36 Patient positioned for panoramic technique. A head holder is available to assist in the correct positioning of the patient's head.

The exposure begins posterior to the mandibular condyle, and as the film is exposed the tube head and film rotate around the patient's head automatically. At mid-

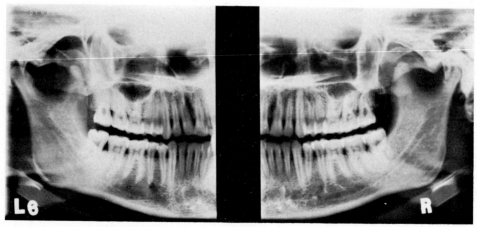

Figure I–37 Panoramic roentgenogram. Center section can be blacked out by pre-exposure of this area or covered by a film mount. Exposure factors vary with the dimensions of the individual patient.

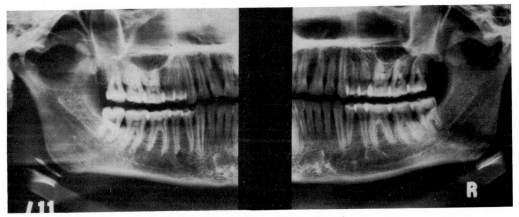

Figure I–38   Distortion. Chin tipped up.

point in the exposure the chair is shifted and the axis of rotation changed in order to place the patient's head near the film for the second half of the exposure, thus minimizing distortion. A significant change in the new Panorex machine has been the stopping of the x-ray emission while the chair is shifted, eliminating unnecessary radiation. Figure I–37 illustrates a typical panoramic film.

It is recognized that there is loss of detail and definition and that there is distortion, which is increased with incorrect positioning of the patient's head, in this type of oral roentgenography (Figs. I–38, I–39, and I–40).

Superimposition of the structures from one side upon the other and superimposition of objects outside of the sharp layer of focus can produce confusing shadows and must be taken into account when interpreting a panoramic film (Figs. I–41 and I–42).

One inadequacy is in definition of interproximal caries. However, by supplementing the panoramic film with posterior or anterior bite-wing films, if indicated, a more complete roentgenographic survey of the patient can be obtained and with less total radiation to the patient than with the standard full-mouth intraoral survey (Jerman et al., 1973).

In addition to the Panorex a variety of machines have been developed: the Panoramix, Status X, Rotagraph, Orthopantomograph, Panoramax, GE-3000, and Panex. Manson-Hing (1973) has pointed out, "In the coming years, clinical evaluations of

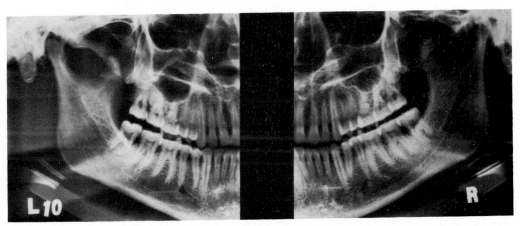

Figure I–39   Distortion. Chin tipped down.

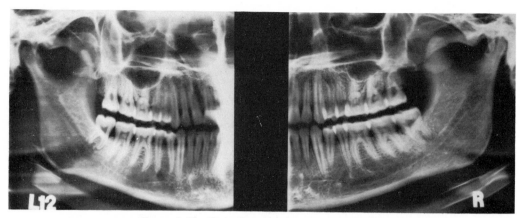

Figure I–40 Distortion. Head turned toward left.

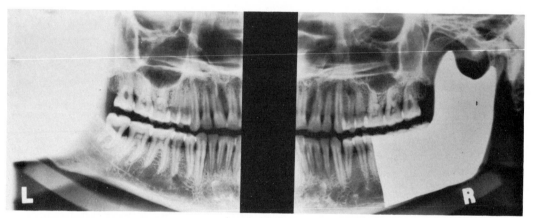

Figure I–41 Right mandible covered with metal. Note area of superimposition on the left.

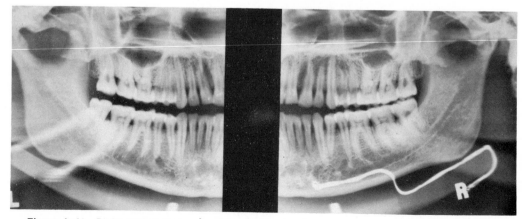

Figure I–42 Right side of chin rest outlined with wire. Note area of superimposition on the left.

these new machines should indicate their specific usefulness; also, new techniques will be developed from innovations built into these new devices."

EXAMINATION OF THE TEMPOROMANDIBULAR JOINT

There are two projections for examination of the temporomandibular joint: the anteroposterior and the lateral.

The anteroposterior projection is not used as frequently as the lateral because of the superimposition of the associated and surrounding structures. Figures I–43 and I–44 illustrate the technique for this projection.

The lateral projection described here is basically the infracranial technique with the central ray directed through the mandibular notch. It is simplified by the use of a "head bow" to facilitate angulation (Hornseth, 1954). Exposures can be made with the mouth closed and open. The

open-mouth view gives a clearer picture of the condylar head.

The procedure is to estimate first the position of the condylar head with the mouth open and closed. The center of the mandibular notch is estimated to be approximately ¾ inch anterior to the condylar head on a line drawn between the incisal edge of the maxillary central incisors and the head of the condyle. These positions may be indicated with a skin-marking pencil for reference (Fig. I–45). The head bow is then positioned with the pointer indicating the condylar head to be examined in either the open or the closed position. The source of radiation is directed through the mandibular notch from the opposite side by means of a short cone with 1 mm of aluminum filtration to protect the patient from low-penetration radiation (Fig. I–46).

As an aid to the clinician a calibrated bite block (Fig. I–47) is placed between the incisal edges of the patient's teeth during the exposure in the open position. The amount of opening is then indicated on the

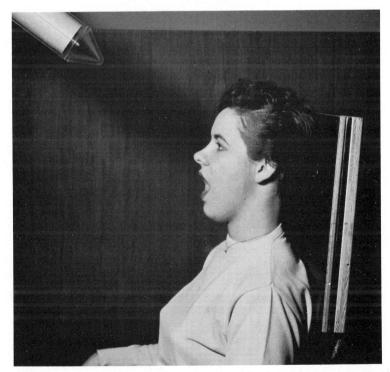

Figure I–43 Patient positioned for anteroposterior projection of temporomandibular joint.

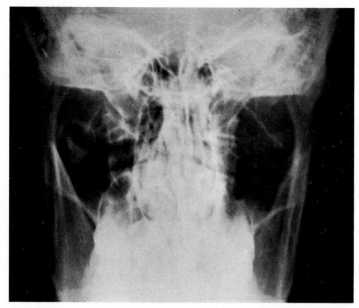

Figure I–44 Anteroposterior projection of temporomandibular joint. Exposure factors: 80 kVp; 10 mA; target-film distance, 27 inches; and 1 second, with intensifying screen.

Figure I–45 Estimated location of condylar head in open and closed positions and outline of mandibular notch.

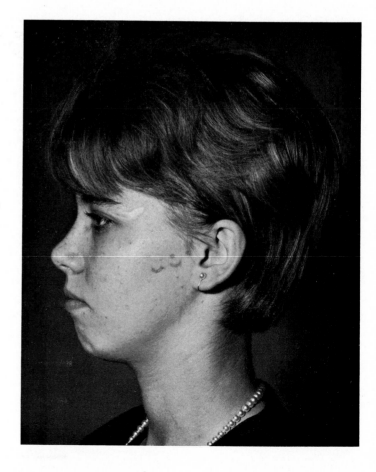

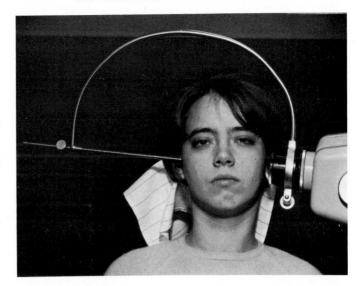

Figure I–46 Position of tube head and head bow for closed projection. Exposure factors: 80 kVp; 15 mA; target-film distance, 12 to 14 inches; and 1/12 second, with intensifying screen.

film along with other identifying information for future reference (Fig. I–48). Figure 19–1 illustrates temporomandibular films of the mouth in the open and the closed position.

Tomograms may be used for a more detailed examination of the temporomandibular joint. In tomography a specified region of the body is examined in layers by diffusion of all structures except the particular plane to be examined. The diffusion is done by a coordinated movement of the tube, grid, and film about the specific plane to be shown. Figure 19–5 illustrates tomograms of the temporomandibular joint.

CEPHALOMETRIC ROENTGENOGRAPHY

Cephalometric roentgenograms are lateral and posteroanterior head films taken while the patient's head is stabilized. The head may be supported in either calibrated (cephalometer or craniometer) or uncalibrated (cephalostat or craniostat) instruments.

The tube head is usually fixed at a distance of 5 feet from the patient. If only one x-ray tube is used, the patient and the film-head holder must be rotated to secure both views. The use of two x-ray tubes eliminates this rotation (Fig. I–49).

For the lateral view the patient is seated with the right side facing the x-ray tube. The chair is raised until the ear rods can be placed in the auditory canals. Thus positioned the ear rods prevent rotation of the head in horizontal plane. The head is then rotated vertically until the left infraorbital ridge is parallel to the ear rods and

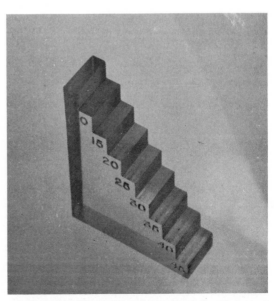

Figure I–47 Calibrated bite block for placement between incisal edges. (Reproduced with permission from Tolman, D. E. and Eppard, D. G.: An Aid to the Roentgenographic Examination of the Temporomandibular Joint. Am. J. Roentgenol. *103*:674 [July] 1968.)

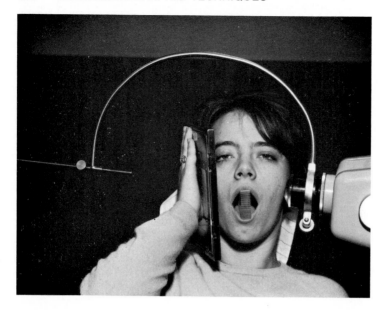

Figure I–48 Position of tube head, film, and bite block for open projection. (Reproduced with permission from Tolman, D. E. and Eppard, D. G.: An Aid to the Roentgenographic Examination of the Temporomandibular Joint. Am. J. Roentgenol. *103*:674 [July] 1968.)

secured in this position by placing the anterior holder against the nasion (Fig. I–50). In this position the central ray is directed at the ear rods and their image will appear as a circle on the film.

For the posteroanterior view the cassette is brought into contact with the nose and the exposure is made from the second x-ray tube positioned behind the patient. If only one tube head is available, the patient is first rotated for the correct position and the cassette is then positioned.

Figures I–51 and I–52 demonstrate lateral and posteroanterior cephalometric films.

SIALOGRAPHY

Sialography is the roentgenographic examination of a salivary gland after injection of a radiopaque substance into the ducts. The radiopaque substance or liquid contrast medium is an iodized oil. The

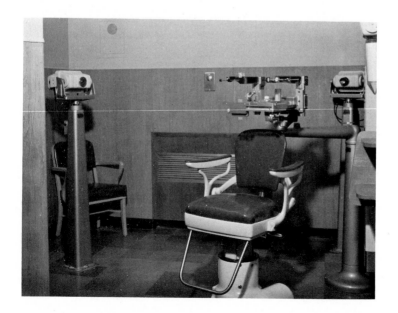

Figure I–49 Cephalometric equipment with two tube heads fixed at a distance of 5 feet from patient.

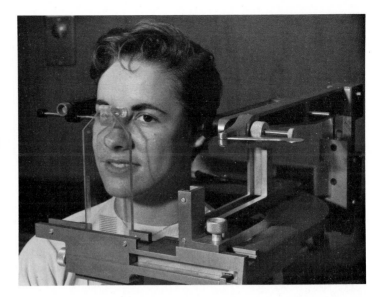

Figure I–50 Patient positioned for cephalometric technique.

amount of contrast medium to inject varies from 0.8 to more than 2 ml for the parotid gland (Ollerenshaw and Rose, 1956; Wainwright, 1965; Cook and Pollack, 1966; Carlin and Seldin, 1967) and from 0.5 to 1.2 ml for the submandibular gland (Wainwright, 1965; Cook and Pollack, 1966).

Prior to injection of the radiopaque fluid a roentgenogram of the gland should be taken. The duct then can be probed and

dilated with lacrimal probes, the mouth rinsed with a mouthwash or antiseptic solution, and an 18- to 22-gauge needle attached to a 5- or 10-ml syringe inserted. The tip of the needle should be blunt and smooth. A drop of solder on the needle acts as a stopper to seal the opening when the needle has been inserted. The needle used for the parotid gland is inserted only a short distance because of the sharp angle of

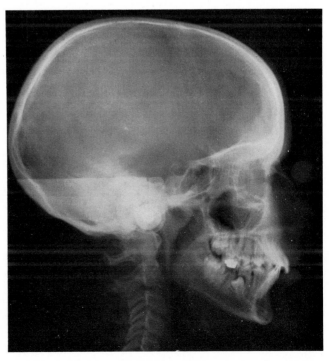

Figure I–51 Lateral cephalometric roentgenogram. Exposure factors: 82 kVp; 15 mA; and 6/10 to 8/10 second.

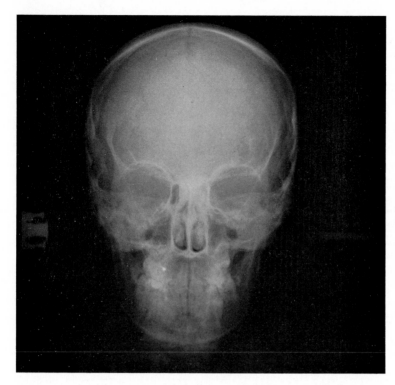

Figure I-52 Posteroanterior cephalometric roentgenogram. Exposure factors: 82 kVp; 15 mA; and 8/10 to 1 second, with intensifying screens.

Stenson's duct as it passes through the buccinator muscle (Fig. I-53).

Insertion of the needle in Wharton's duct may be facilitated by placing traction on this duct. This can be done under local anesthesia with a tissue forceps. Castigliano (1962) has suggested a transverse cut

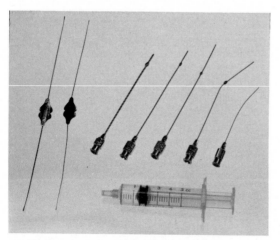

Figure I-53 Lacrimal probes, intravenous needles, and syringe necessary for sialography. Note angulation and position of solder stopper.

halfway through Wharton's duct approximately 1 cm proximal to the opening as an aid to cannulization.

After insertion of the needle or cannula, residual saliva is withdrawn, the syringe is loaded with warm radiopaque solution, and the solution is slowly injected into the gland. A piece of tape can be placed over the handle of the syringe and the needle and syringe left in place to be held by the patient during roentgenographic examination. For the parotid gland the central ray is directed through the opposite side of the mandible in the first molar region toward the gland to be observed. For the submandibular gland the central ray is directed toward the gland to be observed from beneath the opposite side of the mandible.

The cannula is then removed and roentgenograms are taken at varying intervals to study emptying of the gland. Normal glands empty in 30 minutes.

Figures I-54 and I-55 illustrate sialograms for parotid and submandibular glands.

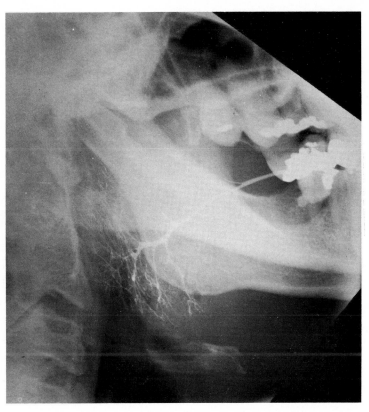

Figure I–54 Parotid sialogram. Exposure factors: 80 kVp; 15 mA; target-film distance, 23 inches; and 1/15 to 1/12 second, with intensifying screen.

OTHER EXTRAORAL EXAMINATIONS

Additional extraoral roentgenograms are valuable in the diagnosis and treatment

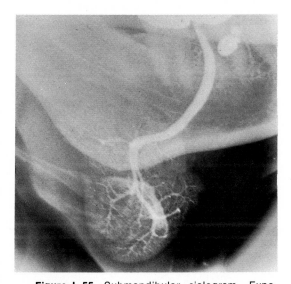

Figure I–55 Submandibular sialogram. Exposure factors: 80 kVp; 15 mA; target-film distance, 23 inches; and 1/15 to 1/12 second, with intensifying screen.

of facial fractures. These include the lateral skull projection, Towne's projection, Waters' projection, submental-vertical projection of zygomatic arches, and lateral projection of nasal bones. Figures I–56, I–57, I–58, I–59, and I–60 illustrate these views.

CINEROENTGENOGRAPHY

Cineroentgenography is motion-picture roentgenography. With the development of the light-intensification tube the amount of radiation required has been reduced, making this a practical roentgenographic procedure.

In dentistry cineroentgenography has been used to study velopharyngeal relationships during phonation and deglutition and movement of the temporomandibular joint (Cooper and Hoffman, 1955; Berry and Hoffman, 1956, 1957; Cleall, 1965; Milne and Cleall, 1970; Sloan et al., 1965, 1967; Hanson et al., 1970). For these procedures the patient is placed in the seated

Text continued on page 421.

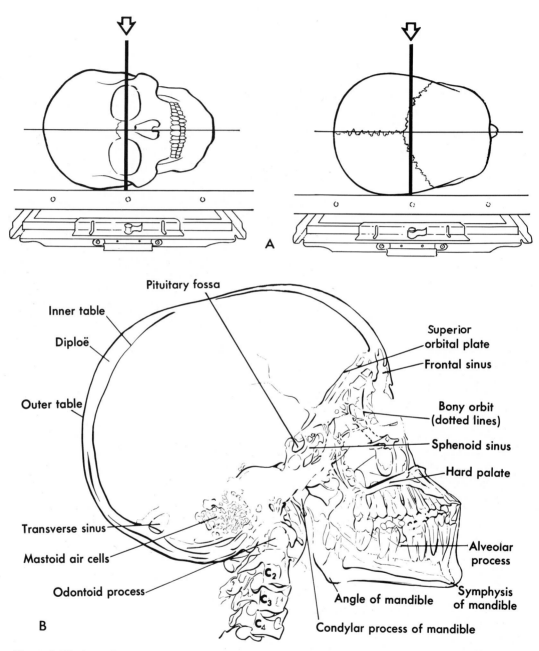

Figure I–56 Lateral projection of skull. *A,* This view is taken with side of head in contact with the table. Midsagittal plane should be parallel to table. The central ray is perpendicular to the center of the film and passes through the sella turcica. *B,* Diagrammatic representation.

Illustration continued on opposite page.

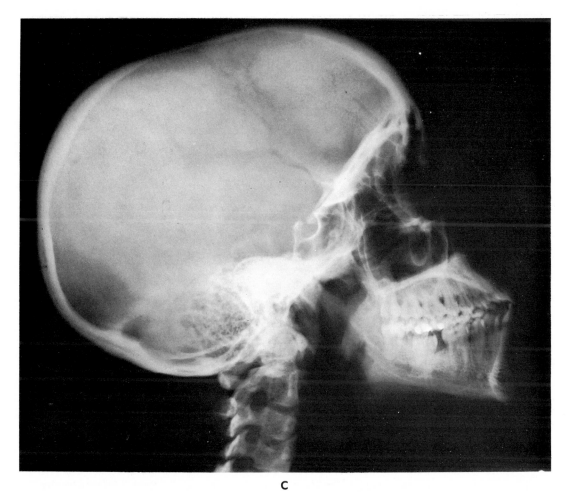

C

Figure I–56 *continued* *C,* This projection shows a direct lateral profile of the facial bones and may show soft tissues of the face. It provides a profile view of the entire skull and is useful in studying fractures of the outer and inner plates of the frontal sinuses, as well as underdevelopment or overdevelopment of the mandible. This view may reveal foreign bodies in the oropharynx. It also demonstrates the relations of the maxilla to the mandible and is useful in evaluating posterior displacement in maxillary fractures. The upper cervical spine is shown on this projection. (Reproduced with permission from Dingman, R. O. and Natvig, P.: Surgery of Facial Fractures. Philadelphia, W. B. Saunders Company, 1964, 380 pp.)

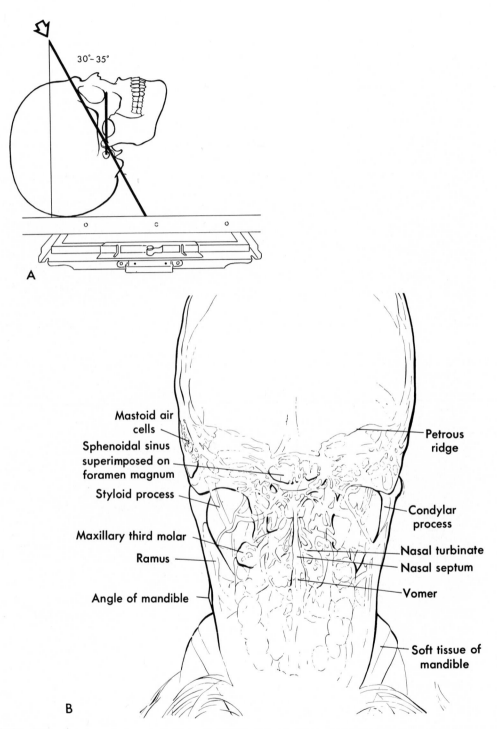

30°– 35°

A

Mastoid air
cells

Sphenoidal sinus
superimposed on
foramen magnum

Styloid process

Maxillary third molar

Ramus

Angle of mandible

Petrous
ridge

Condylar
process

Nasal turbinate

Nasal septum

Vomer

Soft tissue of
mandible

B

Figure I–57 Anteroposterior projection of mandibular condylar processes, including zygomatic arches (modified Towne's projection). *A,* The patient is placed in the supine position with the occiput resting on the table, with Reid's base line at a right angle to the table. The midsagittal plane of the skull is aligned vertically to the midplane of the cassette. The central ray is directed 35° caudad through the frontal bone and the foramen magnum midway between the temporomandibular joints. The position of the cassette is adjusted so that its midpoint coincides with the central ray. Respiration is suspended during exposure of the film. *B,* Diagrammatic representation.

Illustration continued on opposite page.

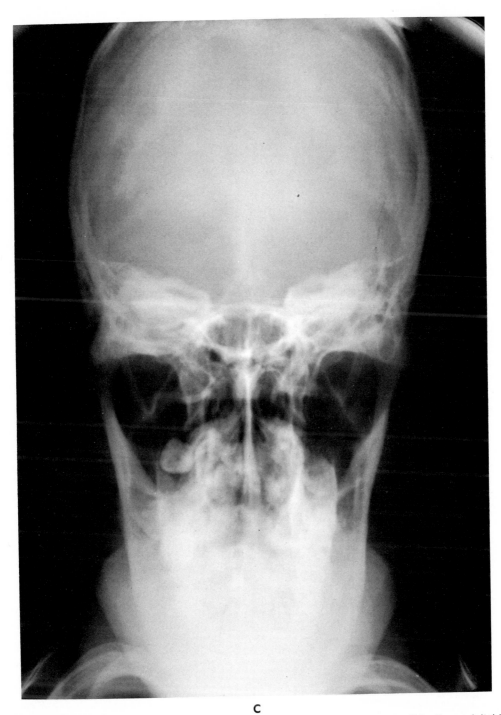

C

Figure I–57 *continued.* C, This view shows the condylar processes of the mandible, the occipital bones, and the posterior cranial fossa. It is one of the best to demonstrate angulation of the condylar processes and may reveal basilar and occipital skull fractures. The nasal septum is well delineated. The zygomatic arches are often seen well by using hyperillumination. (Reproduced with permission from Dingman, R. O. and Natvig, P.: Surgery of Facial Fractures. Philadelphia, W. B. Saunders Company, 1964, 380 pp.)

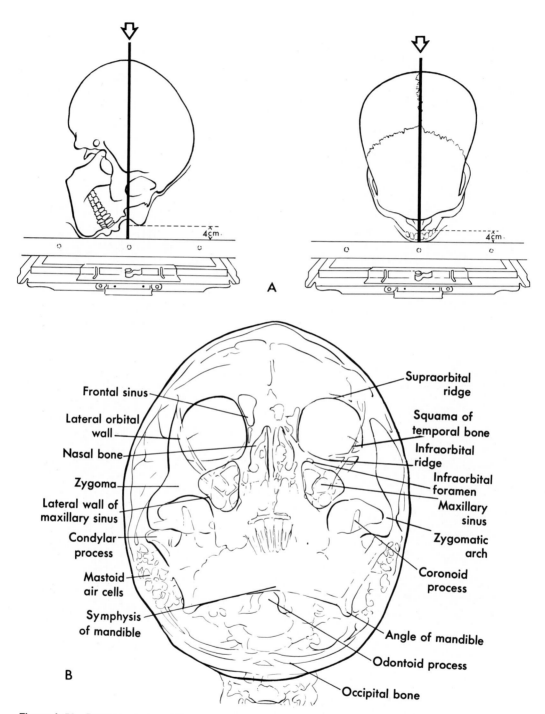

Figure I-58 Posteroanterior oblique projection of face (Waters' projection). *A*, The patient is placed in the prone position with the face against the table. The midsagittal plane of the head is aligned vertically to the vertical midline of the film. The head is rested on the chin with the nasal tip elevated approximately 4 cm from the table. The upper lip is placed directly over the center of the film, and the central ray is directed perpendicular to the midpoint of the film. *B*, Diagrammatic representation.

Illustration continued on opposite page.

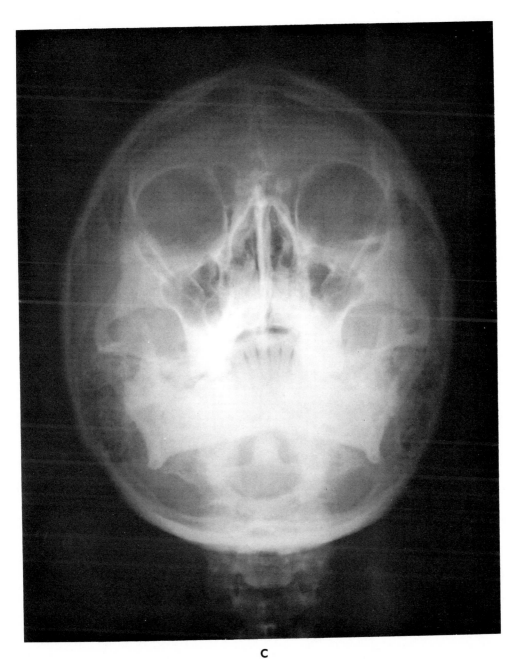

C

Figure I-58 *continued*   *C,* This is the best single view for demonstrating fractures of the maxillae, maxillary sinuses, the floors and inferior rims of the orbits, the zygomatic bones, and the zygomatic arches. It is also helpful in showing fractures of the nasal bones and the frontal processes of the maxillae. In this view there is minimal superimposition of structures. This projection is especially helpful when taken steroscopically. When the patient is severely injured and is unable to assume the prone position, the reverse Waters projection gives almost the same detail, but the structures appear somewhat larger because of the greater distance from the film. (Reproduced with permission from Dingman, R. O. and Natvig, P.: Surgery of Facial Fractures. Philadelphia, W. B. Saunders Company, 1964, 380 pp.)

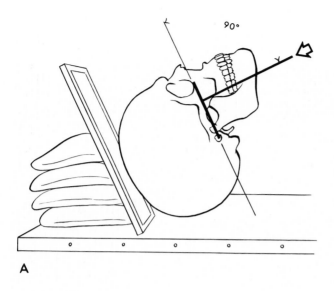

A

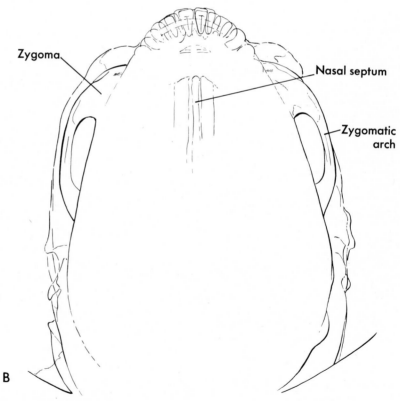

B

Figure I-59 Submental-vertical projection of zygomatic arches. *A,* The patient is placed in the dorsal recumbent position with the shoulders elevated on pillows or sand bags to obtain maximal extension of the neck. The occiput is rested against the table with the midsagittal plane of the skull aligned vertically to the central vertical line of the film. The vertex is rested against the upright cassette. Reid's base line is parallel to the plane of the cassette. The central ray is directed midway between the angles of the jaw, perpendicular to the base line of the skull. *B,* Diagrammatic representation.

Illustration continued on opposite page.

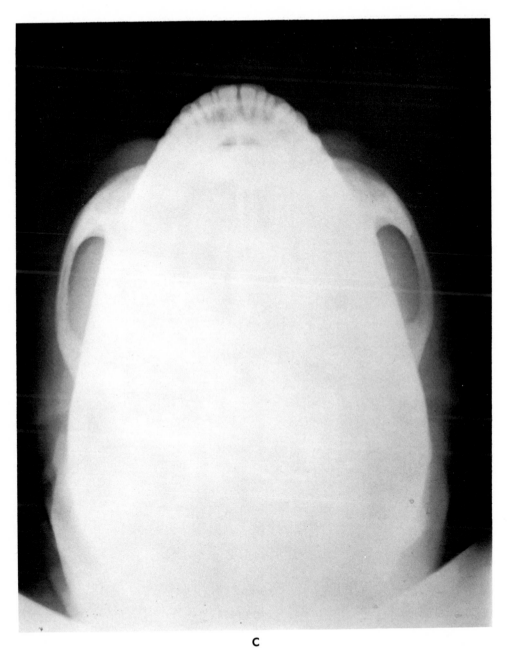

C

Figure I–59 *continued C,* This is an excellent view to demonstrate the zygomatic arches and medial or lateral displacement of fractured segments. If the view is underexposed, it is useful only for outlining the zygomatic arches, but if taken to expose the base of the skull, it may reveal basilar skull fractures. (Reproduced with permission from Dingman, R. O. and Natvig, P.: Surgery of Facial Fractures. Philadelphia, W. B. Saunders Company, 1964, 380 pp.)

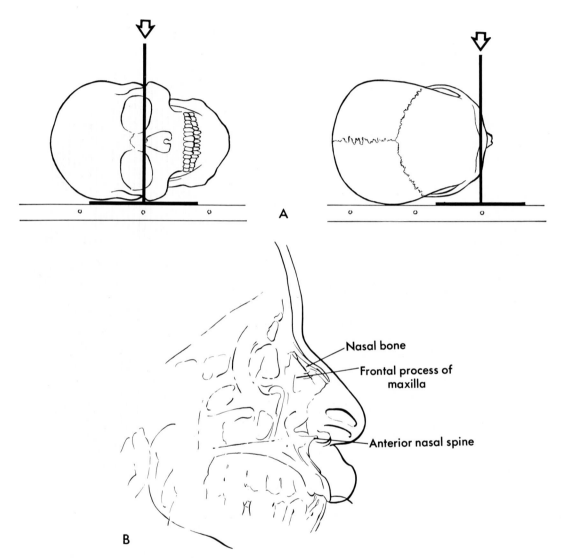

Figure I–60   Lateral projection of nasal bones. *A,* The head is placed in the precise lateral position over a film packet placed below the nose. The central ray is directed through the base of the nose at right angles to the plane of the film. Right and left lateral views should be taken. Respiration is suspended during exposure. *B,* Diagrammatic representation.

Illustration continued on opposite page.

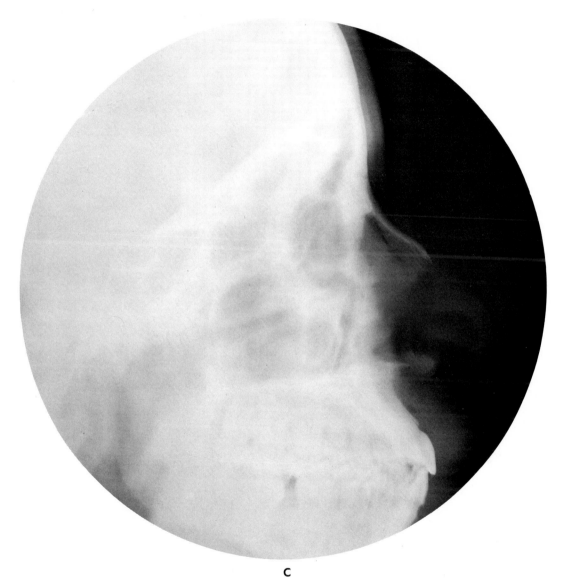

C

Figure I-60 *continued*   C, The nasal bone closest to the film is well demonstrated in the lateral view. Soft tissues and the anterior nasal spine of the maxilla are shown in profile. This view demonstrates fractures of the nasal bones, the anterior nasal spine, and the frontal process of the maxilla. (Reproduced with permission from Dingman, R. O. and Natvig, P.: Surgery of Facial Fractures. Philadelphia, W. B. Saunders Company, 1964, 380 pp.)

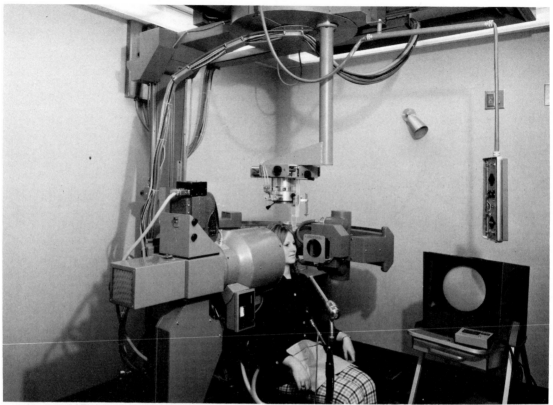

Figure I–61   Patient seated between the x-ray tube and intensifier, with the ''C'' arm adjusted to view the velopharyngeal relationships. Note camera (behind intensifier) and microphone.

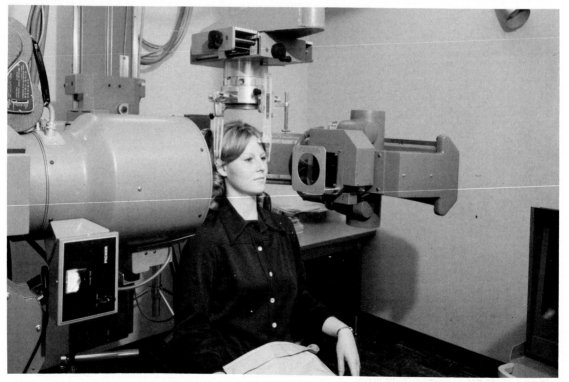

Figure I–62   Patient seated with unit positioned to study the temporomandibular joint.

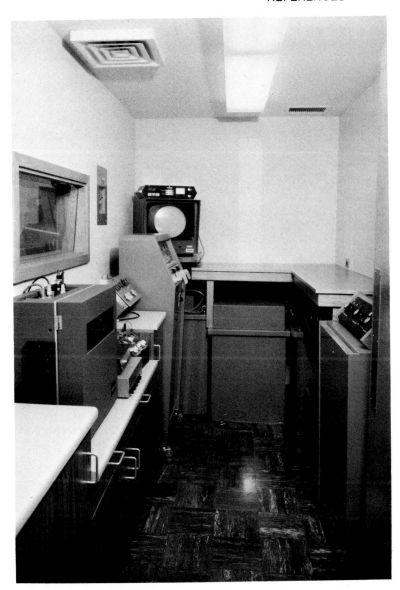

Figure I–63 Control room for cineroentgenography.

position between the x-ray tube and the image intensifier or amplifying tube that orbits on the "C" arm of the machine. The unit permits fluoroscopy from any angle in various planes without moving the patient. In those patients in whom sound recording is desired, the microphone and camera are synchronized with the x-ray tube (Figs. I–61 and I–62). The operator is able to monitor both the patient, through a glass window, and the specific area being studied, via a closed-circuit viewing screen, during the procedure (Fig. I–63). At present a standard technique has not been devel-

oped. However, Sloan and colleagues (1967) wrote that "the standardization of techniques and criteria for diagnostic information is extremely feasible within the next 5 to 10 years."

REFERENCES

Barr, J. H., and Grøn, P.: Palate Contour as a Limiting Factor in Intraoral X-ray Technique. Oral Surg., Oral Med. & Oral Path. *12*:459–472 (Apr.) 1959.

Berry, H. M., Jr. and Hofmann, F. A.: Cinefluorography with Image Intensification for Observing

Temporomandibular Joint Movements. J. Am. Dent. A. 53:517–527 (Nov.) 1956.

Berry, H. M., Jr. and Hofmann, F. A.: Preliminary Work on Cinefluorography, with Image Intensification, in the Study of the Temporomandibular Joint. Oral Surg., Oral Med. & Oral Path. 10:63–68 (Jan.) 1957.

Blackman, S.: Rotational Tomography of the Face. Brit. J. Radiol. 33:408–418 (July) 1960.

Blackman, S.: Panography. Oral Surg., Oral Med. & Oral Path. 14:1178–1189 (Oct.) 1961.

Carlin, R. T. and Seldin, R.: Sialography: A Useful Aid in Diagnosing Parotid Tumors. J. Oral Surg. 25:139–146 (Mar.) 1967.

Castigliano, S. G.: Sialography of the Submaxillary Salivary Gland: A New Technique. Am. J. Roentgenol. 187:385–386 (Feb.) 1962.

Clark, K. C.: Positioning in Radiography. Ed. 9. Chicago, Year Book Publishers, Inc., 1974, 2 vols.

Cleall, J. F.: Deglutition: A Study of Form and Function. Am. J. Orthodontics. 51:566–594 (Aug.) 1965.

Cook, T. J. and Pollack, J.: Sialography: Pathologic-Radiologic Correlation. Oral Surg., Oral Med. & Oral Path. 21:559–573 (May) 1966.

Cooper, H. K. and Hofmann, F. A.: The Application of Cinefluorography with Image Intensification in the Field of Plastic Surgery, Dentistry and Speech. Plast. & Reconstruct. Surg. 16:135–137 (Aug.) 1955.

Dingman, R. O. and Natvig, P.: Surgery of Facial Fractures. Philadelphia, W. B. Saunders Company, 1964, 380 pp.

Eastman Kodak Company: X-rays in Dentistry: A Manual of Procedure for Dental Radiography. Rochester, New York, 1962, 80 pp.

Ennis, L. M. et al.: Dental Roentgenology. Ed. 6. Philadelphia, Lea & Febiger, 1967.

Fitzgerald, G. M.: Dental Roentgenography. II. Vertical Angulation, Film Placement and Increased Object-Film Distance. J. Am. Dent. A. 34:160–170 (Feb. 1) 1947.

Fitzgerald, G. M.: Dental Roentgenography. III. The Roentgenographic Periapical Survey of the Upper Molar Region. J. Am. Dent. A. 38:293–303 (Mar.) 1949.

Fixott, H. C., Jr. and Neely, A. R.: An Outline of Roentgenographic Technical Procedure, as Used in the Department of Oral Roentgenology of the University of Oregon Dental School. 1962. (Duplicated.)

Hanson, M. L., Hilton, L. M., Barnard, L. W., and Case, J. L.: Tongue-Thrust in Preschool Children. Part III. *Cinefluorographic Analysis.* Am. J. Orthodontics. 58:268–275 (Sept.) 1970.

Hornseth, W.: Temporomandibular Roentgenography Through the Coronoid Notch. X-ray Technician. 25:100–101 (Sept.) 1954.

Jacobson, A. F. and Ferguson, J. P.: Evaluation of an S. S. White Panorex X-ray Machine. Oral Surg., Oral Med. & Oral Path. 36:426–442 (Sept.) 1973.

Jerman, A. C., Kinsley, E. L., and Morris, C. R.: Absorbed Radiation from Panoramic plus Bitewing Exposures vs. Full-Mouth Periapical plus Bitewing Exposures. J. Am. Dent. A. 86:420–423 (Feb.) 1973.

Kite, O. W., Swanson, L. T., Levin, S., and Bradbury, E.: Radiation and Image Distortion in the Panorex X-ray Unit. Oral Surg., Oral Med. & Oral Path. 15:1201–1210 (Oct.) 1962.

Kumpula, J. W.: Present Status of Panoramic Roentgenography. J. Am. Dent. A. 63:194–200 (Aug.) 1961.

Laney, W. R. and Tolman, D. E.: The Use of Panoramic Radiography in the Medical Center. Oral Surg., Oral Med. & Oral Path. 26:465–474 (Oct.) 1968.

Lewis, G. R.: Temporomandibular Joint Radiographic Technics: Comparison and Evaluation of Results. Dent. Radiogr. Photogr. 37:8–20, 1964.

Manson-Hing, L. R.: Evaluation of Radiographic Techniques, Including Pantomography. J. Am. Dent. A. 87:145–154 (July) 1973.

McCall, J. O. and Wald, S. S.: Clinical Dental Roentgenology: Technic and Interpretation: Including Roentgen Studies of the Child and the Adolescent. Ed. 4. Philadelphia, W. B. Saunders Company, 1957, 466 pp.

Milne, I. M. and Cleall, J. F.: Cinefluorographic Study of Functional Adaptation of the Oropharyngeal Structures. Angle Orthodont. 40:267–283 (Oct.) 1970.

Mitchell, L. D., Jr.: Panoramic Roentgenography: A Clinical Evaluation. J. Am. Dent. A. 66:777–786 (June) 1963.

O'Grady, C. S. and Reynolds, R. L.: Paralleling Technic with a Short Cone: Shortcomings of This Procedure. Dent. Radiogr. Photogr. 46:15–19, 1973.

Ollerenshaw, R. and Rose, S.: Sialography—a Valuable Diagnostic Method. Dent. Radiogr. Photogr. 29:37–46, 1956.

Paatero, Y. V.: Pantomography and Orthopantomography. Oral Surg., Oral Med. & Oral Path. 14:947–953 (Aug.) 1961.

Raper, H. R.: Practical Clinical Preventive Dentistry Based Upon Periodic Roentgen-Ray Examinations. J. Am. Dent. A. 12:1084–1100 (Sept.) 1925.

Richards, A. G. and Alling, C. C.: Extraoral Radiography: Mandible and Temporomandibular Articulation. Dent. Radiogr. Photogr. 28:1–7, 18–19, 1955.

Ritter Company: A Textbook of Selective X-ray Technique. Ed. 3. Rochester, New York, Ritter Company, Inc., 1951.

Robinson, M. and Lytle, J.: Simplified Method for Office Roentgenograms of the Temporomandibular Joint. J. Oral Surg. 20:217–219 (May) 1962.

Salzmann, J. A.: Practice of Orthodontics. Philadelphia, J. B. Lippincott Company, 1966, vol. 1, 554 pp.

Silha, R. E.: The Versatile Occlusal Dental X-ray Film. Part I. Dent. Radiogr. Photogr. 38:36–38, 43–44, 1965.

Silha, R. E.: The Versatile Occlusal Dental X-ray Film. Part II. Dent. Radiogr. Photogr. 38:51–54, 68–69, 1965.

Sloan, R. F., Brummett, S. W., Westover, J. L., and Mansfield, L.: Cinefluorographic Motion Picture Production Technics Including Cinefluorographic Data Analysis. Dent. Radiogr. Photogr. 40:30–33, 40–44, 1967.

Sloan, R. F., Ricketts, R. M., Brummett, S. W., Bench, R. W., and Westover, J. L.: Quantified Cinefluorographic Techniques Used in Oral Roentgenology. Oral Surg., Oral Med. & Oral Path. 20:456–463 (Oct.) 1965.

Tolman, D. E. and Eppard, D. G.: An Aid to the Roentgenographic Examination of the Temporomandibular Joint. Am. J. Roentgenol. *103*:674 (July) 1968.

Updegrave, W. J.: Simplifying and Improving Intraoral Dental Roentgenography. Oral Surg., Oral Med. & Oral Path. *12*:704–716 (June) 1959.

Updegrave, W. J.: High or Low Kilovoltage. Dent. Radiogr. Photogr. *33*:71–78, 1960.

Updegrave, W. J.: Panoramic Dental Radiography. Dent. Radiogr. Photogr. *36*:75–83, 1963.

Updegrave, W. J.: The Role of Panoramic Radiography in Diagnosis. Oral Surg., Oral Med. & Oral Path. *22*:49–57 (July) 1966.

Waggener, D. T.: Newer Concepts in Dental Roentgenology. Canad. Dent. A. J. *17*:363–370 (July) 1951.

Waggener, D. T.: The Right-Angle Technique Using the Extension Cone. Dent. Clin. North America. November, pp. 783–788, 1960.

Wainwright, W. W.: Dental Radiology. New York, McGraw-Hill Book Company, Inc., 1965, pp. 329–333.

Wuehrmann, A. H.: The Long Cone Technic. Practical Dental Monographs. Chicago, Year Book Publishers, Inc., July, 1957, pp. 1–30.

Wuehrmann, A. H. and Manson-Hing, L. R.: Dental Radiology. St. Louis, The C. V. Mosby Company, 1965, pp. 126–148.

APPENDIX PART II

THE PROCESSING OF X-RAY FILMS

STANLEY A. LOVESTEDT, D.D.S.

Simply stated, the roentgenogram is a photographic record obtained by passage of roentgen rays, or x-rays, through an object, or tissue, with recording of relative density on special x-ray film. Processing of the film then creates a visible image of the latent image created by the x-ray exposure. The finest x-ray equipment and the most exacting exposure techniques are of little avail if the exposed film is not processed correctly. Much thought, effort, and expense may be involved in obtaining the proper equipment and supplies without realizing that many otherwise excellent roentgenograms are ruined in the processing room. It has been stated that 90% of radiographic pitfalls are traceable to the darkroom, where artifacts may develop during some stage of film processing. If the finished roentgenogram is to provide specific data, it must be the product of proper film exposure and proper darkroom procedure.

The effort to improve radiation hygiene has led to the development of faster film speeds, resulting in reduced exposure of film and patient. Directions for film development are furnished by film manufacturers along with the chemicals prepared for film processing. While the basic development techniques remain relatively constant, the prepared chemicals may vary and careful attention should be given to the manufacturer's instructions for their use.

424

X-RAY FILM

X-ray film consists of a clear base, or support, for the gelatin emulsion. The material used for the base must be photographically inert and unaffected by the solutions used in processing; it must be strong, lightweight, and flexible, with desirable storage features such as low inflammability and permanency.

The emulsion coating, usually on both sides of the base, is a gelatin containing countless tiny crystals of silver halide. Over the emulsion a very thin, rather transparent layer of gelatin is employed to help protect the surface of the emulsion containing the silver halide from mechanical damage.

Emulsions on negatives are comparatively thick for the purpose of obtaining adequate latitude of exposure. The emulsions have a certain degree of hardness which determines the rate of penetration of solutions that are used in processing the film. Too much hardening will decrease the swelling and consequently the penetration rate of the different processing solutions used.

Films are prepared in various sizes and shapes for ease of use. Intraoral films are used for periapical, bite-wing, and occlusal applications. Extraoral films are used to obtain profile, lateral jaw, anteroposterior, posteroanterior, full head, submental vertical, cephalometric, panoramic, temporomandibular, sialographic, and other projections. Some sizes of films are individually wrapped for intraoral use; larger sizes come in packages with each sheet protected by paper interleaves. These packages are to be opened only in darkrooms where controlled and filtered light will be used and where cassettes will be loaded and unloaded. In the individually packaged smaller films for intraoral use, a sheet of lead foil is used to protect the film from backscatter or secondary irradiation. The foil also absorbs some of the x-rays that have passed through the object and film; in addition it aids in identifying right and left sides.

The placing of emulsion on both sides of the film base (double-coated film) prevents curling of the film, provides for added contrast when used with intensifying screens, and gives greater blackening for the same exposure.

Undue physical strains from pressure, creasing, buckling, and friction should be avoided. Films should not be drawn rapidly from their packets or cartons, from the exposure holders, or from the cassettes in which they have been placed, nor should they be handled in any manner that causes static electrical discharges.

PROCESSING OF X-RAY FILM

Processing is a chemical treatment that is applied to exposed x-ray film to make the invisible latent image a visible and permanent one. Roentgenographic density increases with duration of development and with the temperature of the developing solution.

Two common ways of developing films are: (1) by the process of inspection and (2) by the time-temperature method. For optimal results, the time-temperature method of development is recommended. This method produces roentgenographic images with maximal speed and contrast. Close attention to the manufacturer's directions for processing of film helps ensure roentgenograms of highest quality.

If one is to take advantage of standardized technique in roentgenography, one cannot trust variations that come about in developing by inspection. The dull illumination of the darkroom, the wet surfaces of the film being inspected, and the necessity for the technician developing the film to appreciate what is needed represent some of the problems attending this method. When the time and temperature are carefully controlled, one may be sure that any variation in the quality of the roentgenograms is due more to the exposure than to the development, and that the results obtained in the finished product are significant and may have value in the interpretation of the finished roentgenogram.

In the time-temperature method of processing, a temperature of 20° C is recommended because the manufacturers have prepared a film that will give optimal quality when it is developed at this temperature. The time required for processing is practical, and the temperature usually is conveniently maintained. Temperatures much below 20° C do not allow chemical action to proceed at the required speed, and there may be danger of underdevelopment and poor fixation. On the other hand, temperatures much above 20° C may cause some fogging of the film or make the emulsion softer and more subject to change.

In the dental office in which film is developed only occasionally, with days on which no film is developed, certain problems arise that are difficult to control; for example, it is difficult to maintain the solutions in the proper state of freshness and free of oxidation. Too often, one encounters a situation wherein the water bath surrounding the developing and fixing tanks is at room temperature and the developer and fixing solutions are at a high temperature, so that the quality of the processed roentgenogram, taken perhaps in an emergency situation, hardly justifies the effort of exposing the film.

It may be practical to turn off the water circulating around the jackets of the developing and fixing tanks each evening. If this is done, the temperature of the circulating water bath must be established at 20° C the first thing when the office is opened in the morning. In addition to this, the person developing the films should realize that the solution must be agitated and stirred before being used, in order to assure a uniform temperature throughout the developing solution and the fixing solution.

ROLE OF DEVELOPING AND FIXING SOLUTIONS

Many dentists are acquainted with developing techniques by virtue of their experience in photography. An awareness of the components of the developing solution and the role they play enables one to appreciate the chemistry of film development. If prepared solutions offered by manufacturers of films and others who specialize in providing solutions for processing x-ray film are used, one need not know all the details involved; however, briefly, one should recognize that the developer contains several basic ingredients such as developing agents, accelerators, preservatives, and restrainers.

The developing agents change the exposed grains of silver halide to metallic silver. They have little influence upon the unexposed grains in the emulsion. An accelerator, an alkali, activates the developing agents. Preservatives are antioxidants, and are included because alkaline developing solutions rapidly oxidize in the air and therefore may stain the gelatin of the emulsion. Restrainers added to developing solutions control the action of the developing agent, so that it does not develop the underexposed silver halide. Rinse baths, or stop baths, used between the developer and the hypo solution, generally are solutions of acetic acid and water, and are used to prevent the alkaline developer retained by the film from neutralizing the acid in the fixing solution.

Fixing solutions usually contain a clearing agent that removes the undeveloped silver halide from the emulsion. They also contain preservatives, which prevent the gelatin from swelling excessively or becoming soft and which also shorten drying time. Acidifiers are used in hypo or fixing solutions in order to correct the action of the other chemicals and to neutralize any alkaline developer that may have been carried over into the fixing solution by the film and film holders.

PROCEDURE FOR FILM PROCESSING

Developing. When the films have been attached properly to the film hanger and the temperature of the developing solution has been determined (the solution being thoroughly stirred to equalize the temperature throughout the tank), by then referring to a time-temperature chart, one can ascertain the time for which the timer should be set. When the proper interval has been determined and the timer set for it, the film is immersed immediately and then raised and lowered several times at a uniform rate, in order to remove any air bells or bubbles from the film surfaces and to wet the film surfaces completely and thoroughly with the developer. Some like to agitate the film about once every minute.

Fixing. When development is complete, the film must be removed from the developing solution. After a few moments of film and hanger drainage, the film either is washed briefly in running water to remove developer or is placed in a stop-bath solution for 30 to 45 seconds. This arrests the action of the developer and reduces contamination of the fixing solution (hypo). Stop-bath solutions are made according to the specifications of the film manufacturer and usually contain acetic acid. After the stop bath and rinsing, the film is placed in the fixing solution. This solution should be at the same temperature as the previously used solutions; if it is too warm, the emulsion will swell abnormally and consequently the film will dry slowly. "Clearing time" refers to the time required for complete disappearance of the white or milky opaqueness of the film after it has been placed in the fixing solution. During the time in the fixing solution the underdeveloped silver halide particles are being removed from the emulsion. The total fixing time should be at least twice the time required for clearing the film.

Film may be removed from the fixing solution after clearing and may be viewed for a limited time in an emergency. However, the film should be returned to the fixing solution as soon as possible to complete the fixation. Adequate fixation is necessary to ensure proper processing, and film-storage properties depend on correct processing. Films should not be left in the fixing solutions for more than an hour, to avoid the danger of losing some of the density of the image. Another reason that fixing is critical is that hardening of the emulsion occurs during this procedure.

Fixing solutions lose their usefulness when the acidity is lost and when fixation requires an unduly long period. Continued use of exhausted fixing solution results in inadequate hardening of the film emulsion, swelling of the emulsion, and an unnecessarily long drying period. Films also become stained, and keeping qualities are altered. Where sufficient films are routinely processed, the solution is easily maintained by fixer replenishment according to the manufacturer's directions, or by periodic replacement of the fixing solution. This allows proper fixation, standardization of technique, and quality control of the finished film.

Washing. After the film has been in the fixing solution for the period specified by the film manufacturer (usually a minimum of 10 minutes in newly prepared solution), it must be properly washed to remove the processing chemicals from the emulsion. This requires an adequate supply of flowing water, which should be at the temperature of the processing solutions. Marked variations in the temperature of processing solutions and wash waters induce dimensional changes of the emulsion coating on the film base and may cause reticulation. Film hangers must be well spaced in the washing tank, as well as completely submersed so that the chemicals may be removed from the developed film. After complete washing of the film (usually 20 minutes), a wetting agent may be used in a final procedure to ensure uniform drying of film and freedom from water spotting.

Drying. Drying is a relatively simple step in the processing of film, but, if improperly done, water marks may result or the gelatin may be altered. After removal from the last wash water, with or without wetting agent, wet-processed films should be allowed to drain for a few seconds and then carefully shaken to remove all possible water from the hangers and films. Whether the films are air-dried over a drip pan or placed in a drying cabinet, care should be taken not to damage the film emulsion, or to allow the film to come into contact with any foreign material or surface. Dust and lint on wet film are almost impossible to remove.

Many drying cabinets have some type of heater and a forced-air system to circulate the warmed air and prevent film damage from the heaters. Such dryers should be vented to prevent an excessive increase in temperature and humidity within the dryer and the processing room. Some dryers remove moisture from the circulating air by the use of chemicals, and some use dehumidified air for circulation through the drying cabinet. If films are left in the drying cabinet too long after becoming dry, they tend to become brittle.

Speed Processing. The use of intraoral films to check operative procedures has given rise to chairside development of films, at higher than usual temperatures, for prompt viewing. Eastman DF7 film—developed for 30 seconds at 33° C, rinsed, and fixed—will provide emergency viewing; however, image quality and record-keeping features will not measure up to those of standard time-temperature processed film.

Monosolution film processing has not been successful, but an interesting processing technique is the chairside two-solution method. The film is in a plastic container (Fig. II-1). After it is exposed, it may be developed immediately by first squeezing the contents of the developer tube down around the film, massaging the fluid about the film for 30 seconds, and then squeezing the tube with fixer and again massaging the solution about the film. After a few seconds

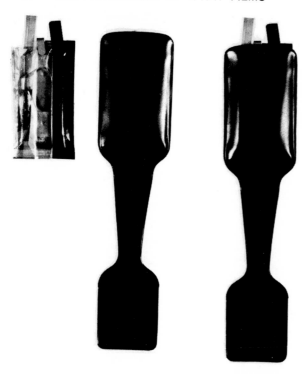

Figure II–1 Self-contained two-solution film packet that may be developed by use of solutions contained in the tubes. Single film is in bottom end and developer and fixer are in top end.

of rinsing, the film can be viewed. This works as a convenience method and could be useful for oral surgery or endodontic purposes, but the picture lacks definition and detail for many restorative applications. After viewing, the film is stored in water until it can be run through an automatic processor or placed on a film hanger and processed. If reprocessing is not considered—for example, the film that has been used as a progress check—this film could be discarded.

In discussing rapid processing, one must include the Polaroid processing technique. The Polaroid-Land method of roentgenography is a one-step, essentially dry photographic process that has a number of applications in diagnostic procedures. Its advantage is primarily the short time required for film processing and viewing. Large-sized films are used and the loading of cassettes and processing may be carried out in fully lighted surroundings. Processing of the film requires only 10 seconds. Polaroid processing is accomplished in a small table-top unit that may be plugged into any convenient 110 to 117 volt, alternating-current electrical outlet. The Polar-

oid principle has not been applied to intraoral films but finds an important place in surgery, for example, where exposures may be made in the operating room with portable x-ray equipment and processing carried out in an adjacent area. This technique is valuable when speed is essential. Machine 90-second automatic processing may be preferable, however, if the processing room is near the surgical area.

Machine, or automatic, film processors are used in many health and medical centers. They produce film ready for reading and storing in about 90 seconds. The practicality of mechanized processing cannot be denied, for the speed with which processed film is made available is a virtue. The features of the large automatic film-processing machines are now being applied to table-top models for intraoral and occlusal films (Fig. II–2). The reduction in processing time is accomplished by the use of higher temperatures and the replenishment of solutions by metering devices. By passing the film through first the developer and then the fixer and washing cycles, time is gained by not having stop baths or washing between development and fixing. Some units are too small to accept 7- by 12-inch, or larger, film. On the other hand, it is possible to place dental films in plastic mounts and pass them through the larger automatic processors designed for medical and industrial use.

Cleanliness is an important feature in operating automatic processors. The gelatin must be carefully wiped from the moving parts of the processor whenever specified, and maybe more often, depending on the use of the equipment. One major consideration in the use of automated processing is matching the capacity against the requirements of a given facility. Another consideration is whether or not the usual processing facilities are still necessary when an automatic technique is used.

In all procedures other than the proven time-temperature development, the long-time keeping qualities of processed film need to be carefully observed. Silver recovery units are available that allow recovery of the silver contained in the fixing solutions. Exhausted fixing solutions are filtered through the silver recovery units before being discarded.

Film Mounting. Mounting of film in folders to facilitate reading may or may not be done in the processing room. The identity of all films must be maintained, and only those belonging to a single patient should be handled at a single time. They should be immediately placed either in film mounts or in labeled envelopes. In either event the name, the file or code number if used, and the date should be properly recorded.

A flush-mounted subsurface-lighted view box assists in the proper identification

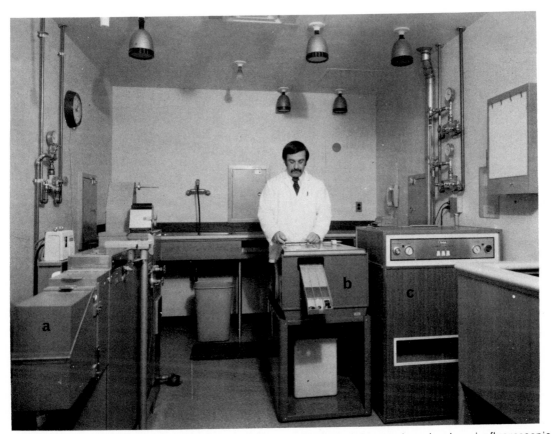

Figure II–2 A well-equipped darkroom designed for high-volume processing, showing cinefluoroscopic movie film developer *(a)*, table-top automated developer *(b)* with replenisher supply below, and automatic large-size film developer *(c)*. Note plumbing with large, easily read gauges and convenient controls, safelight locations, film passes in three walls, large ceiling ventilator, viewbox, and large sink work area for cleaning roller systems of machine processors.

and placement of films in the mount. Care must be exercised to have clean dry areas and to have the hands dry and free of grease or oils.

FILM STORAGE

The film supply should be adequate, yet small enough to provide reasonably rapid turnover of stock. Since all film packages are dated, it is an easy matter to use the oldest film first. Ideally, films should be kept in a cool room (10 to 20°C), and opened packages should be kept at a relative humidity of about 40 to 60%.

Exposed film may be stored by various coding methods for later reference, for educational uses, for illustrations, and for legal reasons. Flexibility and availability are features that need to be built into any film-filing system.

THE FILM-PROCESSING ROOM

In planning the office facilities, special attention should be given to processing-room requirements. The arrangement of the room for convenience and the quality of the processing equipment should not be compromised. The dimensions of the room will be determined, in part, by the number of people expected to use the room, the volume of work that will flow through the area, the size of the processing units to be employed, and the storage space planned. The room should be of adequate size, readily accessible, easily maintained, located near the necessary utilities, and in a radiation-safe relationship to x-ray machines (Fig. II–2).

Right-handed and left-handed people differ in their convenience needs. The arrangement and organization of the work area must be conducive to orderliness and cleanliness so that in the processing of exposed film there will be little or no opportunity for the splashing of chemicals onto the work-bench areas, or onto films that may be mounted on their processing hangers but not yet placed in the developing solutions. Drops of chemical solutions falling onto dry surfaces will evaporate, leaving the dried chemical to be stirred up as dust that will settle on working surfaces as well as on exposed film being readied for processing.

In air-conditioned offices the processing room benefits from the controlled humidity and temperature that air conditioning provides. Special air inlets and exhausts may be required in the processing room if drying cabinets that contain heating elements are used.

The processing unit is the most important part of the darkroom equipment and should be of sufficient dimensions to accept the film sizes employed, or anticipated to be employed, by those who may use the facility. Cephalometric or panoramic films require larger tanks than do periapical or bite-wing films. Plumbing codes control tank installation, and the film-processing units available for installation usually have necessary code features engineered into their design and construction. Where there are no existing processing facilities, or where the building in of such equipment is not advisable for one reason or another, one may consider use of the prefabricated consoles that have the processing tanks and plumbing handily engineered into a single compact unit. For such an installation there are also available many accessories, such as automatic water-temperature control, refrigeration, lights, and dial thermometer.

In most regions of the country the temperature of processing solutions may be controlled manually or automatically by the blending of hot and cold water in a water jacket surrounding the individual processing tanks. Ice cubes are sometimes used to cool the water in jackets of smaller processing tanks. Ice cubes are never placed directly into the solutions, for that dilutes the developer or fixer. Stirring of solutions is necessary to obtain an accurate temperature reading at any given time. Only by controlling the temperature of the processing solutions can one hope to be able to utilize accurately the time-temperature method of film development.

Film holders for processing must be stored where they will be readily available, yet out of the way until needed. Each type of hanger should be kept in its proper place, and necessary repairs should be made before the hanger is returned to its proper storage position. Waste paper should be easily disposed of so that empty film wrappers and film may not become intermixed.

Film hangers and processing tanks need to be cleaned frequently. Care should be exercised not to mar or scratch surfaces. Nylon netting may be suitable for removing the accumulation within processing tanks. Careful rinsing of cleansed tanks should help to eliminate all foreign material.

Developing tanks often need additional cleansing. A diluted solution of commercial hydrochloric acid may be placed in the tank for half an hour. The tank is then emptied and thoroughly rinsed before drying with a cloth. Care should be taken never to place hot water in the hard-rubber containers or tanks. There are also available commercial solutions that may prove convenient for cleansing stainless-steel tanks. One should make certain that all cleansing agents are removed from processing tanks before refilling with processing solutions.

Unclean film hangers may cause spots or streaking artifacts on processed films, because dried fixer may be carried into developing tanks unless the hangers are carefully and thoroughly rinsed or washed after each use. Material collected on the film clips may be removed by soaking the hangers in hot water and then thoroughly brushing the clips and again washing.

SAFELIGHTS

Dental x-ray films are light-sensitive as well as "x-ray"-sensitive, and either will affect the silver halogen in the film emulsion. Lights in the film-processing room require special filters for use when film is being processed. Factors that determine the safety of darkroom lights (safelights) are the type of filter used, the wattage of the bulb employed, the light-film distance, and the length of time film is exposed to the safelight. The Wratten series 6B filter, used with a 7½- or 10-watt bulb at a distance of not less than 4 feet, is a starting point for darkroom illumination. Every dentist should determine for himself whether his safelight is safe.

A simple method of checking the safety of illumination is to use the coin-on-the-film method. A dental x-ray film, or any other film used and processed in the darkroom, is removed from its wrapper and placed on the working surface where film is usually unwrapped and handled beneath the safelight. A coin is placed on the film, and a safelight exposure of 5 minutes is made. The film is processed in the usual manner. If there is an outline of the coin on the film, the safelight is not safe. Correction of the situation suggests either replacing the bulb with one of lower wattage or increasing the safelight-film distance. Following any modification the test should be repeated to determine whether the correction is adequate. In testing, one needs to determine that the correct light filter is being used—that specified by the film manufacturer—and that the safelight is light-tight and that there is no light from any other source.

Leakage of any light into the processing room can fog unprotected film. Fluorescent lights used in a darkroom may cause trouble by their afterglow. The first few films opened after the fluorescent fixture has been turned off may show fogging. Fogging of film may occur after an interruption whereby the film is left on the processing hanger too long before processing is accomplished.

Access to the darkroom should be controlled by the use of interlocking doors, or by a door with an inside lock, so that it may not be opened inadvertently or at an inopportune time during the processing of film. The use of a maze, or baffled entrance, may also be successfully employed as a light-proof entrance to the darkroom. Such an approach, however, may limit the floor area of the processing room, for often the entrance is designed at the expense of processing space.

Proper planning for the processing of film, with care and standardization of the techniques of processing, will help the dentist obtain radiographic films that provide maximal information and record data.

REFERENCES

Alcox, R. W. and Jameson, W. R.: Rapid Dental X-ray Film Processor for Selected Procedures. J. Am. Dent. A. 78:517–519 (Mar.) 1969.

Alcox, R. W. and Waggener, D. T.: Status Report on Rapid Processing Devices for Dental Radiographic Film. J. Am. Dent. A. 83:1330–1333 (Dec.) 1971.

Cahoon, J. B.: Formulating X-ray Technics. Ed. 7. Durham, N.C., Duke University Press, 1970.

Carr, J. D. and Norman, R. D.: Effective Use of the Darkroom. Dent. Clin. North America. July, pp. 363–370, 1961.

Council on Dental Materials and Devices: Revised American Dental Association Specification No. 22 for Intraoral Dental Radiographic Film Adopted. J. Am. Dent. A. 80:1066–1068 (May) 1970.

Crabtree, J. I. and Matthews, G. E.: Photographic Chemicals and Solutions. Boston, American Photographic Publishing Company, 1939, 360 pp.

Eastman Kodak Company, Medical Division: The Fundamentals of Radiography. Rochester, New York, 1960, 76 pp.

Eastman Kodak Company, Radiography Markets Division: X-rays in Dentistry. Rochester, New York, 1972, 84 pp.

Ingle, J. J., Beveridge, E. E., and Olson, C. E.: Rapid Processing of Endodontic "Working" Roentgenograms. Oral Surg., Oral Med. & Oral Path. 19:101–107 (Jan.) 1965.

Meredith, W. J. and Massey, J. B.: Fundamental Physics of Radiology. Ed. 2. Baltimore, Williams & Wilkins Company, 1972, 666 pp.

Richards, A. G.: Technical Factors That Control Radiographic Density. Dent. Clin. North America. July, pp. 371–377, 1961.

Ross, J. A. and Galloway, R. W.: A Handbook of Radiography. Ed. 3. Philadelphia, J. B. Lippincott Company, 1963, p. 191.

United States War Department: Technical Manual (TM 1–219): Basic Photography. 1941, 342 pp.

Webber, R. L., Benton, P. A., and Ryge, G.: Diagnostic Variations in Radiographs. Oral Surg., Oral Med. & Oral Path. 26:800–809 (Dec.) 1968.

Wing, K., Sairenji, E., and Söremark, R.: Extraoral Roentgenography with Polaroid Land Films. Oral Surg., Oral Med. & Oral Path. 28:175–183 (Aug.) 1969.

ROENTGENOGRAPHIC PHYSICS

MARVIN M. D. WILLIAMS, Ph.D.

The field of roentgenographic physics, or the physics of diagnostic roentgenology, is only a part of the broader field of radiologic physics. Roentgenographic physics does not include the physics of radiation therapy or the diagnostic and therapeutic uses of radioisotopes. However, roentgenographic physics and radiologic physics both require a similar background—some knowledge of subjects that are covered in an elementary college physics course, including energy, radiation, atomic structure, electricity, and magnetism. By the time such knowledge is needed in a professional school, some of it may not be remembered; hence some background physics is included in this appendix, but it is not possible to include a discussion of all of the applications of physics to roentgenography, much less a thorough review of basic physics.

RADIATION

Radiation is energy being transferred from one place to another without a material carrier. It is frequently referred to as electromagnetic radiation. Visible radiation is only a minute fraction of the total spectrum of electromagnetic radiation (Fig. III–1). Some of the other parts of the spectrum are known as electric waves, radio waves, infrared radiation, ultraviolet radiation, and x-rays. Gamma rays and cosmic radiation are in the same part of the spectrum as x-rays; they differ from x-rays only in their place of origin.

WAVE THEORY

Associated with this transfer of energy known as radiation are an electric and a magnetic field. The instantaneous strengths of these two fields at a point past which the radiation is traveling vary continuously, and the direction of the fields changes periodically. The variation in strength and the changes in direction can be represented by a curve known as a sine wave (Fig. III–2); the same type of curve is used to represent

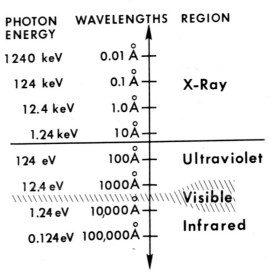

Figure III–1 Part of the spectrum of electromagnetic radiations.

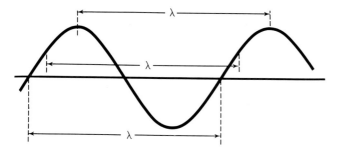

Figure III–2 Sine wave showing the variations in strength and direction of the electric and magnetic fields associated with radiations. Wavelength, λ, is the distance between successive corresponding points on the curve. A sine wave also can represent the variations in value and direction of potential or current for an electric alternating current; the complete sequence of values that occurs in a wavelength is referred to as a cycle.

the transmission of sound through a medium or the variations in current and potential from an alternating-current source of electric power.

A sine wave repeats itself periodically. It may be described in terms of the number of times it repeats itself each second, which is called the *frequency* and is represented by the Greek letter v. The distance between corresponding points on successive waves is called the *wavelength* and is represented by the Greek letter λ. The product of v and λ equals the velocity, represented by c, at which the waves are traveling. In a vacuum, the velocity of all radiations is the same, about 186,000 miles per second or 3×10^{10}* cm/sec. Different kinds of radiation may be specified in terms of either their frequency or, more commonly, their wavelengths.

Radiation of wavelengths of millions of meters is known as electric waves. As the wavelength becomes shorter, approaching a meter in length, the radiation is known as radio waves; still shorter wavelength radiation is known as infrared. Visible radiation has wavelengths measured in a few thousand angstroms (1 angstrom is equal to 1×10^{-8} cm); still shorter wavelength radiation is known as ultraviolet; and when the wavelength is about 12 angstroms, or less, the radiation is known as x-rays (Fig. III–1).

QUANTUM THEORY

Some of the interactions of radiation with matter cannot be explained by the wave theory of radiation but can be explained by the quantum theory. The quantum theory postulates that the energy is transferred in small packets, called photons. The energy contained in a photon is related to the wavelength of the associated electromagnetic wave by an inverse relationship: the energy of a photon in electron volts = 12,400 divided by the wavelength in angstroms.* Hence, the different regions of radiation may also be differentiated by the energy of their photons; the photons of electric waves have extremely small amounts of energy, those of visible radiation have energies from about 1.8 to 3.6 eV, and the photons of x-rays have energies greater than 1000 eV or 1 keV.†

Since the production of x-rays and their interaction with matter can be described much more simply in terms of the quantum theory, little further mention will be made of the wave theory.

PRODUCTION OF X-RAYS

Energy exists in many forms other than radiation, and one kind of energy

---

*Very large or small numbers are conveniently represented by a small number multiplied by a power of 10. A positive exponent of 10 indicates the number of digits that should follow to the right of the decimal point; a negative exponent, the number to the left of the decimal point: thus 3.0×10^{10}=30,000,000,000 and 1.0×10^{-8}=0.000,000,01.

---

*An electron volt, eV, is the energy an electron will have after having been accelerated between two points which differ in potential by 1 volt. A unit 1000 times as great, the kilo-electron volt, keV, is a more convenient unit for this discussion. The constant 12,400 includes Planck's constant, the velocity of light, and factors to convert ergs to electron volts and to convert centimeters to angstroms.

†There is no sharp demarcation between the different regions of radiation. The value of 1 keV for the lower limit of the x-ray region is arbitrary but is satisfactory for this discussion.

frequently changes into another kind. The energy of flowing water in a river may be converted into mechnical energy to drive an electric generator; this electrical energy may be converted into heat, which in turn may be converted into visible radiation; the visible radiation may be converted into electrical energy in a photoelectric cell; and this electrical energy may operate relays to start or stop a motor. The production of radiation is the conversion of some kind of energy* into the kind of energy known as radiation.

ENERGY CONVERSION TO X-RAYS

An x-ray photon is sometimes produced when a high-energy electron loses energy: the energy lost by the electron becomes a photon of that amount of energy. Hence the first step in the production of x-rays is the production of a large number of high-energy electrons, a process that is accomplished practically in an x-ray tube.

An x-ray tube (Fig. III–3) consists of two electrodes in an evacuated glass envelope. One electrode, the cathode, is the source of electrons, and the other electrode, the anode, stops the electrons after they have been accelerated to a high velocity. The x-rays are produced in the anode as the electrons are stopped.

---

*An exception is that under some circumstances mass may be converted into radiation.

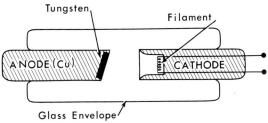

Figure III–3 An x-ray tube consists of a cathode and an anode that extend into the very highly evacuated space inside a glass envelope. The important part of the cathode is the filament, the source of electrons. In the anode is an insert of tungsten, sometimes called the target, which is struck by the electrons from the cathode and in which the x-rays originate.

The electrons emitted by the cathode, actually from the filament in the cathode, are accelerated because of a difference in electrical potential between the two electrodes. Since an electron has mass, it is necessary that work be done on it—a force acting through a distance—to make it travel with high velocity. The amount of kinetic energy—the energy due to the velocity of an object having mass—that the electron obtains will be equal to the work done on it because of the difference in potential. This work, measured in electron volts, is numerically equal to the difference in potential between the electrodes. If the difference in potential is 60 kV, then the kinetic energy of an electron when it reaches the anode will be 60 keV. Thus electrical energy has been converted into kinetic energy.

Most of the kinetic energy of the electrons will be converted into heat and only a small fraction into x-ray photons when the electrons are stopped in the anode. The fraction of the energy of the electrons converted into photons increases as their energy (potential difference between the electrodes) increases and as the atomic number of the material they strike increases. When a potential difference of 100 kV is applied to an x-ray tube that has a tungsten anode, less than 1% of the energy of the electrons is converted into x-rays. This process of producing x-rays may be summarized as:

$$\text{electrical energy} \rightarrow \text{kinetic energy} \begin{cases} \nearrow \text{heat } (99 + \%) \\ \searrow \text{x-rays } (1 - \%) \end{cases}$$

where the arrows mean "is changed to" or "is converted into."

ATOMIC STRUCTURE

An understanding of the production of x-rays (and also of the interaction of x-rays with matter, to be discussed later) requires some knowledge of the structure of atoms. All atoms consist of a nucleus and one or more electrons. The nucleus contains protons and neutrons (except for the most common form of hydrogen, the nucleus of which consists of a single proton). Protons and neutrons have about the same mass (about 6×10^{23} weigh 1 gm). The proton has a positive electric charge, and the neutron has no electric charge. An electron weighs about one-eighteen-hundredth as much as a proton and has a negative electric charge[*] equal in magnitude to the positive charge on a proton. Normally an atom contains the same number of electrons as protons and its net electric charge is zero. Occasionally an atom temporarily will have a few extra electrons or will be minus a few electrons; in such a state the atom is called an ion—a negative ion if it has a surplus of electrons, a positive ion if it is deficient in electrons. A free electron also is called a negative ion.

All of the atoms of an element have the same number of protons in their nuclei and, hence, the same number of electrons in the atom. The number of protons in the nucleus, called the *atomic number,* determines the chemical element to which an atom belongs. The number of neutrons in the nuclei of atoms of the same chemical element may vary.

Bohr Theory. The exact structure of an atom is not known, but a commonly discussed theory, the Bohr theory, postulates that the electrons travel around the nucleus in orbits somewhat as the earth and other planets travel around the sun. The electrons are held in the atom because of the attraction between their negative charge and the positive charge on the nucleus; the electrons are not pulled into the nucleus because the centrifugal force resulting from their traveling in a curved path equals the attractive force between the charges. There may be more than one electron traveling in an orbit; the number of electrons in each orbit is a characteristic of each element. The removal of an electron from an orbit requires that work be done by an outside agent to pull the electron away from the nucleus. If the electron is pulled sufficiently far away, the force of attraction

becomes negligible, the electron is no longer a part of the atom, and two ions have been produced—the free electron is a negative ion and the atom that lost the electron is a positive ion.

Energy Levels. The position of an electron in an atom may be described not only as being in an orbit but also as being in an *energy level.* The value of an energy level is the amount of work that must be done on an electron in that level to free it from the atom—to produce ionization. The amount of work required to remove an electron is frequently called the *ionization potential,* or the *binding energy,* of the electron. The ionization potentials of energy levels in an atom are determined by its atomic number. Figure III–4 shows some of the energy levels for atoms of hydrogen, oxygen, and tungsten.

CHARACTERISTIC RADIATION

If an electron is removed from its normal position in an atom, by being either knocked out of the atom (ionization) or moved to a vacant space in an energy level farther from the nucleus, the atom is said to be in an *excited state.* Generally an atom remains in an excited state for only a short time, perhaps of the order of a fraction of a microsecond. Commonly, the vacancy in the electron configuration is filled by an electron that is pulled into the vacancy from the next outer, or the second outer, or even the third outer energy level. Such a transition involves an acceleration of the electron; the energy it has thus gained when it arrives at the vacancy is lost as a photon. If the excited state also happens to be an ionized state, eventually the atom captures an electron to complete its normal complement of electrons.

The photons produced by electrons, within an atom, which have been accelerated toward the nucleus are characteristic of the element to which the atom belongs; they are spoken of as *characteristic radiations.* They are characteristic of the element because the values of the ionization potentials, and hence the differences between energy levels, are different for all el-

---

[*]When a current of 1 milliampere flows through an x-ray tube, about 6×10^{15} electrons go from the cathode to the anode each second.

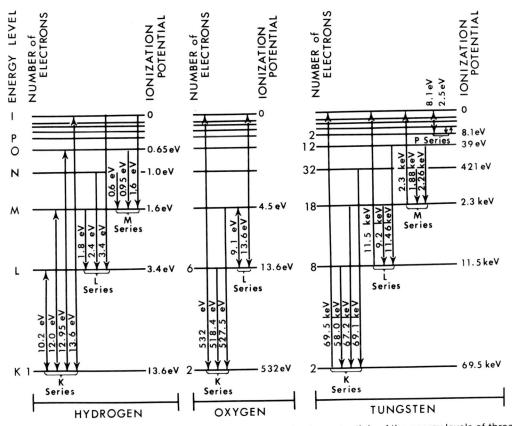

Figure III–4   Number of electrons in and some of the ionization potentials of the energy levels of three elements. A few of the possible transitions of electrons between levels are shown, the arrows indicating the possible directions of the transitions. Characteristic radiation in the visible region occurs in the L series of hydrogen, the M series of oxygen (not shown), and the P series of tungsten. The M series of hydrogen is in the infrared region. The K series of hydrogen and oxygen, the L series of oxygen, and part of the P series of tungsten are in the ultraviolet region. The K, L, and M series of tungsten are in the x-ray region. (Some energy levels consist of several sublevels whose ionization potentials differ slightly. This *fine structure* is not important in a discussion such as this.)

ements but the same for all of the atoms of an element. The ionization potential for a particular energy level—K, L, and so on—increases as the atomic number of the element increases. The energy of a characteristic photon is equal to the difference in the ionization potentials of the two energy levels involved. All elements have characteristic radiation in the infrared, the visible, and the ultraviolet regions of the spectra. Sodium (atomic number 11) is the element of lowest atomic number with characteristic radiation in the x-ray region because it is the element of lowest atomic number with an ionization potential above 1 keV. From the data in Figure III–4 it is evident that the K, L, and M series of tungsten are in the x-ray region.

When a high-energy electron reaches the anode of an x-ray tube, generally tungsten, it may lose a part or all of its energy by causing the atoms in the anode to vibrate more violently, which means the anode is heated. Occasionally the high-energy electron will knock an electron out of its normal position in a tungsten atom; following such an event the atom will emit characteristic radiation. Characteristic x-rays of the M series cannot be produced unless the potential across the tube is at least 2.3 kV, because the incoming electron must have at least 2.3 keV of energy to knock an M electron out of the atom. Similarly, characteristic K radiation cannot be produced unless the potential across the tube is at least 69.5 kV.

BREMSSTRAHLEN

Occasionally an electron that has reached the target of the x-ray tube passes very close to the nucleus of an atom; there, because of the attractive force between the charge on the electron and on the nucleus, the electron is slowed down. The energy lost by the electron, which is the difference between the energy it had when it reached the atom and the energy it had after being slowed down, becomes a photon. The radiation produced by this slowing down of electrons is called *bremsstrahlen*.

An electron may be slowed down only a slight amount or it may be stopped; hence, the energy of the photons comprising the bremsstrahlen spectrum may be of any value from nearly zero up to a maximum equal to the energy of the incoming electrons (Fig. III–5). The energy of the incoming electrons, in turn, is determined by the potential applied to the x-ray tube. The average energy of the photons comprising the spectrum is between one-third and one-half of the maximal energy.

Changing the milliamperage flowing through the tube produces no change in the shape of the spectral curve. For example, if the milliamperage is doubled, there will be twice the number of electrons striking the target each second, but the same fraction of them will lose the same fractions of their energies; the absolute number of photons produced each second will be doubled, but the ratios of those having various energy values will remain the same.

If the potential across the tube is increased, the number of photons of all energies that was present at the lower potential will be increased, the increase will be relatively much greater for the photons of higher energy than for the photons of lower energy, and photons of higher energy than those previously present will be added to the spectrum. These changes resulting from an increased potential produce a beam with a higher average photon energy. If the potential across the tube is high enough, characteristic radiation of the target will be superimposed on the bremsstrahlen spectra; this increases the number of photons of a few specific energy values, but these constitute a negligible fraction of the total number of photons in the x-ray beam. Practically all of the characteristic L and M radiations, as well as the bremsstrahlen photons of similarly low energies, are absorbed by the wall of the x-ray tube and by other filters in the path of the useful beam.

X-RAY MACHINES

For the production of x-rays it is necessary that electrons be accelerated to such a velocity that their energy is high enough to be converted into x-ray photons. For the x-rays used in roentgenography a potential across the x-ray tube of from about 60 kV to 100 kV is necessary.

The operator of the x-ray machine must be able to choose a value of the potential which will produce x-rays of the desired quality — photons having the desired amount of energy. He must be able to control the intensity of the radiation, the intensity depending on the current (rate of flow of electrons) through the x-ray tube.[*] He must be able to control the length of time x-rays are produced.

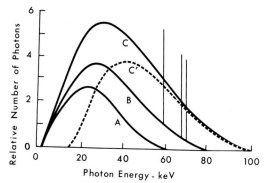

Figure III–5 Bremsstrahlen spectra produced when the potential applied to an x-ray tube is 60 kV *(A)*, 80 kV *(B)*, and 100 kV *(C)*. Characteristic K radiations of the tungsten target are indicated by the three vertical lines on B and C; they are not indicated on A because electrons accelerated by 60 kV do not have sufficient energy to remove tungsten's K electrons. C′ is the spectrum for 100 kV when a filter of 2 mm Al is added.

---

[*]The tube current for most dental x-ray machines is between 5 and 15 milliamperes.

TRANSFORMERS

The high potential necessary for accelerating the electrons and, also, a low potential for the filament of the x-ray tube are obtained by the use of transformers. Most transformers have two coils of wire wound on an iron core. One of these coils is connected to the source of electric power; it is called the *primary coil.* The other coil, called the *secondary coil,* is connected to the apparatus for which power is needed—the electrodes of the x-ray tube or the filament of the x-ray tube, in this instance. The ratio of the potential applied to the primary coil to the potential developed in the secondary coil is equal to the ratio of the number of turns of wire in the two coils.* If the secondary coil has more turns of wire than the primary coil, the potential developed in the secondary will be greater than that applied to the primary; such a transformer is called a *step-up transformer.* If the secondary coil has fewer turns of wire than the primary coil, the potential developed in the secondary will be less than that applied to the primary; such a transformer is called a *step-down transformer.* Such two-coil transformers also isolate the secondary circuits from the primary circuits, a feature that is desirable when the difference in the potentials of the two circuits is large.

Another type of transformer, called an *autotransformer,* consists of a single coil of wire wound on an iron core. Part of the coil is used for the primary and part is used for the secondary; many of the coils of wire are a part of both the primary and secondary circuits. The number of turns of wire included in the secondary can be varied by a switch or by a slider that moves along the coil. The number of turns of wire included in the secondary can be less or a little greater than the number in the primary. An autotransformer is used to obtain a variable voltage supply when the voltage

needed differs little from that supplied to the primary coil and when it is not necessary that the primary and secondary circuits be electrically isolated from each other.

The ratio of the currents flowing in the primary and secondary coils is inversely proportional to the number of turns of wire in the two coils. Hence, in a step-up transformer the current is greater in the primary circuit, and in the step-down transformer the current is greater in the secondary circuit.

MAIN PRIMARY CIRCUIT

The main circuit of an x-ray machine includes a variable voltage supply, commonly an autotransformer, and a step-up transformer to supply the high potential for the x-ray tube (Fig. III–6). The machine is

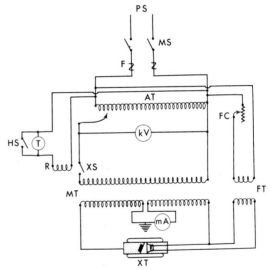

Figure III–6 Circuits of x-ray machines are not all the same, but all contain most of the features shown here. The circuit is connected to its power supply (PS) by a main switch (MS) and is protected by fuses (F). The autotransformer (AT) supplies the desired potential for the main transformer (MT); the potential is measured by the voltmeter (kV), commonly calibrated to indicate the potential to be applied to the x-ray tube (XT). The milliampere meter (mA) in the circuit grounding part of the transformer secondary measures the current flowing through the x-ray tube. The exposure, or x-ray, switch (XS) is part of the relay (R) circuit which is controlled by a timer (T) or by other switches such as a hand switch (HS). Power for the filament of the tube is from the filament transformer (FT) and is controlled by the filament control (FC), here shown as a rheostat.

---

*The ratios of potentials and numbers of turns are not quite equal because a transformer is not a 100% efficient machine; however, for a discussion such as this it is permissible to consider that the ratios are equal.

generally connected to a 110-volt supply line, with the main transformer having a ratio of approximately 1 to 1000 so that the secondary can supply potentials to the x-ray tube of up to about 100 kV. The potential to be supplied to the primary of the main transformer comes from the secondary of the autotransformer. The value of this potential is indicated on a voltmeter. Instead of indicating the volts available for the primary of the main transformer, the reading on this voltmeter generally indicates the kilovolts that will be applied to the x-ray tube; this is possible because there is nearly a constant ratio between the voltage applied to the primary of the main transformer and the kilovolts applied to the x-ray tube.*

X-rays are produced only when the x-ray switch in the primary circuit is closed; when this switch is open no current flows through either coil of the main transformer. A heavy duty switch is required because the current in the primary circuit of the main transformer is large; this switch is commonly operated by a relay. The relay circuit contains a timer that turns the power for the relay on and off, thus controlling the x-ray exposure. Other switches, such as the hand switch in Figure III–6, may be included in the relay circuit to allow the x-rays to be turned on without the use of the timer.

FILAMENT CIRCUIT

The source of electrons in the x-ray tube is a coil of tungsten wire, called the filament, which is part of the cathode. As with most metals, when tungsten is heated to a sufficiently high temperature, electrons are emitted—boiled off, so to speak; the rate at which they are emitted increases

rapidly as the temperature rises above the threshold for emission of electrons. The filament is heated by the passage of a current through it. A greater current through the filament will result in a higher temperature, a greater emission of electrons, and a greater current through the x-ray tube. Because the filament is a part of the cathode and is connected to the high potential, it is necessary that the filament circuit be isolated from the main power supply. This isolation is accomplished by a step-down transformer that supplies a potential of a few (ordinarily between 3 and 5) volts and a current of a few (ordinarily between 1.5 and 2.5) amperes for the filament. The temperature of the filament must be controlled accurately to maintain the desired current through the x-ray tube; the current through the filament is determined by the potential generated in the secondary of the filament transformer, which, in turn, is determined by the potential applied to the primary of this transformer. The control for this primary potential, commonly called the *filament control* or the *milliamperage control*, is a variable resistance, called a *rheostat*, in the primary of the filament circuit. (Occasionally another device, called a *choke coil*, is used instead of a rheostat.)

HIGH-VOLTAGE CIRCUIT

If the high-voltage part of the circuit (secondaries of the main and filament transformers and the x-ray tube) were entirely insulated from other circuits and from ground, it might develop a large potential difference with respect to ground potential. This potential difference would develop because electrical charges gradually flow into the insulating materials from the conductors in the circuit. This potential difference might cause the insulation to break down. To prevent the development of such a potential difference with respect to ground, one point of the high-voltage circuit, either the center or one end of the transformer secondary, is connected to ground (Fig. III–6). This grounding of the second-

---

*Because of power losses in various parts of the circuit, some of which depend on the current flowing through the x-ray tube, the voltmeter, frequently referred to as the kV meter, may not indicate the true kV. The errors are generally constant and small, hence the meter reading may be depended on for the duplication of exposures. Also, some of these power losses cause the reading of the meter to be less during the time x-rays are being produced.

ary circuit permits one of the grounding wires to be connected to a milliampere meter in the control cabinet before being connected to ground. Since this meter is in series with the secondary of the transformer and the x-ray tube, it will measure the current flowing through the tube.

In most dental x-ray equipment, the main transformer, filament transformer, and x-ray tube are housed in a small metal container. This container is filled with oil to insulate the parts of the circuit from one another and from the container, which is connected to ground so that anyone touching it will not receive an electric shock. The container, except for a small area through which the useful beam of x-rays emerges, is lined with lead to prevent x-rays from going out in all directions from the tube. The remaining circuits, including the milliampere meter (Fig. III–6), are located in the control cabinet.

The potential developed in the secondary of the main transformer is an alternating current potential (Fig. III–7), which normally would cause a current to flow in opposite directions during alternate half-cycles. However, a current can flow through the x-ray tube in only one direction, from filament to target,* unless the focal spot becomes hot enough to emit electrons which then could flow from the focal spot to the filament. Such an inverse current would heat the cathode assembly to a very high temperature and ruin it because it is not designed to withstand such high temperatures. If the machine is operated properly the focal spot will not become hot enough to emit electrons. A current flows through the x-ray tube only during those half-cycles when the potential is such that the filament is negative and the target is positive; these half-cycles are called the *useful half-cycles*. During the other half-

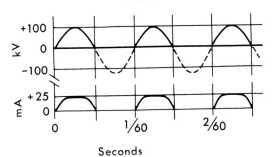

Seconds

Figure III–7 Wave forms of potential applied to and current flowing through the x-ray tube. Current flows only during the alternate half-cycles (the useful half-cycles, labeled +) when the potential applied to the cathode is negative and that to the anode is positive. During the other half-cycles (inverse half-cycles, labeled –), the peak value of the potential is greater than in the useful half-cycle. Because the current flows only half the time and is not constant when it does flow, the average current (reading of the milliampere meter) would be approximately 10 milliamperes for the maximum of 25 as shown here.

cycles, the *inverse half-cycles*, no current flows. The x-ray tube acts as a rectifier; this circuit is said to be a *self-rectified circuit.** When a current is flowing, some of the potential is used to send the current through the various resistances in the circuit; this causes the peak value of the potential during the useful half-cycle to be somewhat less than the peak value during the inverse half-cycle.

Because the potential continuously varies, the value of the potential applied to the x-ray tube is customarily designated as that of the peak value during the useful half-cycle. Hence, if the potential is stated to be 90 kV, it is understood that the maximal, or peak, useful potential applied to the tube is 90 kV, often written as 90 kVp.

X-RAY TUBE

The images on a roentgenogram are shadows cast by structures that have various degrees of transmission of x-rays.

---

*The old conventional description of an electric current indicated that the current flowed from positive to negative, necessitating a flow of positive charges. In most circumstances a current is a flow of negative charges (electrons) which flow from negative to positive.

---

*X-ray equipment used for many diagnostic examinations and for radiation therapy may have more complicated high-voltage circuits.

These shadows will not be sharp enough to show small detail unless the source of x-rays is very small. The actual source of the x-rays is the area of the target struck by the electrons—the *focal spot*. The shape of the cathode surrounding the filament is such that it causes the electrons to strike a very small area on the anode—causes the focal spot to be very small. Because more than 99% of the energy of the electrons is converted into heat, the focal spot must be on a material with a very high melting and vaporization temperature; tungsten satisfies these requirements very well. Also it is necessary that the heat produced in the focal spot area be removed as rapidly as possible, and since copper is a much better conductor of heat than tungsten, the small piece of tungsten is imbedded in a large piece of copper.

The actual size of the focal spot is larger than it appears to be because the angle between the face of the target and the central ray of the useful x-ray beam is small (Fig. III–8). This angle is generally 15 to 20° for roentgenographic tubes. The actual focal spot size is a rectangle about three to four times as long as it is wide. When this rectangle is viewed along the central ray it appears to be a square with dimensions equal to the width—commonly 1 to 2 mm. With the actual size of the focal spot a large rectangle rather than a square, the production of heat is spread over a larger area, thus reducing the rise in temperature. Hence an effectively small focal spot can be used with less danger of its being overheated.

INTERACTION OF X-RAYS AND MATTER

If a beam of x-rays from a source, S, Figure III–9A, falls on a thick sheet of lead with a small hole in it, a detector such as an ionization chamber in position D will indicate a quantity proportional to the amount of radiation falling on it. If the detector is moved to position D', it will indicate no radiation; radiation from S which starts in a direction to reach D' is stopped by the sheet of lead.

If a sheet of material, such as a piece of aluminum, is placed in the beam above the lead, as in Figure III–9B, the detector will indicate less radiation. The sheet of aluminum is said to have *attenuated* the radiation. No radiation will be detected at D'. However, if the sheet of aluminum is placed below the lead, as in Figure III–9C, the amount of radiation reaching D will be about the same as when the aluminum was above the lead, but radiation now will be detected at D'.

Experiments such as have been described show that attenuation of a beam of radiation as it passes through matter is a combination of two processes: (1) some of the energy—radiation—remains in the matter and (2) some of the photons—radiation—have their direction of travel changed. The first of these two processes is called *absorption* and the second *scatter*.*

---

*Some of these terms are frequently used in a less strict sense: what is here called attenuation is sometimes called absorption; what is here called absorption is sometimes called true absorption.

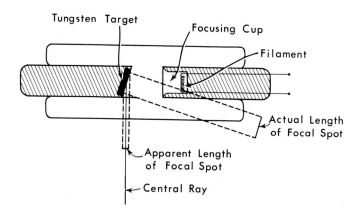

Figure III–8 The focusing cup forces electrons emitted by the filament to strike the anode in a limited rectangular area, the focal spot. Because the angle between the central ray and the face of the target is small, the focal spot appears to be a square when viewed along the central ray.

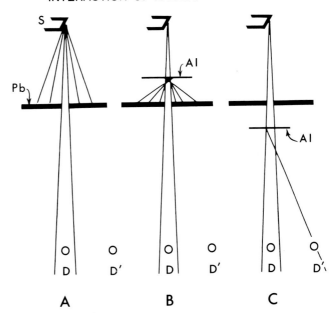

Figure III-9 X-rays from the source (S) are stopped by the thick sheet of lead (Pb) but pass through the small hole. Hence, in *A,* radiation reaches detector D but not D'. In *B* the sheet of aluminum (Al) above the lead absorbs and scatters some of the radiation; the amount reaching D is reduced and none reaches D' because the scattered radiation is stopped by the lead. When the aluminum is below the lead, as in *C,* some of the radiation scattered by it does reach D'.

That energy, or photon, which is absorbed has an effect on the absorber; that energy, or photon, which is scattered has no effect on the scatterer but does decrease the amount of energy, or the number of photons, in the beam of radiation.

The roentgenographic shadow of a tooth is produced because the tooth has attenuated the beam of x-rays by both absorbing and scattering some of the energy. Of that radiation reaching the film, some is absorbed in the film and some is scattered by the film, but only that which is absorbed in the film produces an effect on the film.

When radiation falls on a thin sheet of material, such as aluminum (Fig. III-9), most of the photons pass through unchanged either in the amount of energy they contain or in the direction in which they are traveling. Photons—energy—that pass through unchanged of course have no effect on the material through which they pass.

Absorption or scattering of radiation is the result of a photon having had a collision with an electron. These collisions are not of a particle with a particle—the photon is not a mass particle but only energy—but are an interaction between the electromagnetic field associated with a photon and the electromagnetic field associated with an electron. Three kinds of interactions occur:* (1) *unmodified scatter,* (2) *photoelectric absorption,* and (3) *Compton scatter,* or *modified scatter.* These three kinds of interactions are illustrated in Figure III-10.

UNMODIFIED SCATTER

Unmodified scatter occurs when a photon collides with an electron whose binding energy is greater than the energy of the photon. Since the electron cannot be moved from its position in the atom by this amount of energy, the photon bounces off the electron and travels in a new direction. The scattered photon has the same amount of energy as it had before the collision; therefore no effect has been produced in the scatterer. This kind of interaction is of little importance in the x-ray region.

PHOTOELECTRIC ABSORPTION

Photoelectric absorption occurs when a photon collides with an electron whose binding energy is equal to or less than the

---

*There are other interactions but they occur only with photons of very much higher energy than the photons used in roentgenography.

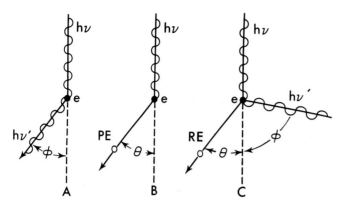

Figure III–10 Three types of interactions between a photon of energy of hν and an electron (e): *A,* Unmodified scatter; the photon is scattered through an angle φ; the energy, hν', of the scattered photon is the same as that of the photon before scattering. *B,* Photoelectric absorption; the photon transfers all of its energy to the electron, the photoelectron (PE), which goes off at some angle θ to the direction the photon had been traveling. *C,* Compton scatter; part of the energy of the photon is given to the recoil electron (RE), which goes off at an angle θ, and the remainder of the energy, hν', goes off as a photon at an angle φ.

energy of the photon. The electron is removed from the atom—ionization has been produced. Any energy of the photon in excess of that necessary to remove the electron from the atom is given to the electron: the electron will have kinetic energy equal to the energy of the photon minus the binding energy of the electron (the energy used to remove the electron from the atom). This electron is called a *photoelectron,* and it may go off in any direction relative to the direction the photon was traveling.

The photoelectron will lose its energy by such processes as producing additional ionization, splitting large molecules, producing heat, and perhaps producing bremsstrahlen. The distance the photoelectron travels will depend on its energy and the medium through which it is traveling; the distance increases as its energy increases, and the distance decreases as the density (grams per cubic centimeter) of the medium increases—an electron with 80 keV of energy will travel about 9 cm in air or 0.1 mm in soft tissue. When the atom from which the photoelectron came captures an electron and returns to normal, characteristic radiation is produced; in tissue most of such characteristic radiation is absorbed close to where it is generated.

Photoelectric absorption results in the disappearance of the photon and in the transference of all of its energy to the medium.

The probability that photoelectric absorption will occur increases very rapidly as the atomic number of the atoms in the medium increases and decreases quite

rapidly as the photon energy increases.* A great deal more photoelectric absorption occurs in teeth and bone than in soft tissues because teeth and bone contain elements of higher atomic number and have greater density (gm/cc).

COMPTON SCATTER

Compton scatter occurs when a photon collides with an electron whose binding energy is very small compared with the energy of the photon. Part of the energy of the photon is used for removing the electron from the atom and giving it kinetic energy, and the rest of the energy continues as a photon traveling in a different direction. This electron is called a *Compton electron* or a *recoil electron* and the new photon, a *scattered photon.* The Compton electron loses its energy by the same processes as does a photoelectron. The scattered photon will eventually interact again, but in a place where it would not have been if it had not been scattered (photons

---

*The decrease with increasing photon energy is true for photons of energies between the ionization potentials of adjacent energy levels of an atom and for photons of energies greater than the K ionization potential of an atom. However, the probability that photoelectric absorption will occur increases suddenly as the photon energy increases from just less than to just more than the ionization potential of an energy level of an atom. The energies of the x-ray photons used in roentgenography are greater than the K ionization potentials of the common elements in body tissues; hence these sudden increases in photoelectric absorption probability do not occur in the range of photon energies used in roentgenography.

scattered from one tooth may interact in a film in the region of the shadow of another tooth; this interaction will reduce the shadow and may obscure some of the detail that should be present in the shadow).

The angle of scatter of the photon may be any angle from 0 to 180°. The average angle of scatter is smaller for photons of high energy than for photons of low energy. The angle of the Compton electron is between 90 and 0°. The angle decreases as the angle of scatter of the photon increases. The energy of the electron—the energy lost by the photon—increases as the angle of scatter of the photon increases, and also increases as photon energy increases.* For those photon energies commonly used in roentgenography, the average angle of scatter of the photons is about 85°, the average angle of the Compton electrons about 47°, and the average energy of the Compton electrons is about 4% to 14% of the energy of the photons.

Compton scatter results in the transference of a part of the energy of the original photon to the medium and the production of a photon of lower energy traveling in another direction.

The probability that Compton scattering will occur decreases slowly as photon energy increases; it is not dependent on the atomic number of the elements in the medium but on the electron density† (number of electrons per cubic centimeter).

For the qualities of radiation used in roentgenography, photoelectric absorption is in general more important than Compton scattering in producing attenuation of the

x-ray beam. However, if a high potential, such as 100 kV, is used for generating the x-rays, Compton scattering may be more important in the soft tissues, but photoelectric absorption still will be more important, or at least as important, in teeth and bone because they contain elements of higher atomic number than do soft tissues.

ATTENUATION

For an x-ray beam containing photons of only one energy value—a monochromatic or monoenergetic beam—a given thickness of a material as a filter will always produce the same percentage of attenuation—will always transmit the same percentage of the radiation falling on it. If one unit of thickness attenuates the beam 10% (transmits 90%), a second thickness will attenuate the beam by 10% of that which is transmitted by the first thickness (9% in this example); thus 81% of the original energy is transmitted by the two thicknesses. A third thickness will produce an additional 10% attenuation of that which was transmitted by the previous two thicknesses, or 10% of 81%, which is 8.1%. This can be stated as: for a monochromatic beam and for a material of constant chemical composition, the rate of attentuation per unit thickness is constant.

The rate at which attenuation occurs is called the *attenuation coefficient* and is expressed as the rate at which attenuation occurs per centimeter thickness of the material.* The attenuation coefficient is represented by the Greek letter μ. The value of μ in general decreases as the photon energy increases and increases as the atomic number of the attenuator increases.

A beam of photons of higher energy is less rapidly attenuated; it is commonly spoken of as a beam of harder quality. Material that has a higher density (gm/cc) generally is composed of higher atomic numbered el-

---

*If a photon of high energy and a photon of low energy are both scattered through the same angle, the Compton electron produced by the photon of high energy will have more energy and its angle will be less.

†The number of electrons per atom does increase with atomic number, but, except for hydrogen, the number of electrons per gram is nearly constant for the elements in body tissues. A gram of hydrogen contains twice as many electrons as a gram of any other element. One of the electrons in an atom of calcium is as likely to produce Compton scattering (if the energy of the photon is high enough) as is an electron in an atom of hydrogen.

---

*This is called the *linear attenuation coefficient.* Another coefficient frequently used is the *mass attenuation coefficient,* that is, the rate of attenuation per gram per square centimeter of surface area.

ements and, hence, is a better attenuator of x-rays. However, a material that is denser because of closer packing of the molecules, such as water as compared with water vapor, will be a better attenuator of a beam of x-rays for equal thicknesses, but different thicknesses having the same cross-sectional area and having the same mass will attenuate a beam by the same amount.

The amount of radiation transmitted by any material can be calculated by the equation

$$I_X = I_0 e^{-\mu X} \text{ where}$$

I_0 is the intensity of the radiation falling on the material, I_X the intensity of the transmitted radiation, e the base of the natural system of logarithms (2.718), μ the attenuation coefficient for the material and for the photon energy, and x the thickness of the material. If the material contains more than one chemical element, it is necessary to calculate an average value for μ by taking into account the relative amounts of each element present. If the beam of x-rays contains photons of more than one energy value (beams used for roentgenography contain photons having a whole spectrum of energy values), it is necessary to calculate separately the transmission for photons of each energy. However, for many practical problems, when approximate values are sufficient, a heterogeneous beam may be considered to be approximately equivalent to a homogeneous beam of some specific photon energy. This equivalent energy value is generally between one-third and one-half of the maximal photon energy.

Figure III–11 is a graph of the values of μ for photon energies from 10 keV to 100 keV for water (which is essentially the same as muscle), bone (which is similar to dentin), and enamel. The values for bone are greater than for water because bone has a greater density and contains large quantities of elements of higher atomic number, for which photoelectric absorption is a

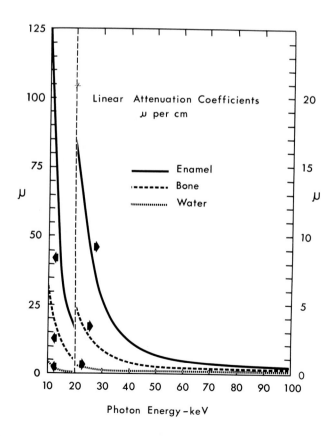

Figure III–11 Linear attenuation coefficients for enamel, bone (similar to dentin), and water (similar to muscle). For photons of low energy, photoelectric absorption predominates and the coefficients differ by large factors; for photons of higher energy, Compton scattering begins to predominate and the variations in the coefficients are small and in about the same ratios as the ratios of the physical densities of the materials.

great deal larger than for the elements of lower atomic number in water. For the same reasons the values of μ are greater for enamel than for bone.

In the region of lower photon energies, Compton scattering accounts for an appreciable fraction of the total attenuation by elements of low atomic number but for a very small fraction of the total attenuation by elements of high atomic number. The probability that Compton scattering will occur decreases slowly with increasing photon energy, whereas the probability that photoelectric absorption will occur decreases very rapidly. For elements of low atomic number, Compton scattering soon becomes more important than photoelectric absorption. For elements of higher atomic number, the initial value of μ is much greater because of the greater photoelectric absorption, and photoelectric absorption continues to be the important part of attenuation to a region of higher photon energy; but eventually Compton scattering also becomes the predominant attenuation factor for these elements of higher atomic number. The value of μ in the region where Compton scattering is the predominant part of attenuation is not greatly different for different elements.

MEASUREMENT OF X-RAYS

Radiation can be measured only by measuring an effect produced by the absorption of energy in a medium.

Many effects that result from the absorption of energy from radiation can be and have been used to measure x-rays. Among these are darkening of photographic material, fluorescence, change of electrical resistance, chemical effects, biological effects such as erythema of the skin, and ionization of air. The magnitude of any of these effects depends primarily on the amount of energy absorbed. The absorption of energy depends on the quality of the radiation and the chemical composition of the absorbing medium.

The absorption of energy in film,

which together with development is responsible for film density, would be a desirable measurement when the primary interest is in roentgenography; but film density is not entirely a measure of energy absorbed because other factors may affect film density. The absorption of energy in tissue would be a most desirable measurement when the primary interest is in biological effects; but such measurements in general are not practical to make. The absorption of energy in air, which produces ionization, is rather easy to measure; air is a universally available medium, and since its chemical composition is similar to that of soft tissue, the absorption of energy in air is similar to that in soft tissue.

The measurement of the ionization produced in air by x-rays forms the basis for their detection and measurement.

EXPOSURE (R)

The amount of ionization produced in a small mass of air by a beam of radiation will depend on such factors as (1) the amount of energy in the beam, (2) the quality of the radiation, (3) whether or not the mass of air, or ionization chamber, is near other objects that are in the beam, and (4) the material and thickness of the wall of the ionization chamber. The first two factors are characteristics of the radiation that must be accepted as they are; the latter two may be controlled. If ionization measurements are made in an ionization chamber with nothing near enough to scatter radiation to the ionization chamber, the measurement is said to have been made in free air. If scattering material is nearby, the conditions are stated; for example, measurements were made with the ionization chamber at the surface or at a specified depth in an irradiated material. The material of the ionization chamber wall commonly is chosen so that it will attenuate the beam to the same degree as an equal mass of air. Such a chamber is said to have an *air-equivalent wall*. The aim of measuring with such a chamber is to determine the amount of energy lost by a beam of radiation in a mass of air, called *exposure.** The unit of exposure is the roentgen,† designated by R.

The R is a measure of the amount of energy transferred from photons to electrons in a mass of air. It does not measure the amount of energy in the beam or the amount of energy that will be absorbed from the beam of radiation by any other material. For the most commonly used qualities of x-rays, measurements in R can be made easily and quite accurately.

The R defines the radiation to which an object may be exposed in terms of the amount of energy that would be transferred to a mass of air placed at that position. An exposure of 1 R means that the amount of energy that will be transferred to 1 gm of air is 87.7 ergs.‡

The exposure rate, R per minute, measured in a beam of x-rays is determined by the milliamperage, the kilovoltage, the filter, and the distance from the source, or focal spot, to the ionization chamber. A change in milliamperage produces a corresponding change in exposure rate because the number of photons produced each second is proportional to the number of electrons striking the target each second (measured in milliamperes). A change in kilovoltage changes the exposure rate because the number of and the relative energies of the photons depend on the kilovoltage; the exposure rate is approximately proportional to the square of the kilovoltage. Increasing the amount of filtration reduces the exposure rate because it reduces the number of photons in the beam (it also changes the average energy of the photons in the beam). The intensity of a beam of x-rays, like that of all radiations, changes inversely as the square of the distance from the source; therefore the exposure rate is reduced to one-fourth if the distance is doubled, to one-ninth if the distance is three times as great, and so on.

If the total exposure, R, to a film remains constant, the effect on the film will be constant* if the quality of the radiation—energies of the photons—remains constant. But exposure is a measure of the amount of interaction of the photons with air, whereas the effect on the film is a measure of the interaction of the photons with the film, particularly the silver in the emulsion. The ratio of the amount of these two interactions changes as the energies of the photons change; hence, equal exposures to different qualities of radiation may not produce the same effect on film.

QUALITY (HVL)

The quality of a beam of radiation is determined by the energy of the photons in a monochromatic beam or by the relative numbers of photons of various energies in a heterogeneous beam. There is no simple method of describing the relative numbers of photons of various energy values in a heterogeneous beam. The quality of a beam of radiation is commonly expressed as half-value layer (HVL), which is the thickness of a material that will reduce the exposure rate to one-half. The HVL in the field of diagnostic roentgenology is generally expressed in millimeters of aluminum. The

---

*Exposure is a measure of the ionization produced in air by x or gamma radiation. It is the sum of the electric charges on all of the ions of one sign produced in air, when all electrons liberated by photons in a volume element of air are completely stopped in air, divided by the mass of the air in the volume element.

†One roentgen equals 2.58×10^{-4} coulombs per kilogram. This definition of the roentgen, like the definition of exposure in the preceding footnote, is in different units from, but has the same meaning as, the older definition, which was: The roentgen shall be the quantity of x or gamma radiation such that the corpuscular emission per 0.001293 gram of air produces, in air, ions carrying 1 esu of quantity of electricity of either sign.

‡The exact number of ergs is uncertain; 87.7 is the value in general use at present.

---

*If the exposure is entirely from x-rays, the effect on the film is independent of the exposure rate. However, if intensifying screens are used, most of the exposure is from visible radiation; for exposures from visible radiation, the effect on the film changes slightly with changes in exposure rate even though the total exposure remains the same. The maximal effect is produced when the exposure time is about 0.1 second.

quality of a beam determines its rate of absorption as it passes through a medium.

ABSORBED DOSE (RADS)

The amount of the exposure, R, of a material to x-rays is not necessarily a measure of the effect that will be produced. The effect that will be produced depends on the actual amount of energy that is absorbed by that material. The amount of energy absorbed, called *absorbed dose,* is expressed in rads. An absorbed dose of 1 rad has been delivered when 100 ergs have been absorbed in 1 gm of irradiated material.*

The amount of energy absorbed (dose) by a material exposed to 1 R may be greater or less than the energy transferred to air exposed to 1 R; it is dependent on the chemical composition of the material and the quality of the radiation. For the qualities of radiation used in roentgenography, 1 gm of muscle exposed to 1 R will absorb from about 92 to 94 ergs, 1 gm of fat from about 50 to 90 ergs, and 1 gm of bone from about 430 to 150 ergs (the second value is for radiation of a higher HVL in each instance).

---

*The present official definition is: The rad is an absorbed dose equal to 0.01 joule/kg. This is equivalent to 100 ergs/gm.

The amount of energy absorbed by 1 gm of enamel exposed to 1 R will be about twice as great as that absorbed by 1 gm of bone. The fact that bone absorbs so much more energy than fat and muscle do is the reason that bone casts a darker shadow in roentgenography. The fact that the absorption in bone decreases as the HVL of the radiation increases, resulting in less difference in the amount of attenuation in bone and in fat and muscle, is one of the reasons that film contrast is less for higher kV.

THE ROENTGENOGRAPHIC IMAGE

The value of a roentgenogram depends on the amount of information—*quality of the radiographic detail*—recorded on the film. Such information is the result of the interaction of x-rays, transmitted by an object, and the emulsion of the film. Hence the available information is determined by the relative transmission of the x-rays by various parts of the object and by the absorption of x-rays in the emulsion of the film. These two factors, transmission of radiation by the object and absorption of radiation in the film, produce varying degrees of blackening of the finished roentgenogram, called *radiographic con-*

Table III-1. Radiographic Detail

RADIOGRAPHIC CONTRAST		RADIOGRAPHIC DEFINITION	
Subject Contrast	*Film Contrast*	*Geometric Factors*	*Graininess and Mottle*

1. Tissues
  a. Thickness
  b. Density
  c. Chemical
    composition
2. Photon energy
3. Scattered radiation
  a. Photon energy
  b. Volume of tissue
    irradiated
4. Contrast agents
	1. Type of film
	2. Intensifying
	  screens
	3. Film processing
	4. Fog
		1. Image sharpness
		  a. Penumbra
		    (1) Focal spot size
		    (2) Source-object distance
		    (3) Object-film distance
		  b. Motion
		    (1) Tube
		    (2) Object
		    (3) Film
		2. Image enlargement
		  a. Object-film distance
		  b. Source-object distance
		3. Image distortion
		  a. Central ray not through center
		    of object
		  b. Angle between central ray and
		    planes of object and/or film
			1. Film
			  a. Grain size
			    (1) Speed
			    (2) Development
			2. Screen
			  a. Speed
			  b. Screen-film
			    contact

trast. The amount of information that can be obtained from a roentgenogram also depends on the sharpness, size, and shape of the shadows, called the *radiographic definition.* The factors that affect radiographic detail are outlined in Table III–1.

RADIOGRAPHIC CONTRAST

The contrast in a radiographic image is determined by the *subject contrast* and the *film contrast.*

Subject Contrast. The variation in the amount of radiation reaching the film that is under various parts of the object, called *subject contrast,* is determined by the thickness, the density (gm/cc), and the chemical composition of the object, by the quality of the radiation, and by the amount of scattered radiation reaching the film.

If the object were of uniform thickness, density, and composition, the amount of radiation transmitted along the paths of all of the rays going through the object would be the same; there would be no subject contrast and the image on the film would be of uniform blackening. But, if along the paths of some rays the thickness of the object is greater, or the density of the object is greater, or there are chemical elements of higher atomic number, then the amount of absorption along these rays will be greater—the transmission less—and there will be subject contrast. The greater the variation in thickness, density, or atomic number, the greater will be the subject contrast.

Sometimes subject contrast can be produced in tissues that normally do not have subject contrast (for example, blood vessels in muscle) by introducing a substance having a different linear attenuation coefficient, called a *contrast agent.* Commonly used contrast agents are air or compounds containing barium or iodine.

Small changes in thickness (Fig. III–12), density, or chemical composition will produce large changes in subject contrast if the radiation consists of photons of low energy, because photoelectric absorption will be the predominant kind of interaction producing attenuation of the radiation. The linear attenuation coefficients for all chemical elements will be relatively large and the coefficients will be very much greater for elements of higher atomic number (Fig. III–11). Small changes in thickness, density, or chemical composition will result in small changes in subject contrast if the radiation consists of photons of only high energy, because much of the attenuation will be due to Compton scattering, particularly for the elements of lower atomic number; the variation in linear attenuation coefficients for all elements will be rather small.

If a large amount of scattered radiation reaches the film, the subject contrast due to variations in thickness, density, and chemical composition will be altered. Scattered radiation tends to produce a uniform exposure over the entire area of the film, thus reducing subject contrast. Scattered radiation increases as photon energy increases

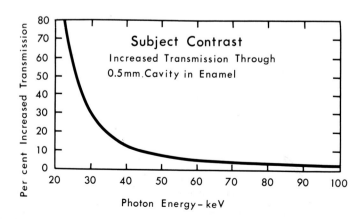

Figure III–12 A small decrease in thickness of an absorber will produce a large increase in x-ray transmission for photons of low energy but only a small increase for photons of high energy. From this graph it is evident that the lower the energy of the photons used to make a roentgenogram, the more easily will a cavity 0.5 mm in diameter in enamel be detected. However, for photons of low energy the attenuation coefficient in enamel is very high (Fig. III–11), and a tremendous exposure would be necessary in order that enough radiation would penetrate the enamel to produce an image on the film. Such large exposures would be likely to produce radiation damage in adjacent tissues.

because more of the interactions are Compton scatter rather than photoelectric absorption.* The amount of scattered radiation reaching the film increases rapidly as the volume of tissue irradiated is increased; therefore, the beam of radiation should always be as small as possible—only large enough to cover the volume of the tissue of interest.†

Film Contrast. Variations in blackness of a roentgenogram resulting from differences in subject contrast are called *film contrast*. Film contrast is determined by the type of film, whether intensifying screens are used, the processing (development, fixing, drying) of the film, and the amount of fog.

Many of the characteristics of film can be illustrated by sensitometric curves, which relate film blackening to exposure. Film blackening is commonly expressed as *film density*, which is the common logarithm of the reciprocal of the visible light transmission (Fig. III–13):

$$\text{density} = \log \frac{\text{incident intensity}}{\text{transmitted intensity}}$$

Sensitometric curves are shown in Figure III–14, in which the film density is plotted against the logarithm of the relative exposure. Under common viewing conditions, the useful range of densities is from about 0.3 to 1.7, but with very strong illumination it can be extended to a density of about 3. The minimal difference in film density that the eye can detect is a difference of 1 or 2% if there is a sharp demarcation between the densities and if there is proper illumination. Curve A of Figure III–14 is for a film

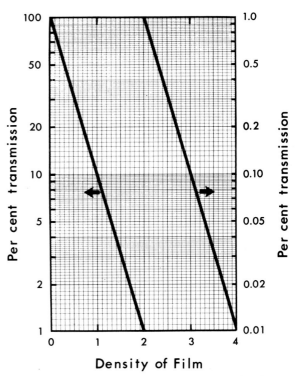

Figure III–13 Relationship between film density and percentage of incident light transmitted by the film.

whose density changes slowly with increasing exposure, whereas curve B is for a film whose density changes rapidly with increasing exposure. Since differences in exposure are determined by subject contrast, it is evident that a small variation in subject contrast will produce a much smaller difference in film density for film A than for film B. However, all of the useful range of film density will be used for a narrow range of subject contrasts for film B, and film A will be capable of showing a much wider range of subject contrasts. Film B will show a much larger difference in film contrast than will film A for a given difference in subject contrast. Film B is said to have more *contrast* than film A, but film A is said to have more *latitude* than film B.

The density of two films exposed to the same quantity (R) and quality of radiation may be different. The one showing the greater density is said to be a faster film. A faster film generally has larger silver bromide crystals in its emulsion than does a

---

*This increase in scattered radiation as the quality of the primary beam becomes harder is of greater importance as the potential across the x-ray tube is increased above about 100 kVp.

†The amount of scattered radiation reaching the film can be reduced by (1) interposing a *grid* (seldom used in dental roentgenography), which consists of strips of lead separated by material of low atomic number, between the object and the film or (2) covering the film with thin lead foil, which removes a greater fraction of the scattered photons (which are of lower energy than the primary photons from which they originated) than of the primary photons.

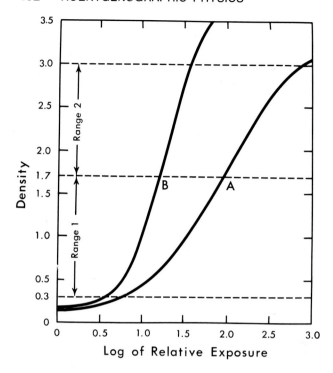

Figure III–14 Sensitometric curves for two films, *A* and *B*. Film *B* is more contrasty, has less latitude, and is faster than film *A*. The densities in range 1 are those that are useful with the illumination commonly used for viewing films; densities in range 2 may be useful with brighter illumination.

slower film. Film speed is occasionally specified as the reciprocal of the number of roentgens required to produce a film density of 1. However, film speed also depends on the quality of the radiation; a film is slower for a harder quality of radiation because the silver absorbs less energy when exposed to 1 R of high energy radiation than when exposed to 1 R of low energy radiation.*

The amount of radiation required to produce useful film densities—apparent speed—can be greatly reduced by the use of *intensifying screens*. Such screens consist of small crystals (commonly of calcium tungstate) embedded in a layer of transparent plastic on a smooth cardboard. They are placed so that the layer is in contact with the film. Many of the atoms in these crystals are excited when exposed to x-rays and, as they return to their normal state, emit characteristic radiation in the visible region. Because film is much more sensitive

to visible radiation than it is to x-rays, satisfactory films are obtained with as little as 1/25 as great an exposure with screens as would be required without the screens. Commonly two intensifying screens, one on each side of the film, are used. Screens are seldom used for intraoral roentgenography, but are commonly used for extraoral roentgenography. Film contrast is greater when intensifying screens are used.

Film contrast is affected also by the processing of the film, particularly the development. If the film is underdeveloped, all of the possible contrast will not be brought out; if it is overdeveloped, there will be some chemical fog that will reduce the contrast. The amount of fog also increases with the age of the film or if the film has been stored at high temperature or in an atmosphere of high humidity.

RADIOGRAPHIC DEFINITION

The definition of the roentgenographic image is determined by *geometric factors* of the equipment and technique and by *graininess* and *mottle* of the film and screen.

---

*To produce the same film densities requires about 10 times as many R of gamma radiation from cobalt-60 as of x-rays generated at 80 kV.

Geometric Factors. The factors that determine the degree to which a roentgenographic image conforms to its object, called *geometric factors*, include the degree of sharpness, enlargement, and distortion of the image.

The sharpness of an image is reduced in part by the *penumbra* of the shadow. The width of the penumbra is determined by the size of the focal spot, or source of the x-rays, the distance from the source to the object, and the distance from the object to the film* (Fig. III–15). The width of the

---

*Commonly the distance from the source to the film is listed as an additional factor; this distance cannot be varied without changing either the source-object distance, or the object-film distance, and it is really the ratio of these last two distances that is significant.

penumbra is decreased—the sharpness or definition of the shadow is increased—by using a tube that has a smaller focal spot, by moving the tube—focal spot—farther away from the object, and by having the object closer to the film. If the penumbra is wide, it is possible that for a narrow object the penumbras from the two sides will overlap and the shadow of the object will not be distinguishable.

There are practical limitations that prevent the use of very small focal spots, very long source-object distances, and very short object-film distances. For a tube with a smaller focal spot, the permissible load (kilovoltage times milliamperage times length of exposure) is decreased because the heat produced would cause too great a rise in temperature in the smaller mass of

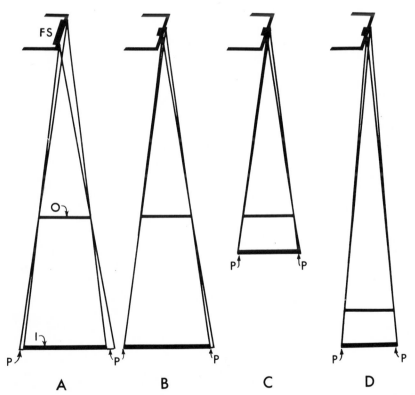

Figure III–15   The sharpness of the image (I) of an object (O) depends partly on the width of the penumbra (P), which is determined by the size of the focal spot (FS) and the relative distances between the source, the object, and the image. The width of the penumbra decreases as the size of the focal spot decreases *(B compared with A),* as the distance between the object and the image decreases *(C compared with B),* and as the distance from the focal spot to the object increases *(D compared with C).* In each instance the width of the penumbra is less on the side of the image under the target (left-hand side) than on the opposite side. The image is always larger than the object, but the amount of enlargement decreases as the distance between the object and the image decreases *(C compared with B)* and as the distance from the source to the object increases *(D compared with C).*

the focal spot. High temperatures may vaporize enough of the tungsten to make the surface of the focal spot pitted; photons produced at the bottom of the pits are likely to be absorbed as they travel through the target material toward the object and film. A very high temperature also may cause the focal spot to emit electrons and thus allow an inverse current to flow through the tube. Increasing the source-object distance decreases the intensity of the x-rays, thus requiring longer exposures or higher milliamperage, which in turn may cause the permissible load on the tube to be exceeded. The shortest distance between the object and film is determined by the size of the object (some parts of a thick object are necessarily farther from the film) and by body structures that may prevent the film from being in contact with the object.

The edge of a shadow will not be sharp—not have good definition—if during the exposure there is motion of the tube, the object, or the film. To reduce the possibility or the amount of motion, the exposure time should be short. However, the exposure time must be long enough to allow some of the heat to travel away from the focal spot so that the focal spot may not become too hot.

The size of a shadow is always larger than the size of the object. From Figure III–15 B, C, and D it is evident that the amount of enlargement increases as the source-object distance decreases and as the object-film distance increases.

The shape of a shadow may not be the same as the shape of the object, a condition called distortion (Fig. III–16). There will be distortion if the planes of the film and of the object are not parallel.

Graininess and Mottle.   Variations in film density at the edge of a shadow may

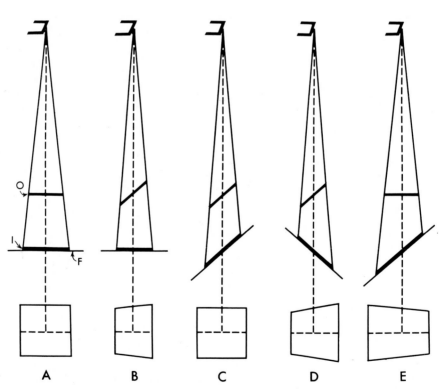

Figure III–16   The shape of an image (I) on a film (F) will be the same as the shape of the object (O), a square in this example, only if the plane of the film is parallel to the plane of the object, as in A and C. When the two planes are not parallel, as in B, D, and E, the image will be distorted—will not be the same shape as the object. The amount of distortion increases as the angle between the two planes increases.

not be sharp because of characteristics of the film or intensifying screen, conditions called *graininess* and *mottle*.

The dark areas in a film are due to grains of silver in the emulsion that have been freed from the molecules of silver bromide by the combined action of the x-rays and the developer. These small grains tend to clump together. When the clumps become large enough to be seen, the film is described as looking grainy. Excessive graininess will reduce the sharpness of the images. Film graininess is more pronounced in fast film than in slow film, and is likely to be increased by overdevelopment.

An image made with the use of intensifying screens will not be as sharp as one made without such screens because a single fluorescing crystal sends light out in all directions, thereby exposing a larger area of the film than the actual area covered by the crystal. If the thickness of the fluorescent layer is increased, the necessary exposure time will be reduced, but the lack of sharpness of the image will be increased. Sharpness of the image will also be reduced if the screen and film are not in good contact.

The image produced by the use of a very fast film or by the film from a fast film-intensifying screen combination may have a mottled appearance. Within a very small area of a film that has a rather high average film density, there may be some very dark spots and some rather light spots. The dark spots may have been produced by the interaction of single photons. On slower film or slower film-screen combinations the interaction of a single photon will not produce as dark a spot. Hence, in order to produce the same average film density, a much larger number of photons will have to interact; the individual spots will be smaller and not so dark but there will be many more of them, and the darkening of the film will be more uniform.

RADIOGRAPHIC QUALITY

A roentgenographic image is never a perfect reproduction of the radiation pat-

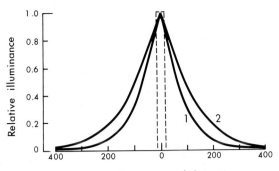

Figure III–17 Normalized line-spread functions of two roentgenographic systems. Curve 1 is for a system with two medium-speed screens; curve 2 is for a system with two high-speed screens. The dotted lines near the center indicate the shape of a perfect image of the slit.

tern of the object being examined, nor is the film contrast ever a perfect reproduction of the subject contrast. Among factors that contribute to the degradation of the image are type of film, intensifying screens, penumbra, and motion (discussed in preceding sections under Radiographic Contrast and Radiographic Definition).

One method of investigating the accuracy of the reproduction is to compare the image of a line with the original line. A very narrow slit, of the order of 10 μm wide, between jaws that are opaque to x-rays, is roentgenographed on a film with intensifying screens positioned immediately behind the jaws. The variation in the density of the film along a line perpendicular to the image of the slit will be as shown in Figure III–17. The spreading of the image of the slit is due mostly to the distance between the film and the fluorescing crystals in the intensifying screen. A film without intensifying screens would show only a little spreading of the image. The higher the speed of the screen—that is, the thicker it is—the greater will be the spreading of the image. If the distance from the slit to the film is increased or if a larger focal spot is used, the spreading of the image will be increased. The observed spreading of the image, as shown in Figure III–17, is referred to as the *line spread function* (LSF).

Because of the spreading of the image—the LSF—an image is never as clearly defined (sharp) as the object. The images of slits that are very close together may not be distinguishable as separate images because the spreading of the images from adjacent slits may cause the density of the film between the images to be essentially the same as the density under the slits. This limits the number of lines per millimeter—the amount of detail—that may be distinguished on a roentgenogram, a feature commonly referred to as the resolving power of the recording medium. The resolving power of a no-screen film is of the order of 20 lines per mm; that of film-screen combinations is from about 8 to 15 lines per mm, depending on the speed of the screens. The resolving power of a system can be determined from its LSF and is expressed in cycles per millimeter (the number of cycles corresponds to the number of lines).

From the LSF one can determine the accuracy with which an imaging system reproduces a radiation pattern, the *modulation transfer function* (MTF).* The MTF can be applied to each factor that influences the LSF, such as the size of the focal spot, source-object-film distances, and type of film; it can be applied to each component of a recording system, such as an image intensifier and television system; and it can be applied to each element of these systems.† The total MTF of a system is equal to the product of the MTF of each component of the system. The MTF of a system or part of a system is always less than 1.0. Thus, every step in the production of an image is accompanied by some loss of sharpness and detail—that is, loss of information.

The choice of a system—size of focal spot, kilovoltage, filter, type of film, processing of film, and the like—always involves compromises. It is desirable to give a patient as small a dose as possible, to use fast film to reduce motion-induced lack of sharpness, to use low kilovoltage for increased contrast, and to use fast processing

techniques so that roentgenograms can be viewed without keeping a patient waiting a long time. A change in a system to improve one feature may be detrimental to another feature: reducing kilovoltage to increase contrast increases the dose to the patient. The system selected must give the maximal useful information with the fewest undesirable features.

REFERENCES

Council on Dental Materials and Devices: Revised American Dental Association Specification No. 22 for Intraoral Dental Radiographic Film Adopted. J. Am. Dent. A. *80*:1066–1069 (May) 1970.

Eastman Kodak Company: X-rays in Dentistry. Rochester, New York, 1964. 64 pp.

Ennis, L. M., Berry, H. M., Jr., and Phillips, J. E.: Dental Roentgenology. Ed. 6. Philadelphia, Lea & Febiger, 1967, 740 pp.

Goodwin, P. N., Quimby, E. H., and Morgan, R. H.: Physical Foundations of Radiology. Ed. 4. New York, Harper & Row, Publishers, 1970, 397 pp.

Johns, H. E. and Cunningham, J. R.: The Physics of Radiology. Ed. 3. Springfield, Illinois, Charles C Thomas, Publisher, 1969, 800 pp.

Radiation Quantities and Units: International Commission on Radiation Units and Measurements. (ICRU Report 19.) July 1, 1971, 21 pp. (Available from ICRU Publications, P. O. Box 30165, Washington, D. C. 20014.)

Richards, A. G.: Quality of an X-ray Beam. Oral Surg., Oral Med. & Oral Path. *17*:739–744 (June) 1964.

Richards, A. G.: New Concepts in Dental X-ray Machines. J. Am. Dent. A. *73*:69–76 (July) 1966.

Richards, A. G., Barbor, G. L., Bader, J. D., and Hale, J. D.: Samarium Filters for Dental Radiography. Oral Surg., Oral Med. & Oral Path. *29*:704–715 (May) 1970.

Ritchey, B., Feldman, A., and Greer, W.: Roentgenography of Enamel: Apatite as a Phantom Material; Contrast as a Function of Exposure Factors. Oral Surg., Oral Med. & Oral Path. *13*:188–193 (Feb.) 1960.

Seeman, H. E.: Physical and Photographic Principles of Medical Radiography. New York, John Wiley & Sons, Inc., 1968, 132 pp.

Shawkat, A. H.: Scattered Radiation Absorbers in Intraoral Radiography. Oral Surg., Oral Med. & Oral Path. *31*:439–446 (Mar.) 1971.

Ter-Pogossian, M. M.: The Physical Aspects of Diagnostic Radiology. New York, Hoeber Medical Division, Harper & Row, Publishers, 1967, 426 pp.

Thomas, J. G. and Graham, W. L.: Rectification and High-Speed Dental Radiography. Oral Surg., Oral Med. & Oral Path. *29*:216–221 (Feb.) 1970.

Wainwright, W. W.: Dental Radiology. New York, McGraw-Hill Book Company, Inc., 1965, 585 pp.

Williams, M. M. D.: Significance of R, Rad, Rem, and Related Units. Am. J. Roentgenol. *96*:794–802 (Mar.) 1966.

Wuehrmann, A. H. and Manson-Hing, L. R.: Dental Radiology. Ed. 3. St. Louis, The C. V. Mosby Company, 1973, 466 pp.

---

*Modulation transfer function is used in many fields other than roentgenology; for example, the quality of a photographic lens is often described in terms of its MTF.

†Image intensifiers and television systems, commonly used in general diagnostic roentgenology, are seldom used in dental roentgenography.

HEALTH PHYSICS

APPENDIX PART IV

MARVIN M. D. WILLIAMS, Ph.D.

The dangers of exposure to radiation* have received widespread publicity during recent years because of radiation associated with nuclear reactions, particularly radiation from the fallout following nuclear weapons testing and from the discharge of radionuclides by nuclear power plants. It is well established that exposure to large quantities of radiation is injurious to health and may be lethal; how injurious exposure to small quantities may be is less well known. Small quantities of radiation, cosmic and that from radioactive materials in the earth, have always been present and cannot be avoided; the intensity of cosmic radiation increases with altitude, and the intensity of radiation from radioactive materials varies severalfold from one locality to another. Some members of the dental and medical professions who have used x-rays and radioactive materials over periods of many years have demonstrated no adverse effects that can be ascribed to the additional radiation. However, there is some evidence that even small exposures to radiation may produce some undesirable results. The opinion of most students of the subject is that no exposure is desirable per se, but that some exposure can be tolerated with very little probability of harmful effects.

The benefits derived from the proper use of radiation far outweigh the possible harm that might be produced. Many abnormal conditions of the teeth, or of other organs of the body, can be detected by the use of small amounts of radiation better or more easily than by other means, and, in some instances, they can be detected by no other means. Somewhat larger exposures at times are valuable therapeutic agents.

The proper use of radiation demands that the dose received by everyone involved in its use be minimal. This requires some understanding of radiation dose, the relation of dose to effect produced, and methods of avoiding unnecessary and unwanted exposure.

DOSE UNITS

Radiation dose is determined by the amount of energy absorbed in a medium and is expressed in rads. An absorbed dose of 1 rad has been delivered when 100 ergs have been absorbed in 1 gm of the irradiated material. Although it is not feasible to measure doses in tissue, approximate values can be calculated if the exposure (R), the quality of the radiation, and the chemical composition of the tissue are known.

The biological effect produced in tissue by a dose measured in rads depends on many factors, such as the quality of the radiation, the tissue irradiated, the biological effect of interest, the dose rate, and the blood supply to the tissue. Of most importance in the field of radiation protection is the factor that depends on the quality of

---

*By radiation, in this chapter, is meant electromagnetic radiation in the x-ray region, and not infrared, visible, or ultraviolet radiation.

457

the radiation; it is called the *quality factor* and has values from 1 to as high as 15 or 20. The product of the rads and the proper quality factor (and at times other modifying factors, such as that due to unequal dose distribution) gives a quantity that should be nearly equivalent to the biological effect; this quantity is called the *dose equivalent,* is measured in *rems,* and is the unit of dose used in the field of protection.

It is the biological effect of irradiation that is of importance in the field of radiation protection, not the exposure or dose. The only way in which doses of different kinds of irradiation can be added so as to have any significance is to add their rem values. This requires a knowledge of the quality factors. Only approximate values for the quality factors are known at present; they have been chosen as the highest probable values so as to allow some factor of safety. In the field of radiation protection, because doses cannot be measured accurately and there are many unknown factors, a number of approximations are justified if it is certain that these will not jeopardize an individual's health.

For the radiation used in dental roentgenology, with one exception, it is sufficiently accurate for protection calculations to assume that an exposure of 1 R will result in an absorbed dose of 1 rad, which will produce a dose equivalent of 1 rem. The exception is that when the bony structures of the head are irradiated, particularly in children, it is preferable to assume that exposure to 1 R may result in an absorbed dose of perhaps 3 rads and a dose equivalent of 3 rems because of the greater absorption of energy in bone than in soft tissues.

BIOLOGICAL EFFECTS OF RADIATION

The only effect radiation itself can produce in any medium is to increase the energy content of the medium by an amount equal to the energy absorbed. The biological effects that follow irradiation and are observed at some later time are second-ary effects in that they are the result of physical, chemical, and biological actions set in motion by the absorption of this energy.

The results that follow irradiation of biological material are not unique to radiation, for similar effects may be produced by other agents or may seem to occur normally. Partly for this reason it is difficult to determine a cause-effect relationship. The first detectable or observable effects of radiation generally occur, if they occur, from within a few days to a few weeks after the irradiation. This latent period tends to decrease as the dose increases. Some effects may not occur for several years; some effects that may be induced by therapeutic irradiation occasionally occur as long as 20 or more years following therapy. At times it is difficult to know whether the observed effect may be the result of the irradiation, associated with the disturbance for which the radiation was given, a combination of these two, or entirely unrelated to either. Some of our "questionable knowledge" about the effects of radiation is derived from observations of patients who have received therapeutic doses to rather small volumes of tissue; these observations are complicated by the abnormality for which the radiation was given, and may have little relationship to the effects that might be produced by other dosage rates, total doses, or irradiation of larger volumes of tissue, or that might be produced in the absence of the abnormality for which the therapy was given. Other "questionable knowledge" has been derived from experimental work on animals, which may or may not be applicable to other species.

Biological effects of radiation are (1) somatic, effects on any of the cells of the individual himself, or (2) genetic, mutations which are not evident in the individual but which are effects on the germ plasma that are passed on to future generations.

SOMATIC EFFECTS

Somatic effects are partly dependent on the rate at which the radiation is given. A total dose that would be lethal if given in a short time, such as a few days, may result in no detectable effect if given in small daily increments over a period of several years. This is owing to the ability of living tissue to repair some of the damage done to it.

There is much evidence which indicates that rather small doses of radiation repeated over long periods may produce irremediable damage to blood-forming organs of the body. If leukemia develops in an individual who has received exposures to radiation, it is possible that it may have developed only because of such exposures, that it would have developed, and just as quickly, if the individual had not received such exposures, that the exposures may have been an added factor—the straw that broke the camel's back—or, which is seldom mentioned, that the exposures may conceivably have postponed its development since radiation is an agent sometimes used for treating leukemia.

Malignancies developed in many of those persons associated with the early use of x-rays; there can be little doubt that these malignancies were radiation induced. For the malignancies that have occurred in luminous-watch-dial painters and in other individuals who have ingested radioactive materials, a cause-effect relationship can hardly be questioned. For those malignancies in the neck that have been reported in individuals who received radiation to the thymus in childhood or radioiodine therapy for hyperthyroidism, a radiation cause-effect relationship, while probable, has not been firmly established.

It has been suggested that chronic irradiation induces aging, but very little is known about the aging process. One published report supposedly showed that radiologists had a shorter life expectancy than other medical specialists. Other statisticians thought the conclusion may not have been justified because the samples compared may not have been otherwise equivalent; no consideration was given to the possibility that perhaps the "chemistry" of the individual that caused him to choose radiology might also have affected his life span. Some experiments on animals have

been reported in which those animals that had received small doses of radiation had a longer life span than their nonirradiated controls.

There is little doubt that radiation in rather small doses may cause skin changes, may be a factor in producing cataracts, and may slow or stop growth of bones and teeth; and there is some evidence that developing tissues are more easily damaged than mature tissues, hence radiation damage is more likely to follow irradiation of children than of older persons.

Although there is much uncertainty regarding radiation cause-effect relationships, enough experience now has been accumulated so that a dose which will not produce any objectionable somatic changes is fairly well known, and permissible exposures established by various agencies are believed to be considerably below this value. While there is no evidence that even small amounts of radiation are beneficial in themselves, it is most likely that they may be no more harmful to an individual than overeating, lack of exercise, too little rest, the fumes from automobiles, smoking, or even coffee.

GENETIC EFFECTS

Genetic mutations in flies, animals, and plants have been found to be much more frequent following irradiation, and a cause-effect relationship can hardly be doubted. There is every reason to believe that the same would be true for man. In this field of investigation, quantitative results are even less certain than for somatic changes, and it is probable that significant doses vary considerably from species to species. Some estimate of the importance of radiation in producing mutations might be obtained from studying their frequency in man, since he always has been subjected to radiation from the earth and sky, and the dose rate of this background radiation varies significantly in different parts of the world and is fairly well known. The two great uncertainties in such studies are (1) the frequency of the occurrence of mutations, since they vary from those easily recognized to those that may not be detected but that affect an individual in such subtle ways as making him less resistant to some diseases, and (2) whether any apparent mutation was caused by radiation or some other agent, and whether in fact it is a mutation or is due to some type of injury to the individual.

Various investigators have estimated the dose of radiation that would cause an eventual doubling of the load of genetic defects carried by man. These estimates vary severalfold. Since it is most probable that background radiation is responsible for only a fraction of the mutations being produced, it is not likely that the total mutation rate would be much increased if in the future exposure were increased, because of man-made radiation, by an amount comparable to that of background radiation.

The load of genetic defects carried by man in the future will be increased by a number of factors other than the probable increased exposure to radiation. Some drugs are capable of producing genetic changes. It is possible that mutations may be produced by some food additives, by some constituents of some cosmetics, and by some of the pollutants of our atmosphere deriving from industrial wastes. The improved medical care of our population is making it possible for many individuals with genetic defects to reproduce, whereas in the past they would not have lived long enough. In the overall picture, the mutations resulting from an increase in the radiation to which man may be exposed in the future may be of rather minor significance, but are within his power to control to a considerable degree.

An individual's attitude toward the importance or necessity of keeping the increase in radiation exposure to an absolute minimum is affected by his moral, religious, and even political beliefs, and by his attitude toward responsibility for the well-being of future generations. The dangers of radiation have been widely publicized in recent years. Some of this publicity has been misleading and has greatly magnified the possible bad effects. Because of the wide interest that has been thus created and the association of radiation with the atomic bomb, radiation has become somewhat of a political football in local, national, and international politics. Attempts to interpret data in this field often are influenced by emotions and religious and political beliefs to such an extent that it is difficult to obtain good scientific evaluations of the data available.

It is almost certain that in the future the use of atomic energy in various ways will intensify and that man's exposure to radiation will increase. Many advances in our civilization have been accompanied by added risks to our health and life. The burgeoning death toll on our highways has little effect on the use of these highways. The scare produced by the suggestion that cigarette smoking causes cancer of the lungs has not resulted in an appreciable decrease in the use of cigarettes. It seems to be a characteristic of man to adjust to changes and to accept new risks to his life and health. So, while at present there is so much agitation against increased exposure to radiation that we are in some danger of losing many of its benefits, a greater danger in the future may result from our becoming so accustomed to it that we will fail to take precautions that should and easily can be taken.

PERMISSIBLE DOSES

The maximum permissible doses (MPD) adopted by the National Council on Radiation Protection and Measurements (NCRP), which are essentially the same as those adopted by various other national and international organizations, are based on assumptions such as these: that no amount of irradiation is beneficial; that there is a dose below which no somatic change will be produced that man will not be willing to accept; that children are more susceptible than older people; and that there is a dose below which, even if it is delivered before the end of the reproductive period, the probability of genetic effects will be slight.

In assuming that no amount of irradiation is beneficial, one is excluding possible benefits from radiation therapy and roentgen (and radioisotope) diagnostic procedures; exposures received for these purposes are not included in determining whether an individual's exposure is within the MPD range. In the use of roentgen therapy, the risk of producing some undesirable radiation effects in the future is considered to be a small price to pay for the immediate benefit and perhaps prolongation of life that may be obtained; however, in recent years there has been an increased feeling that for nonmalignant conditions the benefits may not justify the risks. Before a diagnostic procedure requiring exposure to radiation is ordered, it is assumed that the situation has been carefully evaluated and that the probable benefit to the individual is greater than the probable harm; this involves a consideration of the age of the individual, his past and probable future irradiation history, and the part of the body to be irradiated, as well as the importance to the individual's health of the information that may be obtained from the procedure. While there is no conclusive evidence that exposures to small amounts of radiation are harmful to an individual, there is likewise no evidence that such exposures are beneficial. It seems certain that there will be an increase in unavoidable exposure to manmade radiations in the future, so it is desirable to reduce avoidable exposures to the minimum.

Some peculiar or characteristic dangers to health and life are associated with many occupations. Being a truck driver, a miner, an airplane pilot, or a sailor involves risks that are not present in most other occupations, and there are people who would be unwilling to accept the risks associated with such forms of employment. It is possible that exposures to radiation within the occupational MPD level may produce some detectable changes, such as increased dryness of the skin, or some undetectable changes, such as increased susceptibility to certain diseases. These possibilities are risks that radiation workers must accept; those who are not willing to accept such risks should not be employed where there

is exposure to radiation. It is believed by those responsible for setting the occupational MPD levels that these levels are below those which will produce any somatic changes that the average individual would be unwilling to accept; but there is always a possibility that some detectable changes may be produced.

The possibility of undesirable effects from irradiation of children is greater than from irradiation of older individuals for such reasons as these: more actively growing or developing tissues may be more easily damaged, damaged tissue may cease to grow or develop, and greater life expectancy allows more time for undesirable effects to develop. Rapidly growing or developing tissues may be able to repair damage more quickly than mature tissues, but the repair may not be complete. Injured tissues, such as in bones or teeth, may cease to develop normally, thereby producing a deformity. Some of the undesirable radiation effects have a latent period of up to 20 or more years; such effects have a higher probability of occurrence in persons who have been exposed to radiation as children than in those irradiated as adults. For these reasons it is unlawful in many states to hire persons under 18 years of age for work involving exposure to radiation.

Irradiation received subsequent to an individual's reproductive period cannot produce genetic mutations; hence the important dose from this standpoint is the dose received before the age of about 30 years. The probability of production of genetic mutations may be independent of the dose rate, have no threshold value, and be proportional to the total accumulated dose received before conception. Because of this the MPD rate for those past the reproductive age might be set at a higher value than for younger individuals. This would add complications to protection problems, but it does make radiation exposures for diagnostic purposes in older individuals, for whom more such exposure may be indicated, a less serious problem.

The value for the MPD, or "tolerance dose" as it was called in earlier days, has been reduced periodically. From about

1928 to 1936, the commonly accepted value for whole body irradiation was an exposure of 0.2 R per day, which amounted to 50 R per year.* About 1936 the value was reduced to 0.1 R per day, which amounted to 25 R per year. During these periods no distinction was made between the permissible doses for occupationally and nonoccupationally exposed individuals. In 1948 the MPD was again reduced, this time to 0.3 R a week for occupational exposure and one-tenth of this for individuals whose exposure was not related to their work. The most recent reduction was made in 1957, and at the same time the unit of measurement was changed from the exposure — R — to the biological effectiveness of the dose (or dose equivalent) — rem.

The presently accepted MPD for occupational exposure to the whole body is 3 rem in a calendar quarter, with the added restriction that the accumulated dose at any time should not exceed 5 rem multiplied by the individual's age-minus-18. This means that the average occupational exposure dose should not exceed 5 rem a year, which amounts to an average of 0.1 rem a week.

It would be permissible for an individual several years past age 18, who has received less than 5 rem a year, to receive as much as 12 rem in a year, provided that this does not make his accumulated dose exceed 5 (age − 18). This leeway ordinarily should not be used, however, for one of the cardinal rules in radiation protection is that any exposure, regardless of how small, should be reduced if it is feasible to reduce it; that is, that no amount of exposure is desirable.

The hands, because they contain only a small amount of red bone marrow, are allowed a dose of 75 rem in any 1 year (not more than 25 rem in any 1 quarter). (There are several other modifications to the general MPD values, such as for soft radiations that produce an exposure only to the super-ficial layers of the skin.) It is inexcusable for anyone working in the field of dental roentgenology to receive a whole body dose, or dose to the hands, of more than a small fraction of 5 rem a year.

The present MPD for people in the environs, that is, nonoccupationally exposed individuals, is 0.5 rem a year.

The early values were chosen on the basis of what was believed to be a dose level to which some people had been exposed for periods of many years and had shown no unacceptable effects. So far as is known, no one who has received a dose that did not exceed the earlier tolerance doses has shown any effects that are unacceptable to most individuals. The reductions in the MPD before 1957 were made largely to reduce the probability of producing some effects having a threshold dose that may be less than it was originally thought to be, and to allow a greater factor of safety, particularly for the occasional individual who might be more sensitive to radiation.

The chief reason for the 1957 reduction was a growing concern about the likely increased production of genetic defects. There had been a significant growth in the number of occupationally exposed individuals owing to the augmented use of radiation in nonmedical as well as in medical fields and to the greatly expanded use of atomic energy; and the dose to the entire population from man-made radiation sources had increased and was expected to increase further not only because of more widespread use of atomic energy and growing medical uses but also because of the upsurge in general background radiation from atomic energy installations and their waste products and from fallout following nuclear weapons testing. The ultimate increase in the load of genetic defects in the entire population will depend on the total dose to the total population, regardless of its distribution to individuals. Hence, as the number of occupationally exposed individuals increases, as the medical use of radiation for diagnostic purposes increases,

---

*This is calculated on the basis of 5 working days a week and 2 weeks' vacation a year.

and as the unavoidable background dose increases, it becomes necessary that the MPD values be reduced in order to keep the total dose to the total population at the desired low levels. To maintain these low levels may require such measures as an increase in protection devices for the occupationally employed, greater care in the disposal of radioactive wastes, and legal restrictions on the dental and other medical use of radiation if those responsible for such use do not themselves limit radiation to individuals for whom the benefit outweighs any possible harm.

Another entirely different permissible dose value is that for the protection of radiographic film. Recovery processes in film are negligible, and film darkening from exposure to x-rays is independent of dose rate. A total accumulated exposure of 1.0 mR may produce objectionable fog on x-ray film.

PRACTICAL ASPECTS OF PROTECTION

Protective measures required when a dental x-ray machine is in use are those associated with (1) the exposure of the subject whose teeth, or other anatomic parts, are undergoing x-ray examination, (2) the exposure of the dental personnel, and (3) the exposure of the people in the environs.

The primary source of radiation is the x-ray tube; but, since anything struck by x-rays will scatter some of the radiation reaching it, such an object can be considered as a secondary source of radiation.

Although the tube is enclosed in a radiation-absorbing housing, this housing does transmit some radiation. According to the recommendations of the NCRP, the exposure due to leakage radiation through a diagnostic protective tube housing shall be not more than 0.1 R per hour at a distance of 1 meter from the tube target when the tube is operated at its maximal rated potential and the maximal rated continuous current for this potential. The exposure rate on the surface of the tube housing may be higher than 0.1 R per hour. This leakage radiation has been heavily filtered, so its HVL is high and it has an average penetrating ability greater than that of the useful beam.

The exposure rate in the useful beam will depend on the distance from the target, the kilovoltage applied to the tube, the milliamperes of current through the tube, and the filtration in the beam. The total filtration should be at least 2 mm Al or its equivalent for potentials less than 70 kVp, and at least 2.5 mm Al or its equivalent for potentials of 70 kVp or higher. The target-skin distance should be at least 10 cm (4 inches) for potentials up to 50 kVp, and at least 18 cm (7 inches) for potentials above 50 kVp.

An increase in the kilovoltage across the tube increases the dose rate rapidly and produces a more penetrating beam. All beams initially contain large quantities of soft or nonpenetrating radiation which, if not removed, would all be absorbed in superficial tissues and have no effect on the production of the image on the film. A few millimeters of aluminum as a filter in the beam will remove most of the softer component of the beam while having much less effect on the harder, and more useful, component of the beam (Fig. III–5). An increase in either the potential or the filter produces a beam with a higher HVL and decreases the dose to the patient's skin, but produces a roentgenogram that has less contrast.

Changing the milliamperage produces a nearly corresponding change in dose rate. However, it does not affect the total dose to the patient, since with lower milliamperage the exposure time will have to be correspondingly longer.

The use of a faster film requires less radiation, hence reducing the dose to the patient; but the decrease in image quality may reduce the amount of useful information obtainable from the roentgenogram.

The exposure rate decreases as the distance is increased, following the inverse square law. If the distance is made two times as great, the exposure rate would be reduced to $1/(2)^2$, or to $1/4$. If the distance from the target to the film (TFD) is increased, a greater exposure will be necessary in order that the exposure to the film will remain constant, but the exposure to the skin will have been reduced.* The increased distance also will produce a roentgenogram with less distortion.

The greatest source of scattered radiation is the patient, because the amount of radiation scattered by an object depends on the amount of radiation striking the object. This scattered radiation causes the entire body of the patient, as well as everything else in the room, to receive some radiation. One of the most effective methods of reducing the amount of scattered radiation is to reduce the amount of radiation reaching the patient. This can be accomplished by using a small beam. The beam should be no larger than 7 cm (2.75 inches) in diameter for a target-skin distance (TSD) of 18 cm (7 inches), and no larger than 6 cm (2.4 inches) in diameter for a TSD of less than 18 cm (7 inches); ideally, the size and shape of the beam and of the film should be the same. By decreasing the amount of scatter that is produced, not only is the amount of radiation reaching the body of the patient and other objects in the room reduced but the amount of scattered radiation reaching the film is also reduced, thereby producing a better roentgenogram. The use of shielded open-ended cones results in a smaller dose (less scattered radiation) to the patient than does the use of unshielded cones or cones with plastic tips.

The amount of radiation scattered from other objects is generally small compared with that from the patient because they are farther away from the source and are struck only by the radiation not absorbed as the beam passes through the patient. An approximate rule for estimating the intensity of scattered radiation is to consider that the exposure rate of radiation scattered through 90°, at a distance of 1 meter from the scatterer, is 0.1% of the exposure rate incident on the scatterer. This is definitely only an approximation, because the intensity of the scattered radiation will increase if the size of the field is increased, it will increase if the thickness of tissue or other material through which it must pass after being scattered is decreased, and it will be affected by several other factors. The quality of the scattered radiation is softer than that of the radiation from which it originates; but scatter originates mostly from the harder component of the beams used in diagnostic roentgenology, and the softening is not great. The primary beam contains some very soft radiation that does not contribute to the scattered radiation; hence the HVL of the scattered radiation generally is slightly higher than that of the primary beam.

PATIENT EXPOSURE

Every effort should be made to keep the total dose to the patient as low as is feasible and to irradiate only small volumes of tissue. Each of the following procedures will help to accomplish these aims, and, in addition, several of them will help to produce better quality roentgenograms: (1) using sufficient filtration, (2) using a long target-film distance, (3) using small beams of x-rays, (4) using fast films, fully developed, and (5) using gonadal shielding when there is a possibility that the gonads will be in a useful beam.

PERSONNEL EXPOSURE

The permissible exposure of the dental personnel varies according to their duties: (1) duties of some necessitate their being in areas where exposure to radiation is possible, referred to as "controlled areas," and (2) duties of others require their not being in controlled areas but in adjacent areas, called "the environs." The first group includes those who operate an x-ray machine or who for any reason are near enough to a machine to possibly receive some exposure

---

*Assume a change of TFD from 12 to 16 inches. This will require that the exposure be increased $(16)^2/(12)^2 = 1.78$ times. If the skin is 1½ inches closer to the target, the TSD will have changed from 10½ to 14½ inches; if the exposure were not increased, the skin dose would be reduced to $(10½)^2/(14½)^2 = 52.5\%$, but since the exposure is increased 1.78 times, the skin dose will be $1.78 \times 52.5\% = 93.5\%$ as great as, or 6.5% less than, for a TFD of 12 inches.

when the x-ray equipment is in use; these individuals are "radiation workers," should be 18 years old or older, and are in the group whose maximal permissible accumulated dose is 5 (age − 18) rem. The second group includes such personnel as secretaries and receptionists, whose duties do not involve any exposure to radiation; these individuals are not radiation workers and their MPD is 0.5 rem per year.

Radiation workers among the dental personnel should have no difficulty in keeping their exposure to radiation down to essentially zero; but if easily followed precautions are ignored, their doses may far exceed the MPD values even though the volume of x-ray work is small. The controls for the x-ray machine should be behind a leaded screen and the operator should stand behind this screen when exposures are being made. Even with a screen the exposure may not be zero because some radiation may be scattered from the patient and walls so that it does get behind the screen. Any screen will provide at least some protection, but a properly designed one can provide almost complete protection.

Every effort should be made to keep the dose to radiation workers at a value far below the MPD levels, and this can be accomplished by their (1) never standing in the direct beam of radiation; (2) always standing more than 6 feet from the patient and preferably behind a protective barrier;* (3) never holding a film in the patient's mouth during an exposure (impossible if rule 2 is obeyed); (4) never using an intraoral fluoroscopic mirror (impossible if rule 2 is obeyed); (5) reducing the dose to the patient to as low levels as possible, because the smaller the dose to the patient

the less scattered radiation there will be; and (6) trying to avoid exposure. Protective devices are of no value if not used, and good work habits are essential; *the individual himself must try to avoid exposure to radiation.*

Nonradiation workers among the dental personnel are governed by the same exposure rules as are recommended for all people in the environs.

EXPOSURE IN THE ENVIRONS

The MPD for individuals in the environs is 0.5 rem a year. This level is readily obtained in the environs of dental equipment since the radiation is easily absorbed. Actually, it is feasible to reduce the dose rate in the environs to such a level that its detection is questionable, and such a level should generally be accomplished.

The walls, floor, and ceiling of rooms containing x-ray machines may need to contain lead or other material to absorb the radiation striking them. The amount of protective material will generally need to be greater for a primary than for a secondary barrier. The amount of protective material needed in a barrier will increase as the use of the x-ray equipment increases, as the kVp on the tube increases, as the distance to occupied areas decreases, and as the time spent by an individual in the occupied area increases; also the amount needed will be determined by various other factors.

Exact rules for the protective values of barriers, too extensive to be included in this discussion, are available in many handbooks and books. It is advisable to have the protection for an x-ray installation specified by an individual trained for such work.

RADIATION-PROTECTION SURVEYS

It is the responsibility of the dentist in charge of x-ray equipment to be sure that the exposure to the patients, to the radiation workers, and to people in the environs is at satisfactorily low levels.

In spite of all the protective devices

---

* A *protective barrier* is a wall that reduces the exposure to radiation. A *primary* protective barrier is one that may be struck by the useful beam, and a *secondary* protective barrier is one that cannot be struck by the useful beam but only by leakage and scattered radiation. Barriers very commonly are constructed of lead, but sufficient thicknesses of other materials may be satisfactory. The use of higher kV may require an increase in thickness of barriers because the harder radiation will be more penetrating.

that may be provided, radiation exposures will not be as low as they should be unless the devices are used properly. The only way to be reasonably certain that exposures do not exceed acceptable limits is to have the department and its environs surveyed by a competent individual. Such a survey should include (1) measurements made with a proper survey instrument* while the equipment is in use, and (2) measurements of radiation received by all individuals in the department as determined by appropriate personnel monitoring devices, such as film badges. The exposure received by people in the environs, or the exposure that might be received by people in these areas, also should be determined. The use of personnel monitoring devices in addition to checks with survey instruments is desirable, because such devices can integrate the exposure over periods of up to a month, during which time most of the possible variations in exposure procedures are likely to have occurred.

Because techniques are occasionally changed, the work load may gradually increase, and humans are likely to alter their habits, protection surveying is continually necessary.

The aim in providing protection from radiation is to *prevent undesirable exposures* rather than to learn of their already having occurred. A protection survey of an x-ray installation and its environs should aim to determine whether or not undesirable exposures are possible, and whether limitations on occupancy of areas or on use of equipment are necessary. The use of personnel monitoring devices is a check on the efficiency of surveys that have been made and on the work habits of the personnel.

Blood counts on radiation workers serve no useful purpose in determining the adequacy of protection, because a change in blood count produced by radiation in-

dicates that the undesirable exposure already has occurred and damage, perhaps irremediable, has been done. Blood counts on radiation workers are desirable, however; individuals with pre-employment blood counts that are not entirely normal should not be employed as radiation workers, and those who develop abnormal blood counts, as shown by periodic checks, should not continue as radiation workers, even though the abnormal counts may not be radiation-induced. There is no reason to believe that a change in blood count from normal to abnormal in a radiation worker is a radiation effect if his exposure has been well within the MPD limits; but an individual who tends to have occasional abnormal blood counts should avoid those things that could possibly be a contributing factor.

If one knows what radiation is, how it acts, and what radiation protection is attempting to accomplish, methods of providing proper protection become easy to understand and are often self-evident. If in the future the values for the MPD are again changed, or if changes in equipment and available protective materials alter the specifications of protective devices, the current values for the MPD and specifications of protective barriers can always be obtained from the NCRP. Basic understanding of radiation, its effects, and the philosophy of radiation protection, rather than ungrounded fear or foolish disregard of radiation, is needed in this age when unavoidable exposure to radiation is increasing.

GOVERNMENT REGULATIONS

The United States Food and Drug Administration issued Performance Standards for diagnostic x-ray equipment that became effective on August 1, 1974. All new x-ray diagnostic equipment bought after that date must meet the Standards. However, equipment in use before that date need not be modified to meet the Standards unless the unit requires replacement of major components, is moved and put into use, or is sold and put into use. The Standards

*The sensitivity of most radiation detecting and measuring devices varies with the quality of the radiation to which they are exposed. This is particularly true when the exposure is to soft radiations such as are used in dental roentgenology.

include the ability to reproduce exposures, HVL of the radiation, accuracy of meter readings, minimal source-film distances, length and construction of cones, and maximal size of fields. At present, the Standards are not as specific in some respects for dental machines as for other diagnostic machines, but more specific Standards for dental machines will probably be announced in the future. Specific values for filters, target-skin distances, and size of radiation fields suggested in this chapter satisfy the Standards that became effective on August 1, 1974.

REFERENCES

Publications available from the International Commission on Radiation Units Publications, P.O. Box 30165, Washington, D.C. 20014.
   a. Radiation Dosimetry: X Rays Generated at Potentials of 5 to 150 kV. Report No. 17 (June) 1970, 39 pp.
   b. Radiation Quantities and Units. Report No. 19 (July) 1971, 21 pp.
   c. Dose Equivalent. Supplement to Report 19 (Sept.) 1973, 3 pp.
Publications available from the National Council on Radiation Protection Publications, P.O. Box 4867, Washington, D.C. 20008.
   a. Medical X-ray and Gamma-Ray Protection for Energies up to 10 MeV: Equipment Design and Use; Recommendations. Report No. 33 (Feb.) 1968, 66 pp.
   b. Medical X-ray and Gamma-Ray Protection for Energies up to 10 MeV: Structural Shielding Design and Evaluation Handbook; Recommendations. Report No. 34 (Mar.) 1970, 117 pp.
   c. Dental X-ray Protection. Report No. 35 (Mar.) 1970, 50 pp.
   d. Basic Radiation Protection Criteria: Recommendations. Report No. 39 (Jan.) 1971, 135 pp.
Alcox, R. W.: Exposure and Dose. J. Am. Dent. A. 80:270 (Feb.) 1970.
Barr, J. H.: Dental Radiology: A Perspective on Priorities. Oral Surg., Oral Med. & Oral Path. 34:672–679 (Oct.) 1972.
Baum, A. T. and Morgan, E.: Reduction of X-ray Dose by Variable Rectangular Collimation and Reflex Optical Direction of Dental X-ray Beams and by the Supine Position of the Patient. J. Am. Dent. A. 85:1091–1098 (Nov.) 1972.
Bean, L. R., Jr. and Devore, W. D.: The Effect of Protective Aprons in Dental Roentgenography. Oral Surg., Oral Med. & Oral Path. 28:505–508 (Oct.) 1969.
Bruce, K. W. and Stafne, E. C.: The Effect of Irradiation on the Dental System as Demonstrated by the Roentgenogram. J. Am. Dent. A. 41:684–689 (Dec.) 1950.
Committee on the Biological Effects of Atomic Radiation: A Report to the Public on the Biological Effects of Atomic Radiation. National Academy of Sciences & National Research Council, Washington, D.C., 1960, 19 pp.
Council on Dental Materials and Devices: Recommendations in Radiographic Practices, May 1972. J. Am. Dent. A. 84:1108 (May) 1972.
Council on Dental Materials and Devices: Federal Standard for Diagnostic X-ray Systems and Dental Practice. J. Am. Dent. A. 87:192 (July) 1973.
Ennis, L. M., Berry, H. M., Jr., and Phillips, J. E.: Dental Roentgenology. Ed. 6. Philadelphia, Lea & Febiger, 1967, 740 pp.
Ice, R. D., Updegrave, W. J., and Bogucki, E. I.: Influence of Dental Radiographic Cones on Radiation Exposure. J. Am. Dent. A. 83:1297–1302 (Dec.) 1971.
Jacobson, A. F. and Ferguson, J. P.: Evaluation of an S. S. White Panorex X-ray Machine. Oral Surg., Oral Med. & Oral Path. 36:426–442 (Sept.) 1973.
Jerman, A. C., Kinsley, E. L., and Morris, C. R.: Absorbed Radiation from Panoramic plus Bitewing Exposures vs Full-Mouth Periapical plus Bitewing Exposures. J. Am. Dent. A. 86:420–423 (Feb.) 1973.
Kimball, A. W.: Evaluation of Data Relating Human Leukemia and Ionizing Radiation. J. Nat. Cancer Inst. 21:383–391 (Aug.) 1958.
McMahon, J. J.: Head and Neck Exposures From Panoramix Roentgenography. Oral Surg., Oral Med. & Oral Path. 31:122–132 (Jan.) 1971.
Nelsen, R. J.: Hazards in Roentgenography: A Discussion of the Philosophy of Risk in the Use of Dental X-rays. Dent. Clin. North America. November, pp. 771–778, 1960.
Peller, S. and Pick, P.: Leukemia and Other Malignancies in Physicians. Am. J. M. Sc. 224:154–159 (Aug.) 1952.
Richards, A. G.: How Hazardous Is Dental Roentgenography? Oral Surg., Oral Med. & Oral Path. 14:40–51 (Jan.) 1961.
Richards, A. G.: Quality of an X-ray Beam. Oral Surg., Oral Med. & Oral Path. 17(Suppl. 3):739–744 (June) 1964.
Richards, A. G. and Webber, R. L.: Dental X-ray Exposure of Sites within the Head and Neck. Oral Surg., Oral Med. & Oral Path. 18:752–756 (Dec.) 1964.
Seltser, R. and Sartwell, P. E.: Ionizing Radiation and Longevity of Physicians. J.A.M.A. 166:585–587 (Feb. 8) 1958.
Taylor, L. S.: X Rays and the Dental Profession. J. Am. Dent. A. 79:885–888 (Oct.) 1969.
United States Food and Drug Administration: Performance Standards for Electronic Products: Diagnostic X-ray Systems and Their Major Components. Federal Register 37:16461–16470 (Aug. 15) 1972.
United States Food and Drug Administration: Performance Standards for Electronic Products: Diagnostic X-ray Systems and Their Major Components; Extension of Effective Date. Federal Register 38:15444–15446 (June 12) 1973.
Updegrave, W. J.: Simplified and Standardized Intraoral Radiography with Reduced Tissue Ir-

radiation. J. Am. Dent. A. *85*:861–869 (Oct.) 1972.

Wainwright, W. W.: Filtration for Lowest Patient Dose in Dental Radiography. Oral Surg., Oral Med. & Oral Path. *16*:561–571 (May) 1963.

Wainwright, W. W.: Dental Radiation Dose: Sensitometric Method for Determination of Exposure-Development Factors. Oral Surg., Oral Med. & Oral Path. *16*:674–682 (June) 1963.

Wainwright, W. W.: Dental Radiology. New York, McGraw-Hill Book Company, 1965, 585 pp.

Warren, S.: Longevity and Causes of Death from Irradiation in Physicians. J.A.M.A. *162*:464–468 (Sept. 29) 1956.

Weissman, D. D. and Longhurst, G. E.: Clinical Evaluation of a Rectangular Field Collimating Device for Periapical Radiography. J. Am. Dent. A. *82*:580–582 (Mar.) 1971.

Wuehrmann, A. H., and Manson-Hing, L. R.: Dental Radiology. Ed. 3. St. Louis, The C. V. Mosby Company, 1973.

Yale, S. H.: Radiation Control in the Dental Office. Dent. Clin. North America July, pp. 355–362, 1961.